THE STUDY OF ANOSOGNOSIA

THE STUDY OF ANOSOGNOSIA

Edited by

George P. Prigatano, Ph.D.

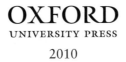

UNIVERSITY PRESS

2010

OXFORD
UNIVERSITY PRESS

Oxford University Press, Inc., publishes works that further
Oxford University's objective of excellence
in research, scholarship, and education.

Oxford   New York
Auckland   Cape Town   Dar es Salaam   Hong Kong   Karachi
Kuala Lumpur   Madrid   Melbourne   Mexico City   Nairobi
New Delhi   Shanghai   Taipei   Toronto

With offices in
Argentina   Austria   Brazil   Chile   Czech Republic   France   Greece
Guatemala   Hungary   Italy   Japan   Poland   Portugal   Singapore
South Korea   Switzerland   Thailand   Turkey   Ukraine   Vietnam

Copyright © 2010 by Oxford University Press, Inc.

Published by Oxford University Press, Inc.
198 Madison Avenue, New York, New York 10016

www.oup.com

Oxford is a registered trademark of Oxford University Press, Inc.

Library of Congress Cataloging-in-Publication Data
The study of anosognosia / George P. Prigatano, editor.
    p.   ;   cm.
Includes bibliographical references and index.
ISBN-13: 978-0-19-537909-9 (alk. paper)
ISBN-10: 0-19-537909-8 (alk. paper)
1. Anosognosia.   2. Nervous system—Degeneration—Rehabilitation.
3. Hemiplegia.   I. Prigatano, George P.
[DNLM: 1. Agnosia—psychology.   2. Agnosia—rehabilitation.
3. Awareness.   4. Hemiplegia.   5. Neurodegenerative Diseases—psychology.
6. Neurodegenerative Diseases—rehabilitation.   WL 340 S9335 2009]
RC553.C64S78 2009
616.8'0471—dc22

                                                            2009024065

9   8   7   6   5   4   3   2   1

Printed in the United States of America
on acid-free paper

To Dagmar, Laura, and Katie

Preface

The study of anosognosia is important for several reasons:

1. Patients with identifiable brain disorders (e.g., cerebrovascular accident [CVA], severe traumatic brain injury [TBI], etc.) may have reduced self-awareness of residual neurological or neuropsychological impairments that negatively impact their clinical care.
2. Understanding the biological and neuropsychological mechanisms responsible for anosognosia in its various forms may reveal important insights into brain organization and how human consciousness (subjective awareness of the self and the environment) is possible.
3. The comparative study of anosognosia in patients with identifiable brain disorders in comparison to patients with psychiatric disorders (e.g., hysterical, conversion disorder) may provide rich insights into the "body–mind" problem.
4. Understanding the basis of how anosognosia changes with time (i.e., "recovers" or "worsens") may provide important insights into mechanisms of "recovery" and "deterioration" after various brain disorders. This has clear implications for treatment and patient management.

It is, therefore, with considerable pleasure that this volume has become a reality. Hopefully, it will encourage clinicians and researchers to continue creative work in this area of investigation. This text is the direct result of a conference held in Phoenix, Arizona, at the Arizona Biltmore Hotel between October 24 and 27, 2008. Prominent clinicians and researchers who have studied anosognosia were willing to prepare chapters prior to meeting at the conference. During the conference they presented their ideas to the various participants. The authors then modified their chapters after the meeting concluded, to help clarify the new findings and review present and old theoretical perspectives. Additional chapters were added after the conference to cover topics not addressed at that time. The expressed goal of the conference and of this book was to summarize advances in the study of anosognosia. It is hopeful that readers and reviewers of this edited text will conclude that this has been achieved.

The text does not cover all possible studies relevant to understanding anosognosia, but it does provide a summary of hundreds of studies that have bearing on this topic. I am indebted to the various authors who have taken seriously the need to summarize important findings relevant to the study of anosognosia. Chapter lengths within this volume vary, but they do so primarily because of the databases that presently exist. Clearly, there is more to say in some areas than in others.

In the initial section of this book, chapters are devoted to the study of anosognosia for hemiplegia (AHP). These chapters repeat certain historical observations and models that have helped explain this phenomenon. This is necessary because each set of authors needed to set the stage for their particular approach to the study of AHP. Repetition can also be valuable insofar as it helps reveal how the same historical observations have impacted individual investigators differentially, thus modifying their focus of attention when conducting research. As is true in all of science, advances represent the unique interests of investigators and the body of research knowledge that they find most relevant.

Other sections of this text have described how the study of anosognosia has expanded over the last several years. This expansion may, in part, have been stimulated by the first book that emanated from a similar conference on anosognosia that was held in Phoenix, Arizona, in October of 1988. That conference resulted in the edited text *Awareness of Deficit after Brain Injury: Clinical and Theoretical Issues* (Prigatano & Schacter, 1991).

Both conferences were made possible by the generous support of the Barrow Neurological Institute at St. Joseph's Hospital and Medical Center in Phoenix, Arizona. I have had the good fortune of being affiliated with the Barrow Neurological Institute (BNI) since 1985, and wish to express to hospital administrators, including Phil Pomeroy, Vice President of Neuroscience and Dr. Robert F. Spetzler, Director of the BNI, my gratitude for their continued support and encouragement. I would also like to explicitly recognize Dr. Spetzler for his continued efforts in providing support to carry out such an important meeting during difficult financial times. Funding from the Barrow Neurological Foundation (BNF) and the Newsome Foundation made this conference possible.

Special recognition and thanks also goes to Lindsey Kerby, conference planning manager for the BNI, and to Mary Henry, administrative assistant in the Department of Clinical Neuropsychology. Ms. Henry's work in preparing this manuscript is especially appreciated. Jennifer Gray, Ph.D., was invaluable in her help editing the chapters of this book.

The continued goal of the Department of Clinical Neuropsychology within the Barrow Neurological Institute at St. Joseph's Hospital and Medical Center is to provide patient care based on our most recent scientific understanding of how various brain disorders affect psychological functioning. This needs to be done, however, in a manner that is sensitive to each individual's personal reaction to his or her neurological and neuropsychological disturbances. This book represents our most recent efforts in this regard.

George P. Prigatano, Ph.D.,
Newsome Chair, Clinical Neuropsychology

Contents

Part VIII

Contributors

Bernhard Baier, M.D.
Department of Neurology
University of Mainz
Mainz, Germany

Anna Berti, M.D., Ph.D.
Department of Psychology
Neuropsychology Research Group
University of Turin
Turin, Italy

Gabriella Bottini, M.D., Ph.D.
Psychology Department
University of Pavia
Pavia, Italy

Richard S. Burns, M.D.
Barrow Neurological Institute
St. Joseph's Hospital and Medical Center
Phoenix, Arizona

Carlo Caltagirone, M.D.
Department of Clinical and Behavioural Neurology
IRCCS S. Lucia Foundation
Rome, Italy

Gianna Cocchini, Ph.D.
Psychology Department
Goldsmiths University of London
London, England

A. D. (Bud) Craig, Ph.D.
Atkinson Research Lab
Barrow Neurological Institute
Phoenix, Arizona

Anthony S. David, M.D.
Department of Psychiatry
Section of Cognitive Neuropsychiatry
Institute of Psychiatry
King's College
London, England

Sergio Della Sala, M.D., Ph.D.
Human Cognitive Neuroscience, Psychology
University of Edinburgh
Edinburgh, Scotland

Emily C. Edmonds, M.A.
Department of Psychology
University of Arizona
Tucson, Arizona

Martina Gandola, M.A., Ph.D.
Psychology Department
University of Pavia
Pavia, Italy

James Gilleen, Ph.D.
Department of Psychiatry
Section of Cognitive Neuropsychiatry
Institute of Psychiatry
King's College
London, England

Kathryn Greenwood, Ph.D.
Department of Psychology
Institute of Psychiatry
King's College London
London, England

Michal Harciarek, Ph.D.
Institute of Psychology
University of Gdańsk
Gdańsk, Poland

Kenneth M. Heilman, M.D.
Department of Neurology
College of Medicine
University of Florida
Veteran's Affairs Medical Center
Gainesville, Florida

Karin F. Hoth, Ph.D.
Division of Psychosocial Medicine
Department of Medicine
National Jewish Health
Department of Psychiatry
University of Colorado Denver
Denver, Colorado

Paola Invernizzi, M.A.
Psychology Department
Univeristy of Milano-Bicocca
Milano, Italy

Sterling C. Johnson, Ph.D.
Geriatric Research Education and Clinical Center
Wm. S. Middleton Memorial Veteran's Hospital
University of Wisconsin School of Medicine and Public Health
Madison, Wisconsin

Ricardo E. Jorge, M.D.
Department of Psychiatry
University of Iowa Hospitals and Clinics
Iowa City, Iowa

Hans-Otto Karnath, M.D., Ph.D.
Section of Neuropsychology
Center of Neurology
Hertie-Institute for Clinical Brain Research
University of Tübingen,
Tübingen, Germany

Alfred W. Kaszniak, Ph.D.
Department of Psychology
University of Arizona
Tucson, Arizona

Andrew Kertesz, M.D., FRCP (C)
Department of Neurology
University of Western Ontario
St. Joseph's Health Center
London, Ontario, Canada

Franziska Maier, M.A.
Movement Disorders and Deep Brain Stimulation
Department of Neurology
University Hospital Cologne
Cologne, Germany

Jeannine Morrone-Strupinsky, Ph.D.
Department of Clinical Neuropsychology
Barrow Neurological Institute
St. Joseph's Hospital and Medical Center
Phoenix, Arizona

M. Donata Orfei, M.A.
Department of Clinical and Behavioural Neurology
IRCCS S. Lucia Foundation
Rome, Italy

Eraldo Paulesu, M.D.
Psychology Department
Univeristy of Milano-Bicocca
Milano, Italy

Jane S. Paulsen, Ph.D.
Departments of Psychiatry, Neurology, and Psychology
College of Medicine
University of Iowa
Iowa City, Iowa

Lorenzo Pia, Ph.D.
Department of Psychology
Neuropsychology Research Group
University of Turin
Turin, Italy

Brian D. Power, M.D.
Lecturer, School of Psychiatry and Neurosciences
University of Western Australia
Fremantle, Australia

George P. Prigatano, Ph.D.
Department of Clinical Neuropsychology
Barrow Neurological Institute
St. Joseph's Hospital and Medical Center
Phoenix, Arizona

Katherine P. Rankin, Ph.D.
Memory and Aging Center
Department of Neurology
University of California San Francisco
San Francisco, California

Michele L. Ries, Ph.D.
Geriatric Research Education and Clinical Center

Wm. S. Middleton Memorial Veteran's Hospital
University of Wisconsin School of Medicine and Public Health
Madison, Wisconsin

Ian H. Robertson, Ph.D., MRIA
School of Psychology and Institute of Neuroscience
Trinity College Dublin
Dublin, Ireland

Gianfranco Spalletta, M.D., Ph.D.
Department of Clinical and Behavioural Neurology
IRCCS S. Lucia Foundation
Rome, Italy

Sergio E. Starkstein, M.D., Ph.D.
School of Psychiatry and Neurosciences
University of Western Australia
Fremantle, Australia

Daniel Tranel, Ph.D.
Departments of Neurology and Psychology
Division of Behavioral Neurology and Cognitive Neuroscience
College of Medicine
University of Iowa
Iowa City, Iowa

Roland Vocat, Ph.D.
Laboratory for Behavioral Neurology and Imaging of Cognition
Department of Neuroscience
University Medical Center & Department of Neurology
University Hospital
Geneva, Switzerland

Patrik Vuilleumier, M.D.
Laboratory for Behavioral Neurology and Imaging of Cognition
Department of Neuroscience
University Medical Center & Department of Neurology
University Hospital
Geneva, Switzerland

Thomas R. Wolf, M.D.
Consultant, Clinical Neuro-ophthalmology
Instructor in Neurology and Visiting Research Scientist in
Aerospace Medicine
Mayo Clinic Arizona
Phoenix, Arizona

I

Historical Overview and Introduction

1

Historical Observations Relevant to the Study of Anosognosia

George P. Prigatano

The Nobel laureate Roger Sperry (1969) proposed that conscious awareness is "...a dynamic emergent property of cerebral excitation" (p. 533) that can have "...causal effects in brain function that control subset events in the flow pattern of neural excitation" (p. 533). He goes on to state that "...the conscious properties of cerebral patterns are directly dependent on the action of the component neural elements" (p. 534).

With these comments, Sperry (1969) elevates conscious awareness to the highest of all integrative brain functions, and he notes that while it is dependent on underlying neural activity, it appears to emerge in such a fashion that it actually exerts some causal effect on other brain regions. If correct, this view suggests that the emergence of consciousness and "normal" self-awareness is an extremely important area of study for neuropsychology and the practice of all brain-related clinical disciplines. Disturbances in consciousness are indeed complex, and they may range from minor alterations to profound unawareness of one's neurological and neuropsychological deficits.

Persistent impairments in self-awareness appear to relate to a variety of cognitive and behavioral problems. They are also linked to poor decision making and may limit a person's engagement in rehabilitation activities that potentially could be helpful to them. Efforts at neuropsychological rehabilitation of brain-dysfunctional patients several years ago emphasize this point (Prigatano et al., 1984). As a result, the study of anosognosia became a central topic for post-acute neuropsychological rehabilitation. It also became a central question for cognitive psychology, as it rediscovered the importance of "consciousness" in psychology (Prigatano & Schacter, 1991; Weiskrantz, 1997).

This book attempts to summarize many of the contributions that have been made over the last 20 years that help advance our understanding of anosognosia. In order to put these advances into perspective, however, it is important that one have a reasonable grasp of both the remote and recent history of the study of anosognosia that impacts our present thinking about this phenomenon. Without such an historical perspective, it is difficult to separate out a "true" advance from an "apparent" advance. The latter is simply a restating of older observations using new terminology. While interesting, these "apparent" advances do not lead to a better, more useful explanation of the phenomenon.

Equating the term "better" with "more useful" is intentional. If the terms used to explain the phenomenon are indeed "better," they lead to more precise predictions and practical methods of intervention. This perspective will, therefore, guide a rather brief review of historical observations concerning the phenomenon of anosognosia that have relevance to the present volume.

Historical Accounts

All historical accounts are shaded by the biases, and at times ignorance, of the historian. Consequently, multiple perspectives from different authors are often needed to get as close as one can to "what really happened in the past" to determine how it influences our present thinking (Prigatano, 2005). In their seminal book *Denial of Illness: Symbolic and Physiologic Aspects*, Edwin Weinstein and Robert Kahn (1955) provided the most comprehensive historical perspective on anosognosia, covering papers written from the late 1800s to the mid-1950s. MacDonald Critchley (1953) also discussed "unawareness of hemiparesis (anosognosia)" (p. 225) in his book *The Parietal Lobes*. His account is also interesting, as it provides an English translation of some of Babinski's actual words when describing anosognosia for hemiplegia (see pp. 231–232). Critchley (1953) makes the important observation that "the patient's attitude toward their inadequate motor performance forms an interesting problem..." (p. 233) that must also be understood in any scientific account of anosognosia (see Heilman & Harciarek, Chapter 5, this volume).

Edoardo Bisiach and Giuliano Geminiani (1991) provide a brief, but valuable historical perspective beginning with observations from antiquity. Prigatano and Schacter (1991) further provide a historical review, which attempts to combine observations made by early neurophysiologists, psychiatrists, and neurologists. Further historical insights have subsequently been made (see Vocat & Vuilleumier,

Chapter 17 and Kertesz, Chapter 6, this volume) that highlight Babinski's observations concerning hysteria and Anton's and Pick's observations concerning anosognosia for hemiplegia. Since the early writings of Anton (1898), Pick (1898, 1908), and Babinski (1914), there have been a number of papers that have described various clinical observations and empirical findings concerning anosognosia. There have also been various models proposed to explain this complicated phenomenon.

The goal of this book is to synthesize knowledge that has been accumulated over many years regarding the study of anosognosia and to specifically highlight advances that have occurred in the field.

What Constitutes an Advance?

Table 1.1 lists the criteria for determining whether advances have occurred in the field. As it relates to the study of anosognosia and impaired self-awareness after brain injury, the first area to consider is whether there have been any new clinical observations that are relevant to the study of anosognosia that must be explained by any theory or model of anosognosia.

The second type of advance to be considered is empirical findings, which use appropriate controlled observations that help enlighten our understanding of the underlying mechanism or mechanisms responsible for this phenomenon. The third area of advance to consider centers around whether new methods of study have emerged that allow the phenomenon to be more thoroughly studied. In this area, revolutionary advances have occurred, particularly over the last 10 years. Finally, we will consider whether there have been advances made in new, testable (and perhaps partially untestable) models/hypotheses that help guide the field to have a more comprehensive and detailed understanding of anosognosia and related disorders.

Chapter 21 of this volume will summarize advances in the study of anosognosia. Before proceeding, however, it is worthwhile to stop and reflect on exactly what we mean by the term *anosognosia*.

Table 1.1 What Constitutes an Advance?

- New, relevant *clinical observations* that must be explained by any theory or model of anosognosia
- New *empirical findings* that clarify the nature of anosognosia and possible underlying mechanism(s) responsible for it
- New *methods of study* of the phenomenon of anosognosia
- New *testable* (and perhaps partially untestable) *models* that are both more comprehensive and specific in their predictions about anosognosia and related disorders

---

Definitions and Early Considerations

If one were to consult the Internet (notably Wikipedia), the following definition of anosognosia is readily available to the public: "*Anosognosia* is a condition in which a person who suffers disability due to brain injury seems unaware of or denies the existence of his or her handicap. This may include unawareness of quite dramatic impairments such as blindness or paralysis. It was first named by neurologist Joseph Babinski in 1914, although relatively little has been discovered about the cause of the condition since its initial identification" ("Anosognosia," 2009, para. 1). As of March 10, 2009, a Google search of articles that include the term *anosognosia* produced 73,200 references. Of those references, 7,030 struggled with a clear definition of exactly what anosognosia means.

Edoardo Bisiach and Giuliano Geminiani (1991) cautioned us about obtaining a truly scientific definition of anosognosia with their following observations: "A satisfactory definition of anosognosia per se is perhaps impossible, attributable to the fact that the term anosognosia, rather than referring to a truly distinct symptom, may be (and has indeed been) used to denote *aspects of patients' behavior in relationship to their illness that are heterogeneous in appearance and unlikely to depend on a specific set of causes* exclusively related to them" (Bisiach & Geminiani, 1991, p. 19; emphasis added).

According to Bisiach and Geminiani (1991), "Anosognosia deserves assessment tailored to each individual case, comprising faithful records of all relevant spontaneous behavior as well as of that instigated by the examiner's queries, the limits to which are set only by the examiner's inventiveness and the patient's mood and intelligence" (p. 20).

In light of these comments, a brief history regarding anosognosia will be presented as follows: observations made before Babinski; what Babinski observed and reported between 1914 and 1918; and observations after Babinski, which have led to the present report.

Anosognosia prior to Babinski

Letters from antiquity provide descriptions of apparent denial or unawareness of profound sensory loss that appeared "incredible" to the observer (see Bisiach & Geminiani, 1991, p. 17). Persons who lose their vision may report the room as "dark," but not self-recognize that they cannot see. Brian Kolb (1990), the noted neuroscientist and neuropsychologist, reported a similar phenomenon after his occipital stroke. He had to "discover" his loss of vision in one visual field. His initial impression that a light bulb had burned out when he attempted to turn on the kitchen light had to be replaced with the self-recognition that something had gone wrong with his own vision.

In 1881 Hermann Munk conducted ablation studies on dogs and discovered a perplexing phenomenon (see Prigatano & Schacter, 1991). Lesions of the association cortex between primary visual and auditory centers produced a situation in which the dog appeared to be able to "see" (i.e., they would not bump into objects when moving), but they failed to recognize their master. He termed this phenomenon "mind blindness." In a sense, it is an early animal model for agnosia and perhaps anosognosia. Recently on YouTube, there is a fascinating video clip of a dog that does not seem to recognize his own (left) hind leg. Could this be even a more striking example of anosognosia in nonprimates? The point of these observations is that for many years, before the formal study of neurology and neuropsychology, anosognosia or anosognostic phenomena were reported, and we continue to see various manifestations of these phenomena today.

Babinski (1914) is credited for introducing the term *anosognosia* to the neurological community when he presented his findings to the French Neurological Society in June of 1914 and then again in December of 1918 (Bisiach & Geminiani, 1991). It has also been reported, however, that Gabriel Anton actually described anosognosia for hemiplegia prior to Babinski in 1893 (see Bisiach & Geminiani, 1991; Karnath & Baier, Chapter 3, this volume). Pick (1898) also reported apparent lack of awareness of left-sided motor deficits.

Constantin von Monakow (1885) described apparent unawareness of cortical blindness, but his patients suffered from Korsakoff's syndrome. It remained unclear whether the lack of awareness of visual loss was secondary to memory impairments, confabulatory tendencies, or a true "isolated" unawareness of visual impairments. Later, Anton (1898) reported cases of patients with visual loss that appeared clearly related to focal cerebral lesions (Weinstein & Friedland, 1977). The patients were not demented or confused.

By providing a name for this phenomenon, Babinski (1914) introduced a whole new study within the field of neurology and later neuropsychology.

Babinski's Observations and Use of the Term *Anosognosia*

For non–French-speaking (and reading) investigators, the writings of Critchley (1953) are informative for understanding Babinski's contributions. When describing "disorders of the body image," Critchley (1953) noted that Babinski first employed the term *anosognosia* to refer to the lack of awareness of left hemiplegia. Critchley makes the following remarks concerning Babinski:

> As Babinski employed the word in 1914, however, the meaning was restricted so as to apply to cases of hemiplegia. In his original communication, Babinski drew attention to a mental disorder he had had the opportunity of observing in cerebral hemiplegia which consisted in the fact that the patients were unaware of, or seemed to be unaware of (*ignorent ou paraissent ignorer*), the existence of the paralysis

with which they were afflicted. His first patient was a woman who had been paralysed down the left side for years, but who never mentioned the fact. If asked to move the affected limb she remained immobile and silent, behaving as though the question had been put to someone else. Babinski's second patient was also a victim of left hemiplegia. Whenever she was asked what was the matter with her, she talked about her backache, or her phlebitis, but never once did she refer to her powerless left arm. When told to move that limb, she did nothing and said nothing, or else a mere, "Voilà, c'est fait!" During a consultation, when her doctors were discussing the merits of physiotherapy in her presence, she broke in... "Why should I have electrical treatment? I am not paralysed." In his second paper on the subject (1918), Babinski drew attention to two clinical points in his cases; both patients had sensory impairment down the affected side, and both had left-sided involvement. "Could it be," wrote Babinski, "that anosognosia is peculiar to lesions of the right hemisphere?"

This remark of Babinski's in 1918 was a shrewd one, for clinical evidence since that date had shown that in the great majority of cases lack of awareness of hemiplegia amounts to a lack of awareness of a left hemiplegia. (p. 231)

Anosognosia after Babinski: Some Key Observations

Critchley's (1953) discussion of Babinski's contribution is followed by a review of several authors' perspectives regarding disorders of body image that were accumulated in the 1920s, 1930s, and 1940s. Critchley (1953) also cites an earlier paper by Weinstein and Kahn (1950), in which they report a patient believing that her left hand actually belonged to the nurse that was involved in her care (p. 236). Couched in the context of body disorders, Critchley felt it was important to separate unawareness of hemiparesis (anosognosia) from denial of hemiparesis in which confabulation was present. The presence of confabulatory tendencies was thought to reveal a psychotic state that rendered the patient's judgment about many things unreliable and not necessarily reflective of an underlying specific neurological disorder of awareness.

Weinstein and Kahn (1955) have championed this latter point of view. They considered denial a form of breakdown in reality testing that had nothing to do with a specific lesion producing a specific awareness deficit. They went on to argue that a lesion in the frontal lobes or parietal lobes will determine what type of deficit a patient may have, but not the mechanism of denial (Weinstein & Kahn, 1955, p. 123) (see Table 1.2).

In speaking with Weinstein a few years before his death, he indicated that he wished that he could retract that statement (personal communication with Ed Weinstein, approximately 1995). The point, however, is that Weinstein and Kahn's (1955) very influential book moved the field of the study of anosognosia out of neurology into psychiatry, and with it, there was a loss of interest in studying the neuropsychological basis of this phenomenon for many years.

Table 1.2 Salient Observations Regarding Anosognosia after Babinski

Nielsen (1938)	"I must believe my feelings."
Sandifer (1946)	"That's my ring on your hand, doctor."
Weinstein & Kahn (1955)	"...various forms of anosognosia are not discrete entities that can be localized in different areas of the brain. Whether a lesion involves the frontal or parietal lobe determines the disability that may be denied, but not the mechanism of denial." (p. 123)
Germann et al. (1964)	"The right side of the car took up too much space on the road." "The right foot failed to come into bed."
Roeser & Daly (1974)	"Something is wrong with the stereo."
Bisiach et al. (1986)	Anosognosia of hemiplegia can be disassociated from anosognosia of hemianopsia in the same patient.

In addition to Babinski's clinical reports, however, a number of other authors have made important clinical observations that need to be kept in mind when evaluating any potential "new observations." Perhaps the first and most poignant observations that were made that are relevant to this volume were those by Nielsen (1938). Nielsen describes a patient who had paralysis of her left arm. When it was brought to her attention that this was, in fact, her arm, she stated that even though she was temporarily convinced that it was her arm, it did not "feel like her arm." Therefore, she could not really accept that it was her arm (see Critchley, 1953, p. 236). This early observation by Nielsen emphasized the importance of feeling states in the phenomenon of anosognosia for hemiplegia.

A few years later, Sandifer (1946) described in detail a case of a patient who was anosognostic for left hemiplegia. Sandifer recorded verbatim statements of what the doctor and patient said to one another, providing a classic description of the phenomenon. In addition to being unaware of the hemiparesis, the patient used a bizarre form of logic to explain apparent discrepancies in perception that may also be related to the phenomenon of anosognosia. At one point, the examining physician asked the patient: "Is this your hand?" The patient responded: "Not mine, doctor." The physician responded: "Whose hand is it then?" The patient responded: "I suppose it's yours, doctor." Later, after several other questions, the physician again asked the patient: "Is this your hand?" Again, the patient responded: "Not mine, doctor." The physician then says: "Yes it is. Look at the ring. Whose is it?" The patient then responded: "That's my ring; you've got my ring, doctor." Instead of recognizing the obvious differences in the hands, the patient focused on the fact that her ring appeared to be on the hand of the physician and not her own hand. These types of phenomena have led both researchers and clinicians to recognize that anosognosia is indeed a complicated phenomenon and has many overlapping symptoms. It seems to involve not only cognitive and perceptual disturbances, but perhaps disturbances in various "belief" systems. Bisiach and Geminiani (1991) also addressed this issue.

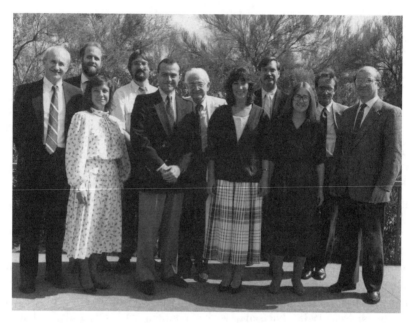

Figure 1.1 Presenters/authors of the initial conference on anosognosia held in 1988 in Phoenix, AZ. Back row, from left to right: David Schacter, Alfred Kaszniak, Edwin Weinstein, John Kihlstrom, Edoardo Bisiach. Front row, from left to right: Kenneth Heilman, Lisa Lewis, George Prigatano, Susan McGlynn, Marcia Johnson, Donald Stuss.

There are, however, other accounts that often are not given adequate attention. One was written by William Germann (Germann, Flanigan, & Davey, 1964), who was a practicing neurosurgeon when he suffered a subdural hematoma secondary to a roller coaster ride at Disneyland in Los Angeles. Germann appeared to have a lack of awareness of right-sided neglect, as opposed to left-sided neglect. His description highlighted that one may have unawareness as a consequence of a left-sided brain injury, as opposed to purely right-sided brain injury. It also emphasized that in very capable individuals who are quite aware of anosognostic phenomena, there is a tendency not to recognize this deficit when it occurs in oneself.

A case report by Roeser and Daly (1974) provides an example of a patient who had a thalamic lesion: the patient was arguing that something was wrong with her stereo, but she was not aware that there was something wrong with her own perception of music. Again, this phenomenon highlights that an impairment or loss of a sensorimotor function is not readily attributed to oneself, but often some form of external explanation is provided to explain an apparent failure.

Finally, in modern times, several insightful observations about anosognosia were made by Edoardo Bisiach and his colleagues. Bisiach et al. (1986) were able to demonstrate for the first time that one could separate anosognosia for hemiplegia from anosognosia for hemianopsia in the very same patient. This was a strong argument for some type of modular representation of awareness of a given function. It also was an argument that conscious awareness may reflect the highest organization of that modular function.

To further discuss modern perspectives of anosognosia, a conference was held in 1988 in Phoenix, Arizona. At the conference, prominent clinicians and researchers discussed varying views concerning the nature of impaired self-awareness in different brain disorders. These discussions led to the book *Awareness of Deficit: Clinical and Theoretical Issues* (Prigatano & Schacter, 1991). At that conference, Edoardo Bisiach, Edwin Weinstein, Kenneth Heilman, and others presented their ideas. Figure 1.1 includes a picture of some of the individual presenters/authors who were involved in the first Phoenix conference on anosognosia.

As noted in the Preface, a second conference was held in Phoenix, Arizona, in 2008. Again, several leaders in the field of impaired self-awareness or anosognosia met to discuss recent research findings and theoretical perspectives. The chapters that follow highlight many of the ideas presented at that meeting. Figure 1.2 is a picture of the individual presenters (authors) that gathered in Phoenix for this second meeting.

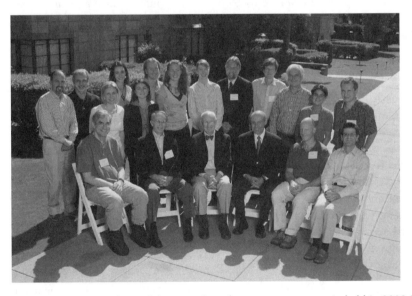

Figure 1.2 Presenters/authors of the second conference on anosognosia held in 2008 in Phoenix, AZ. Back row from left to right: Sergio Starkstein, Ricardo Jorge, Claudia Cacciari, Sterling Johnson, Franziska Maier, Alfred Kaszniak, Hans-Otto Karnath, Ian Robertson, Gabriella Bottini, Patrik Vuilleumier. Middle row from left to right: Gianna Cocchini, Maria Donata Orfei, Katherine Rankin. Front row from left to right: Bud Craig, Andrew Kertesz, Kenneth Heilman, George Prigatano, Daniel Tranel, Anthony David.

"Blindsight:" Does It Have Anything to Tell Us about Anosognosia?

In his profoundly thoughtful and scholarly book *Consciousness Lost and Found*, Larry Weiskrantz (1997) reminds us that there is a "flip side" to the problem of anosognosia. Instead of the patient not being aware of a loss in neurological or neuropsychological functioning, the patient may be unaware of preserved neurological/ neuropsychological functioning following significant brain pathology. The study of patients with profound visual loss who have retained some visual capacity for which they are unaware highlights this point. Understanding the neuroanatomical substrates of blindsight may help us understand the importance of certain anatomical regions that underlie the phenomenon of anosognosia for complete blindness.

Weiskrantz (1997) struggled with the broader problem of what consciousness is and humbly admitted that "the solution to the thorny problem of conscious awareness and its neurological basis" (p. 4) has not been solved by any of us. His observation remains true to this day. As this volume will demonstrate, we have, in fact, made some advances in the scientific study of anosognosia, but we still have a considerable distance to go before we understand the phenomenon. In preparation for reading the chapters that follow, it is important to keep in mind that there are certain questions that, if answered, may in fact advance our knowledge of this important phenomenon.

Questions That Need to Be Answered in Order to Advance the Study of Anosognosia

Advances in science are often unexpected, but detected by the "experienced mind" or the "prepared observer." One cannot say where or when a true advance is most likely to occur. However, keeping in mind certain questions may prepare us to detect important advances. Below are a series of questions worth thinking about when reading the various chapters that follow. At the end of this book, I will refer back to these questions in an effort to consolidate how we presently view the phenomenon of anosognosia and to specifically address the question of whether advances have occurred in our understanding of this phenomenon over the last 20 years.

1. Are we any closer today to a scientific definition of anosognosia for hemiplegia than Babinski was in 1914?
2. What have recent studies revealed regarding the mechanism or mechanisms responsible for anosognosia for hemiplegia?
3. Why does anosognosia for hemiplegia seem to change rapidly for some patients and not for others?
4. Why is anosognosia for hemiplegia frequently associated with anosodiaphoria?
5. Why is anosognosia for hemiplegia at times associated with somatoparaphrenia?

6. What role, if any, does the patient's premorbid personality play in anosognosia for hemiplegia?

7. Why is anosognosia for hemiplegia most commonly observed following large lesions of the brain secondary to stroke, rather than small focal lesions?

8. Is anosognosia for hemiplegia commonly associated with both cortical and subcortical lesions? If so, why?

9. What advances have been made in understanding Anton's syndrome?

10. What have recent studies revealed regarding the mechanism or mechanisms responsible for anosognosia for aphasia?

11. Is there any new information regarding the mechanism or mechanisms of unawareness of auditory perceptual skills, as described by Roeser and Daly (1974), after thalamic lesions?

12. What are the neurological/neuroanatomical, neurophysiological, and neuropsychological changes associated with hysterical sensorimotor loss? Are they different from what is observed in anosognosia for hemiplegia?

13. Do milder forms of anosognosia exist for cognitive, motor, perceptual, emotional, and motivational functioning in different patient groups?

14. Why do some brain-dysfunctional patients show anosognosia or impaired self-awareness, and patients with other disorders do not?

15. Are there neurotransmitter disturbances specifically associated with anosognosia?

16. Is anosognosia a purely cognitive, perceptual dysfunction? What role do emotions or feelings play in anosognostic conditions?

17. How is it possible that a patient can return to consciousness, be oriented to time and place, and remember what is being said, and still be unaware of a neurological or neuropsychological impairment?

18. Why is it that we cannot predict which patients will show anosognosia by just looking at their MRI scans of the brain or reviewing their medical history?

19. Why is anosognosia seldom reported in children?

20. What are the neuroimaging correlates of normal self-awareness in individuals with no neurologic conditions? Do they change in the presence of anosognosia?

21. Do disturbances in self-awareness observed in psychiatric patients have a neurological basis (i.e., a direct effect of brain dysfunction)? Do they represent some type of functional disturbance due to the emotional state of the patient? How does one separate out impaired self-awareness due to a neurological problem versus denial of disability?

22. Can anosognosia or impaired self-awareness coexist with denial of illness?

23. What measurement issues need to be kept in mind when studying anosognosia?

24. Is there any effective way of treating or at least managing anosognosia or impaired self-awareness (ISA) after brain disorder?

References

Anosognosia (2009, March 4). In *Wikipedia, the free encyclopedia*. Retrieved March 10, 2009, from http://en.wikipedia.org/wiki/Anosognosia

Anton, G. (1898). Ueber Herderkrankungen des Gehirnes, welche von Patienten selbst nicht wahrgenommen warden. *Wiener Klinische Wochenschrift, 11*, 227–229.

Babinski, J. (1914). Contribution à l'etude des troubles mentaux dans l'hémiplégie organique cérébrale (Anosognosie). *Revue Neurologique, 27*, 845–847.

Bisiach, E., & Geminiani, G. (1991). Anosognosia related to hemiplegia and hemianopia. In G. P. Prigatano & R. L. Schacter (Eds.), *Awareness of deficit after brain injury: Clinical and theoretical issues* (pp. 17–39). New York: Oxford University Press.

Bisiach, E., Vallar, G., Perani, D., Papagno, C., & Berti, A. (1986). Unawareness of disease following lesions of the right hemisphere: Anosognosia for hemiplegia and anosognosia for hemianopia. *Neuropsychologia, 24*(4), 471–481.

Critchley, M. (1953). *The parietal lobes*. New York: Hafner Press.

Germann, W. J., Flanigan, S., & Davey, L. M. (1964). Remarks on subdural hematoma and aphasia. *Clinical Neurosurgery, 12*, 344–350.

Kolb, B. (1990). Recovery from occipital stroke: A self-report and an inquiry into visual processes. *Canadian Journal of Psychology, 44*, 130–147.

Nielsen, J. M. (1938). Disturbances of the body scheme: Their physiological mechanism. *Bulletin of the Los Angeles Neurology Society, 3*, 127–135.

Pick, A. (1898). *Beiträge zur Pathologie und pathologischen Anatomie des Centralnervensystems*. Berlin: Karger.

Pick, A. (1908). Ueber Störungen der Orientierung am eigenen Körper. Arbeiten aus der psychiatrischen. In *Universtats-klinic in Prag* (pp. 1–19). Berlin: Karger.

Prigatano, G. P. (2005). A history of cognitive rehabilitation. In P. Halligan & D. Wade (Eds.), *The effectiveness of rehabilitation for cognitive deficits* (pp. 3–10). New York: Oxford University Press.

Prigatano, G. P., Fordyce, D. J., Zeiner, H. K., Roueche, J. R., Pepping, M., & Wood, B. (1984). Neuropsychological rehabilitation after closed head injury in young adults. *Journal of Neurology, Neurosurgery and Psychiatry, 47*, 505–513.

Prigatano, G. P., & Schacter, D. L. (1991). *Awareness of deficit after brain injury: Clinical and theoretical issues*. New York: Oxford University Press.

Roeser, R. J., & Daly, D. D. (1974). Auditory cortex disconnection associated with thalamic tumor: A case report. *Neurology, 24*, 555–559.

Sandifer, P. H. (1946). Anosognosia and disorders of body scheme. *Brain, 69*, 122–137.

Sperry, R. W. (1969). A modified concept of consciousness. *Psychological Review, 76*(6), 532–536.

von Monakow, C. (1885). Experimentelle und pathologisch-anatomische Untersuchungen über die Beziehungen der sogentannen Sehsphäre zu den infracorticalen Opticuscentren und zum N. opticus. *Archiv Für Psychiatri, und Nervenkrankheiten, 16*, 151–199.

Weinstein, E. A., & Friedland, R. P. (Eds.) (1977). *Hemi-inattention and hemisphere specialization*. New York: Raven Press.

Weinstein, E. A., & Kahn, R. L. (1950). The syndrome of anosognosia. *Archives of Neurology and Psychiatry, 64*, 772–791.

Weinstein, E. A., & Kahn, R. L. (1955). *Denial of illness: Symbolic and physiological aspects*. Springfield, IL: Charles C. Thomas.

Weiskrantz, L. (1997). *Consciousness Lost and Found: Neuropsychological exploration*. New York: Oxford University Press.

II

Anosognosia of Motor and Language Impairments

2

Anosognosia for Hemiplegia and Models of Motor Control: Insights from Lesional Data

Gabriella Bottini, Eraldo Paulesu, Martina Gandola, Lorenzo Pia, Paola Invernizzi, and Anna Berti

Anosognosia is a term generally used to denote a complete or partial lack of awareness of different neurological (e.g., hemianopia, hemiplegia, cortical blindness, cortical deafness) and/or cognitive dysfunctions, such as, for example, fluent aphasia or memory deficits (see Prigatano & Schacter, 1991, for a review). In 1914, Babinski first introduced the term *anosognosia*, describing in particular the denial of motor deficits contralateral to a brain lesion (Babinski, 1914). Clinically, this disturbance ranges from emotional indifference or anosodiaphoria (Babinski, 1914), in which patients admit the paralysis and simply minimize its severity, to a complete unawareness of the unilateral motor impairment. The classical assessment of anosognosia proposed by Bisiach, Vallar, Perani, Papagno, and Berti (1986), using a 0 to 3 point scale, allows us to discriminate between patients who simply deny the deficit (score: 2/3) but are still able to discover the impairment when an explicit action is requested, from patients who still remain anosognosic despite the obvious inability to perform a specific movement (for example, clapping one's hand) requested by the examiner (score: 3/3). In this last case patients not only deny the impairment but present a false productive belief of having moved in spite of the evidence that a movement did not actually occur ("active" delusional component of anosognosia).

Delusional beliefs concerning the affected limb, such as somatoparaphrenia (Gerstmann, 1942), in which the ownership of the limb is ascribed to another person (e.g., doctor/examiner or a relative), misoplegia (e.g., hatred toward the affected limbs; Critchley, 1974), or personification (e.g., the hemiplegic limb is considered as an entity with an own identity), are usually considered as additional abnormal manifestations linked to anosognosia (referred to as "anosognosic phenomena"; Cutting, 1978). Adopting a more general classification, all these symptoms may be distinguished as defective (anosognosia) or productive (somatoparaphrenia). Due to this dichotomy it has become difficult to consider all these productive manifestations as equally linked to anosognosia, as recently emphasized by Marcel, Tegner, and Nimmo-Smith (2004). This difficulty also derives from the historical definition of anosognosia as a negative/defective manifestation; thus, it becomes quite incoherent to consider the somatoparaphrenic delusion as a consequence of anosognosia. These two symptoms are typically strictly associated.

Furthermore, anosognosia is frequently associated with unilateral neglect (Appelros, Karlsson, & Hennerdal, 2007; Bisiach et al., 1986; Rode et al., 1992; Rode, Perenin, Honore, & Boisson, 1998; Starkstein, Fedoroff, Price, Leiguarda, & Robinson, 1992; Willanger, Danielsen, & Ankerhus, 1981). The coexistence of these disturbances may be due to lesion of adjacent cerebral areas involving spatial processing and body representation. However, the observation of multiple dissociations between neglect, anosognosia, and delusional impairments of body schema suggests that neglect itself does not seem the crucial factor to elicit anosognosia and is not always present when anosognosia occurs (Berti, Ladavas, & Della Corte, 1996; Bisiach et al., 1986; Dauriac-Le Masson et al., 2002).

The clinical manifestations of anosognosia for hemiplegia are of great interest because they may provide indirect information on the cognitive organization of motor control. In this chapter some of the cognitive models on motor control will be considered in order to understand the pathological mechanisms underlying anosognosia for hemiplegia. Furthermore, the anatomical substrates of this symptom will also be taken into account as a contribution to the comprehension of anosognosia for hemiplegia as an impairment of motor control. Finally, recent evidence concerning the intention to move and its role in anosognosia will be discussed.

Interpretations of Anosognosia

The study of patients with anosognosia is of great interest for the comprehension of the neural mechanisms of body representation and motor awareness (review in Bisiach, 1995; Heilman, Barrett, & Adair, 1998; Vallar, Bottini, & Sterzi, 2003). Classically, the interpretations of anosognosia may be categorized into motivational and cognitive theories.

Motivational Theories of Anosognosia

Motivational theories, such as Weinstein and Kahn's (1955) psychodynamic interpretation of unawareness of the deficit, considered anosognosia as a psychological defensive mechanism or reaction aimed to protect the self from the potential distress deriving from suffering from a severe impairment or disease

(Schilder, 1935; Weinstein & Kahn, 1955). On the other hand, cognitive theories interpreted the symptom as a consequence of a specific disorder due to the damage of specific brain regions. The motivational theories, although fascinating, have been abandoned due to mounting evidence that anosognosia is frequently associated with right hemispheric lesions and present during the acute phase of the disease (Berti et al., 1996; Bisiach & Geminiani, 1991). Furthermore, this disturbance may be selective (e.g., a patient may be unaware of his hemiplegia but completely aware of his hemianopia or aphasia; Berti et al., 1996) and could be transiently modulated by different physiological manipulations (Cappa, Sterzi, Vallar, & Bisiach, 1987; Geminiani & Bottini, 1992; Vallar, Sterzi, Bottini, Cappa, & Rusconi, 1990). Collectively, these data suggest that a psychological defensive mechanism explanation of anosognosia is improbable.

Levine's "Discovery Theory"

The fact that anosognosia implies a cognitive impairment has been emphasized by Levine and colleagues' (1991) "discovery" theory. These authors suggest that the loss of a function would not be sufficient to produce by itself an immediate experience of loss; instead, the deficit would need to be discovered or inferred (Levine, Calvanio, & Rinn, 1991), and the lack of proprioceptive information together with additional cognitive defects would not enable the patients to "make the necessary observations and inferences to diagnose the paralysis" (Levine et al., 1991). However, since the first observation of Babinski (1914, 1918) it was emphasized that anosognosia did not seem to be related to global mental confusion or other intellectual deficits and more in general, somatosensory deficit, personal neglect, mental confusion, and global cognitive impairment do not necessarily co-occur with anosognosia (Berti et al., 1996; Bisiach et al., 1986; Marcel et al., 2004; Small & Ellis, 1996; Starkstein et al., 1992; Willanger et al., 1981). Cognitive disturbances cannot be therefore considered a prerequisite for anosognosia to emerge and persist (Bisiach & Geminiani, 1991; McGlynn & Schacter, 1989; Vuilleumier, 2004).

The Disconnection Hypothesis

In 1965, Geschwind (1965a, 1965b) proposed a more neurologically based theory of the anosognosic behavior, suggesting the presence of an interhemispheric disconnection that would isolate speech areas from the sensory and proprioceptive information deriving from the right brain side (Geschwind, 1965a, 1965b). Deprived from any veridical sensory information from the right hemisphere, the left speech areas would produce a verbal confabulation when the patient was questioned about his hemiplegia. This theory attempts to explain the prevalence of anosognosia after right brain damage. However, as noted by Bisiach et al. (1986), patients who verbally deny their deficit should still be able to express it in a nonverbal modality, and no dissociations between verbal and nonverbal response modalities have ever been reported (Berti, Ladavas, Stracciari, Giannarelli, & Ossola, 1998). Moreover, a simple manipulation like placing the left paretic arm into the unaffected right visual field, providing additional and correct sensory feedbacks to the left hemisphere, seems to improve the awareness of the motor deficit only in a few number of patients, for example, in 5 out of 15 patients in the study of Adair et al. (1997).

Anosognosia as a Consequence of a Central Monitoring Mechanism Deficit

Other models are based on the concept that anosognosia derives from a more pervasive awareness impairment, thus to be ascribed to damage of a central monitoring mechanism (Goldberg & Barr, 1991). Similarly, the conscious awareness system (CAS; McGlynn & Schacter, 1989) model explains selective forms of anosognosia with a disconnection of CAS from specific peripheral input modules damaged by the brain lesion.

Anosognosia as a Modality-Specific Monitoring System Impairment

Further studies on the clinical manifestations of anosognosia suggest that this disorder represents the consequence of damage to a modality-specific monitoring system (e.g., a motor monitoring system for anosognosia for hemiplegia) rather than of a central executive system (Bisiach, 1995; Bisiach, Meregalli, & Berti, 1990). This may better explain selective and modality-specific forms of unawareness of neurological deficits and also the presence of "productive" symptoms such as somatoparaphrenia (Bisiach, 1995; Bisiach et al., 1990). This theory inspired the topological representation of egocentric space (TRES) model (Bisiach, 1995; Bisiach & Berti, 1987; Bisiach & Geminiani, 1991; Bisiach et al., 1990), which explains both negative and productive deficits of contralesional space-body representation as a consequence of a more general representational deficit called dyschiria (Bisiach & Berti, 1987; Zingerle, 1913). Layer I of TRES is the terminal of a sensory transducer that carries information about an external object or body parts; layer II is a sensory-driven (veridical) representational network that analyzes and synthesises contents of layer I; layer III is composed of autochthonous (nonveridical), internally driven topologically organized cell assemblies. In normal waking conditions, the activity of layer III is inhibited by layer II cell assemblies so that the nonveridical product of layer III does not arrive to layer IV or is considered as imaginary. Layer IV represents the veridical final output of body-space representation. Inactivation of different components of this model may lead to different deficits: a partial or complete inactivation of one side of layers II and III produces lack of representation in layer IV of half the side of the space causing defective phenomena such as unilateral neglect or anosognosia. On the other hand, when there is damage to one side of only layer II, layer III is free from the inhibitory activity of layer II cell assemblies, so that autochthonous and nonveridical representations reach layer IV and give rise to delusional contents such as somatoparaphrenia (for a review of the model, see Bisiach & Berti, 1995; Bisiach & Geminiani, 1991; Bisiach & Vallar, 2000).

Anosognosia as an Impairment of the "Intention to Move": The Feed-Forward Hypothesis

More recent interpretations have searched for the pathogenetic mechanism of anosognosia in the context of models of motor control (Wolpert & Ghahramani, 2000; Wolpert, Ghahramani, & Jordan, 1995). Heilman (1991) proposed a *feed-forward* theory, which explains anosognosia as a deficit of the intentional system to formulate expectations of movement. This model implies that the intentional system activates at the same time as the motor system to perform the movement and a body representation as it should be after the movement execution. This representation is constantly compared with the afferent information. Heilman (1991) argues that if no expectations of movement are generated, then no failure of the movement itself can be detected. In hemiplegic patients, aware of their motor impairment, the monitor-comparator—or body representation—detects the mismatch between expectations of movement and the failed performance. Conversely, anosognosic patients do not "intend to move or prepare to move" (Heilman et al., 1998) their paretic limb (motor neglect), so that the comparator does not detect any mismatch. The authors proposed that this intentional network is centered on the dorsolateral (Brodmann's areas 6 and 8) and the medial frontal lobe (supplementary motor area and cingulate gyrus), the inferior parietal lobe, the thalamus, and the basal ganglia (Heilman et al., 1998). This interpretation of anosognosia is supported by several studies (Adair et al., 1997; Gold, Adair, Jacobs, & Heilman, 1994). Furthermore, the interpretation of anosognosia as a manifestation of motor neglect is supported by the observation that caloric vestibular and optokinetic stimulations induce the transient remission of both hemiplegia and anosognosia (Vallar et al., 2003; Vallar, Guariglia, Nico, & Pizzamiglio, 1997). This fact suggests that anosognosia, at least in those patients with motor deficit not due to a primary defect, could be unawareness of a "higher-order neglect related disorder", namely the defective intention to execute the movement (Vallar et al., 2003). Although the Heilman model (1991) is extremely convincing, it is not completely clear how anosognosic patients who assert to have performed a movement, for example, clapping their hands, could have lost their intention to move as the unimpaired limb does move.

The Feedback Hypothesis of Anosognosia

Frith, Blakemore, and Wolpert (2000) emphasized that the Heilman (1991; Heilman et al., 1998) model does not completely explain the delusional component of anosognosia, whereby patients affirm to have performed a movement, in spite of evidence that a movement did not actually occur. In response, they proposed an alternative interpretation of anosognosia based on a complex model of motor control (Wolpert & Ghahramani, 2000; Wolpert et al., 1995). This model provides three levels of motor representation: actual, desired, and predicted states. Controllers and predictors are also included in this system: the former provide the motor commands, and the latter provide an internal representation of the future movement. Comparisons between the three levels may signal errors that are adjusted by the means of predictors and controllers. Errors originating by a difference between desired and actual states activate the controllers in order to modify the motor commands. On the other hand, errors generated by discrepancies between predicted and actual states improve the predictors functioning. Finally, errors produced by the comparison between the desired and the predicted states activate the controllers at the level of the mental practice in the absence of real movement. The authors proposed that in anosognosic patients the comparison between desired (i.e., instantaneous goal of the system) and predicted state (i.e., future state of the system) is preserved. The normal functioning of both—controllers, which issued the appropriate motor commands to achieve the desired state, and predictors, which estimated the sensory consequences of the action—induces the normal experience of initiating a movement. On the other hand, denial of the motor deficit would be caused by a failure to register the incongruence between predicted and actual sensory consequences of the action and a failure to use these discrepancies to update the operations of the predictors. This is because information derived from the sensory feedback about the actual state of the system is not available or neglected, due to a lesion in the parietal lobe (Frith et al., 2000).

Clearly, the Heilman theory makes the neurophysiological prediction of a global damage of the system involved in motor planning; on the other hand, the Frith model is consistent with a distributed anatomical system for motor control, with a possible sparing of some specific components.

Anatomy of Anosognosia

Anatomical investigations have the potential to provide information that can be used to test current models of anosognosia. Early studies have associated anosognosia with parietal lobe lesions that classically have been related to spatial unilateral neglect (Critchley, 1953; Gerstmann, 1942; Pia, Neppi-Modona, Ricci, & Berti, 2004). With regard to the problem of the anatomical correlates of anosognosia for hemiplegia, the main outstanding questions relate to the hemispheric lateralization of the lesion and the crucial brain regions, which when damaged induce the symptom (Pia et al., 2004). Regarding the first issue, several studies based on clinical observation (Bisiach et al., 1986), Wada test experiments (Adair, Gilmore, Fennell, Gold, & Heilman, 1995; Breier et al., 1995; Carpenter et al., 1995; Gilmore, Heilman, Schmidt, Fennell, & Quisling, 1992), and a recent meta-analysis (Pia et al., 2004) consider the right hemisphere pivotal for the pathogenesis of anosognosia. However, the role played by damage to the left hemisphere should be taken into account, because of the presence of linguistic deficits that might prevent proper investigation of anosognosia (Pia et al., 2004).

Even more controversial is the issue of the crucial intrahemispheric site of lesion correlated to the genesis of this symptom. Several cortical and subcortical structures have been indicated as having a role in causing unawareness of motor deficits. Historically, right parietal or thalamic damage, including thalamo-parietal connections, has been considered a necessary prerequisite for the presence of anosognosia (Barkman, 1925; Potzl, 1925). The involvement of such areas and other subcortical regions such as the corona radiata, the internal capsule, and the basal ganglia has been confirmed by several studies (Bisiach et al., 1986; Ellis & Small, 1997; Small & Ellis, 1996). A recent meta-analysis of the major studies about the anatomical correlates of anosognosia published between 1983 and 2001 (Pia et al., 2004) concluded that the associated damage of the fronto-parietal or fronto-temporo-parietal cortices is the most frequent combination of lesions linked to the presence of anosognosia. Pia and colleagues (2004) found large involvement of subcortical structures (in particular of the basal ganglia) in 41% of the patients. Therefore, even if anosognosia has often been considered a deficit tightly linked to a parietal lesion, a review of the results of the past studies does not show a clear and sure prevalence of the role of damage in this structure in generating the anosognosic behavior.

Nevertheless, these seminal studies leave several uncertainties. First of all, many of them are single cases. Second, although many of these reports contain very interesting descriptions of patients' behavior, in general there is not clear information about the degree of anosognosia. Third, the severity of the neurological deficit that is denied is usually not detailed, and there is no mention of a standardized neurological exam. And finally, the anatomical conclusions are not based on a systematic exploration including a control group of hemiplegic patients with neglect and without anosognosia.

Recent studies have adopted a more methodologically rigorous approach by enrolling specific control groups (Berti et al., 2005; Karnath, Baier, & Nagele, 2005). The goal is to identify the precise anatomical lesional pattern of anosognosia while considering the complexity of the motor system and motor awareness, as well as the variety of behavioral manifestations.

Anosognosia out of the Parietal Cortex

In a recent paper, Berti et al. (2005) explored the lesional pattern of anosognosia following strict methodological rules for the behavioral profile and anatomical mapping. The authors compared, using a voxel-based statistical analysis, the brain lesion distribution of 12 patients with anosognosia and 17 patients without anosognosia (all with right brain damage). Interestingly, they only enrolled subjects presenting with a complete left hemiplegia that had been investigated by a standardized neurological clinical examination (hemiplegia = complete absence of movement). One patient (case RMA) presented with anosognosia without neglect. All the studied subjects were in the acute clinical phase. The anatomical lesional mapping was performed in the stereotactic space of Talairach and Tournoux (1988) using a standard MRI volume that conformed to that space as redefined by the Montreal Neurological Institute (MNI) space. Image manipulations were performed with the applications Analyze and MRIcro (Rorden & Brett, 2000). The lesion distribution was identified using a probabilistic Brodmann's areas map released with MRIcro. The statistical significance of the occurrence of a brain lesion in a given group was based on two omnibus tests (chi-square test with Yates' correction, and Mann-Whitney U test) and a voxel-by-voxel test, implemented in Matlab 6.5.

The authors found a significant association of unawareness for motor deficit with lesion of the dorsal premotor cortex (Brodmann's area 6), area 44, and the somatosensory and primary motor cortex. Brodmann's area 46 and the insula were also involved (see Figure 2.1). It is interesting to note that the same lesional pattern (Brodmann's area 6, 4, 44, and 3 and in the insula) was also found in patient RMA, who was anosognosic in the absence of neglect, attesting to the specificity of this anatomical correlate with the symptom of motor deficit denial. Conversely, in hemiplegic patients without anosognosia the premotor cerebral cortex was spared while a significant involvement of the subcortical white matter in the depth of the centrum semiovale was found. The fact that the brain damage of motor regions was not complete, as the supplementary motor cortex (SMA) and the pre-SMA were spared (see Figure 2.1; Berti et al., 2005), suggests that a representation of the conscious intention of action could still be available in anosognosic patients (Berti, Spinazzola, Pia, & Rabuffetti, 2007), supporting Frith's interpretation of anosognosia.

Karnath et al. (2005) compared the lesion distribution of 14 anosognosic patients in the acute phase of the disease with 13 patients aware of their motor deficit considered as the control group with a comparable frequency and severity of additional neurological defects, such as spatial neglect, hemianesthesia, and hemianopia. The subtractive anatomical comparison revealed a significant involvement of the posterior insular cortex. This region was less damaged in patients with hemiplegia/hemiparesis without anosognosia. The authors

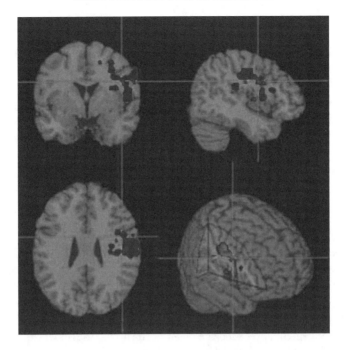

Figure 2.1 Brain areas with lesions associated with anosognosia (From Berti et al., 2005, reprinted with permission from the Association for the Advancement of Science, *Science*, *309*(5733), 488–491.) (See Color Plate 2.1)

proposed that the posterior insula, which integrates different sensory inputs (e.g., sensory, motor, auditory, and vestibular; Mesulam & Mufson, 1985) has an important role in the construction of self-awareness. In our opinion, the main difference between the study conducted by Berti et al. (2005) and this one is that Karnath et al. (2005) enrolled patients with variable severity degree of the contralesional motor deficit ranging from hemiparesis to the complete absence of movement. Although the exploration of unawareness for mild motor impairments may certainly contribute to understanding the organization of motor control, we think that it is important to study anosognosic patients comparable for the degree of motor deficit, as it is not still clear whether there is only one kind of denial of the impairment. In patients showing a residual motor function, the firm belief of having performed a movement could still be ascribed to the left, although defective, motor activity in the contralesional arm.

The Role of the Intention to Move in Anosognosia

As we have just commented, anosognosia can be interpreted in the context of the models of motor control and related to the impairment of some of the processes involved in motor monitoring and execution. Thus, anosognosia may depend on the lack of the intention to move, of the capacity to provide correct motor planning, or to compare different representations of the status of the motor system. Although many studies investigated motor functions in normal subjects, at different levels while performing tasks of explicit motor action, of motor imagery or motor awareness (Ehrsson, Spence, & Passingham, 2004; Jeannerod, 1994; Jeannerod & Decety, 1995; Lau, Rogers, Haggard, & Passingham, 2004; Stephan & Frackowiak, 1996), a systematic study integrating data derived from the investigation of normal subjects and evidence from the exploration of anosognosic patients is still lacking.

A crucial issue for the comprehension of motor deficit denial is about the intactness of the intention to act. The anatomical correlates of motor intention components have been extensively investigated in normal subjects. In a seminal paper published in 1983 (Libet, Gleason, Wright, & Pearl, 1983), healthy subjects were asked to signal the exact moment when they reported the experience of "wanting" to perform a movement (intention/urge/decision to move; "W judgement") and when they become aware to initiate a movement ("M judgement"). These two subjective time judgments were correlated with both the precise onset of the real movement, measured by the EMG, and the readiness potential (RP), recorded by the EEG. The authors found that both W and M judgements preceded the onset of the actual movement (EMG onset), respectively, by about 200 and by 50–80 ms. Even more interesting was the result that the negative readiness potential precedes by several hundred milliseconds the W judgement. Libet and colleagues (1983) concluded that the neural process (RP potential) preceding a voluntary, self-generated action starts before the appearance of conscious intention to initiate a motor action. This signal of cerebral activation recorded by the RP is considered to be arising from the supplementary motor area (SMA; Deecke & Kornhuber, 1978; Lang, Zilch, Koska, Lindinger, & Deecke, 1989). More recently, Haggard and Eimer (1999) recorded both RP and the lateralized readiness potential (LRP) while subjects performed M and W judgements in two different experimental conditions: *(1)* fixed movement (performing movement with the same hand in each experimental block) and *(2)* free choice condition (subjects freely decided in each trial which hand to use to perform the movement). The authors found a covariation between W judgement and the onset of the LRP, while no correlation was found with the onset of RP. This result has been interpreted in the view that the conscious intention to move reflects the neural activity related to the selection of a specific movement and not to an abstract representation of action (prior intention). Following this model, conscious intention occurs after the stage of movement selection (see Figure 2.2; C = urge to move).

In summary, the results of the electrophysiological studies mentioned above suggest that SMA is crucial for the awareness of the intention to move. Functional MRI experiments, in which self-initiated and externally triggered movements were compared, support this hypothesis (Cunnington,

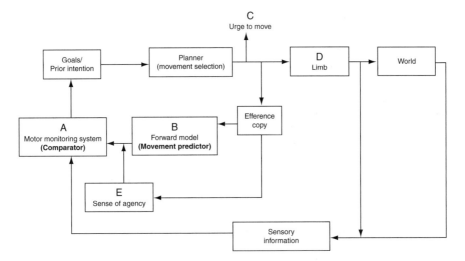

Figure 2.2 A modified version of the forward model of motor production (From Haggard, 2005, with permission from Elsevier, *Trends in Cognitive Science*, 9(6), 290–295.) and motor control (From Berti & Pia, 2006, with permission from Wiley InterScience, *Current Directions in Psychological Science*, 15(5), 245–250.)

Windischberger, Deecke, & Moser, 2002; Jahanshahi et al., 1995; Jenkins, Jahanshahi, Jueptner, Passingham, & Brooks, 2000). More recently, in an fMRI study Lau and colleagues (2004), using Libet's paradigm, found activations in the pre-SMA, the dorsolateral prefrontal cortex (DPFC or Brodmann's area 46), and in the intraparietal sulcus when normal healthy subjects attended to their intentions. The relevance of SMA and pre-SMA is also corroborated by the anatomical lesional data. Berti et al. (2005) found that both these areas are generally spared in hemiplegic patients with anosognosia, suggesting that in such patients representation of the intended motor act it is still possible, although distorted. Thus, in anosognosic patients the intentional system and probably the feed-forward model appear to still be preserved, and possibly unawareness for hemiplegia is caused by a damage of the comparator (see lesion of A in Figure 2.2). To further support this hypothesis, Berti et al. (2007) compared the muscle electric activity (recorded using surface electromyogram: EMG) in the left and right upper trapezius of one patient with hemiplegia (case CR) and a dense anosognosia (Bisiach Standard Neurological Examination score: 3/3), one patient with hemiplegia without anosognosia (case SF), and one healthy control. There were three experimental conditions: *(1)* reaching with the left hemiplegic limb; *(2)* reaching with the right limb; and *(3)* resting condition. Detection of the activation of the proximal muscles on both sides for reaching movement with the left hemiplegic arm could be considered an indirect evidence of the preserved intention to move. This hypothesis was confirmed as in patient CR a preserved activity in the left proximal muscle despite the presence of anosognosia has been found. The authors suggested that the differences between the two patients SF and CR could concern the dysfunctioning comparator in CR, demonstrating that motor intention is still preserved.

To verify the Frith et al. (2000) hypothesis that the nonveridical awareness of action is based on the dominance of motor planning (forward model) on the somatosensory feedback, Fotopoulou et al. (2008) studied four patients with motor anosognosia and four with hemiplegia without anosognosia. They manipulated both intention to move and visual feedback of movement using a rubber hand. The visual feedback could be coherent or incoherent with respect to the intention to move modulated by different instructions: *(1)* perform a self-generated movement; *(2)* patients were told that an experimenter would lift his left arm (externally generated movement); and *(3)* no movement required. Dependent variables were the movement detection and the agency score. Anosognosic patients showed a comparable performance with controls in all conditions with the exception of the first condition (self-generated movement performance) while an incoherent feedback was provided (no rubber hand movement). Anosognosic subjects ignored the incoherent visual feedback (the rubber hand was not moving) only in the condition in which they intended to move. On the other hand, in the externally generated movement they performed correctly, demonstrating that anosognosic patients ignore the visual information (sensory feedback) only in the condition implying the intention to move. These results are compatible with the Frith et al. (2000) hypothesis that the nonveridical awareness of movement "is created on the basis of a comparison between the intended and predicted position of the limbs, and not on the basis of a mismatch between the predicted and actual sensory feedback" (Fotopoulou et al., 2008).

Effect of Caloric Vestibular Stimulation on Neglect and Related Disorders

It is well known that cold caloric vestibular stimulation (CVS) may produce a transient (nearly 15–20 minutes) recovery of extrapersonal (Cappa et al., 1987; Rubens, 1985; Silberpfennig, 1941), personal (Cappa et al., 1987; Rode et al., 1992), representational neglect (Geminiani & Bottini, 1992; Rode & Perenin, 1994) and of several related disorders such as anosognosia for hemiplegia (Cappa et al., 1987; Rode et al., 1992), somatoparaphrenia (Bisiach, Rusconi, & Vallar, 1991; Rode et al., 1992), somatosensory (Vallar, Bottini, Rusconi, & Sterzi, 1993; Vallar et al., 1990), and motor deficits (Rode et al., 1992; see also Rossetti & Rode, 2002 and their Table 1 for a review of the effect of CVS on different neglect symptoms).

Caloric vestibular stimulation consists of an iced water irrigation of the external ear canal contralateral to the brain lesion. The injection determines an ocular reflex (slow-phase nystagmus) toward the stimulated ear and sometimes may induce negative sensations, such as nausea, vomiting, and dizziness.

Table 2.1 Positive and Negative Effects of CVS as a Function of the Side of Stimulation (Left or Right Ear) and Water Temperature (Cold or Warm Water) in RBD Patients

	Left-Ear CVS	Right-Ear CVS
Cold water	Leftward nystagmus improvement of the deficit	Rightward nystagmus worsening of the deficit
Warm water	Rightward nystagmus worsening of the deficit	Leftward nystagmus improvement of the deficit

CVS, Caloric vestibular stimulation; RBD, right brain damaged.

During CVS the experimenter may vary the side of stimulation (ipsilesional or contralesional ear) and the water temperature (cold or warm water). The interaction of these two factors induces different physiological changes (direction of slow-phase nystagmus) and as a consequence positive or negative effects on the deficit. In fact, in right brain–damaged (RBD) patients, the irrigation of the contralesional ear with cold water (left CVS) or the irrigation of the ipsilesional ear with warm water, both producing a leftward slow-phase nystagmus, induces an improvement of neglect. Conversely, the irrigation of the ipsilesional ear (right CVS) with cold water or the irrigation of the contralateral ear (left CVS) with warm water produces a rightward slow phase nystagmus and induces a worsening of these symptoms (Rubens, 1985; see Table 2.1).

As mentioned above, CVS may produce a temporary recovery of some neurological deficits such as hemianesthesia, namely the impaired detection of tactile stimuli delivered on the side of the body contralateral to a brain lesion (Bottini et al., 2005; Vallar et al., 1993; Vallar et al., 1990). The effect of CVS on an apparently elementary deficit suggests that the right hemisphere may have a role on conscious tactile perception. In RBD patients, left CVS (cold vestibular stimulation in the left ear) induces a transient improvement of left tactile perception (Bottini et al., 2005; Vallar et al., 1990; Vallar et al., 1993). Conversely, in left brain–damaged patients (LBD) right CVS (cold vestibular stimulation in the right ear) does not modulate right hemianesthesia. The only exception is represented by the few cases of LBD patients presenting right hemineglect (Vallar et al., 1993; for an extensive review of the effects of CVS on somatosensory processing, see Vallar, 1997). The observation of this hemispheric asymmetry suggested that left hemianesthesia also contains a "nonsensory or perceptual component" (Vallar et al., 1993), responsible for the access to conscious awareness of tactile stimuli, which is strictly related to neglect and may be positively modulated by CVS (Vallar et al., 1993). Conversely, right hemianesthesia associated with lesion of the left hemisphere could reflect a mainly primary (elementary) sensory deficit. This hypothesis has been supported by different neurophysiological (Vallar, Bottini, Sterzi, Passerini, & Rusconi, 1991; Vallar, Sandroni, Rusconi, & Barbieri, 1991) and clinical (Smania & Aglioti, 1995; Sterzi et al., 1993) evidence.

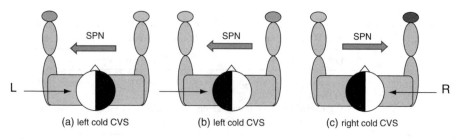

Figure 2.3 Effects of cold caloric vestibular stimulation (CVS) on tactile hemianesthesia in right brain–damaged and left brain–damaged patients as a consequence of the stimulation side (contralesional versus ipsilesional ear stimulation). The damaged hemisphere is colored in black. L, left; R, right; SPN, slow-phase nystagmus; green: positive effect (recovery) of tactile perception; red: no effect on tactile perception. (See Color Plate 2.3)

To better clarify this hemispheric asymmetry, Bottini et al. (2005) systematically studied the effect of CVS on RBD and LBD hemianesthetic patients (Bottini et al., 2005). The authors confirmed previous evidence of an improvement of tactile perception after left cold CVS in RBD patients (a) and the absence of positive effects after right cold CVS on LBD subjects (c). Interestingly, they also described a significant remission of right hemianesthesia when the *left ipsilesional* ear was stimulated in LBD patients (b) (see Figure 2.3).

The authors also studied an LDB patient with fMRI before and after CVS and a group of healthy subjects during a tactile perception task. They found that recovery of tactile perception after CVS was associated with neural activity in patient's right secondary somatosensory cortex (SII). In the control subjects the activation of SII for ipsilateral stimuli was of a greater extent in the right hemisphere for right touches than in the left hemisphere for left touches (right SII–right stimuli, left SII–left stimuli). These results suggest a right hemispheric specialization for the body representation (in particular for the hand representation) and that this hemisphere contains a more complete representation of the whole body space compared with the left hemisphere (Bottini et al., 2005).

Recovery of Anosognosia for Hemiplegia after Caloric Vestibular Stimulation

The effects of caloric vestibular stimulation on RBD patients unaware of their left hemiplegia were first described by Cappa and colleagues (1987), who used this method on four patients with severe neglect and anosognosia for both motor (upper and lower limbs) and visual deficits. In two cases, anosognosia was not affected by the manipulation, while in the other two patients cold left CVS provoked a transient remission of this disorder immediately after the stimulation. Vallar et al. (1990) observed a temporary amelioration of hemianesthesia after CVS in three patients and, in one of these, they also reported a temporary complete remission of extrapersonal, personal neglect and anosognosia. Bisiach et al. (1991) described a patient suffering from a right fronto-temporo-parietal stroke showing anosognosia with somatoparaphrenic delusions who underwent CVS three times; after all the trials he completely recovered from his somatoparaphrenic delusion, which reappeared with the same characteristics in about 2 hours, demonstrating the possible modulation of a body scheme disorder by a peripheral stimulation. Rode et al. (1992) found the same results applying CVS on a somatoparaphrenic and long-lasting anosognosic patient with a severe hemiplegia and hemianopia caused by a large cortico-subcortical infarction in the right brain hemisphere involving the parieto-temporo-occipital carrefour. After the left ear canal irrigation with iced water, a dramatic recovery of both anosognosia and somatoparaphrenia was reported and, surprisingly, CVS also caused a reduction of the left motor deficit.

Geminiani and Bottini (1992) observed the effect of CVS in RBD patients. In one patient with slight personal neglect and moderate anosognosia, vestibular stimulation caused personal neglect to temporarily disappear but anosognosia remained unchanged. In two other cases, CVS produced a temporary amelioration of, respectively, a moderate and severe anosognosia (Geminiani & Bottini, 1992).

Ramachandran (1995) used CVS on a woman with a severe left neglect syndrome and a dense left hemiplegia of which she was totally unaware. Furthermore, when asked about whose hand was her left one, she showed a clear "feeling of non belonging" of her left arm, which she attributed either to the experimenter or to her son (Ramachandran, 1995, p. 27). After the irrigation of the left canal ear with 10cc of iced water and the appearance of the nystagmus, the patient was assessed for the awareness of the motor deficit and the sense of limb ownership, showing a full recovery from both these conditions.

The relationship between recovery of motor deficits and improvement of anosognosia has been more systematically investigated by Rode et al. (1998), who studied the effect of vestibular stimulation comparatively in two groups of hemiplegic patients: *(1)* three RBD patients with neglect without anosognosia and six with neglect and anosognosia; and *(2)* nine LBD patients without neglect. In contrast to the LBD group, motor performance in the RBD group significantly improved after CVS, and a temporary remission of personal neglect and anosognosia was also observed in 5 out of 6 patients (Rode et al., 1998).

Vallar et al. (2003) replicated the same results in a group of four RBD patients with neglect, hemianopia, hemianesthesia, and hemiplegia of the left upper limb showing anosognosia for the motor defect. The stimulation with iced water temporarily improved motor strength together with a recovery from the unawareness deficit (Vallar et al., 2003). Taken together, these observations suggest that CVS can have a positive effect on both motor deficit itself and anosognosia for hemiplegia. This evidence may argue for a nonprimary, higher-order motor neglect component in patients' hemiplegia; furthermore, it is worth noting, even if counterintuitive, that the less severe the deficit, the more aware of it the patient seems to become (Vallar et al., 2003). These findings suggest that anosognosia might not relate to a primary deficit but to a higher-level disorder such as a "deficit of motor intention or planning" (Vallar et al., 2003) and that the positive effects of the stimulation on both hemiplegia and anosognosia could be due to the possible amelioration of this intentional motor deficit (Vallar et al., 2003).

We may speculate that another possible interpretation is that CVS may restore the space and body schema representation and therefore rebalance the predicted and the actual state components of Frith's model of anosognosia (Frith et al., 2000).

Conclusion

In our opinion the main outstanding questions relative to the pathological mechanisms underpinning anosognosia are as follows:

1. The role of the intention to move: in other words is the denial of hemiplegia due to the fact that patients with this symptom do not have the intention to move the plegic limb, not even to trigger the cognitive procedures to plan and perform the movement? In some patients, not all of them anosognosic subjects, the presence of a motor neglect component could explain this deficit denial (Vallar et al., 2003). Nevertheless, recent experiments on anosognosic patients seem to show that the intention to move is still preserved (Berti et al., 2007; Fotopoulou et al., 2008). Furthermore, this theory does not fully explain why there are anosognosic patients that do not show motor neglect, and why there are some patients that claim to have performed the movement when the movement has not actually occurred (Frith et al., 2000). We call this clinical manifestation as a form of delusional/nonveridical awareness/productive anosognosia.

2. The role of damage at different levels of the motor control system. We assume that anosognosia may be generated by a dysfunction of the comparator as described by the Frith et al., model (2000). In this case the patients are still able to compare desired and predicted states, but the discrepancies between predicted and actual states are ignored. Frith proposes that this happens because the sensory feedback is not available or neglected, inducing an overcoming of the prediction on the afferent information. This hypothesis better explains the delusional anosognosia, and it also explains some interesting aspects of the modulation of anosognosia through the vestibular caloric stimulation (Cappa et al., 1987; Vallar et al., 2003). One may speculate that vestibular stimulation transiently recovers the somatosensory afferents, rebalancing the predicted and the actual state components in the model, temporarily resolving the overcoming of the former on the latter. The role of the comparator in generating anosognosia remains to be clarified.

3. Focusing on the anatomical correlates of anosognosia, the feed-forward model and the feedback theory make different anatomical predictions. The debate is still open on the crucial localization of anosognosia in the parietal or in the motor cortices.

Observation of anosognosic patients (Bisiach et al., 1986; Ramachandran, 1995; Vallar et al., 2003) indicates that there are diverse manifestations that suggest not only different degrees of severity of motor denial (quantitative index) but also a qualitative/functional difference among these symptoms (qualitative/functional indexes)—some of them being more negative/defective, others more positive/productive. In the future, a more detailed investigation of these symptoms could probably lead to a multifaceted classification, including different kinds of motor denial.

References

Adair, J. C., Gilmore, R. L., Fennell, E. B., Gold, M., & Heilman, K. M. (1995). Anosognosia during intracarotid barbiturate anesthesia: Unawareness or amnesia for weakness. *Neurology, 45*(2), 241–243.

Adair, J. C., Schwartz, R. L., Na, D. L., Fennell, E., Gilmore, R. L., & Heilman, K. M. (1997). Anosognosia: Examining the disconnection hypothesis. *Journal of Neurology, Neurosurgery and Psychiatry, 63*(6), 798–800.

Appelros, P., Karlsson, G. M., & Hennerdal, S. (2007). Anosognosia versus unilateral neglect. Coexistence and their relations to age, stroke severity, lesion site and cognition. *European Journal of Neurology, 14*(1), 54–59.

Babinski, J. (1914). Contribution à l'étude des troubles mentaux dans l'hémiplégie organique cérébrale (anosognosie). *Revue Neurologique, 27*, 845–848.

Babinski, J. (1918). Anosognosie. *Revue Neurologique (Paris), 31*, 365–367.

Barkman, A. (1925). De l'anosognosie dans l'émiplegie cérébrale: Contribution a l'étude de ce symptome. *Acta Medica Scandinavica, 62*, 235–254.

Berti, A., Bottini, G., Gandola, M., Pia, L., Smania, N., Stracciari, A., et al. (2005). Shared cortical anatomy for motor awareness and motor control. *Science, 309*(5733), 488–491.

Berti, A., Ladavas, E., & Della Corte, M. (1996). Anosognosia for hemiplegia, neglect dyslexia, and drawing neglect: Clinical findings and theoretical considerations. *Journal of the International Neuropsychological Society, 2*(5), 426–440.

Berti, A., Ladavas, E., Stracciari, A., Giannarelli, C., & Ossola, A. (1998). Anosognosia for motor impairment and dissociations with patient's evaluation of the disorders: Theoretical considerations. *Cognitive Neuropsychiatry, 3*, 21–44.

Berti, A., & Pia, L. (2006). Understanding motor awareness through normal and pathological behavior. *Current Directions in Psychological Science, 15*(5), 245–250.

Berti, A., Spinazzola, L., Pia, L., & Rabuffetti, M. (2007). Motor awareness and motor intention in anosognosia for hemiplegia. In P. Haggard, Y. Rossetti, & M. Kawato (Eds.), *Sensorimotor foundations of higher cognition series: Attention and performance number XXII* (pp. 163–182.). New York: Oxford University Press.

Bisiach, E. (1995). Unawareness of unilateral neurological impairment and disordered representation of one side of the body. *Higher Brain Function Research, 15*(2), 113–140.

Bisiach, E., & Berti, A. (1987). Dyschiria: An attempt at its systemic explanation. In M. Jeannerod (Ed.), *Neurophysiological and neuropsychological aspects of spatial neglect* (pp. 183–201). Amsterdam: Elsevier.

Bisiach, E., & Berti, A. (1995). Consciousness in dyschiria. In M. S. Gazzaniga (Ed.), *The cognitive neurosciences* (pp. 1331–1340): MIT Press.

Bisiach, E., & Geminiani, G. (1991). Anosognosia related to hemiplegia and hemianopia. In G. Prigatano & D. Schacter (Eds.), *Awareness of deficit after brain injury: Clinical and theoretical issues* (pp. 17–39). New York: Oxford University Press.

Bisiach, E., Meregalli, S., & Berti, A. (1990). Mechanisms of production control and belief fixation in human visuospatial processing: Clinical evidence from unilateral neglect and misrepresentation. In R. J. Commons, S. M. Hernstein, S. M. Kosslyn, & D. B. Mumford (Eds.), *Quantitative analysis of behavior: Computational and clinical approach to pattern recognition and concept formation* (Vol. IX, pp. 3–21): Hillsdale, NJ: Lawrence Erlbaum Associates.

Bisiach, E., Rusconi, M. L., & Vallar, G. (1991). Remission of somatoparaphrenic delusion through vestibular stimulation. *Neuropsychologia, 29*(10), 1029–1031.

Bisiach, E., & Vallar, G. (2000). Unilateral neglect in humans. In F. Boller, J. Grafman, & G. Rizzolatti (Eds.), *Handbook of neuropsychology* (2nd ed.) (pp. 459–502). Amsterdam: Elsvier Science B.V.

Bisiach, E., Vallar, G., Perani, D., Papagno, C., & Berti, A. (1986). Unawareness of disease following lesions of the right hemisphere: Anosognosia for hemiplegia and anosognosia for hemianopia. *Neuropsychologia, 24*(4), 471–482.

Bottini, G., Paulesu, E., Gandola, M., Loffredo, S., Scarpa, P., Sterzi, R., et al. (2005). Left caloric vestibular stimulation ameliorates right hemianesthesia. *Neurology, 65*(8), 1278–1283.

Breier, J. I., Adair, J. C., Gold, M., Fennell, E. B., Gilmore, R. L., & Heilman, K. M. (1995). Dissociation of anosognosia for hemiplegia and aphasia during left-hemisphere anesthesia. *Neurology, 45*(1), 65–67.

Cappa, S., Sterzi, R., Vallar, G., & Bisiach, E. (1987). Remission of hemineglect and anosognosia during vestibular stimulation. *Neuropsychologia, 25*(5), 775–782.

Carpenter, K., Berti, A., Oxbury, S., Molyneux, A. J., Bisiach, E., & Oxbury, J. M. (1995). Awareness of and memory for arm weakness during intracarotid sodium amytal testing. *Brain, 118 (Pt 1)*, 243–251.

Critchley, M. (1953). *The parietal lobe.* New York: Hafner.

Critchley, M. (1974). Misoplegia, or hatred of hemiplegia. *Mt. Sinai Journal of Medicine, 41*(1), 82–87.

Cunnington, R., Windischberger, C., Deecke, L., & Moser, E. (2002). The preparation and execution of self-initiated and externally-triggered movement: A study of event-related fMRI. *NeuroImage, 15*(2), 373–385.

Cutting, J. (1978). Study of anosognosia. *Journal of Neurology, Neurosurgery and Psychiatry, 41*(6), 548–555.

Dauriac-Le Masson, V., Mailhan, L., Louis-Dreyfus, A., De Montety, G., Denys, P., Bussel, B., et al. (2002). Double dissociation between unilateral neglect and anosognosia. *Revue Neurologique (Paris), 158*(4), 427–430.

Deecke, L., & Kornhuber, H. H. (1978). An electrical sign of participation of the mesial "supplementary" motor cortex in human voluntary finger movement. *Brain Research, 159*(2), 473–476.

Ehrsson, H. H., Spence, C., & Passingham, R. E. (2004). That's my hand! Activity in premotor cortex reflects feeling of ownership of a limb. *Science, 305*(5685), 875–877.

Ellis, S., & Small, M. (1997). Localization of lesion in denial of hemiplegia after acute stroke. *Stroke, 28*(1), 67–71.

Fotopoulou, A., Tsakiris, M., Haggard, P., Vagopoulou, A., Rudd, A., & Kopelman, M. (2008). The role of motor intention in motor awareness: An experimental study on anosognosia for hemiplegia. *Brain.* 131 (Pt 12), 3432–42.

Frith, C. D., Blakemore, S. J., & Wolpert, D. M. (2000). Abnormalities in the awareness and control of action. *Philosophical Transactions of the Royal Society of London B Biological Sciences, 355*(1404), 1771–1788.

Geminiani, G., & Bottini, G. (1992). Mental representation and temporary recovery from unilateral neglect after vestibular stimulation. *Journal of Neurology, Neurosurgery and Psychiatry, 55*(4), 332–333.

Gerstmann, J. (1942). Problem of imperception of disease and of impaired body territories with organic lesions. Relation to body schema and its disorders. *Archives of Neurology and Psychiatry, 48*, 890–913.

Geschwind, N. (1965a). Disconnexion syndromes in animals and man. I. *Brain, 88*(2), 237–294.

Geschwind, N. (1965b). Disconnexion syndromes in animals and man. II. *Brain, 88*(3), 585–644.

Gilmore, R. L., Heilman, K. M., Schmidt, R. P., Fennell, E. M., & Quisling, R. (1992). Anosognosia during Wada testing. *Neurology, 42*(4), 925–927.

Gold, M., Adair, J. C., Jacobs, D. H., & Heilman, K. M. (1994). Anosognosia for hemiplegia: An electrophysiologic investigation of the feed-forward hypothesis. *Neurology, 44*(10), 1804–1808.

Goldberg, E., & Barr, W. B. (1991). Three possible mechanisms of unawareness of deficit. In G. P. Prigatano & D. L. Schacter (Eds.), *Awareness of deficit after brain injury: Clinical and theoretical issues* (pp. 152–175). New York: Oxford University Press.

Haggard, P. (2005). Conscious intention and motor cognition. *Trends in Cognitive Science, 9*(6), 290–295.

Haggard, P., & Eimer, M. (1999). On the relation between brain potentials and the awareness of voluntary movements. *Experimental Brain Research, 126*(1), 128–133.

Heilman, K. M. (1991). Anosognosia: Possible neuropsychological mechanisms. In G. Prigatano & D. Schacter (Eds.), *Awareness of deficit after brain injury: Clinical and theoretical issues* (pp. 53–62). New York: Oxford University Press.

Heilman, K. M., Barrett, A. M., & Adair, J. C. (1998). Possible mechanisms of anosognosia: A defect in self-awareness. *Philosophical Transactions of the Royal Society of London B Biological Sciences, 353*(1377), 1903–1909.

Jahanshahi, M., Jenkins, I. H., Brown, R. G., Marsden, C. D., Passingham, R. E., & Brooks, D. J. (1995). Self-initiated versus externally triggered movements. I. An investigation using measurement of regional cerebral blood flow with PET and movement-related potentials in normal and Parkinson's disease subjects. *Brain, 118*(Pt 4), 913–933.

Jeannerod, M. (1994). The representing brain: Neural correlates of motor intention and imagery. *Behavioral and Brain Sciences, 17*, 187–245.

Jeannerod, M., & Decety, J. (1995). Mental motor imagery: A window into the representational stages of action. *Current Opinion in Neurobiology, 5*(6), 727–732.

Jenkins, I. H., Jahanshahi, M., Jueptner, M., Passingham, R. E., & Brooks, D. J. (2000). Self-initiated versus externally triggered movements. II. The effect of movement predictability on regional cerebral blood flow. *Brain, 123*(Pt 6), 1216–1228.

Karnath, H. O., Baier, B., & Nagele, T. (2005). Awareness of the functioning of one's own limbs mediated by the insular cortex? *Journal of Neuroscience, 25*(31), 7134–7138.

Lang, W., Zilch, O., Koska, C., Lindinger, G., & Deecke, L. (1989). Negative cortical DC shifts preceding and accompanying simple and complex sequential movements. *Experimental Brain Research, 74*(1), 99–104.

Lau, H. C., Rogers, R. D., Haggard, P., & Passingham, R. E. (2004). Attention to intention. *Science, 303*(5661), 1208–1210.

Levine, D. N., Calvanio, R., & Rinn, W. E. (1991). The pathogenesis of anosognosia for hemiplegia. *Neurology, 41*(11), 1770–1781.

Libet, B., Gleason, C. A., Wright, E. W., & Pearl, D. K. (1983). Time of conscious intention to act in relation to onset of cerebral activity (readiness-potential): The unconscious initiation of a freely voluntary act. *Brain, 106*(Pt 3), 623–642.

Marcel, A. J., Tegner, R., & Nimmo-Smith, I. (2004). Anosognosia for plegia: Specificity, extension, partiality and disunity of bodily unawareness. *Cortex, 40*(1), 19–40.

McGlynn, S. M., & Schacter, D. L. (1989). Unawareness of deficits in neuropsychological syndromes. *Journal of Clinical and Experimental Neuropsychology, 11*(2), 143–205.

Mesulam, M. M., & Mufson, E. J. (1985). The Insula of Reil in man and monkey: Architectonics, connectivity, and function. In A. Peters & E. Jones (Eds.), *Cerebral cortex* (Vol. 4, pp. 179–226). New York: Plenum.

Pia, L., Neppi-Modona, M., Ricci, R., & Berti, A. (2004). The anatomy of anosognosia for hemiplegia: A meta-analysis. *Cortex, 40*(2), 367–377.

Potzl, O. (1925). Ueber Storungen der Selbtwahrnehmug bei Linksseitiger Hemiplegie. *Neurologie und Psychiatrie, 93*, 117–168.

Prigatano, G. P., & Schacter, D. L. (Eds.) (1991). *Awareness of deficit after brain injury: Clinical and theoretical issues.* New York: Oxford University Press.

Ramachandran, V. S. (1995). Anosognosia in parietal lobe syndrome. *Consciousness and Cognition, 4*(1), 22–51.

Rode, G., Charles, N., Perenin, M. T., Vighetto, A., Trillet, M., & Aimard, G. (1992). Partial remission of hemiplegia and somatoparaphrenia through vestibular stimulation in a case of unilateral neglect. *Cortex, 28*(2), 203–208.

Rode, G., & Perenin, M. T. (1994). Temporary remission of representational hemineglect through vestibular stimulation. *Neuroreport, 5*(8), 869–872.

Rode, G., Perenin, M. T., Honore, J., & Boisson, D. (1998). Improvement of the motor deficit of neglect patients through vestibular stimulation: Evidence for a motor neglect component. *Cortex, 34*(2), 253–261.

Rorden, C., & Brett, M. (2000). Stereotaxic display of brain lesions. *Behavioural Neurology, 12*(4), 191–200.

Rossetti, Y., & Rode, G. (2002). Reducing spatial neglect by visual and other sensory manipulations: noncognitive (physiological) routes to the rehabilitation of a cognitive disorder. In H. O. Karnath, D. Milner, & G. Vallar (Eds.), *The cognitive and neural bases of spatial neglect* (pp. 375–396). New York: Oxford University Press.

Rubens, A. B. (1985). Caloric stimulation and unilateral visual neglect. *Neurology, 35*(7), 1019–1024.

Schilder, P. (1935). *The image and appearance of the human body.* New York: International Universities Press.

Silberpfennig, J. (1941). Contributions to the problem of eye movements. III. Disturbances of ocular movements with pseudohemianopsia in frontal lobe tumors. *Confinia Neurologica 4*, 1–13.

Small, M., & Ellis, S. (1996). Denial of hemiplegia: An investigation into the theories of causation. *European Neurology, 36*(6), 353–363.

Smania, N., & Aglioti, S. (1995). Sensory and spatial components of somaesthetic deficits following right brain damage. *Neurology, 45*(9), 1725–1730.

Starkstein, S. E., Fedoroff, J. P., Price, T. R., Leiguarda, R., & Robinson, R. G. (1992). Anosognosia in patients with cerebrovascular lesions. A study of causative factors. *Stroke, 23*(10), 1446–1453.

Stephan, K. M., & Frackowiak, R. S. (1996). Motor imagery—anatomical representation and electrophysiological characteristics. *Neurochemical Research, 21*(9), 1105–1116.

Sterzi, R., Bottini, G., Celani, M. G., Righetti, E., Lamassa, M., Ricci, S., et al. (1993). Hemianopia, hemianaesthesia, and hemiplegia after right and left hemisphere damage. A hemispheric difference. *Journal of Neurology, Neurosurgery and Psychiatry, 56*(3), 308–310.

Talairach, J., & Tournoux, P. (1988). *A co-planar stereotactic atlas of the human brain* (Thieme Verlag ed.). Stuttgart, Germany. Thieme Verlag.

Vallar, G. (1997). Spatial frames of reference and somatosensory processing: A neuropsychological perspective. *Philosophical Transactions of the Royal Society of London B Biological Sciences, 352*(1360), 1401–1409.

Vallar, G., Bottini, G., Rusconi, M. L., & Sterzi, R. (1993). Exploring somatosensory hemineglect by vestibular stimulation. *Brain, 116*(Pt 1), 71–86.

Vallar, G., Bottini, G., & Sterzi, R. (2003). Anosognosia for left-sided motor and sensory deficits, motor neglect, and sensory hemiinattention: Is there a relationship? *Progressive Brain Research, 142*, 289–301.

Vallar, G., Bottini, G., Sterzi, R., Passerini, D., & Rusconi, M. L. (1991). Hemianesthesia, sensory neglect, and defective access to conscious experience. *Neurology, 41*(5), 650–652.

Vallar, G., Guariglia, C., Nico, D., & Pizzamiglio, L. (1997). Motor deficits and optokinetic stimulation in patients with left hemineglect. *Neurology, 49*(5), 1364–1370.

Vallar, G., Sandroni, P., Rusconi, M. L., & Barbieri, S. (1991). Hemianopia, hemianesthesia, and spatial neglect: A study with evoked potentials. *Neurology, 41*(12), 1918–1922.

Vallar, G., Sterzi, R., Bottini, G., Cappa, S., & Rusconi, M. L. (1990). Temporary remission of left hemianesthesia after vestibular stimulation. A sensory neglect phenomenon. *Cortex, 26*(1), 123–131.

Vuilleumier, P. (2004). Anosognosia: The neurology of beliefs and uncertainties. *Cortex, 40*(1), 9–17.

Weinstein, E., & Kahn, R. (1955). *Denial of illness: Symbolic and physiological aspects.* Springfield, IL: C. Thomas Charles.

Willanger, R., Danielsen, U. T., & Ankerhus, J. (1981). Denial and neglect of hemiparesis in right-sided apoplectic lesions. *Acta Neurologica Scandinavica, 64*(5), 310–326.

Wolpert, D. M., & Ghahramani, Z. (2000). Computational principles of movement neuroscience. *Nature Neuroscience, 3* (Suppl.), 1212–1217.

Wolpert, D. M., Ghahramani, Z., & Jordan, M. I. (1995). An internal model for sensorimotor integration. *Science, 269*(5232), 1880–1882.

Zingerle, H. (1913). Über Störungen der Wahrnehmung des eigenen Körpers bei organischen Gehirnerkrankungen. *Monatsschrift für Psychiatrie und Neurologie, 34,* 13–36.

3

Anosognosia for Hemiparesis and Hemiplegia: Disturbed Sense of Agency and Body Ownership

Hans-Otto Karnath and Bernhard Baier

Normally, we are aware that our arms and legs belong to us and not to someone else. When resting, we are aware that our limbs do not move, and when moving, we realize that our limbs cause the action. This natural knowledge is based on a self-awareness, a sense of being us. It allows us to discriminate between our own body and the bodies of other people, and to attribute an action to ourselves rather than to another person. Some of the most challenging questions in cognitive science and in philosophy are, How does this sense arise? How does it function? What mechanisms are involved? How can a subject determine the proper origin of an action or a body part? How is one able to attribute the agent of an action or a body part to oneself?

Recent studies addressed these questions experimentally by using different technical approaches. For example, behavioral investigations in healthy subjects studied the mechanisms underlying the rubber hand illusion (Botvinick & Cohen, 1998; Ehrsson, Holmes, & Passingham, 2005; Ehrsson, Spence, & Passingham, 2004; Ehrsson, Wiech, Weiskopf, Dolan, & Passingham, 2007; Moseley et al., 2008; Tsakiris & Haggard, 2005). Watching a rubber hand being stroked synchronously with one's own (unseen) hand causes a phenomenal incorporation of the rubber hand; the rubber hand is experienced as part of one's own body. Studying the conditions evoking the illusion allows insights into the processes related to our feeling of body ownership. The sense of body ownership and the awareness of being causally involved in an action—the sense of agency—have also been investigated by using functional neuroimaging methods (Farrer et al., 2003; Tsakiris, Hesse, Boy, Haggard, & Fink, 2007a). A further approach is the study of neurological patients showing specific disturbances of these senses after brain damage. Stroke patients with so-called anosognosia for hemiparesis or for hemiplegia (AHP) typically deny the weakness of their paretic or plegic limb(s) and are convinced that they move properly. Stroke patients may also show a disturbed sense of ownership (DSO) with respect to the paretic/plegic limb(s). They experience their limb(s) as not belonging to them and may even attribute them to other persons.

This chapter will provide an overview of recent clinical and anatomical findings in patients with AHP. Interestingly, disturbed beliefs about the functioning of one's own limbs (the sense of agency) and disturbed feelings of limb ownership (the sense of ownership) appear to be closely linked, both clinically and anatomically. It appears that the right insula may play a central role for both senses. We will argue that the right insula may be a central node of the network involved in human body scheme representation.

Anosognosia for Hemiparesis/-plegia

Disturbed Sense of Agency

The characteristic feature of stroke patients with AHP is their false belief that they are not paralyzed. Their feeling of being versus not being causally involved in an action—their sense of agency—is dramatically disturbed. Despite the very obvious fact that the contralesional arm, leg, and/or face are plegic or severely paretic, these patients behave as though the disorder does not exist. Anton (1893) was the first to describe a patient, Wilhelm H., with a left-sided hemiparesis who did not recognize his weakness. Patients such as Wilhelm H. are convinced that their paretic/plegic limbs function normally. When asked to move the paretic/plegic arm or leg, they may do nothing or may move the limb of the opposite side. However, in both situations they are either convinced that they have successfully executed the task or may argue that they can move in a generic manner.

Some patients may not even experience their paresis/plegia when confronted with facts that unambiguously prove the disorder. For example, when asked to clap their hands, no sound is heard due to the paresis/plegia of one arm. Even under these conditions, such patients are not able to correct their feeling of being involved in an action. Often, the patients comment on the apparent inability to move their arm or leg with confabulations such as "My leg is tired" or "My arm is lazy." When directly asked for the reason of not having moved the contralesional limb(s), such patients might respond: "I could walk at home, but not here. It's slippery here" (Nathanson, Bergman, & Gordon, 1952). Patients might argue that the arm "is too stiff, due to the cold" or that "somebody having a hold of the arm" keeps the arm from moving (Nathanson et al., 1952).

Disturbed Sense of Ownership

In the normal experience of an action, the sense of agency and the sense of ownership coincide and are inseparable, though different sources generating these senses have been assumed (Gallagher, 2000; Haggard, 2005; Tsakiris, Schütz-Bosbach, & Gallagher, 2007b; Wolpert, 1997). Therefore, it is interesting to know whether in neurological patients with brain damage a disturbed feeling of being causally involved in an action typically is associated or dissociated from a disturbed feeling of body ownership. Are both senses represented in common or rather separate neural systems?

Indeed, previous studies indicated that the false belief of not being paralyzed in patients with AHP may be associated with other abnormal attitudes toward and/or perceptions of the paretic/plegic limb(s) (Cutting, 1978; Feinberg, Roane, & Ali, 2000; Meador, Loring, Feinberg, Lee, & Nichols, 2000; Stone, Halligan, & Greenwood, 1993). Cutting (1978) referred to them as "anosognosic phenomena." Patients may experience their limb(s) as not belonging to them or as missing (asomatognosia), or may even attribute them to other persons (somatoparaphrenia). Both of these misbeliefs have a common characteristic, namely that the subjects experience a disturbed sense of ownership of their contralateral limb(s). They are convinced that this is not their own arm and/or leg. Thus, it has been suggested to unify these phenomena under the term "disturbed sensation of limb ownership" (DSO) (Figure 3.1; see also subsequent paragraphs). Other phenomena observed were "anosodiaphoria" (patients considering their paresis/plegia as harmless, i.e., are not appropriately concerned about it), "misoplegia" (patients expressing negative feelings about their paretic/plegic limbs), "personification" (patients giving names to their limbs), "kinaesthetic hallucinations" (the illusion that the paretic/plegic limb is moving as if controlled by an invisible force), or "supernumerary phantom limb" (patients' belief that a new, intact limb has appeared).

Although "anosognosic phenomena" and the false belief of not being paralyzed were regarded to be associated in some way (Feinberg et al., 2000), it is not clear how tightly these phenomena are linked. Some studies found a strong association between a disturbed feeling of being involved in a limb movement and the experience that this limb is not belonging to one's body (Feinberg et al., 2000; Meador et al., 2000). Meador et al.'s data (2000) revealed an association close to 70% between the two phenomena in patients who underwent diagnostic intracarotid amobarbital inactivation of the right cerebral hemisphere. In contrast, Cutting (1978) observed that 29% of his patients with left hemiplegia showed such "anosognosic phenomena" without having the false belief of not being paralyzed, while only 8% exhibited both phenomena.

A recent study reassessed this issue in a large sample of 79 acute stroke patients with right brain damage and hemiparesis/-plegia (Baier & Karnath, 2008). The authors systematically examined both phenomena, the experience of being involved in an action, as well as the presence of various "anosognosic phenomena." Their particular focus was on the occurrence of a disturbed sensation of limb ownership (DSO). The authors found a false belief of not being paralyzed in about 15% of their patient sample. Interestingly, all but one (92%) of these patients also showed a DSO for their contralesional limb(s) (see Figure 3.1). No other subjects in the sample of 79 patients exhibited DSO. Baier and Karnath (2008) thus concluded that a disturbed sense of limb ownership obviously is a characteristic feature of AHP. If this surprising finding should be confirmed by future work, it would indicate that our sense of being involved in an action and our sense of ownership with respect to this limb not only are tightly linked phenomena in the normal experience of an action but also in the case of their disturbance after brain injury.

Two of the patients with DSO from the sample of Baier and Karnath (2008) attributed their limb to their wife, three to the examiner, and one to their room neighbor. Traditionally, such beliefs were termed "somatoparaphrenia." Five further patients with DSO from this sample neither attributed their limb to

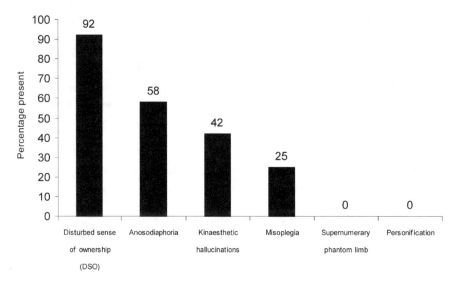

Figure 3.1 Percentage of additional disturbance of sensing limb ownership (DSO) as well as other abnormal attitudes toward and/or perceptions of the paretic/plegic limb(s) found in a continuously admitted sample of patients with anosognosia for hemiparesis/-plegia (AHP). Asomatognosia and somatoparaphrenia have the common characteristic that the subjects experience a disturbed ownership of their contralatateral limb(s). Both misbeliefs thus were combined and illustrated as "disturbed sensation of limb ownership (DSO)." All but one (92%) of the patients with AHP also showed DSO. The finding argued for a tight link between our sense of agency and our sense of limb ownership. (Adapted from Baier & Karnath, 2008, with permission from the American Heart Association, *Stroke, 39,* 486–488.)

themselves nor to somebody else—traditionally labeled as "asomatognosia." Nevertheless, also the latter group of patients had the feeling that their limb somehow belonged to another person. When they were asked whether their limb belonged to another person, none of them clearly denied that it did not belong to somebody else. Answers were given such as "I don't know," "I'm not sure," "I don't think so," etc. On the other hand, the patients with so-called somatoparaphrenia used terms like "perhaps" or "believe" when they attributed their limb to a specific person. This led the authors to suggest that these misbeliefs do not necessarily correspond to two distinct phenomena (Baier & Karnath, 2008). Rather, it seems that there is a continuum of conviction that the limb does not belong to one's own body but to someone else. "Disturbed sensation of limb ownership (DSO)"thus appeared to be a more appropriate term to describe these feelings.

Normal or Pathological? Criteria to Assess the Disturbed Senses

Clinically, AHP and DSO are not trivial problems. A failure to realize a paresis of one's own extremities may delay medical consultation after a stroke (Ghika-Schmid, van Melle, Guex, & Bogousslavsky, 1999). Also, such patients are often reluctant to enroll in rehabilitation programs (Appelros, Karlsson, Seiger, & Nydevik, 2002; Hartman-Maeir, Soroker, & Katz, 2001). Thus, a reliable diagnosis of the disorder as soon as possible after onset is desired.

However, to date some inconsistencies in diagnosing the misbeliefs still seem to exist between different investigators. Consequently, widely varying incidence rates have been reported for AHP in acute stroke patients, ranging from 7% to 77% (for review, see Orfei et al., 2007). This variation points to a central question: What exactly do we mean when we talk about AHP? Shall we already consider a patient as "anosognosic" if he or she does not spontaneously mention the deficit in a conversation with the examiner? Indeed, according to Bisiach et al.'s anosognosia scale (1986) patients should be considered to have "mild anosognosia" when they do not acknowledge their hemiparesis spontaneously following a general question about their complaints. However, the question arises whether there are "normal," that is, nonpathological explanations for not addressing a deficit after such a general question.

A recent study investigated this question (Baier & Karnath, 2005). The authors examined 128 acute stroke patients for AHP by applying the anosognosia scale of Bisiach et al. (1986). They closely analyzed the motives and the explanations given by those patients who did not acknowledge their hemiparesis spontaneously, that is, who traditionally would have been diagnosed showing at least "mild AHP." The authors detected that 94% of these patients suffered from other neurological deficits in addition to their paresis/plegia. Following a general question about their complaints, they mentioned these deficits instead of limb paresis/plegia. However, the same patients immediately acknowledged their paresis/plegia when the examiner addressed the strength of their limbs. Baier and Karnath (2005) thus concluded that a reason for not mentioning a paresis/plegia after a first, general question could be that other, additional deficits have a higher impact for these subjects after stroke. The authors argued that such behavior is reasonable and thus should not be diagnosed as "anosognosia." With respect to the anosognosia scale of Bisiach et al. (1986), they suggested that only patients with grade 2 (the disorder is acknowledged only after demonstrations through routine techniques of neurological examination) and grade 3 (no acknowledgement of the disorder can be obtained) should be labeled as AHP (see Table 3.1). If this criterion is used, comparable incidence rates between 10% and 18% are observed for AHP in unselected samples of acute, hemiparetic stroke patients (Appelros et al., 2002; Baier & Karnath, 2005, 2008; Starkstein, Fedoroff, Price, Leiguarda, & Robinson, 1992).

Since patients with a disturbed sense about the functioning of body parts often exhibit additional DSO for their contralesional limb(s), a clinical exam of stroke patients with hemiparesis/-plegia should combine both aspects (see Tables 3.1 and 3.2). Beyond these aspects, the questionnaire illustrated in Table 3.2 also explores whether a subject has a lack of appropriate concern of the paretic/plegic limbs (*anosodiaphoria*); expresses negative feelings, for example, hatred, for his or her limb (*misoplegia*); gives his or her limbs names (*personification*); feels his or her limbs moving automatically (*kinesthetic hallucinations*); or is convinced that a new, intact limb has appeared (*supernumerary phantom limb*).

Table 3.1 Clinical Scale to Test for a Disturbed Belief about the Functioning of One's Own Limbs (Sense of Agency)

No Anosognosia
- The disorder is spontaneously reported or mentioned by the patient following a general question about his or her complaints.

    (former grade 0 by Bisiach et al., 1986)
- The disorder is reported only following a specific question about the strength of the patient's limbs.

    (former grade 1 by Bisiach et al., 1986)

Anosognosia—Grade I
- The disorder is acknowledged only after demonstrations through routine techniques of neurological examination.

    (former grade 2 by Bisiach et al., 1986)

Anosognosia—Grade II
- No acknowledgement of the disorder is obtained.

    (former grade 3 by Bisiach et al., 1986)

Source: From Baier & Karnath, 2005. This table is a modified version of the anosognosia scale suggested by Bisiach and colleagues (1986).

Table 3.2 Questionnaire to Test for a Disturbed Sense of Limb Ownership (DSO) as Well as for Other Abnormal Attitudes toward and/or Perceptions of Paretic/Plegic Limbs

Disturbed sense of limb ownership (DSO)	Is this your arm/leg? (combined with pointing or elevating the arm/leg) [aspect: asomatognosia]
	To whom belongs this arm/leg? (combined with pointing or elevating the arm/leg) [aspect: somatoparaphrenia]
Anosodiaphoria	Does the weakness of your arm/leg represent a strong impairment or just a minor issue, which is not important to you?
Misoplegia	Do you have any emotions for your arm/leg? Do you hate or deny your arm/leg?
Personification	Does your arm/leg have a name? Have you ever given your leg/arm a name?
Kinesthetic hallucinations	Have you ever had the impression that your arm/leg moves without your own will, i.e., without you having moved it/having initiated the movement? Does your arm/leg move as if controlled by an invisible hand?
Supernumerary phantom limb	How many arms/legs do you have? Do you have the feeling that you have another arm/leg beyond the two arms/legs that you have since birth?

Source: From Baier & Karnath, 2008.

Pathogenetic Models

The pathogenesis of AHP continues to be a subject of controversy. Early investigators like Anton (1893) and Babinski (1914) emphasized the importance of hemisensory loss, particularly the loss of proprioception for the genesis of the disorder. The loss of sensory feedback would induce the patient's unawareness of the contralateral limb function. Levine, Calvanio, and Rinn (1991) postulated that in the absence of somatosensory and proprioceptive input, the patient does not have immediate knowledge that his or her limb has moved or not moved but rather must discover the paresis/plegia by observing his or her own failure in tasks requiring movement of the affected limb. General intellectual impairment or spatial neglect might prevent this discovery. Other models considered AHP as a defect of neural awareness systems (McGlynn & Schacter, 1989), an overestimation of self-performance, lack of mental flexibility, inability to integrate episodic awareness into generic knowledge (Marcel, Tegnér, & Nimmo-Smith, 2004), or a psychological defense mechanism manifesting "the patient's drive to be well" when he or she is facing a sudden and threatening reality such as hemiparesis/-plegia after stroke (Weinstein & Kahn, 1955). Carruthers (2008) claimed that patients with AHP might have an impaired "online" representation of their body (what the body is currently like) due to a lack of access to an updated "offline" representation of the body (the state of what the body is usually like). New information from the body has not been integrated since the patient was paralyzed. The patient's access to the erroneous "offline" representation makes the patient feel embodied as he or she was before the paresis.

Several authors have focused on processes involved in motor planning and motor control to explain the disorder. According to the feed-forward model suggested by Heilman (1991), weakness of a limb is recognized when a mismatch is detected between an intended movement and the actual motor performance. A module comparing intended and observed movements notes possible discrepancies. Patients with AHP do not intend to move. As a consequence, no mismatch is generated in the comparator module and the patient does not recognize his or her paresis. Berti and Pia (2006) proposed a modification of this hypothesis, suggesting that in AHP the comparator module itself is deficient. A further model by Frith, Blakemore, and Wolpert (2000) assumed that awareness of the current and possible states of the motor system are based on sensory information from the muscles, the skin, and the motor command stream. Awareness of initiating a movement is based on a representation of the predicted consequences of making that movement. In patients with AHP, the representations of the desired and the predicted positions of the limb are intact, inducing the normal experience of initiating a movement. However, according to Frith and colleagues, these patients are not aware of the actual limb position. Due to a loss of sensory feedback (by damage of the relevant brain regions or by spatial neglect), information about the actual position of the limb indicating that no motor action has occurred is not available. AHP thus is assumed to result from the lack of experiencing a discrepancy between intended and predicted positions, based on the unawareness of the actual state of the limb. As a result, a successful motor action is pretended and a false experience of movement is induced. A first direct experimental investigation of this hypothesis has recently been undertaken by Fotopoulou et al. (2008).

Anatomy of Anosognosia for Hemiparesis or Hemiplegia: The Neural Correlates of Disturbed Experience of One's Own Limbs and Actions

Disturbed Sense of Agency

The neural correlates of the patient's false belief of not being paralyzed despite obvious hemiparesis/-plegia is also a matter of considerable debate. Lesions of various brain areas such as parietal, temporal and frontal cortex, the thalamus, corona radiate, basal ganglia, internal capsule, and pons were suggested to evoke AHP (Bakchine, Crassard, & Seilhan, 1997; Bisiach et al., 1986; Ellis & Small, 1997; Evyapan & Kumral, 1999; Levine et al., 1991; Maeshima et al., 1997; Starkstein et al., 1992). Consistently, several studies have observed large lesions in the territory of the middle cerebral artery of the nondominant hemisphere to be associated with the disorder. Bisiach and colleagues (1986) assumed that large lesions encompassing the right infero-posterior parietal regions as well as the right thalamus and/or the lenticular nucleus lead to a disturbed feeling of being causally involved in an action. Another group study compared 30 acute stroke patients with AHP and 10 patients with hemiplegia and spatial neglect but no AHP (Ellis & Small, 1997). The patients with AHP had right-sided lesions, in particular in the deep white matter, the basal ganglia, the thalamus, and the insula, whereas both patient groups had lesions of frontal areas, especially the premotor, Rolandic, and paraventricular regions. The authors concluded that AHP is due to damage of neuronal circuits involving the basal ganglia, leading to an inflexibility of the response to the lack of movement in a paretic/plegic limb. A recent review of 23 single case and group studies revealed that among the 83 reported patients with AHP, 44 patients had lesions of the frontal lobe and/or the parietal lobe, 31 patients of the temporal lobe and 12 patients of the occipital lobe (Pia, Neppi-Modona, Ricci, & Berti, 2004). Only 17 patients were reported with a lesion restricted to a single cortical area, whereas in 45 cases more than one cortical lobe was involved. With regard to subcortical structures, 34 out of the 83 patients with AHP had subcortical lesions. The basal ganglia (22 patients), the insula (19 patients), and the internal capsule (18 patients) were the most frequently affected subcortical structures.

Recently, new tools have been developed that allow more precise lesion localization in humans (for a review, see Rorden & Karnath, 2004). These techniques reduce significantly the uncertainty brought in by the procedures used in previous anatomical studies where only rough anatomical landmarks could be taken into consideration, where lesion documentation still was based on a paper-and-pencil basis, where only a rather small number of patients was included, and no direct visual and/or statistical comparisons between patients with and without a disturbed sense of agency was carried out. In contrast, the new techniques can use the entire lesioned area of each individual subject for a high-resolution analysis (Rorden & Karnath, 2004). Different procedures have been developed that allow voxelwise statistical comparisons between anatomical groups. Such voxelwise lesion-behavior mapping (VLBM) techniques differ in major respects but share the idea of comparing the performance of individuals with injury to a voxel to the performance of individuals where that voxel is not injured (Rorden, Fridriksson, & Karnath, 2009; Rorden, Karnath, & Bonilha, 2007). Voxelwise lesion-behavior mapping techniques detect brain regions that predict poor performance when injured and good performance when spared (see Box 3.1).

Box 3.1 An illustration of the importance of using control groups in lesion studies

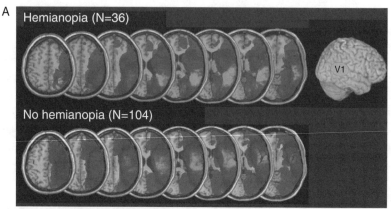

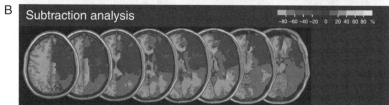

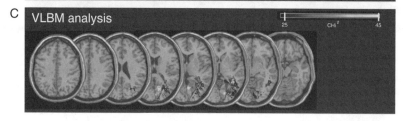

Consider that we are interested in identifying primary visual cortex in humans. In order to identify the relevant brain region, we explore the anatomy correlated with a complete loss of primary vision for the left visual half-field, following a unilateral, right-hemisphere stroke. (A) The top row shows a classical lesion overlay plot for 36 consecutively admitted patients with left-sided visual field cuts following a right-sided lesion. This panel highlights damage to the subcortical white matter extending to the cortical temporoparietal junction (TPJ). The conclusion from this lesion overlay plot would be that primary vision in the left visual half-field is a function of the right subcortical white matter and the surrounding cortical region at the TPJ. The correct location of primary visual cortex is revealed not until the lesion overlay plot of the patient group with hemianopia is contrasted to an adequate control group. The second row demonstrates the distribution of lesion frequency in 104 patients admitted in the same time period who also had right-sided brain lesions but did not show visual field defects (control group). (B) If the overlay plot of this control group is subtracted from the overlay image of the patient group with hemianopia, the subtraction image now accurately highlights the optic radiation and primary visual cortex. (C) A valid result also is obtained by analyzing the same data by voxelwise lesion-behavior mapping (VLBM). VLBM statistically compares the performance of individuals with injury to a voxel to the performance of individuals where that voxel is not injured. Illustrated are all voxels in which a significant difference between the patients with and without hemianopia was revealed (controlled for dependent multiple comparisons using a 1% false discovery rate threshold). (See Color Plate 3.1)

(Adapted with permission from Rorden & Karnath, 2004, with permission from Nature Publishing Group, *Nature Reviews Neuroscience, 5,* 813–819.)

Based on such new analysis techniques, four recent studies compared the location of brain lesions in patients with and without AHP (Baier & Karnath, 2008; Berti et al., 2005; Karnath, Baier, & Nägele, 2005; Vocat & Vuilleumier, Chapter 17, this volume). Karnath and colleagues (2005) investigated 14 consecutively admitted acute stroke patients with right brain damage who showed the false belief that they are not paralyzed. Twelve of these patients showed left-sided plegia and in two patients the left-sided limb(s) were severely paretic. The motor defect thus was homogeneously represented in this group: The majority of the sample (86%) demonstrated complete absence of movement (plegia). Since many of the patients with AHP had additional neurological defects such as spatial neglect, extinction, etc., the control group had to be selected such that all neurological defects were present with the same frequency and severity, except for the critical variable to be investigated: the false belief of not being paralyzed. The authors thus compared the AHP patients with a group of 13 right brain damaged acute stroke patients admitted in the same period who had no AHP but who were comparable with respect to age, acuity of lesion, size of lesion, strength of hemiparesis/-plegia, the frequency of sensory loss, and the frequency of additional spatial neglect, extinction, and visual field defects. Lesion analysis between the groups revealed that the right posterior insula was commonly damaged in patients showing the false belief about the functioning of their own limbs but was significantly less affected in patients without that disorder (see Figure 3.2A). Thus, the authors speculated that the right insular cortex might be a crucial anatomical region in integrating input signals related to self-awareness about the functioning of body parts.

A study by Berti and colleagues (2005) also examined 30 patients with right-sided brain lesions and contralateral hemiplegia. The superimposed lesion plots of 17 patients with AHP and neglect were compared to 12 patients with neglect but without AHP. Their findings revealed that AHP was associated with lesions affecting the dorsal premotor cortex (Broadman's area [BA] 6) and BA 44, motor area BA 4, somatosensory cortex, BA 46, as well as the insula. The authors concluded that, in particular, premotor areas 6 and 44, motor area 4, and the somatosensory cortex are part of a system relevant for motor control as well as self-awareness of motor actions. In our opinion the main difference between their findings and those obtained by Karnath and colleagues (2005) is that Berti et al. (2005) used a very specific selection of subjects for their control group. The control

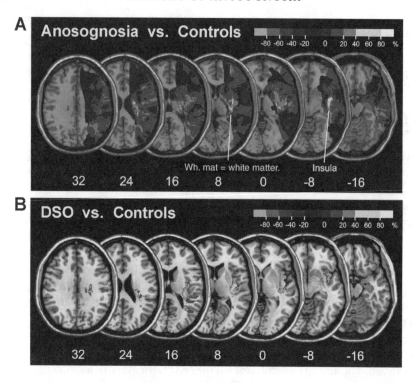

Figure 3.2 *(A)* Overlay plot of the subtracted superimposed lesions of a group of right brain damaged patients with anosognosia for hemiparesis/-plegia (AHP) minus a group of patients without AHP (control group). Wh. mat. = white matter. (Adapted from Karnath et al., 2005, with permission from The Society for Neuroscience, *The Journal of Neuroscience,* 25(31), 7134–7138.) *(B)* Overlay plot of the subtracted superimposed lesions of a patient group showing a disturbed sense of limb ownership (DSO) and AHP minus a control group without the disorder. (From Baier & Karnath, 2008, with permission from the American Heart Association, *Stroke, 39,* 486–488.) In each panel, the percentage of overlapping lesions of the anosognosia patients after subtraction of controls is illustrated by five colors coding increasing frequencies from dark red (difference = 1% to 20%) to white-yellow (difference = 81% to 100%). Each color represents 20% increments. The colors from dark blue (difference = –1% to –20%) to light blue (difference = –81% to –100%) indicate regions damaged more frequently in control patients. MNI z-coordinates of each transverse slice are given. In concordance, the two independent patient samples and analyses *(A and B)* revealed that the right insula is commonly damaged in patients with AHP and DSO but is significantly less affected in patients without these disorders. (See Color Plate 3.2)

subjects, that is, the patients with spatial neglect but without AHP, had mainly lesions of subcortical structures such as the basal ganglia, thalamus, and periventricular white matter (Berti et al., 2005; their Figure 1B). However, more frequently spatial neglect is associated with cortical lesions, involving parietal, temporal, and/ or frontal regions (Buxbaum et al., 2004; Committeri et al., 2007; Heilman, Watson, Valenstein, & Damasio, 1983; Husain & Kennard, 1996; Karnath,

Ferber, & Himmelbach, 2001; Karnath, Fruhmann Berger, Küker, & Rorden, 2004; Vallar & Perani, 1986). A neglect control group, in which the cortical lesion sites associated with spatial neglect are underrepresented, controls only for the subcortical sites of spatial neglect. When such a group is used as a control for a group of patients suffering from both AHP and spatial neglect, the resulting lesion contrast map does not only reveal brain areas related to AHP. In addition, the contrast map shows also those areas that are linked (at the cortical level) with spatial neglect. Part of the cortical brain regions revealed by Berti and colleagues (2005) thus most likely represent neural correlates of spatial neglect rather than of AHP.

Evidence supporting the hypothesis that the right insular cortex might be a crucial anatomical region in integrating input signals related to self-awareness about the functioning of body parts (Karnath et al., 2005) has been reported from two further studies investigating lesion localization in AHP. The first study examined a series of 79 acute stroke patients with right brain damage and hemiparesis/-plegia showing AHP versus not showing AHP (Baier & Karnath, 2008). In correspondence with their earlier findings, in this new patient sample the authors found that the brain area more frequently affected in AHP patients compared to controls was the right insular cortex (Figure 3.2B; for details, see subsequent paragraph). The second study analyzed the structural damage of patients with AHP in relation to their anosognosia scores collected 3 days after the stroke and a second assessment 1 week later (Vocat & Vuilleumier, Chapter 17, this volume). In both phases, the authors found the most distinctive lesion areas in the right insular cortex and adjacent anterior subcortical structures. One week post-stroke, additional regions were observed in the right hemisphere. They included the parieto-temporal junction, premotor areas, and the amygdalo-hippocampal complex. The authors interpret these sites as constituents of a network of interacting cerebral regions involved in the occurrence and persistence of AHP.

Disturbed Sense of Ownership

The studies of Karnath et al. (2005), Berti et al. (2005), as well as Vocat and Vuilleumier (Chapter 17, this volume) concentrated on the phenomenon of a disturbed feeling of being causally involved in an action—the sense of agency. Whether the patients included in these investigations also experienced their paretic/plegic limb(s) as not belonging to them (i.e., whether they had a DSO) was not reported. A recent study addressed this issue, examining the neural correlate of a DSO (Baier & Karnath, 2008). The authors investigated a series of 78 subjects with acute right hemisphere stroke and left-sided hemiparesis/-plegia. They found a "disturbed sensation of ownership" (DSO) for the paretic/plegic limb(s) in 11 subjects, that is, in 14% of their patient sample. Interestingly, all 11 patients suffered from a false belief of not being paralyzed, that is, also showed a disturbed sense of agency. The brain lesions of these patients were contrasted to those of 11 acute right hemisphere stroke patients without such disorder but who were comparable with respect to age, acuity of lesion, size of lesion, strength of hemiparesis/-plegia, and the frequency of additional spatial neglect and visual field defects. Lesion analysis between the groups revealed that the right posterior insula was more frequently affected in patients showing a disturbed experience of own limbs and actions (see Figure 3.2B). The data suggested a tight anatomical relationship between the two phenomena. The authors concluded that the right insula might be involved not only in the genesis of one's belief about limb movement but also in our sense of limb ownership.

Right Insula for Our Sense of Limb Ownership and Self-Awareness of Actions

The Island of Reil, or the insular cortex, is the cortical tissue beneath the frontal and temporal lobe that consists of four to seven oblique gyri encircled by the insular sulcus (Augustine, 1996; Duvernoy, 1999; Mesulam & Mufson, 1985; Naidich et al., 2004; Rhoton, 2007; Türe, Yaşargil, Al-Mefty, & Yaşargil, 1999). The central sulcus of the insula divides the insular cortex into a large anterior part and a posterior part (Naidich et al., 2004). The anterior part is divided by several shallow sulci into three to five short gyri, whereas the posterior insular cortex is formed by the anterior and the posterior long gyri. While the anterior part has more extensive connections with limbic, paralimbic, olfactory, gustatory, and autonomic structures, the major projections of the posterior insula include those with the primary and secondary somatosensory area (SI, SII), the superior and inferior temporal areas, parietal cortices, orbitofrontal, prefrontal, and premotor cortex, auditory cortex (AI, AII), amygdala, thalamus, basal ganglia, and the cingulate gyrus (Augustine, 1996; Flynn, Benson, & Ardila, 1999; Mesulam & Mufson, 1985).

Converging evidence has been reported that the anterior insular cortex is a central structure for pain mechanisms and temperature regulation (Brooks, Nurmikko, Bimson, Singh, & Roberts, 2002; Craig, Chen, Bandy, & Reiman, 2000; Craig, Reiman, Evans, & Bushnell, 1996; Frot & Maugière, 2003; Kong et al., 2006; Maihöfner, Kaltenhäuser, Neundörfer, & Lang, 2002; Schreckenberger et al., 2005). This led to the view that this cortical area might represent an important correlate of human "interoception" (Craig, 2002, 2009). Other interoceptive stimuli that have been shown to be associated with the anterior insula were, for example, taste perception (Faurion, Cerf, Le Bihan, & Pillias, 1998; Ogawa et al., 2005), thirst (Farrell et al., 2006), and autonomic functions such as blood pressure regulation (Kimmerly, O'Leary, Menon, Gati, & Shoemaker, 2005), visceral motor functions (Humbert & Robbins, 2007), and bladder control (Griffiths, Tadic, Schaefer, & Resnick, 2007). Moreover, the anterior insular cortex was suggested to be involved in emotional feelings such as anger or anxiety (Damasio et al., 2000; Ehrsson et al., 2007; Paulus & Stein, 2006; Phillips et al.,

1997; Stein, Simmons, Feinstein, & Paulus, 2007), in craving (Contreras, Ceric, & Torrealba, 2007; Naqvi, Rudrauf, Damasio, & Bechara, 2007), and in visual self-recognition (Devue et al., 2007).

It has been suggested that the posterior insular cortex might represent a somatosensory association area (Augustine, 1996; Mesulam & Mufson, 1985). Neurons in this area showed responsiveness to auditory and to somatosensory stimulation, the latter with large receptive fields covering the limbs, trunk, or entire body (Schneider, Friedman, & Mishkin, 1993). Several investigators also reported a link between the posterior insula and motor processes. In patients with an insular tumor (Fiol, Leppick, Mireles, & Maxwell, 1988) or an aneurysm lying on the insula (Schneider, Calhoun, & Kooi, 1971), an epileptic aura consisting of rotational and circling limb movements was reported. Early stimulation experiments at the posterior insula reported that gross movements (Showers & Laucer, 1961), as well as restricted movements of single muscles or small groups of muscles, could be elicited (Sugar, Chusid, & French, 1948). However, these latter findings lack confirmation using more recent neurophysiological techniques. Lesion and functional imaging studies in humans further suggested that the posterior insula may be part of the human vestibular system (Bense et al., 2004; Brandt, Dieterich, & Danek, 1994; Dieterich & Brandt, 2008) and might be involved in language and articulation processes in the left hemisphere (Cereda, Ghika, Maeder, & Bogousslavsky, 2002; Dronkers, 1996), as well as in processes of spatial exploration and orientation in the right hemisphere (Karnath et al., 2004).

The recent findings (see above) deriving from lesion localization in patients with AHP and DSO suggest that the right insular cortex may also play a crucial role in the genesis of our sense of limb ownership and our self-awareness of limb movement (Baier & Karnath, 2008; Karnath et al., 2005). This hypothesis is supported by other observations. For example, Cereda and colleagues (2002) documented that even a small, isolated lesion of the right insula suffices to induce a DSO for the contralesional limb(s). They screened a total of 4,800 stroke patients from the Lausanne Stroke Registry to identify patients showing a lesion restricted to only the insular cortex. They found four patients and identified five characteristic clinical disturbances of insular strokes: *(1)* somatosensory deficits with contralateral pseudothalamic sensory stroke in three patients; *(2)* taste disorder in a patient with a left posterior insular infarct; *(3)* pseudovestibular syndrome in three patients with posterior insular infarct; *(4)* cardiac disturbance with hypertensive disorder in one patient with right posterior insular infarct; and *(5)* neuropsychological disorders, including aphasia (left posterior insular infarct) and—interesting in the present context—one patient with damage to the insular cortex who showed DSO. This latter patient was one of the two patients with a right-sided insular infarct identified by Cereda and colleagues (2002). The 75-year-old right-handed woman was hospitalized after she woke up in the night with a sensation of being touched by a stranger's hand and alarmed by a foreign body in her bed, not recognizing her own left upper limb.

Further evidence that the right insula is involved in our feeling of body ownership and our self-awareness of limb movement comes from studies using caloric vestibular stimulation. Positron emission tomography (PET) imaging has revealed that vestibular stimulation induces activation predominantly of the right posterior insula as well as the right temporoparietal junction, SI and SII, retroinsular cortex, putamen, and anterior cingulate cortex (Bottini et al., 1994, 2001; Emri et al., 2003). Therefore, it is interesting that such stimulation in patients with right brain damage may induce transitory remission of AHP and of DSO (Bisiach, Rusconi, & Vallar, 1991; Cappa, Sterzi, Vallar, & Bisiach, 1987; Rode et al., 1992; Vallar, Bottini, & Sterzi, 2003).

Spinazzola and colleagues (2008) investigated four right brain damaged patients showing anosognosia for hemianaesthesia. Interestingly, all four subjects presented a lesion including the right insular cortex. This suggests that not only processes linked with AHP but also with anosognosia for hemianaesthesia appear to be associated with the right insula.

Supporting evidence for the role of the right posterior insula for self-awareness of limb actions also comes from recent PET experiments (Farrer et al., 2003; Farrer et al., 2004; Tsakiris et al., 2007a). Farrer et al. (2003) found involvement of the right posterior insula when subjects had to indicate whether movements they saw corresponded to their own executed movements or were controlled by someone else. The authors observed a gradually reduced activity of the right posterior insula with an associated gradual decreased feeling of controlling a movement. The level of activity in the right posterior insula correlated with the experience of controlling an action. Right insular activity was high when the subjects experienced a concordant feeling between the viewed and the actually executed movement. Another PET study by the same group showed that in patients with schizophrenia the subjects' degree of movement control was related to regional cerebral blood flow in the right angular gyrus but not in the insular cortex (Farrer et al., 2004). The authors argued that the differences in activation between normal subjects (Farrer et al., 2003) and patients with schizophrenia (Farrer et al., 2004) might reflect the impaired recognition of one's own actions in patients with schizophrenia.

A recent fMRI study explored the mechanisms of disembodiment (Corradi-Dell'Acqua et al., 2008). The authors presented a movie in which three fictional players were throwing each other a ball. Each subject's key-press could either be synchronous or asynchronous with one of the player's actions. The study revealed that the left posterior insular cortex was activated when the movements of the subjects were synchronous with those of the players in the video game. The finding could suggest that not only the right but also the left insula is involved in mechanisms differentiating between one's own body and the external environment.

An experimental paradigm that allows manipulation of the feeling of body ownership is the rubber hand illusion (Botvinick, 2004; Botvinick & Cohen, 1998). Studies have found that the observation of a rubber hand being stroked

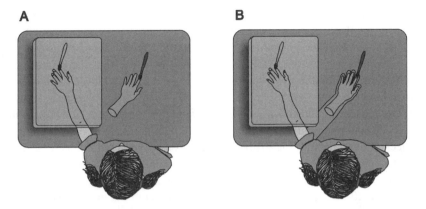

Figure 3.3 The rubber hand illusion. In the illusion, the subjects observe a facsimile of a human hand (the rubber hand) while their own hand is hidden from view *(A)*. Synchronously touching of the subject's hand and of the artificial hand with a probe leads to the illusion that the rubber hand belongs to one's own body *(B)*.

synchronously with one's own hidden hand can cause the rubber hand to be attributed to one's own body (see Figure 3.3). This paradigm was applied in a recent PET study (Tsakiris et al., 2007a). Healthy subjects saw either a right or a left rubber hand being touched either synchronously or asynchronously with respect to their own hidden right hand. Across all conditions, participants judged the felt position of their own hand before and after visuotactile stimulation. The proprioceptive judgment was used as a behavioral measure of the phenomenal incorporation of the rubber hand into one's own body. The authors found that the elicited feeling of ownership for the rubber hand was positively correlated to activity in the right posterior insula and the right frontal operculum. Conversely, when the rubber hand was not attributed to the self, activity was observed in the contralateral parietal cortex, particularly the somatosensory cortex. Tsakiris and colleagues concluded that the posterior insula is active even in the absence of movement and efferent information, that is, when a nonacting subject integrates multisensory information to decide if a body part belongs to one's own body. Based on this finding they proposed that the posterior insula incorporates the sense of body ownership per se.

Craig has argued that the sense of the physiological condition of the body, that is, the "interoception" (see above), which is associated with autonomic control, is engendered in the right anterior insula and might present the basis for our awareness of the "feeling self" (Craig, 2002, 2009). He suggested that this area might represent a polymodal integration zone involved in all human feelings and thus may contain a representation of "me" as a feeling entity, engendering the fundamental phenomenon of human subjective awareness (Craig, Chapter 4, this volume). Evidence for this view comes from the various observations that the insula is involved in pain mechanisms, temperature regulation, in subjective feelings such as anger or anxiety, or in autonomic regulation processes (for a more detailed review, see Craig, 2009). Direct evidence that the interoceptive systems implemented in the insular cortex are associated with the sense of body ownership has come from two recent studies using the rubber hand illusion paradigm. Moseley and colleagues (2008) found that the sense of body ownership and the autonomic regulation of the body are tightly linked. They observed that the feeling of ownership for a rubber hand was associated with a decrease of the skin temperature of the real hand. This effect was limb specific, that is, a decrease of skin temperature only occurred in the aligned, hidden real hand. Ehrsson and colleagues (2007) showed that threat to the rubber hand can induce a similar level of activity in the brain areas associated with anxiety and interoceptive awareness, that is, anterior insular and anterior cingulate cortex, as when the person's real hand is threatened. Their findings thus suggest that incorporated artificial limbs can evoke the same feelings as real limbs. It appears as if indeed our sense of body ownership is tightly linked with the insular interoceptive systems.

Conclusions

In the normal experience of an action, the sense of agency and the sense of ownership coincide. Recent findings have suggested that these two feelings are closely linked in brain-damaged patients as well. In stroke patients with AHP, a disturbed feeling of being causally involved in an action often seems to be associated with a disturbed feeling of body ownership. Also, both senses seem to share common neural structures. New lesion mapping and analysis methods revealed that the false belief about the functioning of one's own limbs, as well as a disturbed sensation of ownership with respect to these limbs, is associated with damage involving particularly the right insula. Functional brain imaging studies supported the role of the right posterior insular cortex in self-awareness of actions and in our sense of limb ownership. Thus, it seems as if the right insula plays a central role for both senses: our sense of limb ownership as well as our sense of agency. The insular cortex is characterized by an extensive spectrum of cortical and subcortical somatosensory and motor connections. The right posterior insula thus may constitute a central node of the network involved in human body scheme representation.

Acknowledgments

This work was supported by the Bundesministerium für Bildung und Forschung (BMBF-Verbundprojekt "Räumliche Orientierung" 01GW0641) and the

Deutsche Forschungsgemeinschaft (KA 1258/10–1). We are grateful to Bud Craig, Aikaterini Fotopoulou, George P. Prigatano, and Patrik Vuilleumier for their insightful comments and discussion. We also would like to thank Andrea Klein for Figure 3.3 illustrating the rubber hand illusion as well as Jennifer Gray for her help with the English language.

References

Anton, G. (1893). Beiträge zur klinischen Beurtheilung und zur Localisation der Muskelsinnstörungen im Grosshirne. *Zeitschrift für Heilkunde, 14,* 313–348.

Appelros, P., Karlsson, G. M., Seiger, A., & Nydevik, I. (2002). Neglect and anosognosia after first-ever stroke: Incidence and relationship to disability. *Journal of Rehabilitation Medicine, 34,* 215–220.

Augustine, J. R. (1996). Circuitry and functional aspects of the insular lobe in primates including humans. *Brain Research Reviews, 22,* 229–244.

Babinski, J. (1914). Contribution à l'étude des troubles mentaux dans l'hémiplégie organique cérébrale (anosognosie). *Revue Neurologique, 27,* 845–848.

Baier, B., & Karnath, H.-O. (2005). Incidence and diagnosis of anosognosia for hemiparesis. *Journal of Neurology, Neurosurgery, and Psychiatry, 76,* 358–361.

Baier, B., & Karnath, H.-O. (2008). Tight link between our sense of limb ownership and self-awareness of actions. *Stroke, 39,* 486–488.

Bakchine, S., Crassard, I., & Seilhan, D. (1997). Anosognosia for hemiplegia after a brainstem haematoma. A pathological case. *Journal of Neurology, Neurosurgery, and Psychiatry, 63,* 686–687.

Bense, S., Bartenstein, P., Lochmann, M., Schlindwein, P., Brandt, T., & Dieterich, M. (2004). Metabolic changes in vestibular and visual cortices in acute vestibular neuritis. *Annals of Neurology, 56,* 624–630.

Berti, A., Bottini, G., Gandola, M., Pia, L., Smania, N., Stracciari, A., Castiglioni, I., Vallar, G., & Paulesu, E. (2005). Shared cortical anatomy for motor awareness and motor control. *Science, 309,* 488–491.

Berti, A., & Pia, L. (2006). Understanding motor awareness through normal and pathological behavior. *Current Directions in Psychological Science, 15,* 245–250.

Bisiach, E., Rusconi, M. L., & Vallar, G. (1991). Remission of somatoparaphrenic delusion through vestibular stimulation. *Neuropsychologia 29,* 1029–1031.

Bisiach, E., Vallar, G., Perani, D., Papagno, C., & Berti, A. (1986). Unawareness of disease following lesions of the right hemisphere: Anosognosia for hemiplegia and anosognosia for hemianopia. *Neuropsychologia, 24,* 471–482.

Bottini, G., Karnath, H.-O., Vallar, G., Sterzi, R., Frith, C. D., Frackowiak, R. S., & Paulesu, E. (2001). Cerebral representations for egocentric space: Functional-anatomical evidence from caloric vestibular stimulation and neck vibration. *Brain, 124,* 1182–1196.

Bottini, G., Sterzi, R., Paulesu, E., Vallar, G., Cappa, S. F., Erminio, F., Passingham, R. E., Frith, C. D., & Frackowiak, R. S. (1994). Identification of the central vestibular projections in man: A positron emission tomography activation study. *Experimental Brain Research, 99,* 164–169.

Botvinick, M. (2004). Probing the neural basis of body ownership. *Science, 305,* 782–783.

Botvinick, M., & Cohen, J. (1998). Rubber hands "feel" touch that eyes see. *Nature, 391,* 756.

Brandt, T., Dieterich, M., & Danek, A. (1994). Vestibular cortex lesions affect the perception of verticality. *Annals of Neurology, 35*, 403–412.

Brooks, J. C., Nurmikko, T. J, Bimson, W. E., Singh, K. D., & Roberts, N. (2002). fMRI of thermal pain: Effects of stimulus laterality and attention. *NeuroImage, 15*, 293–301.

Buxbaum, L. J., Ferraro, M. K., Veramonti, T., Farne, A., Whyte, J., Ladavas, E., Frassinetti, F., & Coslett, H. B. (2004). Hemispatial neglect: Subtypes, neuro-anatomy and disability. *Neurology, 62*, 749–756.

Cappa, S., Sterzi, R., Vallar, G., & Bisiach, E. (1987). Remission of hemineglect and anosognosia during vestibular stimulation. *Neuropsychologia, 25*, 775–783.

Carruthers, G. (2008). Types of body representation and the sense of embodiment. *Consciousness and Cognition, 17*, 1302–1316.

Cereda, C., Ghika, J., Maeder, P., & Bogousslavsky, J. (2002). Strokes restricted to the insular cortex. *Neurology, 59*, 1950–1955.

Committeri, G., Pitzalis, S., Galati, G., Patria, F., Pelle, G., Sabatini, U., Castriota-Scanderbeg, A., Piccardi, L., Guariglia, C., & Pizzamiglio, L. (2007). Neural bases of personal and extrapersonal neglect in humans. *Brain, 130*, 431–441.

Contreras, M., Ceric, F., & Torrealba, F. (2007). Inactivation of the interoceptive insula disrupts drug craving and malaise induced by lithium. *Science, 318*, 655–658.

Corradi-Dell' Acqua, C., Ueno, K., Ogawa, A., Cheng, K., Rumiata, R. I., & Iriki, A. (2008). Effects of shifting perspective of the self: An fMRI study. *NeuroImage, 40*, 1902–1911.

Craig, A. D. (2002). How do you feel? Interoception: The sense of the physiological condition of the body. *Nature Reviews Neuroscience, 3*, 655–666.

Craig, A. D. (2009). How do you feel—now? The anterior insula and human awareness. *Nature Reviews Neuroscience, 10*, 59–70.

Craig, A. D., Chen, K., Bandy, D., & Reiman, E. M. (2000). Thermosensory activation of insular cortex. *Nature Neuroscience, 3*, 184–190.

Craig, A. D., Reiman, E. M., Evans, A., & Bushnell, M. C. (1996). Functional imaging of an illusion of pain. *Nature, 384*, 258–260.

Cutting, J. (1978). Study of anosognosia. *Journal of Neurology, Neurosurgery, and Psychiatry, 41*, 548–555.

Damasio, A. R., Grabowski, T. J., Bechara, A., Damasio, H., Ponto, L. L. B., Parvizi, J., & Hichwa, R. D. (2000). Subcortical and cortical brain activity during the feeling of self-generated emotions. *Nature Neuroscience, 3*, 1049–1056.

Devue, C., Collette, F., Balteau, E., Degueldre, C., Luxen, A., Maquet, P., & Brédart, S. (2007). Here I am: The cortical correlates of visual self-recognition. *Brain Research, 1143*, 169–182.

Dieterich, M., & Brandt, T. (2008). Functional brain imaging of peripheral and central vestibular disorders. *Brain, 131*, 2538–2552.

Dronkers, N. F. (1996). A new brain region for coordinating speech articulation. *Nature, 384*, 159–161.

Duvernoy, H. M. (1999). *The Human Brain: Surface, Three-Dimensional Sectional Anatomy with MRI, and Blood Supply*. New York: Springer.

Ehrsson, H. H., Holmes, N. P., & Passingham, R. E. (2005). Touching a rubber hand: Feeling of body ownership is associated with activity in multisensory brain areas. *Journal of Neuroscience, 25*, 10564–10573.

Ehrsson, H. H., Spence, C., & Passingham, R. E. (2004). That's my hand! Activity in premotor cortex reflects feeling of ownership of a limb. *Science, 305,* 875–877.

Ehrsson, H. H., Wiech, K., Weiskopf, N., Dolan, R. J., & Passingham, R. E. (2007). Threatening a rubber hand that you feel is yours elicits a cortical anxiety response. *Proceedings of the National Academy of Sciences of the USA, 104,* 9828–9833.

Ellis, S., & Small, M. (1997). Localization in denial of hemiplegia after acute stroke. *Stroke, 28,* 67–71.

Emri, M., Kisely, M., Lengyel, Z., Balkay, L., Márián, T., Mikó, L., Berényi, E., Sziklai, I., Trón, L., & Tóth, A. (2003). Cortical projection of peripheral vestibular signaling. *Journal of Neurophysiology, 89,* 2639–2646.

Evyapan, D., & Kumral, E. (1999). Pontine anosognosia for hemiplegia. *Neurology, 53,* 647–649.

Farrell, M. J., Egan, G. F., Zamarripa, F., Shade, R., Blair-West, J., Fox, P., & Denton, D. A. (2006). Unique, common, and interacting cortical correlates of thirst and pain. *Proceedings of the National Academy of Sciences of the USA, 103,* 2416–2421.

Farrer, C., Franck, N., Frith, C. D., Decety, J., Georgieff, N., d'Amato, T., & Jeannerod, M. (2004). Neural correlates of action attribution in schizophrenia. *Psychiatry Research, 131,* 31–44.

Farrer, C., Franck, N., Georgieff, N., Frith, C. D., Decety, J., & Jeannerod, M. (2003). Modulating the experience of agency: A positron emission tomography study. *NeuroImage, 18,* 324–333.

Faurion, A., Cerf, B., Le Bihan, D., & Pillias, A.-M. (1998). fMRI study of taste cortical areas in humans. *Annals of the New York Academy of Sciences, 855,* 535–545.

Feinberg, T. E., Roane, D. M., & Ali, J. (2000). Illusory limb movements in anosognosia for hemiplegia. *Journal of Neurology, Neurosurgery, and Psychiatry, 68,* 511–513.

Fiol, M. E, Leppick, I. E., Mireles, R., & Maxwell, R. (1988). Ictus emeticus and the insular cortex. *Epilepsy Research, 2,* 127–131.

Flynn, F. G., Benson, D. F., & Ardila, A. (1999). Anatomy of the insula—functional and clinical correlates. *Aphasiology, 13,* 55–78.

Fotopoulou, A., Tsakiris, M., Haggard, P., Vagopoulou, A., Rudd, A., & Kopelman, M. (2008). The role of motor intention in motor awareness: An experimental study on anosognosia for hemiplegia. *Brain, 131,* 3432–3442.

Frith, C. D., Blakemore, S. J., & Wolpert, D. M. (2000). Abnormalities in the awareness and control of action. *Philosophical Transactions of the Royal Society B Biological Sciences, 355,* 1771–1788.

Frot, M., & Mauguière, F. (2003). Dual representation of pain in the operculo-insular cortex in humans. *Brain, 126,* 438–450.

Gallagher, S. (2000). Philosophical conceptions of the self: Implications for cognitive science. *Trends in Cognitive Sciences, 4,* 14–21.

Ghika-Schmid, F., van Melle, G., Guex, P., & Bogousslavsky, J. (1999). Subjective experience and behavior in acute stroke: The Lausanne Emotion in Acute Stroke Study. *Neurology, 52,* 22–28.

Griffiths, D., Tadic, S. D., Schaefer, W., & Resnick, N. M. (2007). Cerebral control of the bladder in normal and urge-incontinent women. *NeuroImage, 37,* 1–7.

Haggard, P. (2005). Conscious intention and motor cognition. *Trends in Cognitive Sciences, 9,* 290–295.

Hartman-Maeir, A., Soroker, N., & Katz, N. (2001). Anosognosia for hemiplegia in stroke rehabilitation. *Neurorehabilitation and Neural Repair, 15*, 213–222.

Heilman, K. M. (1991). Anosognosia: Possible neuropsychological mechanisms. In G. P. Prigatano & D. L. Schacter (Eds.), *Awareness of deficit after brain injury: Clinical and theoretical issues* (pp. 53–62). New York: Oxford University Press.

Heilman, K. M., Watson, R. T., Valenstein, E., & Damasio, A. R. (1983). Localization of lesions in neglect. In A. Kertesz (Ed.), *Localization in neuropsychology* (pp. 471–492). New York: Academic Press.

Humbert, I. A., & Robbins, J. (2007). Normal swallowing and functional magnetic resonance imaging: A systematic review. *Dysphagia, 22*, 266–275.

Husain, M., & Kennard, C. (1996). Visual neglect associated with frontal lobe infarction. *Journal of Neurology, 243*, 652–657.

Karnath, H.-O., Baier, B. & Nägele, T. (2005). Awareness of the functioning of one's own limbs mediated by the insular cortex? *Journal of Neuroscience, 25*, 7134–7138.

Karnath, H.-O., Ferber, S., & Himmelbach, M. (2001). Spatial awareness is a function of the temporal not the posterior parietal lobe. *Nature, 411*, 950–953.

Karnath, H.-O., Fruhmann Berger, M., Küker, W., & Rorden, C. (2004). The anatomy of spatial neglect based on voxelwise statistical analysis: A study of 140 patients. *Cerebral Cortex, 14*, 1164–1172.

Kimmerly, D. S., O'Leary, D. D., Menon, R. S., Gati, J. S., & Shoemaker, J. K. (2005). Cortical regions associated with autonomic cardiovascular regulation during lower body negative pressure in humans. *Journal of Physiology, 569*, 331–345.

Kong, J., White, N. S., Kwong, K. K., Vangel, M. G., Rosman, I. S., Gracely, R. H., & Gollub, R. L. (2006). Using fMRI to dissociate sensory encoding from cognitive evaluation of heat pain intensity. *Human Brain Mapping, 27*, 715–721.

Levine, D. N., Calvanio, R., & Rinn, W.E. (1991). The pathogenesis of anosognosia for hemiplegia. *Neurology, 41*, 1770–1781.

Maeshima, S., Dohi, N., Funahashi, K., Nakai, K., Itakura, T., & Komai, N. (1997). Rehabilitation of patients with anosognosia for hemiplegia due to intracerebral hemorrhage. *Brain Injury, 11*, 691–697.

Maihöfner, C., Kaltenhäuser, M., Neundörfer, B., & Lang, E. (2002). Temporo-spatial analysis of cortical activation by phasic innocuous and noxious cold stimuli— a magnetoencephalographic study. *Pain, 100*, 281–290.

Marcel, A., Tegnér, E., & Nimmo-Smith, I. (2004). Anosognosia for plegia: Specifity, extension, partiality and disunity of bodily unawareness. *Cortex, 40*, 19–40.

McGlynn, S. M., & Schacter, D. L. (1989). Unawareness of deficits in neuropsychological syndromes. *Journal of Clinical and Experimental Neuropsychology, 11*, 143–205.

Meador, K. J., Loring, D. W., Feinberg, T. E., Lee, G. P., & Nichols, M. E. (2000). Anosognosia and asomatognosia during intracarotid amobarbital inactivation. *Neurology, 55*, 816–820.

Mesulam, M. M., & Mufson, E. J. (1985). The Insula of Reil in man and monkey. Architectonics, connectivity, and function. In A. Peters & E. G. Jones (Eds.), *Cerebral cortex* (pp. 179–226). New York: Plenum Press.

Moseley, G. L., Olthof, N., Venema, A., Don, S., Wijers, M., Gallace, A., & Spence, C. (2008). Psychologically induced cooling of a specific body part caused by the illusory ownership of an artificial counterpart. *Proceedings of the National Academy of Sciences of the USA, 105*, 13169–13173.

Naidich, T. P., Kang, E., Fatterpekar, G. M., Delman, B. N., Gultekin, S. H., Wolfe, D., Ortiz, O., Yousry, I., Weismann, M., & Yousry, T. A. (2004). The insula: Anatomic study and MR imaging display at 1.5 T. *American Journal of Neuroradiology, 25,* 222–232.

Naqvi, N. H., Rudrauf, D., Damasio, H., & Bechara, A. (2007). Damage to the insula disrupts addiction to cigarette smoking. *Science, 315,* 531–534.

Nathanson, M., Bergman, P., & Gordon, G. (1952). Denial of illness. Its occurrence in one hundred consecutive cases of hemiplegia. *Archives of Neurology and Psychiatry, 68,* 380–387.

Ogawa, H., Wakita, M., Hasegawa, K., Kobayakawa, T., Sakai, N., Hirai, T., Yamashita, Y., & Saito, S. (2005). Functional MRI detection of activation in the primary gustatory cortices in humans. *Chemical Senses, 30,* 583–592.

Orfei, M. D., Robinson, R. G., Prigatano, G. P., Starkstein, S., Rüsch, N., Bria, P., Caltagirone, C., & Spalletta, G. (2007). Anosognosia for hemiplegia after stroke is a multifaceted phenomenon: A systematic review of the literature. *Brain, 130,* 3075—3090.

Paulus, M.P., & Stein, M. B. (2006). An insular view of anxiety. *Biological Psychiatry, 60,* 383–387.

Phillips, M. L., Young, A. W., Senior, C., Brammer, M., Andrew, C., Calder, A. J., Bullmore, E. T., Perrett, D. I., Rowland, D., Williams, S. C. R., Gray, J. A., & David, A. S. (1997). A specific neural substrate for perceiving facial expressions of disgust. *Nature, 389,* 495–498.

Pia, L., Neppi-Modona, M., Ricci, R., & Berti, A. (2004). The anatomy of anosognosia for hemiplegia: A meta-analysis. *Cortex, 40,* 367–377.

Rhoton, A. L. (2007). The Cerebrum. Anatomy. *Neurosurgery, 61*(Suppl. 1), 37–118.

Rode, G., Charles, N., Perenin, M.-T., Vighetto, A., Trillet, M., & Aimard, G. (1992). Partial remission of hemiplegia and somatoparaphrenia through vestibular stimulation in a case of unilateral neglect. *Cortex, 28,* 203–208.

Rorden, C., Fridriksson, J., & Karnath, H. -O. (2009). An evaluation of traditional and novel tools for lesion behavior mapping. *NeuroImage, 44,* 1355–1362.

Rorden, C., & Karnath, H.-O. (2004). Using human brain lesions to infer function: A relic from a past era in the fMRI age? *Nature Reviews Neuroscience, 5,* 813–819.

Rorden, C., Karnath, H.-O., & Bonilha, L. (2007). Improving lesion-symptom mapping. *Journal of Cognitive Neuroscience, 19,* 1081–1088.

Schneider, R. C., Calhoun, H. D., & Kooi, K. A. (1971). Circling and rotational automatisms in patients with frontotemporal cortical and subcortical lesions. *Journal of Neurosurgery, 35,* 554–563.

Schneider, R. J., Friedman, D. P., & Mishkin, M. (1993). A modality-specific somatosensory area within the insula of the rhesus monkey. *Brain Research, 621,* 116–120.

Schreckenberger, M., Siessmeier, T., Viertmann, A., Landvogt, C., Buchholz, H. G., Rolke, R., Treede, R. D., Bartenstein, P., & Birklein, F. (2005). The unpleasantness of tonic pain is encoded by the insular cortex. *Neurology, 64,* 1175–1183.

Showers, M. J. C., & Laucer, E. W. (1961). Somatovisceral motor patterns in the insula. *Journal of Comparative Neurology, 117,* 107–115.

Spinazzola, L., Pia, L., Folegatti, A., Marchetti, C., & Berti, A. (2008). Modular structures of awareness for sensorimotor disorders: Evidence from anosognosia for hemiplegia and anosognosia for hemianaesthesia. *Neuropsychology, 46,* 915–926.

Starkstein, S. E., Fedoroff, J. P., Price, T. R., Leiguarda, R., & Robinson, R. G. (1992). Anosognosia in patients with cerebrovascular lesions. *Stroke, 23*, 1446–1453.

Stein, M. B., Simmons, A. N., Feinstein, J. S., & Paulus, M. P. (2007). Increased amygdala and insula activation during emotion processing in anxiety-prone subjects. *American Journal of Psychiatry, 164*, 318–327.

Stone, S. P., Halligan, P. W., & Greenwood, R. J. (1993). The incidence of neglect phenomena and related disorders in patients with an acute right or left hemisphere stroke. *Age and Aging, 22*, 46–52.

Sugar, O., Chusid, J. G., & French, J. D. (1948). A second motor cortex in the monkey (Macaca mulatta). *Journal of Neuropathology & Experimental Neurology, 7*, 182–189.

Tsakiris, M., & Haggard, P. (2005). The rubber hand illusion revisited: Visuotactile integration and self-attribution. *Journal of Experimental Psychology: Human Perception and Performance, 31*, 80–91.

Tsakiris, M., Hesse, M. D., Boy, C., Haggard, P., & Fink, G. R. (2007a). Neural signatures of body ownership: A sensory network for bodily self-consciousness. *Cerebral Cortex, 17*, 2235–2244.

Tsakiris, M., Schütz-Bosbach, S., & Gallagher, S. (2007b). On agency and body-ownership: Phenomenological and neurocognitive reflections. *Consciousness and Cognition, 16*, 645–660.

Türe, U., Yaşargil, D. C., Al-Mefty, O., & Yaşargil, M. G. (1999). Topographic anatomy of the insular region. *Journal of Neurosurgery, 90*, 720–733.

Vallar, G., Bottini, G., & Sterzi, R. (2003). Anosognosia for left-sided motor and sensory deficits, motor neglect, and sensory hemiinattention: Is there a relationship? In C. Prablanc, D. Pélisson, & Y. Rossetti Y (Eds.), *Progress in brain research, Vol. 142* (pp. 289–301). Amsterdam: Elsevier Science.

Vallar, G., & Perani, D. (1986). The anatomy of unilateral neglect after right-hemisphere stroke lesions. A clinical/CT-scan correlation study in man. *Neuropsychologia, 24*, 609–622.

Weinstein, E. A., & Kahn, R. L. (1955). *Denial of illness: Symbolic and physiological aspects.* Springfield, IL: Charles C. Thomas.

Wolpert, D. M. (1997). Computational approaches to motor control. *Trends in Cognitive Sciences, 1*, 209–216.

4

The Insular Cortex and Subjective Awareness

A. D. (Bud) Craig

In the preceding chapter, Karnath and Baier described clinical documentation for a crucial role of the insular cortex in anosognosia for hemiplegia and hemi-anesthesia, that is, the lack of awareness of feelings of functionally impaired movement or touch in the contralateral body. In this chapter, I present evidence that all feelings from the body are substantialized by an ascending sensory pathway to the posterior insula of primates that represents the physiological condition of the body (Craig, Bushnell, Zhang, & Blomqvist, 1994; Craig, 2002, 2003a). The evidence indicates that integration of this pathway in the mid-insula leads to a polymodal zone in the anterior insular cortex (AIC) of the human brain that is uniquely involved in the subjective perception of feelings from the body (Craig, Chen, Bandy, & Reiman, 2000; Craig, 2002). Further, the AIC is activated in imaging studies of all subjective feelings and emotions in humans, and thus this evidence supports the proposal of the James-Lange theory of emotion (James, 1890) and Damasio's "somatic marker" hypothesis (Damasio, 1993) that the representation of the sentient self is based on the homeostatic condition of the body. Finally, recent observations from a broad range of imaging and clinical studies provide convergent findings that extend this hypothesis to suggest that the AIC and the adjacent frontal operculum may engender the fundamental phenomenon of subjective human awareness of oneself, others, and all salient perceptions (Craig, 2009).

This chapter presents the perspective of a functional neuroanatomist who has studied the neural basis for feelings from the body employing such techniques as single-unit microelectrode recordings, tract-tracing, psychophysics, and functional imaging. First, I will review the functional anatomy of the ascending pathway for feelings from the body. Then I will discuss the integration of such activity with salient environmental, motivational, and social factors, which seems to provide the basis for a coherent representation of all feelings, or the sentient self, in the AIC. The evidence supporting the concept that the AIC engenders phenomenal awareness will be presented next, followed by the outline of a structural model of awareness that could explain these findings. More detailed presentations of these findings and ideas are available elsewhere (Craig, 2002, 2003a, 2009). This chapter concludes with comments on the relevance of these findings for clinicians studying patients with anosognosia or insular damage.

The Interoceptive Pathway to Insular Cortex for Feelings from the Body

Humans perceive feelings from the body that provide a sense of their physical condition and underlie mood and emotional state. In the conventional view presented in most textbooks, the well-discriminated feelings of temperature, itch, and pain are associated with an "exteroceptive" somatosensory system that represents haptic touch and proprioception, whereas the less distinct visceral feelings of vasomotor activity, hunger, thirst, and internal sensations are associated with a separate "interoceptive" system. That categorization, originally espoused by Sherrington (1948), ignores several fundamental discrepancies, such as the fact that lesions or stimulation of the somatosensory cortices rarely affect temperature, itch, or pain sensation, and the fact that all such feelings from the body, in contrast to mechanical touch and proprioception, are endowed with inherent emotional (affective/motivational) qualities and reflexive autonomic effects. The findings I describe here lead to a conceptual shift that resolves these issues by showing that all affective feelings from the body are represented in a novel, unforeseen pathway, phylogenetically unique to primates and well-developed in humans, which evolved from the afferent limb of an evolutionarily ancient, hierarchical homeostatic system that maintains the integrity of the body. These feelings thus represent a sense of the physiological condition of the entire body, which I refer to as "interoception" redefined (Craig, 2002).

Spinal and Brainstem Organization

The neural processes (autonomic, neuroendocrine, and behavioral) that maintain an optimal physiological balance in the body, collectively called homeostasis, must receive sensory inputs that report the condition of the tissues of the entire body (Cannon, 1939). The small-diameter (A-delta and C) sensory fibers that innervate all tissues of the body (including skin, muscle, joints, teeth, bone, and viscera) and respond selectively to all manner of physiological conditions (including mechanical, thermal, and metabolic changes) provide the necessary homeostatic afferent input. Such sensory fibers in parasympathetic nerves (e.g., vagal and glossopharyngeal) send their central terminals to the nucleus of the solitary tract (commonly abbreviated NTS for the Latin name, *nucleus tractus solitarius*) in the brain stem, and the A-delta and C sensory fibers in somatic and sympathetic nerves send their central terminals to the spinal cord, where they terminate monosynaptically on neurons in lamina I of the superficial dorsal horn. The ontogeny of these fibers is intimately linked with the development of lamina I cells, indicating that together they form a coherent homeostatic afferent system. Thus, lamina I cells do not arise from cells of the dorsal placode, but rather from the progenitors of autonomic interneurons in the lateral horn, and they ascend to the top of the dorsal horn (during a ventromedial rotation of the entire dorsal horn) at precisely the right time to meet the ingrowing small-diameter fibers from the small dorsal root ganglion (B) cells (Altman & Bayer, 1984). In contrast, the large-diameter fibers, which arise from a distinct set of large dorsal root ganglion (A) cells, grow into the dorsal horn earlier and contact large cells of the dorsal placode that end up at the base of the dorsal horn (because of the rotation) and connect to ventral horn motoneurons. As described below, this ancient structural pattern of organization, that is, an interoceptive (homeostatic) afferent system in the superficial dorsal horn that controls smooth muscle and an exteroceptive system in the base of the dorsal horn that controls skeletal muscle, is maintained in the organization of regions that receive somatic afferent activity in the cerebral cortex of humans.

The central projections of lamina I cells confirm the view that they provide the central continuation of the small-diameter afferent system and subserve homeostasis. Lamina I neurons project densely to the spinal autonomic cell columns, thus forming a spino-spinal loop for somato-autonomic reflexes, and they project to the cardiorespiratory integration and preautonomic sites in the brain stem, which likewise receive dense input from the NTS (Craig, 1993, 1995). The concept that lamina I serves as a homeostatic afferent integration site is strikingly corroborated by the observation that lamina I and the autonomic cell columns are the only spinal targets of descending fibers from the hypothalamus (Holstege, 1988).

The small-diameter primary afferent fibers selectively signal changes in the physiological condition of the tissues of the body (for references, see Craig, 2003a). For example, one class of C-fibers is sensitive only to itch-producing agents, and another is sensitive only to light (sensual) touch. Accordingly, lamina I neurons comprise several distinct modality-selective classes that receive input from specific subsets of small-diameter primary afferent fibers. The various classes of lamina I cells can be differentiated on the basis of cell shape, afferent responses, electrophysiological properties, axonal projections, descending modulation, and pharmacological properties, and so they can be regarded as virtual "labeled lines" (Craig, 2003a). Their responses correspond very well with the psychophysical characteristics of the several distinct affective feelings from the body that humans perceive, including first (sharp) pain, second (burning) pain, cooling, warm, itch, sensual touch, and muscle burn and cramp.

In contrast to prior descriptions of lamina I as a "pain and temperature" processing stage, a comprehensive view of the evidence suggests that the distinct types of lamina I neurons provide the substrate for the modality-selective somato-autonomic adjustments that support ongoing homeostasis. For example, innocuous thermoreceptive (cool) activity that is conveyed by thermoreceptive-specific lamina I neurons to the brain stem linearly modulates respiratory parameters, consistent with the primordial role of thermoreception in thermoregulation (Diesel et al., 1990). The lamina I neurons that are directly related to human pain sensation are also essentially homeostatic in nature. In particular, consider the multipolar lamina I cells driven by polymodal nociceptive C-fibers, which uniquely correlate with the feeling of second (burning) pain during specific psychophysical paradigms, such as the repeated brief contact heat test or the thermal grill pain illusion (Craig & Andrew, 2002; Craig & Bushnell, 1994). The accelerating response of these neurons to noxious cold does not begin at the cold temperatures we call noxious ($<15°C$), but rather at moderate temperatures that are just below a thermoneutral ambient temperature, that is, $\sim24°C$ ($\sim75°F$), which is both the temperature at which thermoregulatory defense mechanisms actuate and the temperature at which humans begin to feel increasing environmental thermal discomfort. In contrast, the cooling-sensitive thermoreceptive-specific lamina I cells that underlie our sense of innocuous cooling are linearly responsive to temperatures lower than normal skin temperature ($\sim32°C$), and their responses plateau at noxious cold levels ($<15°C$). The generation of a feeling of burning pain in fact depends on a comparison in the forebrain of the polymodal lamina I activity with the cooling-specific lamina I activity (Craig, Reiman, Evans, & Bushnell, 1996) and with core temperature (Mower, 1976), which directly implies that such cells actually signal thermal distress as a homeostatic behavioral motivation. The fundamental role of lamina I in homeostasis is corroborated also by the presence of neurons selectively responsive to the small-diameter afferents from muscle, which are sensitive to muscle work and to metabolic conditions and drive cardiorespiratory adjustments in brainstem nuclei on an ongoing basis, but which generate feelings of muscle ache, burning, and cramping pain when strongly activated.

Thalamo-Cortical Organization

The ascending axons of lamina I neurons course in the lateral spinothalamic tract, precisely where contralateral spinal lesions selectively interrupt pain, temperature, itch, sensual touch, and all affective feelings from the body. The thalamic projections of lamina I neurons in primates terminate topographically in a specific thalamocortical relay nucleus in posterolateral thalamus, the posterior portion of the ventral medial nucleus, VMpo (Craig et al., 1994; Craig, 2004). The VMpo is organized somatotopically in the antero-posterior direction, which is orthogonal to the medio-lateral somatotopic gradient in the neighboring main somatosensory ventral posterior (VP) nuclei, which relay mechanoreceptive and proprioceptive activity to the main somatosensory cortex. The VMpo contains distinct modality-selective components corresponding to distinct feelings (i.e., cooling, first pain, second pain, etc.). The basal portion of the ventral medial nucleus (VMb) that adjoins VMpo anteriorly in primates receives direct input from NTS (i.e., afferent activity from parasympathetic nerves), and thus together these two nuclei represent the physiological condition of all tissues of the body. The primordial input to VMb in all mammals (i.e., activity from the main brainstem homeostatic afferent integration site, the parabrachial nucleus or PB) is also maintained in primates. The VMpo is difficult to distinguish in the thalamus of macaque monkeys, but in the thalamus of hominid primates it is greatly enlarged and clearly distinct. The VMpo and VMb project conjointly and topographically to the dorsal margin of the insular cortex, which I refer to as interoceptive cortex.

The insula is a distinct but hidden lobe of the brain—it is a cortical "island" (hence its name) that is buried within the lateral sulcus. Based on tract-tracing studies in monkeys and other mammals, it is interconnected with the anterior cingulate cortex, the amygdala, the hypothalamus, the ventral striatum, and the orbitofrontal cortex (Augustine, 1996; Mufson, Sobreviela, & Kordower, 1997; Saper, 2002). In monkeys, this cytoarchitectonically distinct cortical area is well-demarcated by in situ labeling for receptors of corticotropin-releasing factor, which some regard as a major marker for homeostasis (Sanchez et al., 1999). In monkeys the interoceptive cortex occupies the entire antero-posterior extent of the insula, but in humans it occupies only the posterior half of the insula (Frank et al., 2008; Stephan et al., 2003); this suggests that the anterior insula of humans has no equivalent in the monkey, which is consistent with the observation that the insula in humans is disproportionately (30%) larger than the monkey's on the basis of body size or brain weight (Semendeferi & Damasio, 2000).

The positron-emission tomography (PET) study we performed of discriminative graded thermal (cool) sensation provided the first identification of interoceptive cortex in humans (Craig et al., 2000), and it validated the tract-tracing work in monkeys. Functional imaging studies in humans reveal that the interoceptive cortex in the dorsal posterior insula is also activated in a graded manner by noxious stimuli (pain) and by itch, warmth, sensual touch, muscle exercise, cardiorespiratory activity, hunger, thirst, taste, and so on, that is, all of the distinct feelings from the body (e.g., Brooks, Nurmikko, Bimson, Singh, & Roberts, 2002; Del Parigi et al., 2002; Drzezga et al., 2001; Keltner et al., 2006; Olausson et al., 2002; Veldhuizen, Bender, Constable, & Small, 2007; for additional references, see Craig, 2002, 2009), and that it is somatotopically organized along an antero-posterior gradient, as predicted from the tract-tracing work in monkeys (Brooks et al., 2005; Henderson, Gandevia, & Macefield, 2007; Hua, Strigo, Baxter, Johnson, & Craig, 2005). Lesion, stimulation, and evoked potential studies in humans confirm the role of the interoceptive cortex as the primary cortical representation for pain, temperature, taste, and so on

(Greenspan, Lee, & Lenz, 1999; Iannetti, Zambreanu, Cruccu, & Tracey, 2005; Ostrowsky et al., 2002; Pritchard, Macaluso, & Eslinger, 1999; Schmahmann & Leifer, 1992). The primordial role of the insular cortex is modulation of brainstem homeostatic afferent integration sites (such as PB), which are the main targets of its descending projections. Thus, the interoceptive cortical image of the physiological condition of the body in humans emerged evolutionarily as an extension of the hierarchical homeostatic afferent system. Consistent with the properties of lamina I neurons described above, these anatomical considerations imply that affective feelings from the body in humans reflect its homeostatic condition. Thus, there are two distinct somatic afferent representations in the human cortex, one in the sensorimotor Rolandic cortex that is involved in the (exteroceptive) control of skeletal muscle and one in the insular cortex that is involved in the (interoceptive) control of smooth muscle, analogous to the organization of the spinal dorsal horn.

There is also a direct, topographic lamina I projection to the ventral caudal portion of the medial dorsal nucleus (MDvc) in primates, which in turn projects to the anterior cingulate cortex (ACC). The primordial input to the ACC (integrated homeostatic information from the brainstem PB by way of medial thalamus) is also present in primates, but in nonprimates lamina I activity is relayed instead to a portion of the orbitofrontal cortex by way of the submedial nucleus. Lesion studies in rats support the primordial role of the ACC in emotional behavior (e.g., Johansen, Fields, & Manning, 2001), and functional imaging evidence in humans substantiates the role of the ACC in affect, motivation, volition, and behavioral agency (see Amodio & Frith, 2006; Craig, 2002). In my view, the insula can be regarded as limbic sensory cortex and the anterior cingulate (ACC) as limbic motor cortex (Craig, 2002; see also Heimer & Van Hoesen, 2006), which must work together in a complementary fashion like the somatosensory and motor cortices do. The direct activation of both the interoceptive cortex in the posterior insula and the motivational cortex in the ACC by the distinct homeostatic sensory modalities represented in the lamina I pathway (e.g., innocuous cooling: Hua et al., 2005) and during all feelings and emotions (see below) corresponds, in my opinion, with the simultaneous generation of both a sensation and a motivation, which is the basic definition of an emotion (Rolls, 1999). Thus, the affective feelings from the body can be viewed as "homeostatic emotions" that drive behavior necessary for the survival and maintenance of the individual and the species (Craig, 2003b).

Association of the Anterior Insular Cortex with Subjective Feelings and Emotions

The PET study we performed of innocuous graded cooling sensation afforded the opportunity to identify sites of brain activation related to subjective feelings, in addition to objective temperatures, because we asked the subjects to report their feelings after each stimulus on an ordinal scale (Craig et al., 2000). We found a robust statistical differentiation of cortical activation that correlated parametrically with subjective feelings first in the homolateral mid-insula, just anterior to the interoceptive representation of objective temperature in the posterior insula, and second in a large region in the AIC and the adjacent orbitofrontal cortex on the right (nondominant) side. This is neurobiologically parsimonious, because progressive re-representations that combine feature abstraction and cross-modality integration are present in serial processing streams that originate in all primary sensory cortical regions. The data from several recent studies confirm the anatomical progression of activity from the interoceptive cortex in the posterior insula to the mid-insula and then to the anterior insula on the left or right side (e.g., Brooks et al., 2002; Olausson et al., 2002, 2005; Stephan et al., 2003). The posterior-to-mid-to-anterior progression of processing in the insular cortex is consistent with the posterior-to-anterior gradient of integration found generally in the frontal cortex (Koechlin & Jubault, 2006) and with the enormous expansion of anterior insula in hominid primates (Allman, Watson, Tetreault, & Hakeem, 2005; Semendeferi & Damasio, 2000).

The middle insula is a region of convergence and integration. Imaging findings support the convergence in the middle insula of activity associated with emotionally salient stimuli of all sensory modalities, probably by way of interconnections with the amygdala, the temporal pole, and frontal cortex, as well as with hedonic input from the ventral striatum (e.g., Burton, Videen, & Raichle, 1993; Menon & Levitin, 2005; Winston, Strange, O'Doherty, & Dolan, 2002). Thus, if homeostatic afferent (interoceptive) activity becomes integrated first in the middle insula with emotionally salient activity in the sensory environment and subcortical homeostatic control regions (hypothalamus and amygdala) and then more anteriorly with emotionally salient activity from other limbic cortical regions (ACC, orbitofrontal cortex) and from cortical regions involved in social and contextual planning (e.g., mid and dorsolateral prefrontal cortex), then this posterior-to-mid-to-anterior progression of integration provides a foundation for the sequential integration of the homeostatic condition of the body with the sensory environment, with internal autonomic state, with motivational conditions, and finally with social and cognitive conditions. I have proposed that this progressive integration culminates in the final representation of a "global emotional moment" that incorporates all salient factors at one immediate moment of time in the most recently evolved portion of the human AIC (see below; Craig 2008, 2009).

Recent functional imaging reports provide strong evidence for a unique association of the AIC with subjective feelings from the body and with all feelings and emotions. The feelings from the body (caused by interoceptive stimuli) associated with activation of the AIC include not only cooling and pain but also warmth, thirst, dyspnea, "air hunger," the Valsalva maneuver, sensual touch, itch, penile stimulation, exercise, heartbeat, wine-tasting by sommeliers, and distension of the bladder, stomach, rectum, or esophagus (e.g., Henderson et al., 2003; Olausson et al., 2002, 2005; Stephan et al., 2003; for additional references, see Craig, 2002, 2009). For example, as we found for temperature stimuli, activation in the posterior insula correlates with the objective intensity of a noxious stimulation, whereas activation in the right AIC is correlated with subjective attention and evaluation of pain (whether cutaneous, muscular, or visceral) (Brooks et al., 2002; Keltner et al., 2006; Kong et al., 2006). Activation associated with the anticipation of pain or with feelings of chronic pain even localize in a more anterior portion of the right AIC than activation during acute experimental pain (Schweinhardt et al., 2006). A study of nonpainful gastric distension that produces a subjective sense of fullness reported activation in bilateral dorsal posterior insula, left mid-insula, and the left AIC (Stephan et al., 2003); this stimulus activates primarily parasympathetic (vagal) afferents, and thus these results conform to the pattern of posterior-to-mid-to-anterior integration but support the presence of an important asymmetry (see further below). A seminal study by Critchley, Wiens, Rotshtein, Ohman, and Dolan (2004) reported functional and morphometric imaging data indicating a specific role of the right AIC in heartbeat awareness, a subjective interoceptive perceptual capability that is correlated with individual subjective awareness of all emotions (Barrett, Quigley, Bliss-Moreau, & Aronson, 2004).

Activation in the AIC is correlated with subjective feelings associated with virtually every emotion, including disgust, trustworthiness, maternal and romantic love, anger, sadness, happiness, lust, disbelief, fear, sexual arousal, and even with imitation or empathic referral of such emotions (Bartels & Zeki, 2004; Damasio et al., 2000; Jabbi, Swart, & Keysers, 2007; Winston et al., 2002; for additional references, see Craig, 2002, 2009). This convergent evidence thus supports the view that the re-representation of the interoceptive image of the body's physiological condition in the AIC provides a basis for the subjective awareness of all emotional feelings. A demonstration of synergistic activation of the AIC by interoceptive feelings and a visually induced emotion (fear) supports the existence of a final integrated representation of the sentient self (Phillips et al., 2003). The conclusion that the subjective image of "the material me" (Sherrington, 1900) is based on the afferent representation of the homeostatic condition of the body is consistent with the essence of the James-Lange theory of emotion and Damasio's somatic marker hypothesis.

Association of the Anterior Insular Cortex with Awareness

A large number of recent functional imaging reports support the hypothesis that the representation of the feeling self in the AIC engenders the fundamental basis of human awareness. Several studies suggest that the AIC has a crucial role in visual and auditory awareness in the immediate moment. For example, transitions in bistable visual or auditory perceptions are directly associated with activation of the AIC and the adjacent inferior frontal gyrus (IFG; Kondo & Kashino, 2007; Sterzer & Kleinschmidt, 2007). A study of the attentional blink paradigm, in which a second target cannot be perceived if it occurs too quickly following a primary target in a rapid series of visual stimuli, concluded that the AIC/IFG is essential for awareness of a visual stimulus (Kranczioch, Debener, Schwarzbach, Goebel, & Engel, 2005). In a study of brief visual stimuli, Deary et al. (2004) reported that subjects' performance in detecting an asymmetric visual stimulus decreased progressively from 100% to chance at presentation times shorter than 100 msec, but activation selectively *increased* in the AIC and the ACC, which I interpret as an indication of focused or heightened awareness (and which, interestingly, they related to psychometric intelligence).

Furthermore, functional imaging studies of activation associated with subjective awareness of cognitive percepts indicate selective AIC activation. For example, Ploran et al. (2007) tracked brain activation while details in a degraded visual image were slowly revealed and found a gradual increase of activation in higher-order visual processing areas involved in object identification, but a sudden burst of activity in the AIC and ACC bilaterally at the "moment-of-recognition," that is, coincident with the subjects' signals of subjective awareness of the percept itself. Thielscher and Pessoa (2007) compared brain activation with behavioral choices and reaction times using a graded visual series of morphed faces expressing two different emotions (fear and disgust) and found that bilateral activation of the AIC/IFG and the ACC correlated parametrically with perceptual decision making. A notable study by Kikyo, Ohki, and Miyashita (2002) examined the "feeling of knowing," the subjective sense of knowing a word before recalling it, and found parametrically graded activation in the AIC bilaterally that was not associated with the actual recall process itself. This finding suggests that the AIC also represents feelings associated with mental processing and cognition.

An especially noteworthy study of eye movement may provide direct evidence that the AIC engenders awareness. Klein et al. (2007) used an antisaccade task with a distractor, which produced occasional erroneous saccades that the subjects were either aware of (and signaled with a button press) or were unaware of. Evidence of slowed reaction times and improved performance on trials following aware errors corroborated the subjects' awareness reports. The activation on error trials occurred in the bilateral AIC and in three small regions near the ACC. Activation during aware errors (but not during unaware errors) occurred only in the left inferior AIC; similar activation in the right AIC was just subthreshold. Activation near the ACC was not modulated by error awareness (see related findings in Robertson, Chapter 15, this volume).

Studies of the act of seeing one's own image also substantiate a role for the AIC in self-awareness. This is equivalent to the mirror test for self-recognition, an operational test for awareness (De Waal, 2008; Gallup, 1970) that is based on the view that emotional identification with movements and expressions visible in a mirror is only possible with a mental representation of a sentient self. For example, Devue et al. (2007) reported that during visual self-recognition of the face or the body (in contrast to images of significant or nonsignificant others) there was selectively enhanced activation of the right AIC, the adjacent IFG, and the ACC. Consistent with this interpretation, studies of the feeling of agency, awareness of body control, or the sense of body ownership during hand movements indicate a strong association with activation in the mid-insula, especially on the right side (Farrer & Frith, 2002; Farrer et al., 2003; Mutschler et al., 2007; Tsakiris, Hesse, Boy, Haggard, & Fink, 2007; see also Karnath & Baier, Chapter 3, this volume). I interpret these findings to indicate that the insular cortex contains a somatotopic representation of the *feelings* of "my" movements in an emotional present.

In addition, studies on risk, uncertainty, anticipation, attention, perceptual transitions, cognitive control, and performance monitoring show selective activation in the AIC that support the hypothesis that it plays a fundamental role in phenomenal awareness and in comparisons of feelings across time (e.g., Brass & Haggard, 2007; Preuschoff, Quartz, & Bossaerts, 2008; Sridharan, Levitin, & Menon, 2008; for additional references, see Craig, 2009). Activation in studies of the enjoyment of music and of time perception is particularly significant from the point of view of the structural model of awareness described below. For example, listening to subjectively selected pleasant music activates the AIC (especially on the left side, see below; Koelsch, Fritz, von Cramon, Muller, & Friederici, 2006), and attention to the rhythm of a well-known melody selectively activates the left AIC (Platel et al., 1997). The AIC is strongly activated in many studies of time perception in the range of seconds to subseconds (especially on the right side; e.g., Coull, 2004; Lewis & Miall, 2006; Rao et al., 2001). For example, Livesay et al. (2007) manipulated task difficulty in order to isolate time estimation from other task-related cognitive demands and found activation in the dorsal putamen (bilaterally), the left inferior parietal cortex, and the AIC (bilaterally) at its junction with the IFG (with no ACC activation). They suggested that the AIC/IFG focus must be "of central importance" in time perception. Synchronization in real time seems to be especially important; Bushara, Grafman, & Hallett (2001) reported that the right AIC and ACC selectively display a graded response to an auditory-visual timing mismatch (using sounds from a moving mouth).

Finally, as noted at several points above, the functional imaging evidence indicates that homeostatic afferent activity and emotional feelings are represented asymmetrically in the AIC on the left and right sides. The right insula is activated predominantly by stimuli that produce sympathetic arousal (such as pain and temperature), whereas the left insula is activated predominantly by parasympathetic afferents (such as gastric distension). These data fit with a psychophysiological model of emotion in which the right forebrain is associated with negative, aversive, withdrawal emotions and the left forebrain is associated with positive, affiliative, approach emotions (Davidson, 2004; for additional references, see Craig, 2005, 2009), which may originate in an evolutionarily ancient pattern (MacNeilage, Rogers, & Vallortigara, 2009). This concept is consistent with the notion that an opponent organization of emotional control would be most energy efficient (note that the brain uses 25% of the body's energy budget). Accordingly, functional imaging studies of positive and affiliative emotional feelings show activation predominantly in the left AIC. For example, Leibenluft, Gobbini, Harrison, and Haxby (2004) reported activation of left AIC and ACC in mothers viewing their own child; Hennenlotter et al. (2005) saw activation in the left AIC while subjects were either seeing or making a smile; Johnstone, van Reekum, Oakes, and Davidson (2006) reported activation of the left AIC while subjects attended to happy voices; Takahashi et al. (2008) reported selective activation of the left AIC while subjects experienced joy; Ortigue, Grafton, and Bianchi-Demicheli (2007) described selective activation of the left AIC in females that correlated with self-reported orgasm ratings; and Kim, Adolphs, O'Doherty, and Shimojo (2007) documented predominant activation of the left insula and orbitofrontal cortex during the late decision phase of choosing a preferred face. Finally, Winston et al. (2002) reported activation of the right insula when a face was judged untrustworthy and the left insula when a face was judged trustworthy. For further discussion of the forebrain asymmetry of emotion, see Craig (2005).

A Structural Model for the Role of the Anterior Insular Cortex in Awareness

The data reviewed above indicate that the phylogenetically novel ascending homeostatic afferent pathway from lamina I and the solitary nucleus in primates provides the basis for the sense of the physiological condition of the entire body in posterior insular cortex; this includes numerous individually mapped and unique "feelings" from the body. These neural constructs are then re-represented and integrated in the mid-insula and again in the AIC (on the left or right side or both, depending on the source of the activity). This anatomical progression provides a foundation for the sequential integration of homeostatic conditions with the sensory environment and with motivational, hedonic, and social conditions represented in other parts of the brain, and importantly, this is all elaborated on a map of the "feelings" from the body. Thus, a refined and integrated image of the state of the body seems to provide the basis for subjective awareness of "the feeling self" and of others and of all salient objects in the environment.

I have proposed a model in which the integration of salience across all conditions culminates in a unified meta-representation of the "global emotional moment" near the junction of the AIC and the frontal operculum (Craig, 2008, 2009). This key processing stage generates an image of "the material me" at one moment of time. The anatomical repetition of this fundamental unit could produce a finite set of repeated meta-representations of global emotional moments that could be indexed across time with the incorporation of an endogenous timebase. Such a structure could provide the basis for the continuity of subjective emotional awareness within a finite present with a cinemascopic representation of the sentient self.

The original insight for this model came from considering the evidence that the AIC is involved not only in all feelings but also in the sense of movement, in time perception, and in music appreciation. This led to a recognition that, if music is defined as the rhythmic temporal progression of emotionally laden moments, then the temporal progression of global emotional moments could instantiate not merely music appreciation and time perception but also a cinemascopically continuous view of the sentient self. Thus, this model provides an emergent basis for the uniquely human faculty of music. As noted above, functional imaging studies indicate that listening to music or covertly singing strongly activates the AIC (Ackermann & Riecker, 2004; Koelsch et al., 2006), and clinical studies indicate that restricted lesions of the AIC can disrupt the ability to appreciate the emotional content of music (Griffiths, Warren, Dean, & Howard, 2004). Music making has the profound capacity to bind us together emotionally and to change both our emotions and our subjective perception of time. The anthropological evidence suggests that music has been a characteristic of humanity almost from the initial appearance of our species (Klein, 2002). If music is defined as the rhythmic temporal progression of emotionally laden moments, then it emerges directly from the core of awareness in this model.

In order to enable comparisons of past, present, and expected feelings, there must also be storage buffers/comparators that can hold a "global emotional moment"; recent observations directly support this inference (Knutson, Rick, Wimmer, Prelec, & Loewenstein, 2007; Preuschoff et al., 2008; Seymour et al., 2004). One interesting feature of this model is that such a comparator could provide a stable representation of successive global emotional moments that might be experienced introspectively as a reflexive observer (or a Cartesian theater) that, however, could not "see" itself, as described for consciousness (James, 1890). That is, the additional step of updating the comparator with the current global emotional moment must require a finite amount of time, and so it cannot contain a representation of the same global emotional moment that represents "now" in the cinemascopic view.

This model also provides a basis for subjective time dilation during an intensely emotional period (Droit-Volet & Meck, 2007). At such a time, for instance, a car accident or a first parachute jump (Campbell & Bryant, 2007), there is a high rate of salience accumulation. In this model, the information capacity of a neural module representing a global emotional moment must be finite, and so during such a time they must "fill up" and accumulate rapidly.

Accordingly, objective time would appear to pass more slowly, or even "stand still," to the subjective observer.

Finally, in this model the AIC is closely integrated with the ACC, and so the feelings of awareness can incorporate the motivations and urges of the volitional agent (such as cravings; see Pelchat, Johnson, Chan, Valdez, & Raglund, 2004; Wang et al., 2007), and in addition, the feelings represented in the AIC can be modulated by the agent (as in placebo analgesia; see Petrovic, Kalso, Petersson, & Ingvar, 2002; see Figure 4.1). Thus, each global emotional moment includes both feelings and motivations. The close integration of the AIC and the ACC (which I believe could be provided by the unique Von Economo neurons they contain; see Craig, 2008, 2009) supports the direct representation of the active behavioral agent ("I") within the sentient self, which supplies a component that was deemed "illusory" in the "somatic marker" hypothesis (Damasio, 1993) and challenges a major

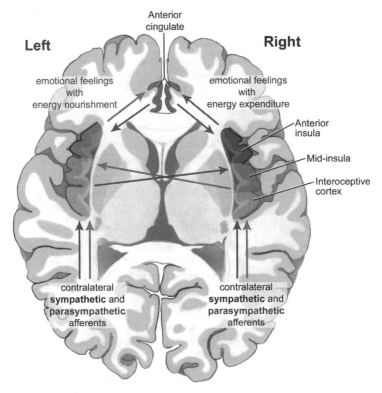

Figure 4.1 A schematic view of the integration of sympathetic (from lamina I) and parasympathetic (from NTS) afferent activity from the contralateral side of the body in the posterior (interoceptive) and middle portions of the insula, each of which becomes lateralized in the right (sympathetic) and left (parasympathetic) anterior insula of the human brain. The "core network" formed by the anterior insular cortex (AIC) and the anterior cingulate cortex (ACC) on both sides is also indicated. Drawing produced by the Neuroscience Publication office of Barrow Neurological Institute ©. (See Color Plate 4.1)

criticism of the James-Lange theory of emotion—that it did not allow for awareness of feelings associated with internally generated emotions.

Conclusions

The evidence reviewed in this chapter indicates that the AIC is associated not just
with all subjective feelings but unmistakably with awareness of sensations and
movements, of visual and auditory percepts, of the visual image of the self, of the
reliability of subjective sensory images and expectations of events and other
individuals, and also with attention, cognitive choice, decision making, music,
and time. In several crucial experiments noted above, the AIC was activated
without activation in the ACC. No other region of the brain is activated in all of
these tasks, and the only feature common to all of the reviewed studies is that
they engaged the awareness of the subjects. Thus, in my opinion, the available
evidence compels the hypothesis that the AIC engenders human awareness.

Awareness can be defined as knowing that one exists ("I am"). A living
organism must be able to experience its own existence as a sentient being before
it can experience the existence and salience of anything else in the surrounding
environment, including portions of its body or its abilities. Thus, the phenomenon
of awareness requires first a neural (mental) representation of "me" as a feeling
(sentient) entity and then a representation of the salience that anything else has for
"me." This view is similar to the proposal that awareness of any object requires a
mental representation of the feeling self, a mental representation of the object, and
a mental representation of the salient interrelationship between me and that object
(Frith, Perry, & Lumer, 1999; Lewis, 2008). This formulation obviates discussion
of a "ghost in the machine": it inherently creates a subjective (or "personal"; see
Damasio, 1993) perspective that differentiates inner and outer realms with separate representations, because the inner feelings that underlie the representation of
the sentient self are only accessible from the owner's body and brain (Churchland,
2002; Damasio, 1993). From this perspective, an individual can lose the ability to
perceive a portion of the surrounding environment, a missing limb, or a functional
impairment—that is, display clinical anosognosia—and yet maintain phenomenal
emotional awareness of his/her own existence as a sentient being. On the other
hand, loss of the ability to know that one exists, of subjective awareness itself,
would result in the loss of emotional awareness of the existence of everything,
although such loss in a mature adult human might be camouflaged by well-
practiced behaviors and verbal abilities that still remain. It has also been suggested
that the evolution of intentional emotional interactions between conspecific individuals—which was probably crucial for hominid primates (Dunbar & Schultz,
2007)— required an awareness of "me" across time that would enable comparisons of the effects of my actions now, in the past, and in the future (Frith & Frith,
2007).

The brain is evolutionarily and reproducibly well organized into hierarchical networks that distribute functionality across multiple sites. The ability of humans to report their behavioral and perceptual abilities or their emotional feelings depends on different cascades of neural mechanisms, and any particular deficit could result from damage to one or more of several levels in these networks; this is particularly relevant for anosognosia (Spinazzola, Pia, Folegatti, Marchetti, & Berti, 2008). Accordingly, different investigators have different views on the causes of anosognosia and the brain regions involved (Orfei et al., 2007). These views are well represented in this book. Similarly, the localization of phenomenal awareness in a single neural substrate, as postulated here, might seem unlikely to many investigators. Nevertheless, the evidence reviewed in this chapter is clearly consistent with the view that there is an ultimate representation of the sentient self in the AIC and the adjoining frontal operculum that is uniquely involved in all human behaviors and perceptions. The proposed structural model is consistent with all available evidence, including the role of the AIC in music and time perception, and it provides a theoretical explanation for the integrative processing in the insula that matches the working definition of awareness. In my opinion, the AIC fulfills the requirements of a neural correlate of awareness.

Clinical observations offer corroborative evidence for the hypothesis that the AIC engenders subjective awareness. For example, Manes, Paradiso, and Robinson (1999) reported that infarcts of the right AIC produced anergia, or complete listlessness; Sterzer, Stadler, Poustka, and Kleinschmidt (2007) reported that adolescents with conduct disorder had a significant decrease in gray matter volume in bilateral AIC that correlated parametrically with lack of empathy and with aggressive behavior; King-Casas et al. (2008) reported that graded activation of the AIC is associated with awareness of social gestures in normal subjects, but that patients with borderline personality disorder (who are incapable of cooperating with others) do not display such activation; Silani et al. (2008) reported reduced activation in the AIC of high-functioning autistics in a task in which the subjects assessed their feelings about unpleasant images, which correlated with measures of increased alexithymia and decreased empathy; and, congenital malformation of the bilateral insula reportedly underlies Smith-Magenis syndrome, which is characterized by mental retardation and the disruption of self-guided behavior in children (Boddaert et al., 2004). Most significantly, it has been reported that fronto-temporal dementia (FTD) patients with degenerate fronto-insular and cingulate cortices display a selective loss of emotional awareness of self and others and a loss of self-conscious behaviors (Sturm, Rosen, Allison, Miller, & Levenson, 2006) that is specifically associated with the degeneration of Von Economo neurons (Seeley et al., 2006, 2007), a unique type of neuron that occurs in the AIC and the ACC of hominid primates with phylogenetically increasing density (Allman et al., 2005; Nimchinsky et al., 1999; for further comments, see Craig, 2008, 2009).

The evidence and the model presented above suggest that damage in the AIC could result in several neurological deficits, including a loss of emotional awareness, empathy, self-conscious behaviors, and personal presence in the "here and now." These characteristics are consistent with the observations made in FTD patients and Smith-Magenis patients with bilateral degeneration of the AIC. Nevertheless, in most instances, an infarct occurs on only one side of the brain, and the loss of a portion or all of the AIC on one side only might have variable results. It is common medical knowledge that a patient with a right-sided stroke is often unjustifiably happy and pleasant, whereas a patient with a left-sided stroke is often angry and depressed (as reviewed in the chapter by Heilman and Harciarek); this is consistent with the homeostatic/psychophysiological model of emotional asymmetry described above. However, it is unknown how the AIC on the two sides of the brain interact in order to generate a unified, coherent self, and thus it is not possible to predict how damage on one side might affect the functional capacity of the remaining AIC on the other side. Does the right side lead (Sridharan et al., 2008) and the left side monitor (Brass & Haggard, 2007; Klein et al., 2007) most of the time, and is that why there are more Von Economo neurons in the right AIC than the left (Allman et al., 2005) and why a large right-sided lesion can produce anergia but a large left-sided lesion cannot (Manes et al., 1999)? Studies of split-brain patients are needed that incorporate the asymmetric findings described above (e.g., Uddin, Rayman, & Zaidel, 2005), although the issue of neural compensation over time also confounds such analyses (Orfei et al., 2007; see also the chapter in this volume by Prigatano). Nevertheless, recent evidence that associates auditory hallucinations in schizophrenics with hyperactivity in the *right* AIC and the *left* ACC (Sommer et al., 2008) is consistent with the possibility that imbalanced coordination between the two sides of the AIC/ACC "core network" (Cole & Schneider, 2007; Sridharan et al., 2008; Thielscher & Pessoa, 2007) may underlie dysfunctional awareness of any sort.

The clinical literature on anosognosia suggests that damage to the insula on the right side in particular may be most apparent clinically. For example, Karnath and colleagues reported that damage to the right mid-insula was a common factor in anosognosia patients who displayed a lack of awareness of movement disability (Baier & Karnath, 2008; Karnath, Baier, & Nagele, 2005; and see Chapter 3 in this volume). Similarly, Spinazzola et al. (2008) reported that damage to the right insula could produce anosognosia for hemiplegia or alternatively anosognosia for hemianesthesia. The modular arrangement of self-monitoring comparators hypothesized by Spinazzola and colleagues (2008) to process separate neural functions is entirely consistent with the model for the integration of awareness in the insular cortex described above and the evidence reviewed in this chapter; partial damage in the insula could certainly result in the independent loss of different functions without a total loss of subjective awareness.

On the other hand, damage to the left AIC is known to produce aphasia (speech apraxia) (Dronkers, 1996), and the recent documentation of concomitant anosognosia and aphasia in patients with left-sided insular lesions (see Chapter 7, Cocchini & Della Sala, this volume) is more consistent with the bilateral activation of the insula in functional imaging studies of the sense of movement (Farrer & Frith, 2002; Farrer et al., 2003). The activation of the right angular gyrus in the inferior posterior parietal cortex in such imaging studies (see also Farrer et al., 2008) is consistent with a putative right-sided asymmetry in the representation of extrapersonal coordinate-based space (Karnath, Ferber, & Himmelbach, 2001; Sterzi et al., 1993), although that may be an earlier stage in the processing cascade, as suggested by Spinazzola et al. (2008). Such integration must be invoked to explain reports that caloric vestibular stimulation by infusion of cold water in the external auditory meatus on the left but not the right side (thus affecting integration predominantly in the right side of the brain) can temporarily alleviate anosognosia or neglect (Cappa, Sterzi, Vallar, & Bisiach, 1987).

The available clinical literature does indeed indicate a variety of other neurological and psychological deficits subsequent to insular infarcts, including pain asymbolia, ageusia, and loss of craving for cigarettes (Berthier, Starkstein, & Leiguarda, 1988; Naqvi, Rudrauf, Damasio, & Bechara, 2007; Pritchard et al., 1999; for additional references, see Craig, 2009), and work in the rat suggests that both negative and positive incentive behavior can be affected (Contreras, Ceric, & Torrealba, 2007). However, in many studies a narrow set of behavioral tests was used or a single characteristic deficit was reported. A comprehensive clinical overview of the effects of insular damage has yet to be published. The evidence certainly suggests that many patients with insular damage could have several significant clinical symptoms, as noted above, and that damage to different portions of the insula could produce different sets of symptoms. Any such study will be hampered by the enormous variability in the gross morphology of the AIC, which even differs between the left and right sides of most individuals (Naidich et al., 2004). The use of high-resolution contrast imaging and perfusion scans, in addition to sophisticated subtraction methods (see Karnath & Baier, Chapter 3, this volume), will be important.

Finally, a crucial role of the AIC in major clinical syndromes in addition to anosognosia and FTD is suggested by converging imaging and clinical findings, such as schizophrenia, post-traumatic stress syndrome, anxiety and panic disorders, alexithymia, functional gastrointestinal disorders, fibromyalgia, and so on (e.g., Giesecke et al., 2005; Moriguchi et al., 2007; Nagai, Kishi, & Kato, 2007; Paulus & Stein, 2006; Takahashi et al., 2004; see Craig, 2009). If the AIC is the seat of human awareness, with an organization based on the homeostatic condition of the body, as these considerations suggest, then it could be involved in a wide variety of somatic and psychic disorders. The integration of this perspective with the knowledge and experience of clinical observers that is needed should prove enlightening.

References

Ackermann, H., & Riecker, A. (2004). The contribution of the insula to motor aspects of speech production: A review and a hypothesis. *Brain and Language, 89,* 320–328.

Allman, J. M., Watson, K. K., Tetreault, N. A., & Hakeem, A. Y. (2005). Intuition and autism: A possible role for Von Economo neurons. *Trends in Cognitive Science, 9,* 367–373.

Altman, J., & Bayer, S. A. (1984). The development of the rat spinal cord. *Advances in Anatomy, Embryology, and Cell Biology, 85,* 1–164.

Amodio, D. M., & Frith, C. D. (2006). Meeting of minds: The medial frontal cortex and social cognition. *Nature Reviews Neuroscience, 7,* 268–277.

Augustine, J. R. (1996). Circuitry and functional aspects of the insular lobe in primates including humans. *Brain Research Reviews, 22,* 229–244.

Baier, B., & Karnath, H. O. (2008). Tight link between our sense of limb ownership and self-awareness of actions. *Stroke, 39,* 486–488.

Barrett, L. F., Quigley, K. S., Bliss-Moreau, E., & Aronson, K. R. (2004). Interoceptive sensitivity and self-reports of emotional experience. *Journal of Personality and Social Psychology, 87,* 684–697.

Bartels, A., & Zeki, S. (2004). The neural correlates of maternal and romantic love. *NeuroImage, 21,* 1155–1166.

Berthier, M. L., Starkstein, S. E., & Leiguarda, R. C. (1988). Asymbolia for pain: A sensory-limbic disconnection syndrome. *Annals of Neurology, 24,* 41–49.

Boddaert, N., De Leersnyder, H., Bourgeois, M., Munnich, A., Brunelle, F., & Zilbovicius, M. (2004). Anatomical and functional brain imaging evidence of lenticulo-insular anomalies in Smith Magenis syndrome. *NeuroImage, 21,* 1021–1025.

Brass, M., & Haggard, P. (2007). To do or not to do: The neural signature of self-control. *Journal of Neuroscience, 27,* 9141–9145.

Brooks, J. C., Nurmikko, T. J., Bimson, W. E., Singh, K. D., & Roberts, N. (2002). fMRI of thermal pain: Effects of stimulus laterality and attention. *NeuroImage, 15,* 293–301.

Brooks, J. C., Zambreanu, L., Godinez, A., Craig, A. D., & Tracey, I. (2005). Somatotopic organisation of the human insula to painful heat studied with high resolution functional imaging. *NeuroImage* 27 (1):201–209.

Burton, H., Videen, T. O., & Raichle, M. E. (1993). Tactile-vibration-activated foci in insular and parietal-opercular cortex studied with positron emission tomography: Mapping the second somatosensory area in humans. *Somatosensory and Motor Research, 10,* 297–308.

Bushara, K. O., Grafman, J., & Hallett, M. (2001). Neural correlates of auditory-visual stimulus onset asynchrony detection. *Journal of Neuroscience, 21,* 300–304.

Campbell, L. A., & Bryant, R. A. (2007). How time flies: A study of novice skydivers. *Behavior Research and Therapy, 45,* 1389–1392.

Cannon, W. B. (1939). *The wisdom of the body.* New York: Norton & Co.

Cappa, S., Sterzi, R., Vallar, G., & Bisiach, E. (1987). Remission of hemineglect and anosognosia during vestibular stimulation. *Neuropsychologia, 25,* 775–782.

Churchland, P. S. (2002). Self-representation in nervous systems. *Science, 296,* 308–310.

Cole, M. W., & Schneider, W. (2007). The cognitive control network: Integrated cortical regions with dissociable functions. *NeuroImage, 37,* 343–360.

Contreras, M., Ceric, F., & Torrealba, F. (2007). Inactivation of the interoceptive insula disrupts drug craving and malaise induced by lithium. *Science, 318,* 655–658.

Coull, J. T. (2004). fMRI studies of temporal attention: Allocating attention within, or towards, time. *Brain Research Cognitive Brain Research, 21*, 216–226.

Craig, A. D. (1993). Propriospinal input to thoracolumbar sympathetic nuclei from cervical and lumbar lamina I neurons in the cat and the monkey. *The Journal of Comparative Neurology, 331*, 517–530.

Craig, A. D. (1995). Distribution of brainstem projections from spinal lamina I neurons in the cat and the monkey. *The Journal of Comparative Neurology, 361*, 225–248.

Craig, A. D. (2002). How do you feel? Interoception: The sense of the physiological condition of the body. *Nature Reviews Neuroscience, 3*, 655–666.

Craig, A. D. (2003a). Pain mechanisms: Labeled lines versus convergence in central processing. *Annual Review of Neuroscience, 26*, 1–30.

Craig, A. D. (2003b). A new view of pain as a homeostatic emotion. *Trends in Neurosciences, 26*, 303–307.

Craig, A. D. (2004). Distribution of trigeminothalamic and spinothalamic lamina I terminations in the macaque monkey. *The Journal of Comparative Neurology, 477*, 119–148.

Craig, A. D. (2005). Forebrain emotional asymmetry: A neuroanatomical basis? *Trends in Cognitive Sciences, 9*, 566–571.

Craig, A. D. (2008). Interoception and emotion. In M. Lewis, J. M. Haviland-Jones, & L. F. Barrett (Eds.), *Handbook of emotions* (3rd edition) (pp. 272–288). New York: Guilford Publications.

Craig, A. D. (2009). How do you feel—now? The anterior insula and human awareness. *Nature Reviews Neuroscience, 10*, 59–70.

Craig, A. D., & Andrew, D. (2002). Responses of spinothalamic lamina I neurons to repeated brief contact heat stimulation in the cat. *Journal of Neurophysiology, 87*, 1902–1914.

Craig, A. D., & Bushnell, M. C. (1994). The thermal grill illusion: Unmasking the burn of cold pain. *Science, 265*, 252–255.

Craig, A. D., Bushnell, M. C., Zhang, E.-T., & Blomqvist, A. (1994). A thalamic nucleus specific for pain and temperature sensation. *Nature, 372*, 770–773.

Craig, A. D., Chen, K., Bandy, D., & Reiman, E. M. (2000). Thermosensory activation of insular cortex. *Nature Neuroscience, 3*, 184–190.

Craig, A. D., Reiman, E. M., Evans, A., & Bushnell, M. C. (1996). Functional imaging of an illusion of pain. *Nature, 384*, 258–260.

Critchley, H. D., Wiens, S., Rotshtein, P., Ohman, A., & Dolan, R. J. (2004). Neural systems supporting interoceptive awareness. *Nature Neuroscience, 7*, 189–195.

Damasio, A. R. (1993). Descartes' error: Emotion, reason, and the human brain. New York: Putnam.

Damasio, A. R., Grabowski, T. J., Bechara, A., Damasio, H., Ponto, L. L., Parvizi, J., & Hichwa, R. D. (2000). Subcortical and cortical brain activity during the feeling of self-generated emotions. *Nature Neuroscience, 3*, 1049–1056.

Davidson, R. J. (2004). Well-being and affective style: Neural substrates and biobehavioural correlates. *Philosophical Transactions of the Royal Society* B: *Biological Sciences, 359*, 1395–1411.

Deary, I. J., Simonotto, E., Meyer, M., Marshall, A., Marshall, I., Goddard, N., & Wardlaw, J. M. (2004). The functional anatomy of inspection time: An event-related fMRI study. *NeuroImage, 22*, 1466–1479.

Del Parigi, A., Chen, K., Salbe, A. D., Gautier, J. F., Ravussin, E., Reiman, E. M., & Tataranni, P. A. (2002). Tasting a liquid meal after a prolonged fast is associated with preferential activation of the left hemisphere. *NeuroReport, 13*, 1141–1145.

Devue, C., Collette, F., Balteau, E., Degueldre, C., Luxen, A., Maquet, P., & Bredart, S. (2007). Here I am: The cortical correlates of visual self-recognition. *Brain Research, 1143*, 169–182.

De Waal, F. B. (2008). The thief in the mirror. *Public Library of Science Biology, 19*, e201.

Diesel, D. A., Tucker, A., & Robertshaw, D. (1990) Cold-induced changes in breathing pattern as a strategy to reduce respiratory heat loss. *Journal of Applied Physiology,* 69:1946–1952.

Droit-Volet, S., & Meck, W. H. (2007). How emotions colour our perception of time. *Trends in Cognitive Science, 11*, 504–513.

Dronkers, N. F. (1996). A new brain region for coordinating speech articulation. *Nature, 384*, 159–161.

Drzezga, A., Darsow, U., Treede, R., Siebner, H., Frisch, M., Munz, F., Weilke, F., Ring, J., Schwaiger, M., & Bartenstein, P. (2001). Central activation by histamine-induced itch: Analogies to pain processing: A correlational analysis of O-15 H(2)O positron emission tomography studies. *Pain, 92*, 295–305.

Dunbar, R. I., & Shultz, S. (2007). Evolution in the social brain. *Science, 317*, 1344–1347.

Farrer, C., Franck, N., Georgieff, N., Frith, C. D., Decety, J., & Jeannerod, M. (2003). Modulating the experience of agency: A positron emission tomography study. *NeuroImage, 18*, 324–333.

Farrer, C., Frey, S. H., Van Horn, J. D., Tunik, E., Turk, D., Inati, S., & Grafton, S. T. (2008). The angular gyrus computes action awareness representations. *Cerebral Cortex, 18*, 254–261.

Farrer, C., & Frith, C. D. (2002). Experiencing oneself vs another person as being the cause of an action: The neural correlates of the experience of agency. *NeuroImage, 15*, 596–603.

Frank, G. K., Oberndorfer, T. A., Simmons, A. N., Paulus, M. P., Fudge, J. L., Yang, T. T., & Kaye, W. H. (2008). Sucrose activates human taste pathways differently from artificial sweetener. *NeuroImage, 39*, 1559–1569.

Frith, C. D., & Frith, U. (2007). Social cognition in humans. *Current Biology, 17*, R724–R732.

Frith, C., Perry, R., & Lumer, E. (1999). The neural correlates of conscious experience: An experimental framework. *Trends in Cognitive Science, 3*, 105–114.

Gallop, G. G., Jr. (1970). Chimpanzees: Self-recognition. *Science, 167*, 86–87.

Giesecke, T., Gracely, R. H., Williams, D. A., Geisser, M. E., Petzke, F. W., & Clauw, D. J. (2005). The relationship between depression, clinical pain, and experimental pain in a chronic pain cohort. *Arthritis and Rheumatism, 52*, 1577–1584.

Greenspan, J. D., Lee, R. R., & Lenz, F. A. (1999). Pain sensitivity alterations as a function of lesion location in the parasylvian cortex. *Pain, 81*, 273–282.

Griffiths, T. D., Warren, J. D., Dean, J. L., & Howard, D. (2004). "When the feeling's gone": A selective loss of musical emotion. *Journal of Neurology, Neurosurgery, and Psychiatry, 75*, 344–345.

Heimer, L., & Van Hoesen, G. W. (2006). The limbic lobe and its output channels: Implications for emotional functions and adaptive behavior. *Neuroscience and Biobehavioral Reviews, 30*, 126–147.

Henderson, L. A., Gandevia, S. C., & Macefield, V. G. (2007). Somatotopic organization of the processing of muscle and cutaneous pain in the left and right insula cortex: A single-trial fMRI study. *Pain, 128*, 20–30.

Henderson, L. A., Woo, M. A., Macey, P. M., Macey, K. E., Frysinger, R. C., Alger, J. R., Yan-Go, F., & Harper, R. M. (2003). Neural responses during Valsalva maneuvers in obstructive sleep apnea syndrome. *Journal of Applied Physiology, 94*, 1063–1074.

Hennenlotter, A., Schroeder, U., Erhard, P., Castrop, F., Haslinger, B., Stoecker, D., Lange, K. W., & Ceballos-Baumann, A. O. (2005). A common neural basis for receptive and expressive communication of pleasant facial affect. *NeuroImage, 26*, 581–591.

Holstege, G. (1988). Direct and indirect pathways to lamina I in the medulla oblongata and spinal cord of the cat. In H. L. Fields & J. M. Besson (Eds.), *Progress in brain research* (pp. 47–94). Amsterdam: Elsevier.

Hua, L. H., Strigo, I. A., Baxter, L. C., Johnson, S. C., & Craig, A. D. (2005). Anteroposterior somatotopy of innocuous cooling activation focus in human dorsal posterior insular cortex. *American Journal of Physiology Regulatory, Integrative and Comparative Physiology, 289*, R319–R325.

Iannetti, G. D., Zambreanu, L., Cruccu, G., & Tracey, I. (2005). Operculoinsular cortex encodes pain intensity at the earliest stages of cortical processing as indicated by amplitude of laser-evoked potentials in humans. *Neuroscience, 131*, 199–208.

Jabbi, M., Swart, M., & Keysers, C. (2007). Empathy for positive and negative emotions in the gustatory cortex. *NeuroImage, 34*, 1744–1753.

James, W. (1890). *The principles of psychology.* Retrieved July 9, 2009, from http://psychclassics.yorku.ca.James/Principles/index.htm.

Johansen, J. P., Fields, H. L., & Manning, B. H. (2001). The affective component of pain in rodents: Direct evidence for a contribution of the anterior cingulate cortex. *Proceedings of the National Academy of Sciences USA, 98*, 8077–8082.

Johnstone, T., van Reekum, C. M., Oakes, T. R., & Davidson, R. J. (2006). The voice of emotion: An FMRI study of neural responses to angry and happy vocal expressions. *Social Cognitive and Affective Neuroscience, 1*, 242–249.

Karnath, H. O., Baier, B., & Nagele, T. (2005). Awareness of the functioning of one's own limbs mediated by the insular cortex? *Journal of Neuroscience, 25*, 7134–7138.

Karnath, H. O., Ferber, S., & Himmelbach, M. (2001). Spatial awareness is a function of the temporal not the posterior parietal lobe. *Nature, 411*, 950–953.

Keltner, J. R., Furst, A., Fan, C., Redfern, R., Inglis, B., & Fields, H. L. (2006). Isolating the modulatory effect of expectation on pain transmission: A functional magnetic resonance imaging study. *Journal of Neuroscience, 26*, 4437–4443.

Kikyo, H., Ohki, K., & Miyashita, Y. (2002). Neural correlates for feeling-of-knowing: An fMRI parametric analysis. *Neuron, 36*, 177–186.

Kim, H., Adolphs, R., O'Doherty, J. P., & Shimojo, S. (2007). Temporal isolation of neural processes underlying face preference decisions. *Proceedings of the National Academy of Sciences USA, 104*, 18253–18258.

King-Casas, B., Sharp, C., Lomax-Bream, L., Lohrenz, T., Fonagy, P., & Montague, P. R. (2008). The rupture and repair of cooperation in borderline personality disorder. *Science, 321*, 806–810.

Klein, R. G. (2002). *The dawn of human culture.* New York: Wiley.

Klein, T. A., Endrass, T., Kathmann, N., Neumann, J., von Cramon, D. Y., & Ullsperger, M. (2007). Neural correlates of error awareness. *NeuroImage, 34*, 1774–1781.

Knutson, B., Rick, S., Wimmer, G. E., Prelec, D., & Loewenstein, G. (2007). Neural predictors of purchases. *Neuron, 53*, 147–156.

Koechlin, E., & Jubault, T. (2006). Broca's area and the hierarchical organization of human behavior. *Neuron, 50,* 963–974.

Koelsch, S., Fritz, T., von Cramon, D. Y., Muller, K., & Friederici, A. D. (2006). Investigating emotion with music: An fMRI study. *Human Brain Mapping, 27,* 239–250.

Kondo, H. M., & Kashino, M. (2007). Neural mechanisms of auditory awareness underlying verbal transformations. *NeuroImage, 36,* 123–130.

Kong, J., White, N. S., Kwong, K. K., Vangel, M. G., Rosman, I. S., Gracely, R. H., & Gollub, R. L. (2006). Using fMRI to dissociate sensory encoding from cognitive evaluation of heat pain intensity. *Human Brain Mapping, 27,* 715–721.

Kranczioch, C., Debener, S., Schwarzbach, J., Goebel, R., & Engel, A. K. (2005). Neural correlates of conscious perception in the attentional blink. *NeuroImage, 24,* 704–714.

Leibenluft, E., Gobbini, M. I., Harrison, T., & Haxby, J. V. (2004). Mothers' neural activation in response to pictures of their children and other children. *Biological Psychiatry, 56,* 225–232.

Lewis, M. (2008). The emergence of human emotions. In M. Lewis, J. M. Haviland-Jones, & L. F. Barrett (Eds.), *Handbook of emotions* (3rd edition) (pp. 304–319). New York: Guilford Press.

Lewis, P. A. & Miall, R. C. (2006) A right hemispheric prefrontal system for cognitive time measurement. *Behavioural Processes,* 71 (2–3):226–234.

Livesey, A. C., Wall, M.B., & Smith, A. T. (2007). Time perception: Manipulation of task difficulty dissociates clock functions from other cognitive demands. *Neuropsychologia, 45,* 321–331.

MacNeilage, P.F., Rogers, L.J., Vallortigara, G. (2009). Origins of the left & right brain. *Scientific American, 301:* 60–67.

Manes, F., Paradiso, S., & Robinson, R. G. (1999). Neuropsychiatric effects of insular stroke. *Journal of Nervous and Mental Disorders, 187,* 707–712.

Menon, V., & Levitin, D. J. (2005). The rewards of music listening: Response and physiological connectivity of the mesolimbic system. *NeuroImage, 28,* 175–184.

Moriguchi, Y., Decety, J., Ohnishi, T., Maeda, M., Mori, T., Nemoto, K., Matsuda, H., & Komaki, G. (2007). Empathy and judging other's pain: An fMRI study of alexithymia. *Cerebral Cortex, 17,* 2223–2234.

Mower, G. (1976). Perceived intensity of peripheral thermal stimuli is independent of internal body temperature. *Journal of Comparative and Physiological Psychology, 90,* 1152–1155.

Mufson, E. J., Sobreviela, T., & Kordower, J. H. (1997). Chemical neuroanatomy of the primate insula cortex: Relationship to cytoarchitectonics, connectivity, function and neurodegeneration. In F. E. Bloom, A. Bjorklund, & T. Hokfelt (Eds.), *Handbook of chemical neuroanatomy, vol. 13: The primate nervous system, Part I* (pp. 377–454). New York: Elsevier Science.

Mutschler, I., Schulze-Bonhage, A., Glauche, V., Demandt, E., Speck, O., & Ball, T. (2007). A rapid sound-action association effect in human insular cortex. *Public Library of Science ONE, 2,* e259.

Nagai, M., Kishi, K., & Kato, S. (2007). Insular cortex and neuropsychiatric disorders: A review of recent literature. *European Psychiatry, 22,* 387–394.

Naidich, T. P., Kang, E., Fatterpekar, G. M., Delman, B. N., Gultekin, S. H., Wolfe, D., Ortiz, O., Yousry, I., Weismann, M., & Yousry, T. A. (2004). The insula: Anatomic study and MR imaging display at 1.5 T. *AJNR American Journal of Neuroradiology, 25*, 222–232.

Naqvi, N. H., Rudrauf, D., Damasio, H., & Bechara, A. (2007). Damage to the insula disrupts addiction to cigarette smoking. *Science, 315*, 531–534.

Nimchinsky, E. A., Gilissen, E., Allman, J. M., Perl, D. P., Erwin, J. M., & Hof, P. R. (1999). A neuronal morphologic type unique to humans and great apes. *Proceedings of the National Academy of Sciences USA, 96*, 5268–5273.

Olausson, H., Charron, J., Marchand, S., Villemure, C., Strigo, I. A., & Bushnell, M. C. (2005). Feelings of warmth correlate with neural activity in right anterior insular cortex. *Neuroscience Letters, 389*, 1–5.

Olausson, H., Lamarre, Y., Backlund, H., Morin, C., Wallin, B. G., Starck, G., Ekholm, S., Strigo, I., Worsley, K., Vallbo, A. B., & Bushnell, M. C. (2002). Unmyelinated tactile afferents signal touch and project to insular cortex. *Nature Neuroscience, 5*, 900–904.

Orfei, M. D., Robinson, R. G., Prigatano, G. P., Starkstein, S., Rusch, N., Bria, P., Caltagirone, C., & Spalletta, G. (2007). Anosognosia for hemiplegia after stroke is a multifaceted phenomenon: A systematic review of the literature. *Brain, 130*, 3075–3090.

Ortigue, S., Grafton, S. T., & Bianchi-Demicheli, F. (2007). Correlation between insula activation and self-reported quality of orgasm in women. *NeuroImage, 37*, 551–560.

Ostrowsky, K., Magnin, M., Ryvlin, P., Isnard, J., Guenot, M., & Mauguière, F. (2002). Representation of pain and somatic sensation in the human insula: A study of responses to direct electrical cortical stimulation. *Cerebral Cortex, 12*, 376–385.

Paulus, M. P., & Stein, M. B. (2006). An insular view of anxiety. *Biological Psychiatry, 60*, 383–387.

Pelchat, M. L., Johnson, A., Chan, R., Valdez, J., & Ragland, J. D. (2004). Images of desire: Food-craving activation during fMRI. *NeuroImage, 23*, 1486–1493.

Petrovic, P., Kalso, E., Petersson, K. M., & Ingvar, M. (2002). Placebo and opioid analgesia—imaging a shared neuronal network. *Science, 295*, 1737–1740.

Phillips, M. L., Gregory, L. J., Cullen, S., Cohen, S., Ng, V., Andrew, C., Giampietro, V., Bullmore, E., Zelaya, F., Amaro, E., Thompson, D. G., Hobson, A. R., Williams, S. C., Brammer, M., & Aziz, Q. (2003). The effect of negative emotional context on neural and behavioural responses to oesophageal stimulation. *Brain, 126*, 669–684.

Platel, H., Price, C., Baron, J. C., Wise, R., Lambert, J., Frackowiak, R. S., Lechevalier, B., & Eustache, F. (1997). The structural components of music perception. A functional anatomical study. *Brain, 120*, 229–243.

Ploran, E. J., Nelson, S. M., Velanova, K., Donaldson, D. I., Petersen, S. E., & Wheeler, M. E. (2007). Evidence accumulation and the moment of recognition: Dissociating perceptual recognition processes using fMRI. *Journal of Neuroscience, 27*, 11912–11924.

Preuschoff, K., Quartz, S. R., & Bossaerts, P. (2008). Human insula activation reflects risk prediction errors as well as risk. *Journal of Neuroscience, 28*, 2745–2752.

Pritchard, T. C., Macaluso, D. A., & Eslinger, P. J. (1999). Taste perception in patients with insular cortex lesions. *Behavioral Neuroscience, 113*, 663–671.

Rao, S. M., Mayer, A. R. & Harrington, D. L. (2001). The evolution of brain activation during temporal processing. *Nature Neuroscience, 4* (3):317–323.

Rolls, E. T. (1999). *The brain and emotion.* Oxford, England: Oxford University Press.

Sanchez, M. M., Young, L. J., Plotsky, P. M., & Insel, T. R. (1999). Autoradiographic and in situ hybridization localization of corticotropin-releasing factor 1 and 2 receptors in nonhuman primate brain. *The Journal of Comparative Neurology, 408,* 365–377.

Saper, C. B. (2002). The central autonomic nervous system: Conscious visceral perception and autonomic pattern generation. *Annual Review of Neuroscience, 25,* 433–469.

Schmahmann, J. D., & Leifer, D. (1992). Parietal pseudothalamic pain syndrome: Clinical features and anatomic correlates. *Archives of Neurology, 49,* 1032–1037.

Schweinhardt, P., Glynn, C., Brooks, J., McQuay, H., Jack, T., Chessell, I., Bountra, C., & Tracey, I. (2006). An fMRI study of cerebral processing of brush-evoked allodynia in neuropathic pain patients. *NeuroImage, 32,* 256–265.

Seeley, W. W., Allman, J. M., Carlin, D. A., Crawford, R. K., Macedo, M. N., Greicius, M. D., Dearmond, S. J., & Miller, B. L. (2007). Divergent social functioning in behavioral variant frontotemporal dementia and Alzheimer disease: Reciprocal networks and neuronal evolution. *Alzheimer Disease and Associated Disorders, 21,* S50–S57.

Seeley, W. W., Carlin, D. A., Allman, J. M., Macedo, M. N., Bush, C., Miller, B. L., & Dearmond, S. J. (2006). Early frontotemporal dementia targets neurons unique to apes and humans. *Annals of Neurology, 60,* 660–667.

Semendeferi, K., & Damasio, H. (2000). The brain and its main anatomical subdivisions in living hominoids using magnetic resonance imaging. *Journal of Human Evolution, 38,* 317–332.

Seymour, B., O'Doherty, J. P., Dayan, P., Koltzenburg, M., Jones, A. K., Dolan, R. J., Friston, K. J., & Frackowiak, R. S. (2004). Temporal difference models describe higher-order learning in humans. *Nature, 429,* 664–667.

Sherrington, C. S. (1900). Cutaneous sensations. In E. A. Schäfer (Ed.), *Text-book of physiology* (pp. 920–1001). Edinburgh: Pentland.

Sherrington, C. S. (1948). *The integrative action of the nervous system.* Cambridge, England: University Press.

Silani, G., Bird, G., Brindley, R., Singer, T., Frith, C., & Frith, U. (2008). Levels of emotional awareness and autism: An fMRI study. *Social Neuroscience, 3,* 97–112.

Sommer, I. E., Diederen, K. M., Blom, J. D., Willems, A., Kushan, L., Slotema, K., Boks, M. P., Daalman, K., Hoek, H. W., Neggers, S. F., & Kahn, R. S. (2008). Auditory verbal hallucinations predominantly activate the right inferior frontal area. *Brain, 131,* 3169–3177.

Spinazzola, L., Pia, L., Folegatti, A., Marchetti, C., & Berti, A. (2008). Modular structure of awareness for sensorimotor disorders: Evidence from anosognosia for hemiplegia and anosognosia for hemianaesthesia. *Neuropsychologia, 46,* 915–926.

Sridharan, D., Levitin, D. J., & Menon, V. (2008). A critical role for the right fronto-insular cortex in switching between central-executive and default-mode networks. *Proceedings of the National Academy of Sciences USA, 105,* 12569–12574.

Stephan, E., Pardo, J. V., Faris, P. L., Hartman, B. K., Kim, S. W., Ivanov, E. H., Daughters, R. S., Costello, P. A., & Goodale, R. L. (2003). Functional neuroimaging of gastric distention. *Journal of Gastrointestinal Surgery, 7,* 740–749.

Sterzer, P., & Kleinschmidt, A. (2007). A neural basis for inference in perceptual ambiguity. *Proceedings of the National Academy of Sciences USA, 104,* 323–328.

Sterzer, P., Stadler, C., Poustka, F., & Kleinschmidt, A. (2007). A structural neural deficit in adolescents with conduct disorder and its association with lack of empathy. *NeuroImage, 37*, 335–342.

Sterzi, R., Bottini, G., Celani, M. G., Righetti, E., Lamassa, M., Ricci, S., & Vallar, G. (1993). Hemianopia, hemianaesthesia, and hemiplegia after right and left hemisphere damage. A hemispheric difference. *Journal of Neurology, Neurosurgery, and Psychiatry, 56*, 308–310.

Sturm, V. E., Rosen, H. J., Allison, S., Miller, B. L., & Levenson, R. W. (2006). Self-conscious emotion deficits in frontotemporal lobar degeneration. *Brain, 129*, 2508–2516.

Takahashi, H., Matsuura, M., Koeda, M., Yahata, N., Suhara, T., Kato, M., & Okubo, Y. (2008). Brain activations during judgments of positive self-conscious emotion and positive basic emotion: Pride and joy. *Cerebral Cortex, 18*, 898–903.

Takahashi, T., Suzuki, M., Hagino, H., Zhou, S. Y., Kawasaki, Y., Nohara, S., Nakamura, K., Yamashita, I., Seto, H., & Kurachi, M. (2004). Bilateral volume reduction of the insular cortex in patients with schizophrenia: a volumetric MRI Study. *Psychiatry Research, 132*, 187–196.

Thielscher, A., & Pessoa, L. (2007). Neural correlates of perceptual choice and decision making during fear-disgust discrimination. *Journal of Neuroscience, 27*, 2908–2917.

Tsakiris, M., Hesse, M. D., Boy, C., Haggard, P., & Fink, G. R. (2007). Neural signatures of body ownership: A sensory network for bodily self-consciousness. *Cerebral Cortex, 17*, 2235–2244.

Uddin, L. Q., Rayman, J., & Zaidel, E. (2005). Split-brain reveals separate but equal self-recognition in the two cerebral hemispheres. *Consciousness and Cognition, 14*, 633–640.

Veldhuizen, M. G., Bender, G., Constable, R. T., & Small, D. M. (2007). Trying to detect taste in a tasteless solution: Modulation of early gustatory cortex by attention to taste. *Chemical Senses, 32*, 569–581.

Wang, Z., Faith, M., Patterson, F., Tang, K., Kerrin, K., Wileyto, E. P., Detre, J. A., & Lerman, C. (2007). Neural substrates of abstinence-induced cigarette cravings in chronic smokers. *Journal of Neuroscience, 27*, 14035–14040.

Winston, J. S., Strange, B. A., O'Doherty, J., & Dolan, R. J. (2002). Automatic and intentional brain responses during evaluation of trustworthiness of faces. *Nature Neuroscience, 5*, 277–283.

5

Anosognosia and Anosodiaphoria of Weakness

Kenneth M. Heilman and Michal Harciarek

Patients with a variety of neurological diseases might be unaware of their deficits. For example, patients with blindness from an infarction of visual cortex (Brodmann's area 17) might not be aware they are blind (Anton, 1896), and patients with a cognitive decline from diseases such as Alzheimer's disease (AD) are often unaware of their deficits (Barrett, Eslinger, Ballentine, & Heilman, 2005). Even patients with an isolated episodic memory loss or amnesia that is associated with either Korsakoff's syndrome or basal forebrain injury can be unaware of their deficits. Some of the most dramatic examples of unawareness of a disease or disability, however, are those patients who cannot move one of their arms but are unaware of their hemiplegia. Although unawareness of illness was first described by Von Monakow in 1885, it was Babinski (1914) who called this lack of awareness or explicit denial of weakness "anosognosia." The term *anosognosia* derives from three classical roots: "a" = without, "noso" = disease, and "gnosis" = knowledge.

Many of the patients who originally have anosognosia for hemiplegia appear to learn that they are weak and thus when asked if they have some form of disability they will not deny their weakness. Although they verbally appear to be aware of their disability, they demonstrate little concern about their illness or disability. Babinski (1914) called this diminished concern of illness or disability *anosodiaphoria*, a term that was later disseminated by Critchley (1953, 1957).

Anosognosia is an important medical problem. There are now treatments that might help reduce the extent of brain damage and disability induced by stroke, but these treatments have to be given shortly after the onset of symptoms (e.g., intravenous thrombolytic therapy). Failure to be aware of a neurological deficit may delay and interfere with a person seeking medical help. When patients have a disability, the presence of anosognosia might interfere with their seeking rehabilitation and if they receive rehabilitation they might not be strongly motivated to "give it their all." In addition, patients who do not recognize their disability may engage in activities, such as driving, that could endanger their and other peoples' well-being. Patients who are unaware of their disabilities are often difficult to manage and, thus, the presence of anosognosia often induces caregiver stress.

In addition to the medical implications of anosognosia, self-awareness (self-consciousness) has been studied, analyzed, and discussed from ancient to current times, but it remains poorly understood. Anosognosia is a deficit of self-awareness, and studies of anosognosia might provide knowledge as to how the brain mediates self-awareness.

In the first section of this chapter, we will focus on what Babinski (1914) termed *anosognosia*, namely, unawareness of hemiplegia. We will present some major hypotheses that have been advanced to explain this disorder and discuss the strengths as well as weaknesses of these hypotheses. In the second section of this chapter, we will discuss the possible mechanisms of anosodiaphoria.

Anosognosia

Psychological Denial Hypothesis

Woody Allen said, "It's not that I am afraid to die, I just do not want to be there when it happens." If he were not there, he would be unaware of his impending death and unawareness would prevent suffering. Denial is a psychological means of eliminating awareness. Dr. Edwin Weinstein, who died in 1998, wrote a book with Robert Kahn entitled *Denial of Illness* (1955). In this book Weinstein and Kahn proposed and provided evidence that patients with severe disabilities, such as hemiplegia, deny their illness because denial is a powerful psychological defense mechanism that helps attenuate the distress and anxiety that can be induced by a catastrophic event such as a hemiplegia. In support of this denial hypothesis, Weinstein and Kahn (1953, 1955) studied the premorbid personality of those individuals who demonstrated denial of their illness and found that these participants often used denial as a coping strategy even before their stroke. That Weinstein posited a psychodynamic approach is consistent with his training; he was trained as both a psychiatrist and as a neurologist. Throughout his life he had a strong interest in psychiatry and even worked at the Virgin Islands Bureau of Mental Health and the Washington School of Psychiatry.

Babinski (1918), when he first used the term *anosognosia*, noted that the two patients he reported with this disorder both had a left hemiparesis. Although not statistically significant, Babinski asked, "Could it be that anosognosia is peculiar to lesions of the right hemisphere?" Subsequently, many clinicians have noted that unawareness or denial of hemiplegia appears to be more frequently associated with right than left hemisphere lesions. If a psychological defense mechanism was inducing denial, and if these patients with anosognosia used denial as a defense strategy before the onset of their strokes, there should be no hemispheric asymmetries in the incidence of anosognosia. Weinstein and Kahn (1955), however, noted that in order for patients to explicitly deny the presence of a hemiparesis, a person has to both understand speech and be able to communicate that he or she is unaware of the disability. In more than 90% of people, it is the left hemisphere that mediates language-speech. Thus, whereas right hemisphere injury would allow a patient to understand speech and to express denial, patients with left hemisphere lesions might be aphasic and have disorders of expression and/or comprehension. These patients with left hemisphere injury might, thus, be incapable of either understanding the question or providing an answer. Weinstein and Kahn (1955) concluded that the high rate of patients with left hemisphere strokes who could not be tested might have induced a sampling bias that led to the incorrect conclusion that anosognosia for hemiplegia is primarily induced by right hemisphere damage.

Nardone, Ward, Fotopoulou, and Turnbull (2007) attempted to test the psychological denial theory by testing patients with anosognosia for hemiplegia and patients who had hemiplegia but were aware of their weakness, as well as normal subjects. The participants were presented with words that were or were not related to their deficit and attempted to learn how the presentation of these words influenced participants' response time to neutral imperative stimuli. They found that the patients who did not have anosognosia when presented with these relevant words reduced the latency of their responses, but the patients with anosognosia increased their latency. The authors suggest that the patients who were aware of their deficits reduced their response times because they were aroused by these words and the patients with anosognosia lengthened their response times because of repression and that this delay is evidence of their implicit knowledge. Although these investigators' conclusions might be valid, patients with right hemisphere damage are often repeatedly told by others that they indeed have deficits. Thus, the increased latency might be related to implicit knowledge. Nevertheless, this knowledge might not be related to their ability to self-discover limb weakness or paralysis but rather to what they have been told by others and the conflict of supplied versus self-discovered information.

As a means of testing this psychological denial hypothesis, my colleagues and I decided to study patients who were undergoing selective hemispheric anesthesia (the Wada procedure). Patients with medically intractable seizures often respond to ablative surgery such as temporal lobectomy. Prior to surgery, selective hemispheric anesthesia is used to learn which hemisphere is dominant for mediating language and verbal memory so that surgery can avoid ablating these critical areas. Just before the barbiturate is injected into the carotid artery, the patient is asked to raise both arms at the shoulders and to keep his or her arms straight out in front of the body. After the barbiturate is injected into the carotid artery, the hemisphere on the same side as the injection stops functioning, and the arm on the opposite side falls. During left hemisphere anesthesia, most patients who are left-hemisphere dominant for language are unable to communicate and, therefore, we would be unable to learn if they are aware or unaware of their weakness during the time their left hemisphere is anesthetized. Thus, we asked these patients if their left or right arm was weak after they recovered from the left and right hemispheric anesthesia. After recovery they were no longer weak and were able to communicate normally.

Gilmore, Heilman, Schmidt, Fennell, and Quisling (1992) studied a group of right-handed patients who underwent Wada testing. When their left hemisphere was anesthetized with the barbiturate, these epileptic patients became globally aphasic and all developed a right hemiplegia. After this anesthesia cleared, they were again able to verbally communicate and were no longer weak. When asked what happened during this procedure, all these patients knew that their right arm became weak. The same patients also had their right hemisphere anesthetized using the same procedure. During their right hemisphere anesthesia, their left arm became weak, but they were not aphasic. After their right hemisphere recovered from the anesthesia, they were asked what they recalled about the procedure and, in contrast to when their left hemisphere was anesthetized, none of these patients recalled their left arm being weak.

During the Wada procedure some patients lose consciousness, but none of these patients lost consciousness and when questioned about their weakness none of them showed evidence for a confusional state. In additional studies from our health center, we continued to observe these overall results. Nonetheless, occasionally we also do observe patients who with left hemisphere anesthesia do not appear to be aware of their weakness and others who are aware of their weakness after their right hemisphere is anesthetized. In one study, investigators were unable to replicate our results (Dywan, McGlone, & Fox, 1995), but several other groups of investigators did replicate these findings (Carpenter et al., 1995; Durkin, Meador, Nichols, Lee, & Loring, 1994).

When the patients who underwent Wada testing were questioned about their hemiplegia, they were no longer hemiplegic. The procedure was over and they did not need a psychological defense mechanism to protect themselves from a catastrophic event. In addition, in these Wada studies, where subjects were unaware of hemiplegia after right but not left hemispheric anesthesia, it was the same people who underwent anesthesia of both hemispheres. Thus, these results fail to support Weinstein and Kahn's (1953, 1955) postulate that it was the patients' premorbid personality with their propensity for denial that accounts for anosognosia of hemiplegia. However, studies performed by Gazzaniga (2000, 2005) on patients with callosal disconnection did appear to reveal that the two hemispheres might have "different personalities." In this study they presented stimuli to either the subjects' right or left hemifield. In patients with callosal disconnection the stimuli that come into the left hemifield only go to the right hemisphere and stimuli that come into the right hemifield only go to the left hemisphere. Two different types of stimuli could come on either side. However, one type of stimulus would come on much more frequently than the other and the subject's left or right hemisphere had to predict which of the two stimuli were most likely to come on to the screen. The right hemisphere always predicted the more common one would appear, but the left hemisphere tried to predict when the less common stimulus would appear. Because the left hemisphere tried to predict the onset of the infrequent stimulus and this stimulus came on randomly, overall the right hemisphere was more accurate than the left. Based on these results, it appears that the left hemisphere attempts to find order, but the right just goes with the odds or is unaware of oddities or unlawful events. More research addressing these types of hemispheric dichotomies needs to be conducted.

There are people who when intoxicated by alcohol or drugs do and say things which when they become sober they do not recall. Animal research has replicated these findings and this phenomena has been called "state-dependent learning or memory." During the time the patients were undergoing Wada testing, they were in a different state than during the time they were asked about their weakness and thus it is possible that following right hemisphere anesthesia there was a selective state-dependent amnesia and the patients were aware of their weakness during the time they were weak but could not recall this weakness after they recovered from anesthesia. To learn if what appeared to be unawareness was actually a problem of amnesia, we asked patients during right hemisphere anesthesia if they were weak and also asked these same subjects after they recovered from anesthesia if they experienced weakness (Adair, Gilmore, Fennell, Gold, & Heilman, 1995a). We learned that the proportion of subjects who were unaware of their weakness during right hemisphere anesthesia was the same as the proportion of patients who demonstrated unawareness of weakness after they recovered from right hemisphere anesthesia. Thus, their postanesthesia anosognosia was not being induced by state-dependent learning and the hemispheric asymmetry could not be explained by the observation that aphasia more commonly occurs with left than right hemispheric injury.

After the Gilmore et al. (1992) study, we observed several patients during the Wada procedure who after having recovered from left hemisphere anesthesia would be unaware of their right arm weakness. Interestingly, though, some of these patients who were unaware of their right arm weakness were aware that they were unable to speak normally (Breier et al., 1995) and other patients who were unaware of their aphasia were aware of their weakness. The hypothesis that anosognosia is caused by psychologically motivated denial is not compatible with this dissociation between knowledge of aphasia and weakness. Many people suffer with weakness from nerve and spinal cord damage and if denial does occur with these disorders it must be extremely rare. When weakness is caused by either nerve or spinal cord damage, it still can be a catastrophic event and the denial hypothesis can also not account for the observation that anosognosia, for the most part, only occurs with injury to the central nervous system.

Whereas the results of the Wada studies and dissociation between injury to the brain versus spinal cord or nerves do not support the denial theory of anosognosia, it does not mean that there are not people who deny catastrophic illness, so that these illnesses do not further impair these peoples' adaptive capacities. However, since the denial hypothesis cannot fully account for anosognosia, we discuss some alternate hypotheses below.

Confusion

Critchley (1953) claimed that following a stroke, anosognosia usually lasted only for a few days. Hecaen and Albert (1978) also suggested that anosognosia may be related to confusion. Mesulam, Waxman, Geschwind, and Sabin (1976) reported that an acute confusional state might occur more frequently with right compared to left hemisphere strokes. Heilman and Van Den Abell (1980) demonstrated that the right hemisphere is dominant for mediating attention. The term *confusion* has many definitions, including disorientation and a lack of orderly thinking. However, if patients with right hemisphere strokes or right hemisphere anesthesia were very inattentive, especially to left-sided stimuli, it is possible that they could be unaware of their weakness. Left-sided inattentions (neglect) will be discussed below. Many patients with anosognosia of hemiplegia are oriented and many do not appear to have confusional states. During the Wada testing of the right hemisphere, many of the patients who have anosognosia for left arm weakness undergo memory and other forms of cognitive testing. We observed that they performed relatively normally on these tests, providing evidence that a confusional state cannot fully account for anosognosia.

Impaired Sensory Feedback

Critchley (1953) wrote that a loss of postural (position) sense plays a significant role in determining the patient's mental attitude toward his or her own disability, and he stated that it was Barre, Morin and Kaiser (1923) who thought this failure of feedback was a critical element in anosognosia for hemiplegia. Even Babinski (1918) noted that the two patients he reported with this disorder had sensory impairments. More recently, Levine, Calvanio, and Rinn (1991) again suggested that anosognosia was being caused by a failure of sensory feedback.

There are several possible means by which a person might learn that he or she is weak. One, as discussed, is proprioceptive feedback, but a person might also view his or her limb and see if it moves. Limb movements also induce alterations in the environment, and a failure to see, hear (e.g., "Clap your hands!"), or feel these alterations in the environment should alert a person that his or her limb is not properly working. Thus, a failure in postural feedback could not fully account for anosognosia.

As mentioned, during the Wada procedure we had subjects raise their arms at the shoulder, and with anesthesia their deltoids became weak and the arms fell down. To learn if these patients with anosognosia during right hemisphere anesthesia had a loss of shoulder position sense, we passively moved their arms at the shoulder or their fingers either up or down and asked each subject to report if his or her arm was moved up or down. During the hemispheric anesthesia, the subjects could not detect whether their contralateral finger was moved up or down, but they could determine if their arm at the shoulder joint was moved up or down (Lu, Barrett, Cibula, Gilmore, & Heilman, 2000). These results suggest that, whereas the proprioceptive information from the distal portion (e.g., finger) of an extremity (e.g., left) projects primarily to the opposite (e.g., right) hemisphere, proprioceptive information from the more proximal joints, such as at the shoulder, project to both hemispheres. The finding that our subjects with anosognosia for left shoulder weakness had intact proprioceptive feedback provides evidence against the sensory feedback hypothesis.

Another means of determining that an extremity is weak is by looking at that extremity. It is possible that people with a left hemianopia are unable to see that their arm is not working. If patients have a hemianopia, they should be able to move their eyes leftward, so that they can see their left arm in their right visual field. However, in order to use this compensatory eye movement strategy, a person would have to know or be aware that he or she has a hemianopia. Studies of patients with hemianopia have revealed that many patients with hemianopia are unaware of their hemianopia (Celesia, Brigell, & Vaphiades, 1997), and if patients are unaware of their hemianopia, then they might not use eye movement to compensate for this loss of left-sided vision.

To learn if a left hemianopia, together with unawareness of this hemianopia can help explain anosognosia of left hemiplegia, during the Wada test when the right hemisphere was anesthetized, we wrote numbers on patients' left hand and moved their weak left arm rightward so that it was in the patients' right visual field. After these patients' left hands were moved to the right side of their body so that their hand was in the right visual field, subjects were asked to name the number written in their hand. If they could see this number and tell the examiner its name, we could be certain that they saw their hand. Using this procedure, there were some patients who discovered their weakness, but the majority of patients remained unaware that their left hand was paralyzed.

Many patients with right hemispheric anesthesia who were able to receive proprioceptive feedback and even were able to see their weak left hand in their right visual field remained unaware of their weakness, and therefore their anosognosia cannot be entirely explained by a failure of sensory feedback.

Hemispatial Neglect

Hemispatial neglect is defined by a failure to be fully aware or interact with novel or meaningful stimuli in the contralesional viewer-centered space when this failure cannot be attributed to elemental sensory or motor defects. Thus, when patients fail to be aware of stimuli in contralesional hemispace it might be related to neglect rather than a hemianopia. Hemispatial neglect is much more commonly associated with right than left hemisphere dysfunction (see Heilman, Watson, & Valenstein, 2003). Thus, it is possible that the patients with hemianopia we mentioned above, who discovered that their hand was weak when it was brought from left to right hemispace, were suffering from hemispatial neglect. Unfortunately, we did not test these individuals for hemispatial neglect and therefore cannot be certain that the lack of feedback, secondary to the severe inattention that is associated with spatial neglect, induced their anosognosia. In addition, even if hemispatial neglect did account for these patients' unawareness, neglect-hemispatial inattention would only be able to explain anosognosia for hemiplegia in a small proportion of subjects. Most subjects after recognizing their left hand placed on their right side of their body and in the right visual field never learned that their hand was paralyzed. In addition, there have been several studies of patients that showed a dissociation between the presence of neglect and anosognosia for hemiplegia (Bisiach, Vallar, Perani, Papagno, & Berti, 1986; Marcel, Tegner, & Nimmo-Smith, 2004).

Personal Neglect and Asomatognosia

Patients with right hemisphere dysfunction might be inattentive to the left side of the body. For example, they might fail to dress the left side of the body and, thus, when they put on a jacket they might not attempt to put their left arm in the left sleeve of their jacket. When grooming they might fail to shave the left side of their face, and after they eat they might not clean food off the left side of their mouth. Some patients with right hemisphere stroke also do not recognize that parts of their body that are on the left belong to them. For example, as a medical student I saw a patient who tried to throw his left arm out of his bed and wanted to know why this hospital put two people in the same bed.

We mentioned earlier that during Wada testing when the right hemisphere was anesthetized, we carried the patient's left arm over to the right side of the body and to the right visual field. To make certain that they were able to see their hand we wrote a number on their hand and had them identify the number. In spite of these maneuvers many of our patients remained unaware that their arm/hand was weak. Since patients with right hemisphere dysfunction can have personal neglect or asomatognosia, it is possible that they did not think they were weak because they did not recognize that the hand with the number was their own. Therefore, to determine if personal neglect or asomatognosia can account for anosognosia, we performed another experiment (Adair et al., 1995b). After the barbiturate was injected into the right carotid artery and the patient developed a left hemiplegia, the examiner either put his or her own hand or the patient's hand into a restrictive viewing space, where the patient could only see this hand. We selected examiners who were about the same age and were the same race and sex as the subjects.

We did have subjects who had anosognosia for the weakness and who also could not discriminate between their hand and the examiner's hand (asomatognosia), but the majority of subjects who were unaware of their hemiparesis were able to recognize their own hand (Adair et al., 1997). The results suggest that there are some patients who might be unaware of their weakness because they do not recognize that their upper limb belongs to them, but they are a minority.

Phantom Movements

People who have a limb amputated often have the perception that the limb is still present and some people, when they attempt to move this limb, actually can feel the limb moving. It is possible that patients with anosognosia are not aware of their weakness because when they attempt to move they feel their limb moving, even though it is not moving. However, to be unaware that phantom movements are not real movements a person would also need to have a failure of feedback. To learn if phantom limb movement could account for anosognosia (Lu, Barrett, Cibula, Gilmore, & Heilman, 1997a), we blindfolded our subjects and again used the Wada procedure. After the right hemisphere was anesthetized, we asked our blindfolded patients to attempt to lift their left upper extremity and then to demonstrate their left limb's position by placing their right upper extremity in the same position as their left. During right hemispheric anesthesia, we also tested left shoulder proprioception by lifting the paretic arm and having the blindfolded patient demonstrate the position of the left limb by raising his or her right upper extremity to the same position as the left limb. Results of this study revealed that there was no significant relationship between phantom movements and anosognosia.

Confabulation

When a person lies, he or she has a desire to mislead. By confabulation we mean a response that is not rooted in reality or a false idea that a person believes to be true. Patients with anosognosia for hemiplegia have a false idea that they are not weak, even though this idea is not rooted in reality. Feinberg, Roane, Kwan, Schindler, and Haber (1994) wanted to learn if patients with anosognosia have a propensity to confabulate and therefore tested subjects with anosognosia to learn if these patients, when compared to controls, had false ideas in other domains. These investigators tested patients' ability to identify stimuli presented in the contralesional (e.g., left) visual field. These investigators found that patients with anosognosia were significantly more likely to confabulate seeing objects in this contralateral visual field than those subjects without anosognosia.

Using the selective hemisphere anesthesia paradigm (the Wada test), we wanted to learn whether patients with anosognosia for hemiplegia would confabulate tactilely presented stimuli (Lu et al., 1997b). During hemispheric anesthesia, we presented one of three different tactile stimuli or no stimuli to the finger tips of the contralateral hand of our blindfolded patient's fingertips. After these patients were or were not stimulated, their blindfold was removed and they were presented with a response card that had the three different textured materials as well as a question mark to indicate if they were uncertain whether they had been touched or what texture they had touched. Pointing to a texture when they were not touched was considered a confabulatory response. If they pointed to a blank or question mark when touched with the textured material, it was considered a failure to perceive. If they pointed to the wrong texture when touched, it was considered a perceptual error. We had patients who did confabulate their responses but did not have anosognosia. We also had patients with anosognosia who did not confabulate their responses and patients who both confabulated and had anosognosia. Overall, we found no significant relationship between anosognosia and confabulation in the tactile domain, but we did not test the visual domain.

Disconnection

If in some patients anosognosia is a form of confabulation, what could be the underlying mechanism? It has repeatedly been demonstrated that when patients with a complete callosal disconnection, who are left hemisphere dominant for speech-language, are presented stimuli on their left side and asked about the nature of these stimuli, they often confabulate a response. In his classic paper "Disconnexion syndromes," Geschwind (1965) suggested that confabulation may be related to hemispheric disconnection and that anosognosia may be related to hemispheric disconnection. Geschwind noted callosal connections start in the cortex in one hemisphere and connect to the cortex in the other hemisphere. Thus, large lesions of the right hemisphere may not only destroy cortical networks and intrahemispheric connections in that hemisphere, but these lesions may also induce an interhemispheric disconnection. With callosal disconnection, information collected by the right hemisphere cannot be transmitted to the left hemisphere and with the absence of information the undamaged left hemisphere fabricates responses to functions mediated and monitored by the injured right hemisphere. Geschwind's disconnection hypothesis can explain why patients with anosognosia confabulate that their arm is not weak. This hypothesis might also explain why anosognosia is more frequently associated with right than left hemisphere lesions.

As mentioned above, to test the feedback hypothesis during right hemisphere anesthesia, we moved patients' left paretic hand into their right visual field, such that the left hemisphere could now see the left arm. In this condition, if there was an interhemispheric disconnection, the left hemisphere would be able to directly view the left hemiplegic extremity. Of 15 patients who had anosognosia for their left hemiplegia, this maneuver allowed only five subjects to recognize their weakness (Adair et al., 1997). That these five subjects discovered weakness when their left hand was brought into their right body space and visual field might have been related to bypassing the hemispheric disconnection. Nonetheless, as discussed, this maneuver could have also bypassed a feedback deficit induced by deafferentation or inattention-neglect. Future research will have to be designed to learn which of these possible mechanisms was responsible for these patients' anosognosia and improvement with visual input into the left hemisphere.

Intentional Feed-Forward Hypothesis

Weakness and Akinesia

Imagine if I were to make the following request: "Let your left arm hang down by your side and do not attempt to move this arm." I then ask, "Is your arm weak?" Unknown to you, I injured the nerves going into your arm by a beam of radiation, which you could not feel. If you did not attempt to move this arm, you would probably respond, "No, it's not weak." In order for a person to learn that he or she has a disability, the person must test himself or herself. Thus, if a person does not attempt to move, he or she might not discover that a weakness is present.

Akinesia is defined as the failure to initiate a movement in the absence of a motor disability that can account for this failure to move. This has also been called motor neglect. In these patients with akinesia, the failure to move is not being caused by dysfunction of the motor cortex (Brodmann's area 4), the corticospinal system, or the motor units. The failure to move in these patients is being induced by dysfunction in the systems that are important for activating the corticospinal system. Studies of patients with akinesia suggest that it can be caused by injury to several regions, including the medial thalamus, the striatum, the premotor areas in the frontal lobes, and the dopaminergic neurotransmitter system. Patients with large lesions of their hemisphere might injure both the corticospinal system and a portion or portions of the network important in activating the corticospinal system. Thus, while difficult to clinically diagnose, an akinesia can coexist with a hemiplegia.

There are some patients with a form of akinesia who will not move sponta-neously (e.g., initiate goal-oriented behaviors) but will move in response to imperative external stimuli (akinesia paradoxica). In one of the experiments described above, there were some patients who with right hemisphere anesthesia were anosognosic for their hemiplegia but who, when their hand was brought into the right body space and the right visual field, discovered their paresis after they were asked to move their left hand and found that it would not move. These observations suggest that these patients did not spontaneously attempt to move their hand and only when asked did they attempt to move it. Not being able to move their hand as requested by the examiner together with intact right-sided feedback allowed them to learn that they were weak. These observations led to the feed-forward hypothesis as one of the causes of anosognosia for hemiplegia (Heilman, 1991, Heilman, Barrett, & Adair, 1998).

As mentioned, the feed-forward theory of anosognosia posits that in order to detect motor deficits a person needs to have expectations and when performance does not match expectations the person becomes aware that something is wrong. In addition to networks that mediate goal-oriented behaviors (the frontal executive systems) that activate the premotor (the premotor-basal ganglia network) and then the motor networks, this feed-forward hypothesis suggests that somewhere in the brain there is a "comparator." The plan for movements, mediated by the frontal-executive and the premotor basal ganglia systems, must set this comparator such that when expectations do not match feedback the person is alerted that there is a performance failure.

We tested this feed-forward model with a patient who was unaware of his left-sided weakness, as well as hemiplegic controls that were without anosognosia. We measured the activation of proximal muscles, using an electromyogram (EMG) in the anosognosic and control subjects during the time they were asked to squeeze a dynamometer with their right and left hands (Gold, Adair, Jacobs, & Heilman, 1994). We found that when the patient with anosognosia squeezed the dynamometer with his normal ipsilesional hand, the pectoralis on both the left and right side of his body contracted. However, when this patient was asked to squeeze the dynamometer with the contralateral paretic hand, he barely contracted either pectoralis muscles. Control patients with hemiplegia who did not have anosognosia, and even a patient with spatial neglect, when attempting to squeeze the dynamometer with their left paretic hand, contracted both their right and left pectoralis muscles. These results suggest that in this patient with anosognosia, his hemiplegia was associated with a loss of motor intention and, according to the feed-forward model, in the absence of motor intention he had no expectancy to move, and without expectancy there is no mismatch and no recognition that there was a failure.

In the beginning of this chapter we discussed the evidence that injury to the right hemisphere is more likely to induce anosognosia than injury to the left hemisphere. Our study using the Wada procedure (Glimore et al., 1992) has more recently been supported by a lesion meta-analysis performed by Pia, Neppi-Modona, Ricci, and Berti (2004). When discussing the feedback hypothesis, we did note that some subjects who were unaware that their left arm was weak when it was in left space learned that it was weak when it was in right space and the right visual field, suggesting that neglect of body or space might be an important factor in some, but not all patients with anosognosia, and it has been well established that neglect is much more common with right than left hemisphere damage (Heilman et al., 2003). Although left-right asymmetries of neglect might in part account for the hemispheric asymmetries of anosognosia, the feedback or motor intention hypothesis of anosognosia may also help to account for this hemispheric asymmetry.

Coslett and Heilman (1989) examined patients with right and left hemisphere strokes for the presence of a limb akinesia (motor neglect) and found that limb akinesia was more commonly associated with right than left hemisphere lesions. Warning stimuli can reduce the time it takes to initiate a motor response (reaction time). Warning stimuli produce this effect because they activate the premotor and motor systems. To learn whether there are hemispheric asymmetries in the ability of each hemisphere to activate the motor system of the opposite hemisphere, Heilman and Van Den Abell (1979) performed a warning stimulus-reaction time task with normal subjects. Warning stimuli that preceded imperative stimuli were delivered to either the left visual field (right hemisphere) or to the right visual field (left hemisphere). We found that warning stimuli directed to the right hemisphere reduced reaction times for both hands, but warning stimuli directed to the left hemisphere primarily reduced the reaction time of the right hand.

These results suggest that the right hemisphere's premotor intentional systems can help activate motor systems for both the right and left hands. In contrast, the left hemisphere's intentional motor systems, for the most part, can only activate the left hemisphere's motor system. Thus, with left hemisphere injury the right hemisphere can usually compensate for the left but with right hemisphere injury, the left hemisphere cannot compensate for the right and this asymmetry results in a higher frequency of motor intentional deficits with damage of the right than of the left hemisphere. In addition, Berti et al. (2005) found that anosognosia /denial was primarily associated with injury to the frontal premotor cortex known to be important in motor intention and activation. Patients with anosognosia, however, also frequently have parietal damage. Lau, Rogers, Haggard, and Passingham (2004), using fMRI, studied the parts of the brain that activated when the subject intended actions. In addition to activation of the preSMA, these investigators found the region of the intraparietal sulcus also activated and this region of the cortex is frequently damaged in patients with anosognosia for hemiplegia.

The location of the hypothetical comparator is not known. Initially Heilman (1991) suggested that the network that represents the body schema might be the comparator. Asomatognosia, which is thought to be induced by alterations of the body schema, might also be associated with comparator deficits. Berti, Spanazzola, Pia, and Rabbuffeti (2007), however, studied one patient with anosognosia using a technique similar to that used by Gold et al. (1994). Unlike Gold et al. (1994), who found that their patient with anosognosia was not attempting to move, Berti et al. (2007) found that their patient did have EMG-muscle activation in proximal muscles when attempting to use the paretic left arm. Thus, Berti et al. (2007) posited that this patient's deficit was not in the feed-forward component of discovery, but rather thought there was damage to the comparator. However, it was not clear that the patient reported by these investigators was fully investigated for a failure of feedback, by having the patient identify and observe her arm in her right visual field and right side of the body. This procedure would have enabled Berti et al. (2007) to learn whether this patient had asomatognosia, personal neglect, or spatial neglect.

Hyperkinetic Movement Disorders

Many patients with hyperkinetic movement disorders such as choreiform movements and hemiballismus are unaware that they are making these abnormal movements. For example, patents with Huntington's disease are often unaware of their chorea (Snowden, Craufurd, Griffiths, & Neary, 1998) and many patients with Parkinson's disease, who when treated with dopaminergic agents develop chorea, are unaware or unconcerned about their abnormal movements. These are other forms of motor anosognosia.

We reported one patient with chorea of unknown etiology who was unaware of his chorea when it was actually occurring (online), but he could easily recognize this chorea when he viewed a video-recording of himself (Shenker, Wylie, Fuchs, Manning, & Heilman, 2004). Investigation of this man revealed that intellectual impairment, loss of position or vision sense, spatial and personal neglect, disconnection, or asomatognosia could not account for his failure of online recognition.

Although the feed-forward hypothesis discussed above was developed to help account for the anosognosia associated with hemiplegia, it is possible that the feed-forward hypothesis might also help explain anosognosia for hyperkinetic movement disorders such as chorea. Unlike other movement disorders, such as tremor, the neural system that programs choreiform movements might be performed by the same basal-ganglia, premotor networks that are responsible for making voluntary movements. These networks might program the comparator to expect these movements and because the comparator, on line, does not detect a mismatch between expectations and performance, the patient remains unaware of his abnormal movements. When watching a videotape of himself, our patient did not expect abnormal movements and when seeing these unexpected movements he became aware of his disability.

Conclusions about Anosognosia

Based on the research studies reported above, we have not identified a single mechanism that can entirely account for anosognosia for hemiplegia in all patients. There is little question that for psychological defense, people do deny their symptoms and disabilities. There are, however, many observations for which this hypothesis cannot account, including why patients will deny one disability but not another and why anosognosia of hemiplegia is more frequently associated with right than left hemisphere dysfunction. Discovery is dependent on feedback and we noted that there are some patients with anosognosia who recognize their hemiparesis when feedback is improved by moving the paretic hand into right body and visual hemispace. Some patients with asomatognosia do not recognize that their left arm belongs to them and if they see that the arm does not move they will not recognize that they have a deficit. Thus, asomatognosia may be another factor in anosognosia. Some patients have phantom movements and some may confabulate because they have a hemispheric disconnection, but these mechanisms do not appear to be prominent causes of anosognosia. A person must have a plan to move and attempt to initiate movements. If a person does not attempt to move, he or she will have no expectations of movement and when he or she fails to move there will be no discord that leads to discovery. Because there are patients who do attempt to move, but are anosognosic for their failure to move, the feed-forward hypothesis cannot be the entire explanation of anosognosia for all patients. Although Berti et al. (2007) posit a defect in the comparator where expectations are compared to feedback, further evidence is needed to support this postulate. Overall, based on the studies of anosognosia for hemiplegia we have reviewed in this section we would suggest that normal self-awareness depends on several modular systems. A summary of the possible lesions that might induce anosognosia are represented in the cartoon figure at the end of this chapter (see Figure 5.1).

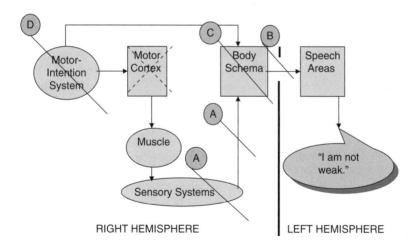

A = sensory feedback and/or neglect anosognosia; B = verbal disconnection anosognosia; C = asomatognosia agnosia; D = action-intentional (feed-forward) anosognosia.

Figure 5.1 Anosognosia for hemiplegia: Cartoon model of the injuries that might induce anosognosia. *(A)* Sensory feedback and/or neglect anosognosia. *(B)* Verbal disconnection anosognosia. *(C)* Asomatognosia agnosia. *(D)* Action-intentional (feed-forward) anosognosia.

Anosodiaphoria

Babinski (1914) stated, "...I have seen some hemiplegics who without being ignorant of the existence of their paralysis, seem to attach no importance to it. Such a state might be called *anosodiaphoria*." Subsequently, Critchley (1953, 1957) noted that usually after right hemisphere strokes, patients have only transient anosognosia and after several days to weeks develop anosodiaphoria. However, neither Babinski nor Critchley discusses the possible mechanisms of this lack of concern. Thus, in this section we will briefly discuss several possible mechanisms of this disorder, which unlike anosognosia is often persistent and also frequently interferes with rehabilitation efforts.

Impaired Emotional Communication

One of the possible explanations for anosodiaphoria is that patients who have right hemisphere injury might have impaired emotional communication. Whereas the left hemisphere appears to be important in what Hughlings Jackson called propositional speech, starting with the reports by Heilman, Scholes, and Watson (1975), Tucker, Watson, and Heilman (1977), and Ross (1981), it has been repeatedly demonstrated that the right hemisphere is involved in expressing the prosody important in communicating emotions. In addition, patients with right hemisphere strokes might also have problems understanding (Bowers, Bauer, Coslett, & Heilman, 1985; DeKosky, Heilman, Bowers, & Valenstein, 1980) and expressing emotions using facial expressions (Blonder, Burns, Bowers, Moore, & Heilman, 1993; Buck & Duffy, 1980).

At a different level, it has been demonstrated that, perhaps due to mirror neurons, people's emotional states are often "contagious" (McIntosh, Reichmann-Decker, Winkielman, & Wilbarger, 2006), and our perception of a particular situation depends on how others behave in this situation. Thus, it is possible that patients with multimodal defective comprehension of emotions induced by the right hemisphere stroke, although at least partially aware of their illness, may feel less concerned about their condition due to misinterpretation or inability to correctly read emotions of others, particularly those of negative valence.

Partial support for the postulate that anosodiaphoria may be related to impaired emotional communication comes from studies by Starkstein, Federoff, Price, Leiguarda, and Robinson (1992, 1994; see also Robinson, 1998). These investigators compared patients with brain injury who subsequently developed anosognosia with those without anosognosia on their ability to recognize facial affect as well as emotional prosody. They found that patients with anosognosia made significantly more errors when identifying facial expressions as well as emotional intonations. Thus, these results suggest that anosodiaphoria might be associated with the inability to recognize the emotions in other people. Future studies are needed, however, to better understand the relationship between impaired emotional processing and anosodiaphoria.

Reduced Emotional Experience

A critical element in emotional experience is arousal. Multiple studies have revealed that patients with right hemisphere injury often have reduced arousal (Heilman, Schwartz, & Watson, 1978), and this reduction of arousal can even involve the uninjured left hemisphere (Morrow, Vrtunski, Kim, & Boller, 1981; Perani, Vallar, Paulesu, Alberoni, & Fazio, 1993). In addition, many (Gainotti, 1972; Robinson & Szetela, 1981), but not all (House, Dennis, Warlow, Hawton, & Molyneux, 1990), studies suggest that with left hemisphere lesions, especially in the frontal region, there is what has been termed the "catastrophic reaction" by Goldstein (1948). In contrast, with right hemisphere strokes patients are often described as euphoric or emotionally flat. This hemispheric asymmetry might be related to knowing that one is impaired from a stroke versus not knowing. Nonetheless, in a series of studies with normal subjects, using measures such as EEG, Davidson, Schwartz, Saron, Bennett, and Goldman (1979; see also Davidson, Ekman, Saron, Senulis, & Friesen, 1990) have suggested that whereas the left hemisphere normally mediates emotions with positive valence (e.g., happiness), the right normally mediates emotions with a negative valence (e.g., sadness). Thus, the anosodiaphoria observed with right hemisphere injury might be related to these changes in arousal and emotion.

Although to our knowledge there are no studies examining the relation between anosodiaphoria and reduced emotional experience, it is well documented that patients with anosognosia due to the right hemisphere damage, particularly to frontal regions, often do not show negative emotions (see Turnbull, Evans, & Owen, 2005). These patients are frequently unreasonably optimistic about the condition of their health and often over-emphasize their abilities (Ramachandran & Blakslee, 1998). Thus, together with the clinical observations mentioned above and the valence approach/withdrawal-related emotion hypothesis posited by Davidson et al. (1979, 1990), it could be suggested that anosodiaphoria would result from a disruption of negative (withdrawal-related) emotions.

Nevertheless, the association between impaired processing of negative emotion and anosodiaphoria seems to be vague and controversial. For example, some researchers have shown that right hemisphere damage may also lead to a negative emotion; for example, "misoplegia," which is the explicit dislike or obsessional hatred of the paretic limb (Critchley, 1974). In addition, the finding that depression has been found in anosognosic patients with right hemisphere lesions (see Robinson, 1998) is also discordant with the absence of negative emotion notion. For instance, Starkstein and co-workers (1992), using the Hamilton Depression Scale, found that depression was equally frequent among patients with and without anosognosia. Turnbull and co-workers (2005) also described a patient with a right convexity hemispheric lesion and anosognosia who reported being frequently overcome by powerful emotions, especially sadness. Thus, anosognosia, and anosodiaphoria cannot be fully explained by an inability to process negative emotions and the development of depression.

Alexithymia

The term *alexithymia* comes from three Greek *morphemes*, "a" = without, "lexi" = word, and "thymia" = mood or emotions. Thus, patients with alexithymia experience emotions but cannot find the words to express the emotions they are experiencing.

In an attempt to treat people with intractable seizures that spread between the cerebral hemispheres, surgeons have treated these patients by sectioning their corpus callosum, the structure that is primary responsible for interhemispheric communication. Hoppe and Bogen (1977) studied 12 patients who had a surgical section of their corpus callosum and noted that these patients had trouble finding words needed to express emotional feeling. As we discussed earlier, large right hemisphere lesions not only destroy cerebral cortex and interrupt intrahemispheric communications but also impair interhemispheric communications. When a subject with an interhemispheric disconnection sees something in his or her left visual field or feels something with her or his left hand, he might not be able to name this object because the percept or concept formed in the right hemisphere cannot access the left hemisphere that performs the verbal labeling (naming). Thus, it is possible that what appears to be a lack of concern is a form of alexithymia.

Partial support for this hypothesis comes from a recent study by Spalletta et al. (2007), who investigated the relationship between anosognosia, alexithymia, neglect, and cognition. They examined 50 right hemisphere stroke inpatients that were within the first 3 months from the acute event. Anosognosia was measured with the Bisiach scale and alexithymia with the TAS-20 scale. A multivariate logistic regression model revealed that the more difficulty the participants had in describing feelings was a significant predictor of anosognosia. However, what still remains unclear is what type of emotional information is not being communicated.

Self-Discovery

A fourth possible mechanism that might account for the presence of anosodiaphoria after anosognosia abates has to do with the means of learning or "knowing." Since the work of Sigmund Freud, it has been repeatedly demonstrated that being told about yourself leads to a more superficial form of self-knowledge than does self-discovery.

After a right hemisphere stroke, patients with anosognosia are repeatedly told that they are weak and, eventually, their left hemisphere learns to say "yes" when someone asks them if they are weak. Nevertheless, this "being told knowledge" is superficial and might be the reason patients who have recovered from anosognosia often demonstrate anosodiaphoria. From a methodological point of view, however, this hypothesis is very difficult to test and, to our knowledge, no studies have attempted to approach it.

Behavioral Abnormalities, Dysexecutive Syndrome, and the Frontal Lobes

As described above, anosodiaphoria, similarly to anosognosia, has been particularly linked to the right hemisphere damage. Nevertheless, there is evidence to suggest that anosodiaphoria might be specifically associated with defective functioning of the frontal (cortical and subcortical) regions of the right hemisphere. The support for this idea comes, for example, from the studies of behavioral variant of frontotemporal dementia (bvFTD), a neurodegenerative disease with atrophy predominantly in orbitofrontal regions that is characterized by disinhibition, inappropriateness, impulsivity, irresponsibility, indifference, and apathy, as well as loss of insight (Kertesz, Davidson, & Fox, 1997). Mendez and Shapira (2005) have suggested that the loss of insight, as well as apathy in FTD may result from the right frontal pathology and that a loss of concern for their condition or their behavioral changes represents anosodiaphoria rather than a true anosognosia. The results of a recent study by Salmon and co-workers (2008) also imply that both FTD and AD patients might be anosodiaphoric rather than anosognosic, at least at the beginning of their disease. These authors have shown that, although caregivers generally tend to assess symptoms more severely than do patients, patient with FTD and AD often do report changes in most clinical domains. Nevertheless, loss of awareness seems to be significantly greater in subjects with FTD. This supports previous research findings suggesting that the impaired awareness of the disease manifests faster and is more pronounced in FTD than in AD (see Gustafson, 1993).

Although anosodiaphoria has not been extensively investigated in AD and FTD, many studies have provided evidence for the association between anosognosia and executive deficits—abilities relying mainly on frontal lobes, basal ganglia, and their reciprocal connections. For example, Mangone and co-workers (1991) demonstrated a relationship between the performance on the Continuous Performance Test as well as a sequencing and word generation test and anosognosia. Also, Lopez, Becker, Somsak, Dew, and DeKosky (1994) found that Choice Reaction Time and Trail Making Test were the best predictors of anosognosia in patients with AD. Thus, anosognosia or even more likely anosodiaphoria may be a result of executive dysfunction like impaired self-monitoring or problems with conflict resolution. For example, patients with lesions to the frontal lobes may know they are ill but at the same time they are unable to apply this knowledge to their behavior.

There is a frequent overlap between behavioral changes and results of tests of executive function (Kertesz, Davidson, McCabe, & Munoz, 2003), as well as the presence of anosognosia/anosodiaphoria. Future research should attempt to better understand the mechanism that underlies the relationship between behavioral changes, executive deficits, and anosognosia/anosodiaphoria.

The hypothesis that lesions of the right frontal lobe can lead to anosodiaphoria are consistent with some of the other explanations of this phenomenon that have been described above. First, although right hemisphere injury is associated with impaired emotional communication and, as suggested, this impairment may at least in part account for anosodiaphoria, it has been shown that these deficits are often induced by lesions of the anterior regions of the right hemisphere (Adolphs, Tranel, Damasio, & Damasio, 1994; Cancelliere & Kertesz, 1990; Harciarek & Heilman, 2008; Jacobs, Shuren, Bowers, & Heilman, 1995). Second, the hemispheric asymmetries in mediating emotional valence (left-positive vs. right-negative) proposed by Davidson and co-workers (1979, 1990) also refer to the frontal lobes. Finally, Spalletta and colleagues (2007) have shown that patients with anosognosia with alexithymia have particular difficulties with frontal lobe functions. Thus, although there are several possible mechanisms that may account for anosodiaphoria, the systems that are impaired might share the same anatomic substrate, the right frontal lobe.

Conclusions about Anosodiaphoria

The possible explanations of anosodiaphoria discussed here are not mutually exclusive, and anosodiaphoria could be in part influenced by one or more of these mechanisms. Future research will have to test these mechanisms to discern their relative importance. Alternatively, these mechanisms may not fully account for anosodiaphoria and investigators might need to develop and test new a priori hypotheses.

References

Adair, J. C., Gilmore, R. L., Fennell, E. B., Gold, M., & Heilman, K. M. (1995a). Anosognosia during intraoperative barbiturate anesthesia: Unawareness or amnesia for weakness. *Neurology, 45*, 241–243.

Adair, J. C., Na, D. L., Schwartz, R. L., Fennell, E. M., Gilmore, R. L., & Heilman, K. M. (1995b). Anosognosia for hemiplegia: Test of the personal neglect hypothesis. *Neurology, 45*, 2195–2199.

Adair, J. C., Schwartz R. L., Na, D. L., Fennell, E. M., Gilmore, R. L., & Heilman, K. M. (1997). Anosognosia: Examining the disconnection hypothesis. *Journal of Neurology, Neurosurgery, and Psychiatry, 63*, 798–800.

Adolphs, R., Tranel, D., Damasio, H., & Damasio, A. (1994). Impaired recognition of emotion in facial expressions following bilateral damage to the human amygdala. *Nature, 372*, 669–672.

Anton, G. (1896). Blindheit nach beiderseitiger Gehirnerkrankung mit Verlust der Orienterung in Raume. *Mitt. Ver. Arzte Steirmark, 33*, 41–46.

Babinski, J. (1914). Contribution à l'etude des troubles mentaux dans l'hémiplégie organique cérébrale (anosognosie). *Revue Neurologique, 27*, 845–847.

Babinski, J. (1918). Anosognosie, *Revue Neurologique, 31*, 365–367.

Barre, J., Morin, L., Kaiser (1923) Etude clinique d'un noveau cas d'Anosognosie de Babinski, *Revue Neurologique, 39*, 500–504.

Barrett, A. M., Eslinger, P. J., Ballentine, N. H., & Heilman, K. M. (2005). Unawareness of cognitive deficit (cognitive anosognosia) in probable AD and control subjects. *Neurology, 64*, 693–699.

Berti, A., Bottini, G., Gandola, M., Pia, L., Smania, N., Stracciari, A., Castiglioni, I., Vallar, G., & Paulesu, E. (2005). Shared cortical anatomy for motor awareness and motor control. *Science, 309*, 488–491.

Berti, A., Spanazzola, L., Pia, L., & Rabbuffeti, M. (2007). Motor awareness and motor intentions in anosognosia for hemiplegia. In P. Haggard, Y. Rossetti, & M. Kawato (Eds.), *Sensorimotor foundations of higher cognition series: Attention and performance XXII* (pp. 163–182). New York: Oxford University Press.

Bisiach, E., Vallar, G., Perani, D., Papagno, C., & Berti, A. (1986). Unawareness of disease following lesions of the right hemisphere: Anosognosia for hemiplegia and anosognosia for hemianopia. *Neuropsychologia, 24*, 471–482.

Blonder, L. X., Burns, A. F., Bowers, D., Moore, R. W., & Heilman, K. M. (1993). Right hemisphere facial expressivity during natural conversation. *Brain and Cognition, 21*, 44–56.

Bowers, D., Bauer, R. M., Coslett, H. B., & Heilman, K. M. (1985). Processing of faces by patients with unilateral, hemispheric lesions. I. Dissociation between judgements of facial affect and facial identity. *Brain and Cognition, 4*, 258–272.

Breier, J. I., Adair, J. C., Gold, M., Fennell, E. B., Gilmore, R. L., & Heilman, K. M. (1995). Dissociation of anosognosia for hemiplegia and aphasia during left-hemisphere anesthesia. *Neurology, 45*, 65–67.

Buck, R. & Duffy, R. J. (1980). Nonverbal communication of affect in brain-damaged patients. *Cortex, 16*, 351–362.

Cancelliere, A. E., & Kertesz, A. (1990). Lesion localization in acquired deficits of emotional expression and comprehension. *Brain and Cognition, 13*, 133–147.

Carpenter, K., Berti, A., Oxbury, S., Molyneux, A. J., Bisiach, E., & Oxbury, J. M. (1995). Awareness of and memory for arm weakness during intracarotid sodium amytal testing. *Brain, 118*, 243–251.

Celesia, G. G., Brigell, M. G., & Vaphiades, M. S. (1997). Hemianopic anosognosia. *Neurology, 49*, 88–97.

Coslett, H. B., & Heilman, K. M. (1989). Hemihypokinesia after right hemisphere strokes. *Brain and Cognition, 9*, 267–278.

Critchley, M. (1953). *The parietal lobes*. London: Hafner Press.

Critchley, M. (1957). Observations on anosodiaphoria. *Encephale, 46*, 540–546.

Critchley, M. (1974). Misoplegia, or hatred of hemiplegia. *Mount Sinai Journal of Medicine, 41*, 82–87.

Davidson, R. J., Ekman, P., Saron, C. D., Senulis, J. A., & Friesen, W. V. (1990). Approach-withdrawal and cerebral asymmetry: Emotional expression and brain physiology. I. *Journal of Personality and Social Psychology, 58*, 330–341.

Davidson, R. J., Schwartz, G. E., Saron, C., Bennett, J., & Goldman, D. J. (1979). Frontal versus parietal EEG asymmetry during positive and negative affect. *Psychophysiology, 16*, 202–203.

DeKosky, S., Heilman, K. M., Bowers, D., & Valenstein, E. (1980). Recognition and discrimination of emotional faces and pictures. *Brain and Language, 9*, 206–214.

Durkin, M. W., Meador, K. J., Nichols, M. E., Lee, G. P., & Loring, D. W. (1994). Anosognosia and the intracarotid amobarbital procedure (Wada test). *Neurology, 44*, 978–979.

Dywan, C. A., McGlone, J., & Fox, A. (1995). Do intracarotid barbiturate injections offer a way to investigate hemispheric models of anosognosia? *Journal of Clinical and Experimental Neuropsychology, 17*, 431–438.

Feinberg, T. E., Roane, D. M., Kwan, P. C., Schindler, R. J., & Haber, L. D. (1994). Anosognosia and visuoverbal confabulation. *Archives of Neurology, 51*, 468–473.

Gainotti, G. (1972). Emotional behavior and hemispheric side of the lesion. *Cortex, 8*, 41–55.

Gazzaniga, M. S. (2000). Cerebral specialization and interhemispheric communication: Does the corpus callosum enable the human condition? *Brain, 123*, 1293–1326.

Gazzaniga, M. S. (2005). Forty-five years of split-brain research and still going strong. *Nature Review of Neuroscience, 6*, 653–659.

Geschwind, N. (1965). Disconnexion syndromes in animals and man. *Brain, 88*, 237–294, 585–644.

Gilmore, R. L., Heilman, K. M., Schmidt, R. P., Fennell, E. M., & Quisling, R. (1992). Anosognosia during Wada testing. *Neurology, 42*, 925–927.

Gold, M., Adair, J. C., Jacobs, D. H., & Heilman, K. M. (1994). Anosognosia for hemiplegia: An electrophysiologic investigation of the feed-forward hypothesis. *Neurology, 44*, 1804–1808.

Goldstein, K. (1948). *Language and language disturbances*. New York: Grune and Stratton.

Gustafson, L. (1993). Clinical picture of frontal lobe degeneration of non-Alzheimer type. *Dementia, 4*, 143–148.

Harciarek, M., & Heilman, K. M. (2008). The contribution of anterior and posterior regions of the right hemisphere to the recognition of emotional faces. *Journal of Clinical Experimental Neuropsychology* (published online), June 9:1–9.

Hecaen, H., & Albert, M. (1978). *Human neuropsychology*. New York: Wiley.

Heilman, K. M. (1991). Anosognosia: Possible neuropsychological mechanisms. In G. P. Prigatano & D. L. Schacter (Eds.), *Awareness of deficit after brain injury: Clinical and theoretical issues* (pp. 53–62). New York: Oxford University Press.

Heilman, K. M., Barrett, A. M., & Adair, J. C. (1998). Possible mechanisms of anosognosia: A defect in self-awareness. *Philosophical Transactions of the Royal Society of London Biological Sciences, 353*, 1903–1909.

Heilman, K. M., Scholes, R., & Watson, R. T. (1975). Auditory affective agnosia. Disturbed comprehension of affective speech. *Journal of Neurology, Neurosurgery, and Psychiatry, 38*, 69–72.

Heilman, K. M., Schwartz, H. D., Watson, R. T. (1978). Hypoarousal in patients with the neglect syndrome and emotional indifference. *Neurology, 28*, 229–232.

Heilman, K. M., & Van Den Abell, T. (1979). Right hemispheric dominance for mediating cerebral activation. *Neuropsychologia, 17*, 315–321.

Heilman, K. M., & Van Den Abell, T. (1980). Right hemispheric dominance for attention: The mechanisms underlying hemispheric asymmetries of inattention (neglect). *Neurology, 30*, 327–330.

Heilman, K. M., Watson, R. T., & Valenstein, E. (2003). Neglect and related disorders. In K. M. Heilman & E. Valenstein (Eds.), *Clinical neuropsychology* (pp. 296–346). New York: Oxford University Press.

Hoppe, K. D., & Bogen, J. E. (1977). Alexithymia in twelve commissurotomized patients. *Psychotherapy and Psychosomatics, 28*, 148–155.

House, A., Dennis, M., Warlow, C., Hawton, K., & Molyneux, A. (1990). Mood disorders after stroke and their relation to lesion location. A CT scan study. *Brain, 113*, 1113–1129.

Jacobs, D. H., Shuren, J., Bowers, D., & Heilman, K. M. (1995). Emotional facial imagery, perception, and expression in Parkinson's disease. *Neurology, 45*, 1696–1702.

Kertesz, A., Davidson, W., & Fox, H. (1997). Frontal behavioral inventory: Diagnostic criteria for frontal lobe dementia. *Canadian Journal of Neurological Sciences, 24*, 29–36.

Kertesz, A., Davidson, W., McCabe, P., & Munoz, D. (2003). Behavioral quantitation is more sensitive than cognitive testing in frontotemporal dementia. *Alzheimer Disease and Associated Disorders, 17*, 223–229.

Lau, H. C., Rogers, R. D., Haggard, P., & Passingham, R. E. (2004). Attention to intention. *Science, 303*, 1208–1210.

Levine, D. N., Calvanio, R., & Rinn, W. E. (1991). The pathogenesis of anosognosia for hemiplegia. *Neurology, 41*, 1770–1781.

Lopez, O. L., Becker, J. T., Somsak, D., Dew, M. A., & DeKosky, S. R. (1994). Awareness of cognitive deficits and anosognosia in probable Alzheimer's disease. *European Neurology, 34*, 277–282.

Lu, L., Barrett, A. M., Cibula, J., Gilmore, R. L., & Heilman, K. M. (1997a). Phantom movement during the Wada test. *Epilepsia, 38*(Suppl. 8), 156.

Lu, L., Barrett, A. M., Cibula, J., Gilmore, R. L., & Heilman, K. M. (2000). Proprioception more impaired distally than proximally in subjects with hemispheric dysfunction. *Neurology, 55*, 596–597.

Lu, L., Barrett, A. M., Schwartz, R. L., Cibula, J., Gilmore, R. L., & Heilman, K. M. (1997b). Anosognosia and confabulation during the Wada test. *Neurology, 49*, 1316–1322.

Mangone, C. A., Hier, D. B., Gorelick, P. B., Ganellen, R. J., Langenberg, P., Boarman, R., & Dollear, W. C. (1991). Impaired insight in Alzheimer's disease. *Journal of Geriatric Psychiatry and Neurology, 4*, 189–193.

Marcel, A. J., Tegner, R., & Nimmo-Smith, I. (2004). Anosognosia for plegia: Specificity, extension, partiality and disunity of bodily unawareness. *Cortex, 40*, 19–40.

McIntosh, D. N., Reichmann-Decker, A., Winkielman, P., & Wilbarger, J. L. (2006). When the social mirror breaks: Deficits in automatic, but not voluntary mimicry of emotional facial expressions in autism. *Developmental Sciences, 9*, 295–302.

Mendez, M. F., & Shapira, J. S. (2005). Loss of insight and functional neuroimaging in frontotemporal dementia. *The Journal of Neuropsychiatry and Clinical Neurosciences, 17*, 413–416.

Mesulam, M. M., Waxman, S. G., Geschwind, N., & Sabin, T. D. (1976). Acute confusional states with right middle cerebral artery infarctions. *Journal of Neurology, Neurosurgery, & Psychiatry, 39*, 84–89.

Morrow, L., Vrtunski, P. B., Kim, Y., & Boller, F. (1981). Arousal responses to emotional stimuli and laterality of lesion. *Neuropsychologia, 19*, 65–71.

Nardone, I. B., Ward, R., Fotopoulou, A., & Turnbull, O. H. (2007). Attention and emotion in anosognosia: Evidence of implicit awareness and repression? *Neurocase, 13*, 438–445.

Perani, D., Vallar, G., Paulesu, E., Alberoni, M., & Fazio, F. (1993). Left and right hemisphere contribution to recovery from neglect after right hemisphere damage— An [18F]FDG pet study of two cases. *Neuropsychologia, 31*, 115–125.

Pia, L., Neppi-Modona, M., Ricci, R., & Berti, A. (2004). The anatomy of anosognosia for hemiplegia: A meta-analysis. *Cortex, 40*, 367–377.

Ramachandran, V. S., & Blakslee, S. (1998). *Phantoms in the brain: Human nature and the architecture of the mind.* London: Fourth Estate.

Robinson, R. G. (1998). *The clinical neuropsychology of stroke: Cognitive, behavioral and emotional disorders following vascular brain injury.* Cambridge, England: Cambridge University Press.

Robinson, R. G., & Szetela, B. (1981). Mood change following left hemispheric brain injury. *Annals of Neurology, 9*, 447–453.

Ross, E. D. (1981). The aprosodias: Functional-anatomic organization of the affective components of language in the right hemisphere. *Annals of Neurology, 38*, 561–589.

Salmon, E., Perani, D., Collette, F., Feyers, D., Kalbe, E., Holthoff, V., Sorbi, S., & Herholz, K. (2008). A comparison of unawareness in frontotemporal dementia and Alzheimer's disease. *Journal of Neurology, Neurosurgery, & Psychiatry, 79*, 176–179.

Shenker, J. I., Wylie, S. A., Fuchs, K., Manning, C. A., & Heilman, K. M. (2004). On-line anosognosia: Unawareness for chorea in real time but not on videotape delay. *Neurology, 63*, 159–160.

Snowden, J., Craufurd, D., Griffiths, H., & Neary, D. (1998). Awareness of involuntary movements in Huntington disease. *Archives of Neurology, 55*, 801–805.

Spalletta, G., Serra, L., Fadda, L., Ripa, A., Bria, P., & Caltagirone, C. (2007). Unawareness of motor impairment and emotions in right hemispheric stroke: A preliminary investigation. *International Journal of Geriatric Psychiatry, 22*, 1241–1246.

Starkstein, S. E., Fedoroff, J. P., Price, T. R., Leiguarda, R., & Robinson, R. G. (1992). Anosognosia in patients with cerebrovascular lesions. A study of causative factors. *Stroke, 23*, 1446–1453.

Starkstein, S. E., Fedoroff, J. P., Price, T. R., Leiguarda, R., & Robinson R. G. (1994). Neuropsychological and neuroradiologic correlates of emotional prosody comprehension. *Neurology, 44*, 515–522.

Tucker, D. M., Watson, R. T., & Heilman, K. M. (1977). Affective discrimination and evocation in patients with right parietal disease. *Neurology, 17*, 947–950.

Turnbull, O. H., Evans, C. E., & Owen, V. (2005). Negative emotions and anosognosia. *Cortex, 41*, 67–75.

Von Monakow, C. (1885). Experimentelle und pathologisch-anatomische Untersuchungen über die Beziehungen der sogenannten Sehphäre zu den infrakorticalen Opticuscentren und zum N. opticus. *Archiv fur Psychiatrie und Nervenkrankheiten, 16*, 151–199.

Weinstein, E. A., & Kahn, R. L. (1953). Personality factors in denial of illness. *American Medical Association Archives of Neurology and Psychiatry, 69*, 355–367.

Weinstein, E. A., & Kahn, R. L. (1955). *Denial of illness. Symbolic and physiological aspects.* Springfield, IL: Charles C. Thomas.

6

Anosognosia in Aphasia

Andrew Kertesz

Anosognosia is literally the lack of recognition of illness observed in a wide variety of neurological conditions. Babinski (1914) first introduced the term to common use in neurology, referring to the nonrecognition or denial of hemiplegia. The term has been extended to other areas, such as denial of amnesia or heart disease (Gerstmann, 1942; Weinstein & Kahn, 1950). Prior to Babinski, this phenomena was documented in aphasia (Wernicke, 1874) and in blindness, such as Anton's syndrome (1898). Anosognosia takes different forms at varying degrees of severity, and it is defined in diverse ways. Some authors include sensory or attentional neglect, while other authors will count only explicit denial of illness or deficit. A patient may deny that anything is wrong or may assign the disability to some trivial cause. Some awareness is often indicated in humor, metaphors, nonaphasic misnaming, confabulations, and delusions about the illness or diseased part, even if there is implicit or explicit denial (Weinstein & Kahn, 1955).

The Mechanisms and Processes in Anosognosia in Aphasia

Anosognosia in aphasia has often been described in association with or intrinsic to jargonaphasia (Alajouanine, 1956; Bay, 1964; Brain, 1961; Cohn & Neumann, 1958; Kinsbourne & Warrington, 1963; Weinstein, Cole, Mitchell, & Lyerly, 1964). Weinstein examined the topic in detail in several articles and chapters (Weinstein & Kahn, 1950, 1955; Weinstein et al., 1964, 1966). Weinstein and colleagues thought of anosognosia in mainly psychiatric terms such as denial as coping mechanism and also as a consequence of weakening of the critical faculties of the brain due to diffuse, general brain impairment. They also noted that improvement in awareness is often associated with depression and that somewhat paradoxically, the more severe the aphasia, the less anosognosia is seen. On the other hand, they confirmed that severe jargon aphasia is

frequently associated with anosognosia. They asserted that jargon and associated anosognosia is most often seen with bilateral lesions or large lesions
with disturbance of consciousness. However, Kertesz and Benson (1970) and
Gainotti (1972) have demonstrated that jargon and accompanying anosognosia
occurs with well-circumscribed lesions in the left hemisphere without diffuse
impairment or contralateral lesions. In our series, 9 out of 10 of the clinically and
structurally documented neologistic jargon patients had significant unawareness
as observed from their behavior and in reply to standard interview questions of
the Boston and the Western Aphasia Battery (WAB): "Why are you here? What
seems to be the trouble?" (Kertesz & Benson, 1970).

Weinstein et al. (1964) emphasized the impairment of social interaction in the
communication of jargon aphasics. He felt that jargon could not be explained on
the basis of impaired phonetic, syntactic, and verbal organization of language.
Jargon, nonaphasic misnaming, and verbal stereotypy involve both language
breakdown and adaptation to the disability and are analogous to the metaphoric
and confabulatory adaptation to hemiplegia with nondominant, nonaphasic
lesions (Weinstein et al., 1964). Neologistic jargon aphasic patients are less
likely to have enough intelligible output to detect metaphor or referential allu-
sions, but patients with semantic jargon often circumlocute and have referential
language. Patients with jargon are often described as euphoric and characteristically unconcerned about their speech defects. Logorrhea with a stream of
unchecked nonsense often under pressure and the lack of self-correction indirectly indicates unawareness. Patients who are unaware of their aphasic errors
seem to expect their listeners to understand their jargon and may show anger if
they do not (Alajouanine, 1956; Weinstein et al., 1964). They often show ludic
(playful, childish, jocular; Piaget's term) behavior, sing, alliterate, and rhyme.
This kind of disinhibited behavior is also common in the behavioral variant
frontotemporal degeneration (bvFTD) without aphasia and semantic dementia
or semantic aphasia (Kertesz et al., in press). Semantic jargon patients may use
"officialese," stilted, ornate, and pedantic language, and often use lower frequency
words in common usage. More severe neologistic jargon is interpreted as a
combination of phonological paraphasia and anomia with semantic substitutions.
Excessive speech or logorrhoea, with normal prosody with the preservation of
grammatical connecting words and grammatical morphemes sounding like
normal English is a characteristic feature. We and others (Kinsbourne &
Warrington 1963, Kertesz, 1982) played back their jargon to several jargonaphasics, who seemed to become animated and gesture approvingly as if they just heard
meaningful communication, suggesting significant unawareness is part of this
animated logorrheic behavior. Others (Shuren, Hammond, Maher, Rothi, &
Heilman, 1995) have found during a similar experiment that jargonaphasics
were critical of their jargon only when it was played back to them in someone
else's voice, and another patient did the same with writing. Kinsbourne and
Warrington (1963) considered this implicit denial.

Anosognosia for the language deficit is commonly seen in Wernicke's aphasia without jargon and transcortical sensory aphasics, in addition to jargon aphasia with severe comprehension deficit. Wernicke (1874) hypothesized that impaired auditory input was responsible for the paraphasias and the lack of corrections. It appeared as if the patients did not hear themselves, and therefore could not correct their errors. Goldstein (1948) objected to this idea, because he thought external auditory input would come too late. Subsequently "inner speech" or physiological rather than physical auditory input was postulated. However, there are case reports of jargonaphasics with good comprehension and anosognosia (Maher, Rothi, & Heilman, 1994; Shuren et al., 1995). Unfortunately, the classification of some fluent aphasics as jargonaphasics is often arbitrary. Some patients with conduction aphasia and copious paraphasias may have relatively good comprehension.

Delayed auditory feedback, a condition thought to interfere with internal monitoring, produces phonological errors and decay in output in controls. Some studies showed the absence of this effect in patients with phonological jargon, suggesting faulty auditory monitoring (Alajouanine & Lhermitte 1957; Boller, Vrtunski, Kim, & Mack, 1978). The methodology measures speech errors, which are difficult to quantify in patients who have such errors already. This remains a controversial territory. There is also a case where severe comprehension impairment is reported with self-correction (Marshall, Rappaport, & Garcia-Bunuel, 1985), indicating that comprehension and auditory monitoring may not be the underlying mechanism for anosognosia. It is difficult to make much of this exception, but internal auditory monitoring without explicit comprehension may still be the explanation.

Lebrun (1987) conceptualized anosognosia in aphasia as possibly related to comprehension deficit or disturbed feedback, echoing the prevailing ideas, but citing many exceptions. He considered the stereotypies of "monophasics" (global aphasics in other, commonly used classifications) as indicative of unawareness. These patients often repeat a single word or phoneme cluster with the prosody, emphasis, and rhythm of conversational speech. Nevertheless, they also have severe comprehension deficit underlying their unawareness. In fact, global aphasics are not only unaware of their speech deficit, they are also usually amnestic for long periods until they recover comprehension (Kertesz & McCabe, 1977). Lebrun (1987) postulated that the limited attentional capacity of aphasics results in defective monitoring, although this is not far from the specific auditory monitoring deficit postulated by Wernicke and many others. Lebrun (1987) thought that aphasics are unable to carry out the task of monitoring at the same time as their linguistic operations.

Visual agnosia and optic aphasia are particularly noteworthy, because of the frequent confabulation and unawareness of the nonsensical responses by the patient, even though there is no auditory comprehension deficit (Kertesz 1979; Lhermitte & Boueavois, 1973). It is possible that a verbal visual disconnection would result in a compensatory run of unchecked visual imagery activating a disinhibited verbal system in the absence of the normal visual cascade of recognition. They rarely complain of visual problems and they rarely have insight or say they can not recognise objects or people.

Others thought that jargonaphasia's impaired lexical access or impaired lexical selection allowed the unimpaired, but uncontrolled phonemic selector to produce the profusion of paraphasias and associated unawareness. Later authors (Shuren et al., 1995) used the computer analogy of impaired "feedback and feed forward" for the phenomenon of paraphasic jargon and anosognosia. Patients with good comprehension such as in Broca's aphasia are typically painfully aware and bitterly frustrated by their deficit, but there are exceptions to both dictums. Some of these exceptions are related to variable definitions of aphasia types or not using standard aphasia test scores to classify patients. Although many aphasics have a degree of awareness of the language deficit many, even nonfluent aphasics, may not be aware of the specific linguistic deficits or errors (Rubens & Garrett, 1991). Furthermore, metacognitive analysis showed that some nonfluent aphasics may not be aware of all their errors. Lebrun's (1987) "monophasic" patients were closer to Global aphasia than Broca's aphasia, the difference being the deficit in comprehension.

Maher et al. (1994) and Shuren and colleagues (1995) published accounts of a man with undifferentiated jargonaphasia and preserved auditory comprehension, unaware of his speech production errors when he had to both speak and listen simultaneously. However, when listening to a recording of his speech, he could detect the speech errors he had made. They, like Lebrun (1987) attributed this patient's unawareness of his speech production errors to a reduced attentional capacity for simultaneous linguistic tasks. Some attempts have been made to quantify anosognosia, such as counting uncorrected speech errors versus corrections (Schlenk, Huber, & Willmes, 1987). Others actually asked the patients to rate their own responses as correct or not (Shuren et al., 1995).

The Relationship of Anosognosia in Aphasia and Hemiplegia

Anosognosia in aphasia often extends to the associated hemiplegia, although there are instances of dissociations. Of course, there are many aphasics who are not hemiplegic, the most common being anomic or Wernicke's aphasia without hemiplegia. There is a large literature discussing the proportion of left versus right hemiplegics with anosognosia and this varies with the definition of anosognosia. Most reports will show a larger proportion of anosognosia with left sided paralysis or nondominant hemisphere lesions, but aphasic and nonaphasic exceptions are probably more often published. The proportion of patients with anosognosia for right hemiplegia was actually smaller in hemiplegic aphasic patients than nonaphasic patients if jargonaphasia was excluded (Weinstein et al., 1964). Anosognosia and aphasia were inversely related outside of jargon aphasia.

The stroke literature indicates that the explicit denial of hemiplegia, a form of anosognosia, is associated more commonly with right- than left-hemisphere lesions (Weinstein et al., 1964). Some investigators have suggested that this asymmetry may be an artifact and that the aphasia that often accompanies left-hemisphere dysfunction may mask some instances of anosognosia (Lebrun, 1987; Weinstein et al., 1964). The issue of anosognosia being "global" or "modular" in nature has been revisited in recent studies. Mechanisms of global explanations include psychological denial and general mental deterioration; modular explanations include feedback and feed-forward theories. Videotapes of 54 patients with medically intractable seizures who had selective barbiturate anesthesia (Wada test) as part of their evaluation for seizure surgery were assessed for anosognosia of hemiplegia and aphasia after hemispheric anesthesia had worn off (Breier et al., 1995). The results suggest that, although aphasia may confound the reported rate of anosognosia for hemiplegia following left-hemisphere dysfunction, the frequency of this is still higher with transient left- than right-sided hemiplegia. Anosognosia for hemiplegia and aphasia were dissociable, providing support for the theory that awareness of the deficit is modular. This is supported by other case reports with more persistent lesions (Breier et al., 1995).

Neglect has been described with subcortical lesions, but Godefroy, Rousseaux, Pruvo, Cabaret, and Leys (1994) demonstrated that patients with pure lenticulostriate infarcts on MRI may exhibit aphasia of moderate severity, but hemineglect, gestural apraxia, and anosognosia were only seen in the subgroup with associated cortical lesions. Therapeutic effects on anosognosia in aphasia such as speech therapy (Lebrun, 1987) or vestibular stimulation have not been particularly successful, even though vestibular stimulation helps temporarily to diminish anosognosia for hemiplegia (Vallar, Papagno, Rusconi, & Bisiach, 1995).

Anosognosia in Frontotemporal Disease and Progressive Aphasia

Loss of insight is one of the core features of FTD (Neary et al., 1998). Impairments in self-awareness and self-monitoring occur in patients with frontotemporal degeneration (FTD), particularly among those with prominent social and executive impairments. Patients with FTD show significantly less behavioral self-awareness and self-knowledge than Alzheimer's disease (AD) and healthy control samples. Patients with FTD with prominent social and executive impairments demonstrate the most extensive loss of self-awareness and self-knowledge, significantly overrating themselves in multiple social, emotional, and cognitive domains, and failing to acknowledge that any behavioral change had occurred in most areas (Eslinger, Dennis, Moore et al., 2005).

Frontotemporal degeneration shares many clinical and pathological features with corticobasal degeneration (CBD) and progressive supranuclear palsy (PSP). O'Keefe and colleagues (2007) recruited 35 patients (14 FTD, 11 CBD, and 10 PSP) and 20 controls. Results indicated that loss of insight was a feature of each of the three patient groups. Patients with FTD were most impaired on monitoring of errors compared to the other two patient groups. Linear regression analysis demonstrated that different patterns of neuropsychological performance and behavioral rating scores predicted insight deficits across three awareness categories. Furthermore, higher levels of depression were associated with poor anticipatory awareness. Reduced empathy was related to impaired metacognitive awareness. Impaired recognition of emotional expression in faces was associated with both metacognitive and anticipatory awareness (ability to accurately predict performance on future tasks) deficits (O'Keefe et al., 2007).

We have recently studied insight and the behavior of four groups of patients with the Frontal Behavioral Inventory, a caregiver-based quantitative instrument. The Frontal Behavioral Inventory (FBI) was developed and standardized with the purpose of being able to differentiate behavioural variety of FTD (bv FTD) from other dementias, such as AD and vascular dementia (VAD) and to quantify the severity of bvFTD (Kertesz, Davidson, & Fox, 1997).

We analyzed lack of insight as a specific behavior as observed by the caregiver. The specific question for one of the items was loss of insight: Is s/he aware of any problems or changes in behavior, or language, or is s/he unaware of them or denies them when discussed? The instruction and the scoring included an explanation to the caregiver that s/he should look for a change from before the illness. The questions are asked in the absence of the patient, and at the end of each question, the caregiver is asked about the extent of the behavioral change and scores it according to the following: 0 = none, 1 = mild, occasional, 2 = moderate, and 3 = severe, most of the time. In addition to recording a yes-no response and a scoring of the severity, the caregiver should be encouraged to provide examples of the abnormal behavior. In this scale, 12 items assess deficit (negative) behaviors (i.e., apathy, aspontaneity, indifference, inflexibility, personal neglect, disorganization, inattention, loss of insight, logopenia, verbal apraxia, loss of comprehension, and alien hand), and 12 items assess disinhibition (positive) behaviors (i.e., perseverations/obsessions, irritability, excessive jocularity, social inappropriateness, impulsivity, restlessness, aggression, hyperorality, hypersexuality, utilization behavior, and incontinence). Some of the negative items are aimed at language and motor behaviors.

The four groups of participants were diagnosed as (1) the behavioral variety of Pick complex/Pick's disease (bvFTD), (2) primary progressive aphasia, including the anomic, logopenic, and nonfluent varieties (further fractionation between these varieties is possible, but they all had relatively preserved comprehension), *(3)* semantic (aphasia) dementia with fluent output, semantic paraphasias, and significant difficulty with semantic processing, particularly comprehension of nouns, and *(4)* AD. The groups were evenly matched for their dementia severity on their Mini Mental Status Examination (MMSE), but differences were found on the behavioral inventory and their language behavior.

The results of the insight measure showed that the bvFTD group had the least awareness of their behavioral and language deficit, and the next most affected group was Semantic Dementia (SD) with often oblivious semantic jargon or at least fluent, tangential, often irrelevant conversational speech. Patients with AD were less affected, but had more anosognosia than patients with Primary Progressive Aphasia (PPA) (also called Progressive Nonfluent Aphasia or PNFA), which resembles Broca or transcortical motor aphasia.

There are frequent observations of the unawareness of behavioral or language change, such as FTD and SD patients, who often argue with the caregiver; "There is nothing wrong with that," or "I am all right." One caregiver complained: "His childish stubbornness and single-mindedness seemed like a 'tunnel vision.'" Other caregivers in our support group ask: "How come he does not realize the consequences of his actions and what he says? He is not deaf or blind; he can hear himself and see how people react with disbelief and rejection, why can't he learn from his social mistakes and foul-ups?" This is often considered impulsivity or a lack of judgement. Recently, it has been emphasized that patients who act as if they have no insight into the consequence of their action lack a "theory of mind" regarding what "others would think" (Stone, Baron-Cohen, & Knight, 1998). Patients with frontal lobe damage do not appear to learn from mistakes and fail to benefit from punishment or rewards. They also tend to make erroneous and inappropriate decisions for immediate rather than long-term gain.

Impaired Pragmatics as a Form of Anosognosia

Semantic dementia patients and FTD patients often violate the rules of effective communication, as they are unable to maintain conversation, frequently go off on tangents, and interrupt others (Kertesz, Davidson, & Fox, 1997; Kertesz et al., 2009). Problems in communication include unawareness of the needs of the interlocutor. This is an impairment of an important component of language called "pragmatics," which is beyond syntax, phonology, and semantics, which are affected in aphasic disturbances. Pragmatics is a systematic study of the give and take of communication, relevance, topic maintenance, and contextual coherence through discourse analysis. Pragmatic rules of language are often violated early in FTD, even though other aspects of language are not yet affected. The following are quotes from caregivers about different FTD/Pick patients that illustrate disturbances in communication, revealing unawareness:

> ...Sometimes he just ignored questions and kept talking about something else...She only had a few topics she was interested in, and repeatedly returned to these regardless of what the other person wanted to talk about...He had stereotypic, circumstantial thinking, and inability to answer questions directly...She had difficulty staying on the topic discussed, if other questions were asked...He was fixated on certain topics...She interrupted people and interjected her comments...He made a lot of out context, irrelevant remarks...She did not seem to know when to stop and perseverated with the same topics, the same jokes...The content of her conversation is corny, nonsensical, or inappropriate...Sometimes he said things that were completely irrelevant to the questions asked...(Kertesz, 2006)

Anosognosia in Aphasic Alzheimer's Disease

Anosognosia for the extent of memory impairment and aphasia is frequent in AD, although initially they often acknowledge their forgetfulness or word finding difficulty. A common defensive rationalization is to attribute these to normal aging. In some patients the evolution of illness elicits an increasingly irrational defensiveness and resistance to help or interference with activities, such as driving, associated with the denial of illness or anosognosia. Some are frustrated by their word finding difficulties, while others compensate by circumlocutions and semantic substitutions, with variable awareness. Formal inquiry into their insight confirms decreasing awareness as the illness progresses. Later the aphasic impairment resembles conduction aphasia and at that stage there is still some awareness and frustration, but at a further stage with increasing comprehension deficit (resembling Wernicke's aphasia) there is total loss of awareness for the deficit (Appell, Kertesz, & Fisman, 1982).

Conclusion

Anosognosia in aphasia is a common and well-described phenomenon. It is clearly independent from anosognosia for hemiplegia, although they may be associated. The major association is with jargon aphasia and comprehension loss, and this supports the prevailing theory of the underlying mechanism of anosognosia of aphasia as impaired auditory feedback. Other theories such as the overloading of multiple processing and lack of self-monitoring are variations on the same theme. In this chapter, we discuss the incidence and variety of anosognosia in degenerative disease, particularly in the behavioral variety of FTD and semantic aphasia/dementia and AD.

References

Alajouanine, T. (1956). Verbal realization in aphasia. *Brain, 79*(1), 1–28.

Alajouanine, T., & Lhermitte, F. (1957). Elective anosognosia: Ignorance of certain functional dissolutions caused by focal cerebral lesions. *Encephale, 46*(5–6), 505–519.

Anton, G. (1898). Uber Herderkrankungen des Gehirns, welche vom Patienten selbst nicht wahrgenommen werden. *Wiener Klinische Wochenschrift, 11*, 227–229.

Appell, J., Kertesz, A., & Fisman, M. (1982). A study of language functioning in Alzheimer patients. *Brain and Language, 17*(1), 73–91.

Babinski, J. (1914). Contribution a l'etude des troubles mentaux dans l'hemiplegie organique cerebrale (anosognosis). *Revue Neurologique* (Paris), *27*, 845–848.

Bay, E. (1964). Present concepts of aphasia. *Geriatrics, 19*, 319–331.

Boller, F., Vrtunski, P. B., Kim, Y., & Mack, J. L. (1978). Delayed auditory feedback and aphasia. *Cortex, 14*, 212–226.

Brain, W. R. (1961). *Speech disorders*. Washington, DC: Butterworth, Inc.

Breier, J. I., Adair, J. C., Gold, M., Fennell, E. B., Gilmore, R. L., & Heilman, K. M. (1995). Dissociation of anosognosia for hemiplegia and aphasia during left-hemisphere anesthesia. *Neurology, 45*(1), 65–67.

Cohn, R., & Neumann, M. A. (1958). Jargon aphasia. *Journal of Nervous and Mental Disease, 127*(5), 381–399.

Eslinger, P. J., Dennis, K., Moore, P., Antani, S., Hauck, R., & Grossman, M. (2005). Metacognitive deficits in frontotemporal dementia. *Journal of Neurology, Neurosurgery, and Psychiatry, 76*(12), 1630–1635.

Gainotti, G. (1972). Emotional behavior and hemispheric side of the lesion. *Cortex, 8*(1), 41–55.

Gerstmann, J. (1942). Problem of imperception of disease and of impaired body territories with organic lesions. *Archives of Neurology and Psychiatry, 48*, 890–913.

Godefroy, O., Rousseaux, M., Pruvo, J.P., Cabaret, M., & Leys, D. (1994). Neuropsychological changes related to unilateral lenticulostriate infarcts. *Journal of Neurology, Neurosurgery, and Psychiatry, 57*(4), 480–485.

Goldstein, K. (1948). *Language and language disturbances*. New York: Grune and Stratton.

Kertesz, A. (1979). Visual agnosia: The dual deficit of perception and recognition. *Cortex, 15*(3), 403–419.

Kertesz, A. Two case studies: Broca's and Wernicke's Aphasia (1982) in Neural Models of Language Processes. Eds. Arbib, M A et al., New York, Academic Press pp, 25–44.

Kertesz, A. (2006). *The banana lady and other stories of curious behaviour and speech*. Victoria, Canada: Trafford Publishing.

Kertesz, A., & Benson, D. F. (1970). Neologistic jargon: A clinicopathological study. *Cortex, 6*(4), 362–386.

Kertesz, A., Davidson, W., & Fox, H. (1997). Frontal Behavioral Inventory: Diagnostic criteria for frontal lobe dementia. *Canadian Journal of Neurological Sciences, 24*, 29–36.

Kertesz, A., & McCabe, P. (1977). Recovery patterns and prognosis in aphasia. *Brain, 100* (Pt. 1), 1–18.

Kertesz, A., Jesso, S., Blair, M., McMonagle, P. (in press). What is Semantic Dementia? *Archives of Neurology*.

Kinsbourne, M., & Warrington, E. K. (1963). Jargonaphasia. *Neuropsychologia, 1,* 27–37.

Lebrun, Y. (1987). Anosognosia in aphasia. *Cortex, 23,* 251–263.

Lhermitte, F., & Beauvois, M. F. (1973). A visual-speech disconnexion syndrome. Report of a case with optic aphasia, agnosic alexia and colour agnosia. *Brain, 96*(4), 695–714.

Maher, L. M., Rothi, L. J., & Heilman, K. M. (1994). Lack of error awareness in an aphasic patient with relatively preserved auditory comprehension. *Brain and Language, 46*(3), 402–418.

Marshall, R. C., Rappaport, B. Z., & Garcia-Bunuel, L. (1985). Self-monitoring behavior in a case of severe auditory agnosia with aphasia. *Brain and Language, 24*(2), 297–313.

Neary, D., Snowden, J. S., Gustafson, L., Passant, U., Stuss, D., Black, S., et al. (1998). Frontotemporal lobar degeneration: A consensus on clinical diagnostic criteria. *Neurology, 51*(6), 1546–1554.

O'Keeffe, F. M., Murray, B., Coen, R. F., Dockree, P. M., Bellgrove, M. A., Garavan H., et al. (2007). Loss of insight in frontotemporal dementia, corticobasal degeneration and progressive supranuclear palsy. *Brain, 130*(3), 753–764.

Rubens, A. B., & Garrett, M. F. (1991). Anosognosia of linguistic deficits in patients with neurological deficits. In G. P. Prigatano & D. L. Schacter (Eds.), *Awareness of deficit after brain injury: Clinical and theoretical issues* (pp. 40–52). Oxford, England: Oxford University Press.

Schlenck, K. J., Huber, W., & Willmes, K. (1987). "Prepairs" and repairs: Different monitoring functions in aphasic language production. *Brain and Language, 30,* 226–244.

Shuren, J. E., Hammond, C. S., Maher, L. M., Rothi, L. J., & Heilman, K. M. (1995). Attention and anosognosia: The case of a jargon aphasic patient with unawareness of language deficit. *Neurology, 45*(2), 376–378.

Stone, V. E., Baron-Cohen, S., & Knight, R. T. (1998) Does frontal lobe damage produce theory of mind impairment? *Journal of Cognitive Neuroscience, 10,* 640–656.

Vallar, G., Papagno, C., Rusconi, M. L., & Bisiach, E. (1995). Vestibular stimulation, spatial hemineglect and dysphasia, selective effects. *Cortex, 31*(3), 589–593.

Weinstein, E. A., Cole, M., Mitchell, M. S., & Lyerly, O. G. (1964). Anosognosia and aphasia. *Archives of Neurology, 10,* 376–386.

Weinstein, E. A., & Kahn, R. L. (1950). The syndrome of anosognosia. *American Medical Association Archives of Neurology and Psychiatry, 64*(6), 772–791.

Weinstein, E. A., & Kahn, R. L. (1955). *Denial of illness: Symbolic and physiological aspects.* Springfield, IL: Charles C. Thomas.

Weinstein, E. A., Lyerly, O. G., Cole, M. & Ozer, M. (1966). Meaning in jargon aphasia. *Transactions of the American Neurological Association, 89,* 266–268.

Wernicke, C. (1874). *Der aphasische symptomen komplex.* Breslau, Germany: Cohn & Weigert.

7

Assessing Anosognosia for Motor and Language Impairments

Gianna Cocchini and Sergio Della Sala

Babinski introduced the term *anosognosie* to describe a state in which brain-damaged patients deny their hemiplegia. The term has since been used more broadly to encompass also unawareness for sensory or cognitive impairments, such as aphasia (for recent reviews, see Adair, Schwartz, & Barrett, 2003; Orfei et al., 2007; Vuilleumier, 2000). Despite this apparently simple definition, anosognosia is an extremely complex syndrome, whose clinical manifestations can vary considerably from patient to patient. Some patients may deny their hemiplegia and attempt walking (e.g., Bisiach & Geminiani, 1991); others may partially admit their impairment but ascribe it to other causes, such as arthritis, or manifest delusions, such as denying that the paretic limb is their own (*somatoparaphrenia*; e.g., Ramachandran & Blakesee, 1998); and others may still acknowledge their deficit but show indifference to it (*anosodiaphoria*; another term coined by Babinski in 1914). Furthermore, some patients may recognize their deficits only if attributed to other people in the same condition (e.g., Maher, Rothi, & Heilman, 1994, for aphasia; Marcel, Tegnér, & Nimmo-Smith, 2004, for hemiplegia). Finally, anosognosia can be deficit specific; that is, some patients may acknowledge their hemiplegia but not their aphasia, or vice versa (e.g., Breier et al., 1995; Kinsbourne & Warrington, 1963, case 1). Dissociations have been observed even for the same type of impairment; for instance, patients may acknowledge motor impairment of their arm but deny the paresis of their leg, or vice versa (Berti, Làdavas, & Della Corte, 1996; Bisiach, Vallar, Perani, Papagno, & Berti, 1986; Della Sala, Cocchini, Beschin, & Cameron, 2009). Similarly, aphasic patients have been observed acknowledging their written mistakes but not their speech errors (e.g., Marshall, Robson, Pring, & Chiat, 1998, case RMM).

Theoretical Accounts

Several theoretical interpretations have been proposed to account for the multiple manifestations of anosognosia for motor impairments. These accounts range from considering anosognosia as a psychological mechanism of defense (e.g., Weinstein, 1991; see also Turnbull & Solms, 2007) to conceiving of it as a failure of the error-monitoring process (e.g., Goldberg & Barr, 1991; see Heilman & Harciarek, Chapter 5, this volume for a recent overview of theoretical accounts of anosognosia for hemiplegia).

Several interpretations have also been put forward to account for anosognosia for language disorders (see Kertesz, Chapter 6, this volume for a recent overview of theoretical accounts of anosognosia for aphasia). Some of these, including the motivational interpretation (Kinsbourne & Warrington, 1963) and the inability to compare the expected with the actual outcome (Heilman, 1991; Rubens & Garrett, 1991), overlap with those proposed for motor impairment.

The different theoretical attempts to account for anosognosia may have arisen from the heterogeneity of the syndrome, which encompasses a variety of signs and symptoms. Indeed, there is accruing agreement among researchers to consider anosognosia as a multifactorial phenomenon (Cocchini, Beschin, Cameron, Fotopoulou, & Della Sala, 2009; Cocchini, Beschin, & Della Sala, 2002; Davies, Davies, & Colheart, 2005; Goldberg & Barr, 1991; Marcel et al., 2004; McGlynn & Kaszniak, 1991; McGlynn & Schacter, 1989; Orfei et al., 2007; Spalletta et al., 2007; Vulleimeur, 2004). This implies that different cognitive steps and processes are involved in this syndrome, but also that similar causes may underlie aspects of anosognosia for motor and language disorders, as suggested by some theoreticians (e.g., McGlynn & Schacter, 1989; Rubens & Garrett, 1991; Weinstein, 1991).

Assessment of Anosognosia

Considering the complexity of anosognosia, relatively little attention has been paid to its assessment. Prigatano (see Chapter 12, this volume) pointed out that questionnaires or structured interviews are an indirect measure of awareness, and the method of comparing the patient's self-evaluation on questionnaires to personal or professional caregivers (Prigatano & Altman, 1990; Prigatano, Ogano, & Amakusa, 1997) may hide methodological bias (see Orfei, Caltagirone, & Spalletta, Chapter 19, this volume).

Some authors have also pointed out that the lack of consensus among researchers and clinicians about methods of assessment could result in contrasting data, making comparisons across studies very difficult (Adair et al., 2003; Baier & Karnath, 2005; Jehkonen, Laihosalo, & Kettunen, 2006; Orfei et al., 2007; Vallar & Ronchi, 2006; Vuilleumier, 2000, 2004). Differences in methods may also induce false contrasting findings across different types of anosognosia. For example, anosognosia for motor impairment and anosognosia for language impairment are reported to dissociate (e.g., Breier et al., 1995); however, anosognosia for these two deficits shows some interesting overlap and shares similar assessment concerns, which will be considered in this chapter.

Anosognosia for Motor Impairment

Frequency of Anosognosia following Brain Damage

A few epidemiological studies have addressed the issue of the incidence of anosognosia for left hemiplegia (see Orfei et al., 2007, for a recent review). Their outcome is extremely varied, ranging from 14% (Baier & Karnath, 2005) to 51% (Nathanson, Bergman, & Gordon, 1952). Baier and Karnath (2005) suggested that a poor agreement on diagnostic criteria may be responsible for such variability. In particular, anosognosia is assessed by means of structured interviews whereby the patient's lack of awareness is rated by the examiner on the basis of the patient's answers to a set of questions (see Table 7.1; Bisiach et al., 1986). However, these answers are not interpreted in the light of norms and, therefore, some borderline values may be considered differently by different researchers.

According to Baier and Karnath (2005), when mild forms of anosognosia are included in the count, the percentage of right brain–damaged patients showing the syndrome within 15 days after brain lesion is about 24%, but it drops to 14% if stricter criteria are used. The different criteria have an even more dramatic effect on the presence/absence of anosognosia in left brain–damaged patients, ranging from about 21% (using the lax criteria) to only 4% (with the strict criteria). The challenge of interpreting the data from the literature is further complicated by the fact that there is disagreement even about which features define the presence of (mild) anosognosia. For example, in Bisiach et al.'s (1986) structured interview mild anosognosia is diagnosed when the patient fails to acknowledge his or her motor deficits spontaneously in response to a nonleading

Table 7.1 Structured Interview

Score:
0—The disorder is spontaneously reported or mentioned by the patient following a general question about his or her complaints.
1—The disorder is reported only following a specific question about the strength of the patient's left limb.
2— The disorder is acknowledged only after its demonstration through routine techniques of neurological examination.
3—No acknowledgement of the disorder can be obtained.

From Bisiach et al., 1986.

question. This criterion has been widely used in the literature of anosognosia for motor impairment (e.g., Appelros, Karlsson, & Hennerdal, 2007; Appelros, Karlsson, Seiger, & Nydevik, 2002; Davies et al., 2005; Marcel et al., 2004; Spinazzola, Pia, Folegatti, Marchetti, & Berti, 2008; Starkstein, Fedoroff, Price, Leiguarda, & Robinson, 1992). Similarly, Cutting (1978) considered the lack of spontaneous reference to one's own motor impairments as evidence of anosognosia without distinction of severity. However, Baier and Karnath (2005) posited that the patient might not report his or her motor impairment spontaneously as it may be subjectively considered less relevant than other ailments. This can be particularly true in the case of patients with no complete paresis. Therefore, some authors have suggested that it would be better to ask direct questions about the deficits. However, some discrepancy persists. Considering Baier and Karnath's (2005) strict criterion, Spalletta et al. (2007) have recently reported that 26% of a group of 50 right brain–damaged patients were still showing evidence of anosognosia about a month after the brain lesion; while Baier and Karnath (2008) themselves found that only 15% of a group of 79 acute (less than 10 days from the lesion) right brain–damaged patients were showing anosognosia. Even using the same diagnostic criterion the frequency of anosognosia is still unsettled.

Orfei et al. (2007) maintained that the length of time from the accident can be another confounding variable in establishing the frequency of anosognosia. Anosognosia often resolves or attenuates within a few weeks from brain damage, and its recorded frequency varies accordingly. Some studies (e.g., Baier & Karnath, 2005, 2008; Cutting, 1978; Starkstein et al., 1992; Stone, Halligan, & Greenwood, 1993) investigated the presence of anosognosia in large samples of patients in the acute phase (i.e., less than 1 month; Levine, Calvanio, & Rinn, 1991). Other studies considered more heterogeneous groups of patients, including both acute and chronic patients (e.g., Berti et al., 1996; Della Sala et al., 2009; Marcel et al., 2004; Nathanson, Bergman, & Gordon, 1952; Spalletta et al., 2007). Moreover, some authors investigated anosognosia for motor deficits in patients with complete paresis or severe motor impairments (e.g., Marcel et al., 2004), while others considered the full range of possible degrees of motor impairment (e.g., Della Sala et al., 2009). This variability about time since lesion onset and degree of motor impairment may have contributed to the contrasting data on the frequency of anosognosia.

Hemispheric Asymmetry

A second relevant issue related to anosognosia for hemiplegia is the respective role of each hemisphere. It is accrued opinion among researchers and clinicians that anosognosia is strongly associated with damage to the right hemisphere. Recent studies have identified the right posterior insular cortex as a crucial area for awareness (e.g., Karnath, Baier, & Nägele, 2005). This hemispheric asymmetry is an important issue for both theoretical and clinical reasons. Theories have been tailored around this belief (for a discussion, see, e.g., Turnbull & Solms, 2007) and clinicians assess anosognosia for hemiplegia mainly in right brain–damaged patients. Some theories (e.g., motivational interpretations or theories suggesting an impairment in monitoring processes) account for unawareness for different deficits, implying that anosognosia for all of them should be subsumed by the impairment of the same mechanisms and the same anatomical substrate located in the right hemisphere. However, available data do not support this view unanimously. A recent review of the literature by Morin (2007) has pointed out how the role of the left hemisphere in self-awareness has been underestimated. Recent neuroimaging studies have confirmed the crucial role of the left hemisphere in awareness (e.g., Farrer & Frith, 2002; Goldberg, Harel, & Malach, 2006). Craig (see Chapter 4, this volume) reported that evidence in literature strongly suggests a crucial role of the anterior insular cortex; however, he also pointed out that it is still unclear how the right and left sides interact and that ". . . it is not possible to predict how damage on one side might affect the functional capacity of the remaining AIC on the other side." Indeed, Appelros and colleagues (2007) found that only 54% of their 46 anosognosic patients were showing right hemisphere damage. Despite this evidence, anosognosia for motor impairment following left hemisphere damage has been neglected and considered a rare occurrence (e.g., Baier & Karnath, 2005).

THE WADA TEST   Some support for the dominant role of the right hemisphere in awareness for motor impairment comes from a stream of studies that used the Wada methodology (see Table 7.2). Gilmore, Heilman, Schmidt, Fennell, & Quisling (1992) investigated the presence of anosognosia in a group of eight presurgery epileptic patients. Each hemisphere was inactivated in turn by means of the barbiturate injected into the patient's carotid artery. Then, when the effect of the drug was wiped out, the patients were asked whether they noticed anything wrong with their limbs during the test. All of them failed to recollect their induced left paresis only (i.e., when the right hemisphere was inactivated). This study is often cited as an emblematic finding when people argue for the dominant role of the right hemisphere in awareness (e.g., Spinazzola et al., 2008). However, a few years later Breier et al. (1995) reported anosognosia in nearly half of their sample following left hemispheric inactivation. Other authors reported exactly the same occurrence of anosognosia following inactivation of either hemisphere (Dywan, McGlone, & Fox, 1995), or a much reduced hemispheric asymmetry when the site of epileptic seizure was considered (Durkin, Meador, Nichols, Lee, & Loring, 1994). In line with Gilmore et al.'s findings, Carpenter et al. (1995) reported that anosognosia following left limb weakness was significantly associated with right temporal lobe pathology. However, when Dywan and colleagues (1995) considered only the 32 patients showing

Table 7.2 Percentage of Participants Showing Evidence of Unawareness following the Wada Test

	Hemiphere Anaesthetized		No. of participants
	Right	Left	
Gilmore et al., 1992	100	0	8
Buchtel et al., 1992	92	57	48
Kaplan et al., 1993	100	71	15*
Durkin et al., 1994	94	86	115†
Dywan et al., 1995	66	66	83
Breier et al., 1995	89	49	54
Carpenter et al., 1995	87	38	31
Lu et al., 1997	80	59	17

* Of these 15 patients, 8 had right and 7 had left intracarotid injection.
† All 115 participants were right handed with left-hemisphere dominance for language. On a larger sample of 150 participants (regardless of hemisphere dominance for language), anosognosia for motor impairment was found in 95% and 89% of the cases after right and left hemisphere injections, respectively.
Modified from Cocchini et al., 2009.

unawareness following either right or left injection, they found that exactly half of them showed unawareness for right hemiplegia after left side injection *only*.

Despite the general trend of the data gathered by means of the Wada methodology suggesting a key function of the right hemisphere in awareness, the role of the left hemisphere cannot be easily dismissed and its role is still open to debate.

ASYMMETRY IN CLINICAL DATA Several clinical studies reported a much higher rate of anosognosia following right rather than left hemisphere damage (e.g., Appelros et al., 2007; Baier & Karnath, 2005; Cutting, 1978; Marcel et al., 2004; Stone et al., 1993). However, with the exclusion of Marcel et al.'s (2004) study whereby different diagnostic tools were used, the typical assessment measure utilized in most of these studies is the Structured Interview typified in Table 7.1, which requires the patients to engage in a conversation about their deficits. This type of diagnostic tool heavily relies on the patient's verbal competence. Unfortunately, no information can be gathered about the exclusion rate of patients with language impairment in some of the relevant studies (Baier & Karnath, 2005; Berti et al., 1996; Bisiach et al., 1986; Marcel et al., 2004). When this information is reported, it is clear that most left hemisphere–damaged patients had to be excluded from the assessment. Nathanson, Bergman, and Gordon (1952) excluded 38%, Cutting (1978) up to 58%, and Stone et al. (1993) up to 45% of right hemiplegics due to their comprehension deficits. The high exclusion rate led to a possible underestimation of anosognosia among left brain–damaged patients due to the consideration that "right hemiplegics at risk for developing anosognosia were the very patients in whom aphasia precluded its determination" (Cutting, 1978, p. 548).

THE VISUAL-ANALOGUE TEST FOR ANOSOGNOSIA FOR MOTOR DEFICIT We have recently investigated whether some methodological issues may have led to an artificially lower percentage of anosognosia for motor impairment among left brain–damaged patients (Cocchini et al., 2009). We assessed the presence of anosognosia in a group of left brain–damaged patients by means of two diagnostic tools: a structured interview similar to those used in previous studies (see Table 7.1), which relies heavily on language and enquires about a general motor impairment, and a newly devised instrument—the VATAm (Visual-Analogue Test for Anosognosia for motor deficit; Della Sala et al., 2009)—which is less dependent on language abilities and enquires about specific motor skills. The VATAm consists of 1 example and 12 questions about difficulty in performing bimanual (e.g., opening a jar; see Figure 7.1a) or bipedal tasks (e.g., climbing the stairs). To account for verbal communication difficulties, each question is illustrated by a drawing. Moreover, a four-point visual-analogue Likert scale is used to obtain the patients' ratings (see Figure 7.1b). Finally the patient's reliability is monitored by means of four "check questions," which require expected ratings regardless of the impairment (e.g., waving, see Figure 7.1c; jumping over a lorry, see Figure 7.1d). Patients who do not provide the expected answer to check questions should be excluded. Patients' ratings are then compared with those of their carergiver(s) and normative data allow interpretation of possible discrepancies (for full test, see http://homepages.gold.ac.uk/gcocchini). We observed that with the VATAm less than 30% of the patients were excluded. This improved inclusion rate led to the finding that about 40% of the left brain–damaged patients showed some evidence of anosognosia. On the contrary, with the classic Structured Interview over half of the same sample of left brain–damaged patients could not be assessed and evidence of anosognosia was found only in about 10% of those patients who could be assessed. Our findings suggest that the impact of left hemisphere damage on awareness may indeed have been underestimated for methodological reasons. This does not necessarily imply a similar frequency of anosognosia across the two hemispheres, but it suggests that anosognosia following left-sided lesions may be more frequent than previously thought.

Is Anosognosia Solely an Acute Phenomenon?

Anosognosia is usually described as a syndrome that spontaneously recovers within a few weeks (e.g., Levine et al., 1991). Some authors have suggested that chronic anosognosia can only be observed in association with general cognitive impairment (Goldberg & Barr, 1991; Levine, 1990; Levine, et al., 1991; McGlynn & Schacter, 1989). However, in reviewing the literature, we pointed out that anosognosia in the chronic phase is not as rare as textbooks would have it (see Cocchini et al., 2002 and Table 1 in that publication). No less than 42

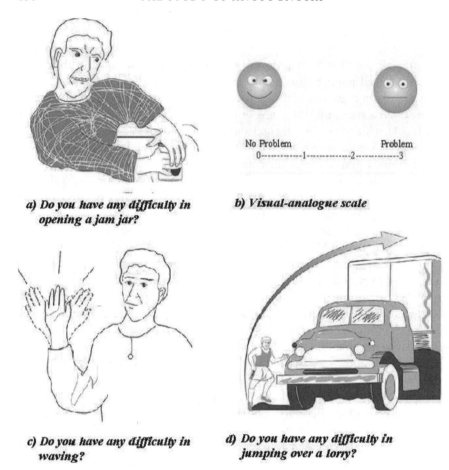

a) Do you have any difficulty in opening a jam jar?

b) Visual-analogue scale

c) Do you have any difficulty in waving?

d) Do you have any difficulty in jumping over a lorry?

Figure 7.1 Examples of Visual-Analogue Test for Anosognosia for motor deficit (VATAm) questions and the visual-analogue scale. See text for details.

cases of chronic or subacute anosognosia could be culled from the literature, and nearly half of them (19 cases) were not presenting with a general cognitive impairment. The relevant issue is whether chronic anosognosia is indeed rare or whether it could have been underestimated because of the diagnostic tools used. We suggested that patients in subacute or chronic phases may have been overexposed to some of the questions used to assess anosognosia (Cocchini et al., 2009). Thus, patients may provide the "correct" response based on what they have "learned" rather than on their actual awareness of their deficit. Interestingly, in a further study (Della Sala et al., 2009) we observed that the questions that best predicted the presence of anosognosia in the less acute phases were those enquiring about activities such as "washing dishes" or "opening bottles," whereas the worst predictors were questions about "walking" or "clapping hands," both recurrent questions in classical assessment of anosognosia. Marcel and colleagues (2004) also observed that more anosognosic cases were reported when questionnaires enquiring about specific bimanual and bipedal tasks were used rather than a general interview about motor impairment. Similarly, Berti and colleagues (1996) described two patients (cases LO and AP) who appeared aware of their hemiplegia during the Structured Interview but subsequently grossly overestimated their ability to perform bimanual actions. However, the opposite dissociation between verbal report and self-evaluation of bimanual tasks was also observed in another two patients (cases MA and IM), who showed mild and severe anosognosia during the Structured Interview but later rated their ability in performing bimanual tasks as rather poor. Data obtained using the Structured Interview could be biased by the patients' exposure to direct and indirect information regarding their motor impairment, yet this form of assessment may provide valuable information about some aspects of this multifactorial syndrome.

Severity of Motor Impairment

Motor deficits improve over time (Bonita & Beaglehole, 1988), and some tools assessing unawareness may be inappropriate with patients showing only a mild or moderate paresis. Nathanson and colleagues (1952) suggested that patients with mild paresis may also show anosognosia, "but in order that the significance of responses to specific questions, such as 'Can you move your hand?' should be interpreted more accurately, the criterion of complete paralysis was necessary" (p. 381). Indeed, structured interviews rely on the fact that the patient is claiming to be able to move a paretic limb. In some cases, the patient is also asked to move the limb and forced to face the ensuing contradiction (see Table 7.1, criteria 2). However, some patients may actually be able to perform some movement. Data collected from patients with partially preserved or recovered motor skills may be particularly difficult to interpret, especially if norms are not available. As a consequence, many studies on anosognosia constrain their recruitment among acute stroke patients presenting with complete paresis (e.g., Baier & Karnath, 2008).

Implicit Awareness

Given the heterogeneity of anosognosia, different measures should be devised in order to assess different aspects of unawareness. The most common diagnostic tools are structured interviews and questionnaires (Orfei et al.'s Chapter 19 of this volume. See also Table 1 in Jehkonen et al., 2006, and Table 2 in Orfei et al., 2007). Invariably, these are based on the patient's verbal report of his or her own deficits, which relies on meta-cognitive processes. Very little is known about other, less explicit, aspects of anosognosia. For example, House and Hodges (1988) described a hemiplegic patient who was asked to look at pictures of people showing motor impairment. While she denied her own motor problem, she identified the person in the wheelchair as most similar to herself. Similarly, a few studies (Berti et al., 1996; Marcel et al., 2004) reported that patients unaware of their motor impairments were more inclined to recognize a motor deficit when asked to rate the examiner's potential ability to perform a series of bimanual and bipedal activities had the examiner had the same condition as the one suffered by the patient.

Berti and colleagues (1996) observed that only two of six anosognosic patients acquired some insight into their deficits when asked to actually perform bimanual actions. An even stronger effect of actual performance of a task was found by Marcel et al. (2004). These authors found that between 47% and 67%, depending on the type of task, of the right brain–damaged patients acquired better knowledge of their condition when asked to actually perform bimanual tasks which they maintained they could perform with no problems only minutes earlier. The effect of actual performance on self-evaluation, which we could label "empirical learning" (i.e., learning through experience), leads to some theoretical and clinical implications. The evidence of empirical learning implies that, in these cases, lack of awareness cannot be due to a general poor ability to perform an appropriate reality check. Rather it is due to the lack of information or appropriate feedback about one's own motor impairment. Exposed to this information, the patients with this type of anosognosia should regain, or increase, awareness about their motor impairment.

The assessment of anosognosia is usually based on meta-cognitive tasks, whereby a patient is asked to reflect upon his or her own condition and provide some type of self-evaluation. Little is known about the less explicit awareness. For example, some patients may acknowledge their hemiplegia but then attempt to stand up or walk with high risk of falling; whereas other patients may deny their deficits but then accept to stay at the hospital and undergo rehabilitation trainings (e.g., Bisiach & Geminiani, 1991; McGlynn & Schacter, 1989). As Prigatano (see Chapter 12, this volume) pointed out, answers to questionnaires or structured interviews are not the best instruments to reveal phenomenological experience. These considerations suggest that there may be an important discrepancy between what is verbally acknowledged and what is less consciously believed by the patient and responsible for the patient's actual behavior.

In a recent study we investigated the implicit aspects of anosognosia examining patients' behavior under particular experimental conditions and the impact of empirical learning on actual performance (Cocchini, & Della Sala, 2008; Cocchini, Beschin, Fotopoulou, & Della Sala, unpublished data). Capitalizing on an anecdotal observation of a patient by Ramachandran and Blakesee (1998), we have assessed anosognosia based on the actual behavior of the patient and with minimal use of verbal communication. We identified a series of eight simple everyday bimanual tasks, which are usually better performed using both hands (e.g., crack a nut with a nutcracker holding the nut in one hand and the nutcracker in the other hand) but can also be performed using one hand if the motor action is reorganized ("aware strategy"; e.g., cracking the nut with the unimpaired hand while the nut is resting on the table). In order to adopt the "aware strategy," patients have to acknowledge their motor impairments. In fact, if they are unaware of their motor difficulties, they would not adopt the correct strategy and behave as if they could use both hands ("Anosognosia"; e.g., holding the nut or the nutcracker as if the patient could use both hands), hence failing to perform the task. A group of brain-damaged patients showing severe upper limb motor impairment were considered and their performance was compared with those of a group of patients with motor difficulties caused by noncerebral impediments, such as a bone fracture or peripheral nerve damage. We observed that about 25% of the patients showed evidence of anosognosia for their motor impairment, and that most of them adopted more aware strategies if they were asked to perform the same tasks a second time. This suggests that empirical learning may not just modify the patient's verbal evaluations, as reported by Marcel et al. (2004) and by Berti et al. (1996; cases CF and CG), but also the patients' behavior. Interestingly, two patients appeared fully aware of their motor deficit when explicitly enquired about (i.e., by means of the Structured Interview and VATAm), but they approached the Bimanual Task as if they could use both hands normally, showing severe "behavioral" anosognosia. These patients may resemble those anecdotes reported by clinicians in charge of patients who, despite being fully aware of their motor deficits, experience recurrent falls as they attempt risky behaviors for hemiplegics. We also observed the opposite dissociation, that is, showing anosognosia on more explicit diagnostic measures but then adopting aware strategies to perform bimanual motor tasks (i.e. "behaviorally" aware). This may imply the existence of quite different types of anosognosia and probably different mechanisms responsible for these patients' anosognosia. Limiting the assessment to one aspect, the more explicit one, of anosognosia could have led researchers to neglect other forms of anosognosia.

We emphasized differences among anosognosic patients; however, it is also important to keep in mind possible overlaps and similarities across unawareness for different impairments, such as unawareness for motor and language deficits. Indeed, it is possible that while different mechanisms underlie different aspects of anosognosia for motor impairment, similar causes may be responsible for the lack of awareness across different deficits.

Assessment of Anosognosia for Language Disorders

Typically aphasics showing anosognosia are unaware of their difficulties in verbal communication (Adair et al., 2003; Rubens & Garrett, 1991; Vuilleumier, 2000). As a result, some aphasics deny language difficulties or do not engage in self-correcting their speech errors (Wernicke, 1874). In 1956, Alajounine was probably the first to underscore that unawareness for one's own language disorder was "one of the major phenomena" (p. 23) of jargon aphasia. In particular, jargon aphasics, or more generally patients with sensory aphasia, may hold conversations with little, if any, attempt to correct their errors so that their communication is largely incomprehensible (e.g., Alajouanine, 1956; Kinsbourne & Warrington, 1963; Levelt, 1983; Maher, Rothi, & Heilman, 1994; Marshall, Rappaport & Garcia-Bunuel, 1985; Weinstein, Lyerly, Cole, & Ozer, 1966).

The assessment process of anosognosia for language deficits is particularly complex, as it is influenced by the difficulty in interpreting aphasics' responses to questions related to their deficits (Lebrun, 1987). For this reason, researchers have relied on forms of assessment such as self-correction and error detection methods. These types of assessment provide valuable data, but they often consist of ad hoc tests tailored around the patient's performance. In this context, information about the patient's explicit self-evaluation, which is the central issue in the literature of anosognosia for motor impairment, is rarely considered (e.g., Breier et al., 1995; Kertesz, Chapter 6, this volume) or it is reported anecdotally (e.g., Kinsbourne & Warrington, 1963).

The Self-Correction Method

Weinstein et al. (1966) found that 78% of a sample of patients with large bilateral brain lesions and jargon aphasia denied their difficulty with verbal communication; these authors defined jargon aphasia as "a mixture of aphasia and anosognosia" (p. 187). Kertesz and Benson (1970) and later Gainotti (1972) also observed that lack of awareness in aphasic patients can be associated with lesions confined to the left hemisphere. In particular, Gainotti (1972) reported that none of the 19 nonfluent and 24 amnesic aphasic patients showed unawareness of their language difficulties, whereas 4 out of 16 fluent aphasics appeared unaware. Therefore, the association of unawareness with jargon and sensory aphasia, and the fact that monitoring relies on intact comprehension, has led researchers to maintain that a lack of understanding could be responsible for unawareness (e.g., Heilman, 1991). However, a number of studies that analyzed the proportion and type of self-corrections produced by aphasics constitute a consistent body of evidence against the emphasis on comprehension failure as the main factor leading to unawareness.

The basic assumption of the self-correction method is that if aphasics are not aware of their language errors, they will not attempt to correct them. Hence, lack of self-corrections has been considered as evidence of anosognosia for language impairments (e.g., Adair et al., 2003, for a review; Rubens & Garrett, 1991). To further complicate the issue, however, Poeck (1972), and later Schlenck, Huber, and Willmes (1987), did not find a clear association between self-correction efforts and sensory aphasia. Marshall and Tompkins (1982) investigated self-corrections in 42 aphasics. They observed that fluent and nonfluent aphasic patients did not differ in terms of proportion of self-corrections. Differences according to severity and fluency were observed only when success in self-correcting errors was considered. In particular, these authors observed that successful self-correction efforts favored patients with high verbal ability regardless of fluency.

More detailed analyses of self-corrections were introduced by Hofmann and Cohen (1979), who noticed that latencies preceding an error were more frequent than actual corrections of previous errors, and that self-corrections were of different natures and implied different mechanisms. This distinction was further considered by Schlenck and colleagues (1987), who, also capitalizing on previous studies by Buckingham and Kertesz (1974), Butterworth (1979), and Keller (1979), proposed a technique to classify self-corrections in the language productions of aphasics. Schlenck and colleagues (1987) distinguished between "repairs," defined as attempts to correct errors that just occurred, and "prepairs," which consist of various searching behaviors (such as pauses) that are not preceded by an error. This distinction is quite important, as these two types of self-corrections seem to act as indexes of good functioning of post-articulatory and pre-articulatory monitoring systems, respectively. Schlenck and colleagues investigated the presence of these types of self-corrections in a sample of 60 aphasic patients. In line with Hofmann and Cohen's (1979) findings, Schlenck and colleagues noticed that repairs were far less frequent than prepairs, suggesting an impairment of the post-articulatory monitor system. Importantly, the proportion of prepairs did not differ between Wernicke and Broca aphasics, leading the author to suggest that "the monitoring process is not exclusively based on language comprehension" (p. 241).

Even if the use of the self-correction method to assess awareness for language disorders provides a considerable contribution towards a better understanding of anosognosia for aphasia, it represents an indirect form of assessment. Maher and colleagues (1994) suggested that aphasics may be fully aware yet fail to correct themselves for other reasons. For example, patients may just decide, more or less intentionally, to withdraw from any further effort when convinced that they will never find the correct word. Therefore, the presence of self-corrections could be reasonably considered as evidence of awareness of one's own language difficulties, whereas their lack does not necessarily imply unawareness.

Error Detection Method

Self-correction of errors implies some preserved ability to identify (repairs) or predict (prepairs) one's own speech errors, which in turn should be a prerequisite of awareness (but see Lecours & Joanette, 1980). Some authors have proposed error detection analysis as an alternative or additional means to the self-correction method. By means of error detection, patients are typically asked to detect their errors during the description of a picture or when performing a naming task (e.g., Marshall et al., 1998). Analyzing the types of error that are more likely to be explicitly detected by patients, researchers have aimed to understand at which stage the monitoring process has been disrupted, and in turn identify different types of anosognosia (see Adair et al., 2003, for a review).

The ability to correctly process feedback information is part of the monitoring system. This has been investigated by means of the delayed auditory feedback procedure, which usually induces a speech disruption in healthy volunteers (Fairbanks & Guttman, 1955). Interestingly, jargon aphasics showed little disruption of speech if delayed feedback was provided, suggesting that for these patients a malfunction of the feedback mechanism may account for their inability to detect their own errors (Boller, Vrtunski, Kim, & Mack, 1978; Peuser & Temp, 1981). However, Marshall et al. (1998) suggested that monitoring failures may not be linked to comprehension or feedback disorders per se. They posited that such failures resulted from the patients' inability to accurately compare the actual with the intended output. This hypothesis was supported by experimental data collected on four aphasic patients. One patient (case CM) failed to detect half of his errors during a naming task, but his performance in detecting his own errors was far better when he was asked to identify errors during repetition or while listening to his own tape-recorded output. Other authors (e.g., Shuren, Hammond, Maher, Rothi, & Heilman, 1995) reported on patients whose detection of speech errors was better when they were asked to listen to their previous recorded performance than they did while speaking. In particular, Maher and colleagues (1994) systematically investigated error detection ability in one aphasic (case AS) while the patient was speaking (online condition) and while he was listening to his own previously recorded performance (offline condition). The patient recognized only about 25% of his own errors in the online condition, but he identified as many as 65% of his errors in the offline condition. This discrepancy between online and offline performance in detecting his own errors has been interpreted as a reduced attentional capacity that would jeopardize the patient's ability to perform two tasks (i.e., speaking and monitoring) simultaneously (Lebrun, 1987; Shuren et al., 1995). Importantly, this type of interpretation is qualitatively different from the others as it implies that the monitoring process is *not* directly linked to the language deficit per se.

However, this interpretation does not account for a few jargon aphasics who acknowledged their oral and written mistakes only when these were believed to be another person's errors (Alajouanine, 1956; Kinsbourne & Warrington, 1963; Maher et al., 1994). Maher and colleagues (1994) also considered a condition when AS was asked to detect errors, which were the same as those previously committed by the patient, in the examiner's recorded performance. AS correctly identified a higher percentage (88%) of the "examiner's errors" than of his own recorded errors, suggesting a higher sensitivity in detecting others' errors than their own. Despite Maher and colleagues (1994) concluding that a reduced attentional capacity could be considered as the most likely cause of AS's unawareness for speech errors, they could not rule out other possible causes, such as adaptive denial mechanisms or auditory processing failures. The authors themselves mentioned that, since successful monitoring of speech depends upon a number of intact processes, "a deficit in any of these mechanisms may be sufficient to cause an anosognosia for aphasia" (p. 415).

This statement suggests also that anosognosia for aphasia should be considered as a multifactorial phenomenon, which may require different diagnostic tools tapping into different aspects of awareness. The error detection method provides valuable information, but it is mainly limited to the analysis of the post-articulatory component (i.e., errors already committed), whereas previous studies on self-corrections (see previous section) have indicated the pre-articulatory component as more sensitive to awareness disorders.

Patients' Self-Report of Aphasia

While patients' self-reports of their deficits have played a crucial role in the literature of anosognosia for motor impairment, this method has rarely been used to assess unawareness for aphasia. Indeed, it can be hard to interpret aphasics' verbal responses, and there is little certainty about the patients' comprehension of the questions. Hence, only very crude and oversimplified measures can be used to investigate the patients' explicit knowledge of their own language deficits. For example, evidence of anosognosia for aphasia following the Wada test was based on a "clear negative response to the question, Did you notice any difficulty with speech after the medicine went in?" (Breier et al., 1995, p. 66). As suggested by McGlynn and Schacter (1989), this method is open to subjective interpretation and "development of methods for investigating unawareness in different aphasic groups is clearly necessary" (p. 180). Some authors have developed clinical scales to assess lack of awareness in patients showing language difficulties mainly based on caregivers' evaluations (e.g., Kertesz, Nadkarni, Davidson, & Thomas, 2000).

Despite other methods (i.e., self-correction, error detection methods, and clinical scales) used to assess anosognosia for aphasia remaining a valuable resource of information about patients' awareness for aphasia, the self-evaluation method may provide further information about a relatively neglected aspect of anosognosia for aphasia, and it could facilitate a more direct comparison between unawareness for motor and language impairment.

The Visual-Analogue Test for Anosognosia for Language Disorders

Recently, we have developed a questionnaire named VATA-L (Visual-Analogue Test for Anosognosia for Language Disorders -L; Gregg et al., 2008). This instrument enquires about typical language tasks that aphasics may fail. Similar to the

VATAm previously discussed, the VATA-L consists of 1 example and 14 questions about the patients' ability to perform common verbal tasks requiring language production (e.g., finding the right word; see Figure 7.2a), language comprehension (e.g., reading the newspaper), or both production and comprehension (e.g., talking on the phone). Each question is illustrated by a drawing to facilitate comprehension for people with aphasia. Patients rate their difficulty in performing these tasks using a four-point visual-analogue Likert scale (see Figure 7.2b). Response reliability is monitored by means of four "check questions," which require expected ratings regardless of the impairment (e.g., hearing a fire engine with its sirens on, see Figure 7.2c; speaking Russian, see Figure 7.2d). The performance of patients who do not provide the expected answer to check questions should be considered unreliable. The patients' ratings are then compared to those of their caregiver/s and normative data allow interpretation of possible discrepancies (for full test and procedures, see http://homepages.gold.ac.uk/gcocchini).

Preliminary data gathered using this instrument suggest that reliable information can be obtained by over 60% of the aphasics tested, and that even patients

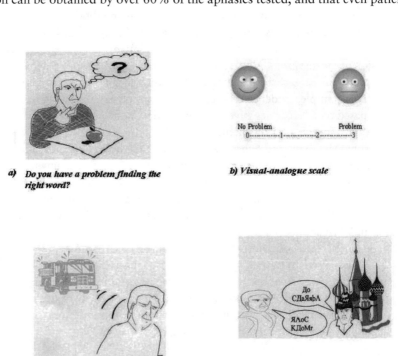

a) *Do you have a problem finding the right word?*

b) *Visual-analogue scale*

c) *Would you have a problem hearing a fire engine with its sirens on?*

d) *Would you have a problem speaking Russian?*

Figure 7.2 Examples of Visual-Analogue Test for Anosognosia for Language Disorders (VATA-L) questions and the visual-analogue scale. See text for details.

with severe aphasia were able to reliably complete the questionnaire. Importantly, 30% of the patients reliably tested showed some degree of anosognosia for their language problems. Moreover, when awareness for motor impairment was assessed by means of the VATAm in a subgroup of 21 aphasics showing associated motor impairment, we observed that 9 (43%) were showing anosognosia, and 3 (33%) of them showed unawareness for both motor and language deficits (Gregg et al., 2008). These findings suggest that impairment of common mechanisms may underline unawareness for motor and language disorders in some patients showing unawareness. This has clear theoretical implications and it contributes to the debate about the role of the left hemisphere in self-awareness.

The VATA-L adds to the array of tools investigating a relatively neglected aspect (patient's self-evaluation) of awareness for language disorders, and it fills a methodological gap in the literature. Moreover, (together with the VATAm), it allows the comparison between anosognosia for motor and language disorders.

Anosognosia as a Multifactorial Phenomenon

As for anosognosia for hemiplegia, a unitary explanation for anosognosia for aphasia seems unlikely. It is interesting to notice how often similar interpretations (e.g., motivational and monitoring hypotheses) have been considered to account for unawareness for motor or language impairment without a direct comparison of the data from the two literatures. A possible reason for this overlooking is the profoundly different method of assessment used to diagnose anosognosia for motor and language impairments. While anosognosia for motor impairment is mainly assessed relying on the patient's verbal report, anosognosia for aphasia is assessed indirectly, inferring level of awareness from the frequency and type of self-corrections or error detections. These methods can provide crucial information, but they may tap into different aspects of awareness (McGlynn & Kaszniak, 1991), whereas similar methods of assessment may improve the comparison between unawareness for different deficits.

Conclusions

There is accruing consensus that deficits in different mechanisms may cause unawareness for hemiplegia (e.g., Marcel et al., 2004) and aphasia (e.g., Maher et al., 1994). In line with some theoretical interpretations (e.g., Goldberg & Barr, 1991; Levine, 1990; McGlynn & Schacter, 1989; Weinstein & Kahn, 1955), anosognosia for different deficits may share similar causes and similar manifestations, and different levels of awareness could be affected differently by brain damage (McGlynn & Schacter, 1989). Developing appropriate assessment procedures to investigate different aspects and severities of unawareness is crucial for future studies on anosognosia. The understanding of anosognosia cannot progress without a parallel improvement of diagnostic tools aimed at facilitating the comparison across studies, at assisting clinicians and researchers to identify different aspects of anosognosia, and at allowing the examination of patients with communication difficulties.

Acknowledgments

The work reported in this chapter has been carried out in collaboration with N. Beschin, N. Gregg, A. Cameron, M. Dean, K. Broomfield, and A. Fotopoulou. We are also grateful to N. Gregg for commenting on a first draft of this chapter. G. C. and S. D. S.'s work on anosognosia has been funded by the Stroke Association (grant no. TSA 06/02) and by the Wellcome Trust (grant no.078580).

References

Adair, J. C., Schwartz, R. L., & Barrett, A. M. (2003). Anosognosia. In K. M. Heilman & E. Valenstein (Eds.), *Clinical Neuropsychology* (pp. 185–214). Oxford, England: Oxford University Press.

Alajouanine, T. (1956). Verbalization in aphasia. *Brain, 79,* 1–28.

Appelros, P., Karlsson, G. M., & Hennerdal, S. (2007). Anosognosia versus unilateral neglect. Coexistence and their relations to age, stroke severity, lesion site and cognition. *European Journal of Neurology, 14,* 54–59.

Appelros, P., Karlsson, G. M., Seiger, A., & Nydevik, I. (2002). Neglect and anosognosia after first-ever stroke: Incidence and relationship to disability. *Journal of Rehabilitation Medicine, 34,* 215–220.

Babinski, M. J. (1914). Contribution à l'étude des troubles mentaux dans l'hémiplégir organique cérébrale (Anosognosie). *Revue Neurologique, 27,* 845–848.

Baier, B., & Karnath, H. O. (2005). Incidence and diagnosis of anosognosia for hemiparesis revised. *Journal of Neurology, Neurosurgery, and Psychiatry, 76,* 358–361.

Baier, B., & Karnath, H. O. (2008). Tight link between our sense of limb ownership and self-awareness of actions. *Stroke, 39,* 486–488.

Berti, A., Làdavas, E., & Della Corte, M. (1996). Anosognosia for hemiplegia, neglect dyslexia and drawing neglect: Clinical findings and theoretical considerations. *Journal of International Neuropsychological Society, 2,* 426–440.

Bisiach, E., & Geminiani, G. (1991). Anosognosia related to hemiplegia and hemianopia. In G. P. Prigatano & D. L. Schacter (Eds.), *Awareness of deficit after brain injury: Clinical and theoretical issues* (pp. 17–39). Oxford, England: Oxford University Press.

Bisiach, E., Vallar, G., Perani D., Papagno, C., & Berti, A. (1986). Unawareness of disease following lesions of the right hemisphere: Anosognosia for hemiplegia and anosognosia for hemianopia. *Neuropsychologia, 24,* 471–482.

Boller, F., Vrtunski, P. B., Kim, Y., & Mack, J. L. (1978). Delayed auditory feedback and aphasia. *Cortex, 14,* 212–226.

Bonita, R., & Beaglehole, R. (1988). Recovery of motor function after stroke. *Stroke, 19,* 1497–1500.

Breier, J. L, Adair, J. C., Gold, M., Fennell, E. B., Gilmore, R. L., & Heilman, K. M. (1995). Dissociation of anosognosia for hemiplegia and aphasia during left-hemisphere anesthesia. *Neurology, 45,* 65–67.

Buchtel, H., Henry, T., & Abou-Khalil, B. (1992). Memory for neurological deficits during the intracarotid amytal procedure: A hemispheric difference. *Journal of Clinical Experimental Neuropsychology, 14,* 96–97.

Buckingham, H. W., & Kertesz, A. (1974). A linguistic analysis of fluent aphasia. *Brain and Language, 1,* 43–62.

Butterworth, B. (1979). Hesitation and the production of verbal paraphasias and neologisms in jargon aphasia. *Brain and Language, 8,* 133–161.

Carpenter, K., Berti, A., Oxbury, S., Molyneux, A. J., Bisiach, E., & Oxbury, J. M. (1995). Awareness of and memory for arm weakness during intracarotid sodium amytal testing. *Brain, 118,* 243–251.

Cocchini, G., Beschin, N., & Della Sala, S. (2002). Chronic anosognosia: A case report and theoretical account. *Neuropsychologia, 40,* 2030–2038.

Cocchini, G., Beschin, N., Cameron, A., Fotopoulou A., & Della Sala, S. (2009). Anosognosia for motor impairment following left brain damage. *Neuropsychology, 23,* 223–230.

Cocchini, G., & Della Sala, S. (2008). Unawareness for illness (anosognosia): A frequent occurrence following brain damage. *Proceeding of Stroke Association,* Harrogate, p. 13.

Cutting, J. (1978). Study of anosognosia. *Journal of Neurology, Neurosurgery, and Psychiatry, 41,* 548–555.

Davies, M. D., Davies, A. A., & Coltheart, M. (2005). Anosognosia and the two-factor theory of delusions. *Mind & Language, 20,* 209–236.

Della Sala, S., Cocchini, G., Beschin, N., & Cameron, A. (2009). VATAm: Visual-analogue test for anosognosia for motor impairment: A new test to assess awareness for motor impairment. *The Clinical Neuropsychologist, 11,* 1–22.

Durkin, M. W., Meador, K. J., Nichols, M. E., Lee, G. P., & Loring, D. W. (1994). Anosognosia and the intracarotid amobarbital procedure (Wada Test). *Neurology, 44,* 978–979.

Dywan, C., McGlone, J., & Fox, A. (1995). Do intracarotid barbiturate injections offer a way to investigate hemispheric models of anosognosia? *Journal of Clinical and Experimental Neuropsychology, 17,* 431–438.

Fairbanks, G., & Guttman, N. (1955). Effects of delayed auditory feedback upon articulation. *Journal of Speech and Hearing Research, 1,* 12–22.

Farrer, C., & Frith, C. D. (2002). Experiencing oneself vs another person as being the cause of an action: The neural correlates of the experience of agency. *NeuroImage, 15,* 596–603.

Gainotti, G. (1972). Emotional behavior and hemispheric side of the lesion. *Cortex, 8,* 41–55.

Gilmore, R. L., Heilman, K. M., Schmidt, R. P., Fennell, E. M., & Quisling, R. (1992). Anosognosia during Wada testing. *Neurology, 42,* 925–927.

Goldberg, E., & Barr, W. B. (1991). Three possible mechanisms of unawareness of deficit. In G. P. Prigatano & D. L. Schacter (Eds.), *Awareness of deficit after brain injury: Clinical and theoretical issues* (pp. 152–176). Oxford, England: Oxford University Press.

Goldberg, I. I., Harel, M., & Malach, R. (2006). When the brain loses its self: Prefrontal inactivation during sensorimotor processing. *Neuron, 50,* 329–339.

Gregg, N., Beschin, N., Cocchini, G., Rado, T., Dean, M., Broomfield, K., & Della Sala, S. (2008). Unawareness for language disorders in brain damaged patients. *Proceedings of the British Psychology Society–Cognitive Division, Southampton.*

Heilman, K. M. (1991). Anosognosia: Possible neuropsychological mechanisms. In G. P. Prigatano & D. L. Schacter (Eds.), *Awareness of deficit after brain injury: Clinical and theoretical issues* (pp. 53–62). Oxford, England: Oxford University Press.

Hofmann, E., & Cohen, R. (1979). Kontrollmechanismen aphatischer patienten bei verbalen und phonemischen paraphasien. *Archiv für Psychiatrie und Nervenkrankheiten, 226,* 325–340.

House, A., & Hodges, J. R. (1988). Persistent denial of handicap after infarction of the right basal ganglia: A case study. *Journal of Neurology, Neurosurgery, and Psychiatry, 51,* 112–115.

Jehkonen, M., Laihosalo M., & Kettunen, J. (2006). Anosognosia after stroke: Assessment, occurrence, subtypes and impact on functional outcome reviewed. *Acta Neurologica Scandinavica, 114,* 293–306.

Kaplan, R. F., Meadows, M. E., Cohen, R. A., Bromfield, E. B., & Ehrenberg, B. L. (1993). Awareness of deficit after the sodium amobarbital (Wada) test. *Journal of Clinical Experimental Neuropsychology, 15,* 383.

Karnath, H.-O., Baier, B., & Nägele, T. (2005). Awareness of the functioning of one's own limbs mediated by the insular cortex? *Journal of Neuroscience, 25,* 7134–7138.

Keller, E. (1979). Planning and execution in speech production. *Recherches linguistiques á Montrèal, 13,* 34–51.

Kertesz, A. & Benson, D. F. (1970). Neologistic jargon: A clinicopathological study. *Cortex, 6,* 362–386.

Kertesz, A., Nadkarni, N., Davidson, W., & Thomas A. W. (2000). The frontal behavioral inventory in the differential diagnosis of frontotemporal dementia. *Journal of the International Neuropsychological Society, 6,* 460–468.

Kinsbourne, M., & Warrington, E. K. (1963). Jargon aphasia. *Neuropsychologia, 1,* 27–37.

Lebrun, Y. (1987) Anosognosia in aphasics. *Cortex, 23,* 251–263.

Lecours, R., & Joanette, Y. (1980). Linguistic and other psychological aspects of paroxysmal aphasia. *Brain and Language, 10,* 1–23.

Levelt, W. J. M. (1983). Monitoring and self-repair in speech. *Cognition, 14,* 41–104.

Levine, D. N., Calvanio, R., & Rinn, W. E. (1991). The pathogenesis of anosognosia for hemiplegia. *Neurology, 41,* 1770–1781.

Levine, N. (1990). Unawareness of visual and sensorimotor defects: A hypothesis. *Brain and Cognition, 13,* 233–281.

Lu, L. H., Barrett, A. M., Schwartz, R. L., Cibula, J. E., Gilmore, R. L., Uthman, B. M., & Heilman, K. M. (1997). Anosognosia and confabulation during the Wada test. *Neurology, 49,* 1316–1322.

Maher, L., Rothi, L., & Heilman, K. (1994). Lack of error awareness in an aphasic patient with relatively preserved auditory comprehension. *Brain and Language, 46,* 402–418.

Marcel, A., Tegnér, R., & Nimmo-Smith, I. (2004). Anosognosia for plegia: Specificity, extension, partiality and disunity of bodily unawareness. *Cortex, 40,* 19–40.

Marshall, R., Rappaport, B., & Garcia-Bunuel, L. (1985). Self-monitoring behavior in a case of severe auditory agnosia with aphasia. *Brain and Language, 24,* 297–313.

Marshall, J., Robson, J., Pring, T., & Chiat, S. (1998). Why does monitoring fail in jargon aphasia? Comprehension, judgment, and therapy evidence. *Brain and Language, 63,* 79–107.

Marshall, R. C., & Tompkins, C. A. (1982). Verbal self-correction behaviors of fluent and nonfluent aphasic subjects. *Brain and Language, 15,* 292–306.

McGlynn, S. M., & Kaszniak, A. W. (1991). Unawareness of deficits in dementia and schizophrenia. In G. P. Prigatano & D. L. Schacter (Eds.), *Awareness of deficit after brain injury: Clinical and theoretical issues* (pp. 84–110). Oxford, England: Oxford University Press.

McGlynn, S. M., & Schacter, D. L. (1989). Unawareness of deficits in neuropsychological syndromes. *Journal of Clinical and Experimental Neuropsychology, 11,* 143–205.

Morin, A. (2007). Self-awareness and the left hemisphere: The dark side of selectively reviewing the literature. *Cortex, 43,* 1068–1073.

Nathanson, M., Bergman, P. S., & Gordon, C. G. (1952). Denial of illness: Its occurrence in one hundred consecutive cases of hemiplegia. *Archives of Neurology and Psychiatry, 68,* 380–387.

Orfei, M. D., Robinson, R. G., Prigatano, G. P., Starkstein, S., Rüsch, N., Bria, P., Caltagirone, C., & Spalletta, G. (2007). Anosognosia for hemiplegia after stroke is a multifaceted phenomenon: A systematic review of the literature. Brain, 130, 3075–3090.

Peuser, B., & Temp, K. (1981). The evolution of jargon aphasia. In J. Brown (Ed.) *Jargon aphasia.* Orlando, FL: Academic Press.

Poeck, K. (1972). Stimmung und krankheitseinsicht bei aphasien. *Archiv für Psychiatrie und Nervenkrankheiten, 216,* 246–254.

Prigatano, G. P., & Altman, I. M. (1990). Impaired awareness of behavioral limitations after traumatic brain injury *Archives of Physical Medicine and Rehabilitation, 71,* 1058–1064.

Prigatano, G. P., Ogano, M., & Amakusa, B. (1997). A cross-cultural study on impaired self-awareness in Japanese patients with brain dysfunction. *Neuropsychiatry, Neuropsychology, and Behavioral Neurology, 10,* 135–143.

Ramachandran, V. S., & Blakesee, S. (1998). *Phantoms in the brain: The sound of one hand clapping.* New York: William and Co.

Rubens, A. B., & Garrett, M. F. (1991). Anosognosia of linguistic deficits in patients with neurological deficits. In G. P. Prigatano & D. L. Schacter (Eds.), *Awareness of deficit after brain injury: Clinical and theoretical issues* (pp. 40–52). Oxford, England: Oxford University Press.

Schlenck, K. J., Huber, W., & Willmes, K. (1987). "Prepairs" and repairs: Different monitoring functions in aphasic language production. *Brain and Language, 30,* 226–244.

Shuren, J. E., Hammond, C. S., Maher, L. M., Rothi, L. J. G., & Heilman, K. M. (1995). Attention and anosognosia: The case of a jargon aphasic patient with unawareness of language deficit. *Neurology, 45,* 376–378.

Spalletta, G., Serra, L., Fadda, L., Ripa, A., Bria, P., & Caltagirone, C. (2007). Unawareness of motor impairment and emotions in right hemispheric stroke: a preliminary investigation. *International Journal of Geriatric Psychiatry, 22,* 1241–1246.

Spinazzola, L., Pia, L., Folegatti, A., Marchetti, C., & Berti, A. (2008). Modular structure of awareness for sensorimotor disorders: Evidence from anosognosia for hemiplegia and anosognosia for hemianaesthesia. *Neuropsychologia, 46,* 915–926.

Starkstein, S. E., Fedoroff, J. P., Price, T. R., Leiguarda, R., & Robinson, R. G. (1992). Anosognosia in patients with cerebrovascular lesions. A study of causative factors. *Stroke, 23,* 1446–1453.

Stone, S. P., Halligan, P. W., & Greenwood, R. J. (1993). The incidence of neglect phenomena and related disorders in patients with an acute right or left hemisphere stroke. *Age and Ageing, 22,* 46–52.

Turnbull, O. H., & Solms, M. (2007). Awareness, desire, and false beliefs: Freud in the light of modern neuropsychology. *Cortex, 43,* 1083–1090.

Vallar, G., & Ronchi, R. (2006). Anosognosia for motor and sensory deficits after unilateral brain damage: A review. *Restorative Neurology and Neuroscience, 24,* 247–257.

Vuilleumier, P. (2000). Anosognosia. In J. Bogousslausky & J. L. Cummings (Eds.), *Behavior and mood disorders in focal brain lesions* (pp. 465–519). Cambridge, England: Cambridge University Press.

Vuilleumier, P. (2004). Anosognosia: The neurology of beliefs and uncertainties. *Cortex, 40,* 9–17.

Weinstein, E. A. (1991). Anosognosia and denial of illness. In G. P. Prigatano & D. L. Schacter (Eds.), *Awareness of deficit after brain injury: Clinical and theoretical issues* (pp. 240–257). Oxford, England: Oxford University Press.

Weinstein, E. A., & Kahn, R. L. (1955). *Denial of illness: Symbolic and physiological aspects.* Springfield, IL: Charles C. Thomas.

Weinstein, E. A., Lyerly, O. G., Cole, M., & Ozer, M. N. (1966). Meaning in jargon aphasia. *Cortex, 2,* 165–187.

Wernicke, C. (1874). *Der aphasische symptomen komplex.* Breslau, Germany: Cohn & Weigert.

III

Anosognosia Observed in Various Brain Disorders

8

Anosognosia in Huntington's Disease

Daniel Tranel, Jane S. Paulsen, and Karin F. Hoth

The term *anosognosia* was coined by Babinski in 1914 to denote the phenomenon whereby a patient seemed to lack awareness of a specific (and often blatantly obvious) neurological impairment, such as hemiplegia. Over time, the connotation of the term has broadened extensively to subsume all manner of neurological, neuropsychological, and psychiatric symptomatology (e.g., Adair, Schwartz, & Barrett, 2003; Prigatano & Schacter, 1991). Adair et al. (2003) defined anosognosia as "a state in which patients with brain injury deny their disabilities or lack awareness of their deficits" (p. 185). This is a general but accurate description of the condition, and one that can be applied to many different types of symptoms and defects. In fact, Adair et al. (2003) organized their presentation of anosognosia around neurological and/or neuropsychological defects (e.g., "anosognosia for hemiparesis," "anosognosia for visual defects," "anosognosia for amnesia," etc.), much akin to the organizational principle for the chapters that make up the current book. Our own empirical work has contributed to and encouraged this broader approach to the phenomenon, and we pointed out in an early study that the conditions of unawareness and/or denial of illness can occur in regard to cognitive and behavioral abnormalities in much the same way that they have traditionally been observed to occur in regard to basic neurological disabilities (Anderson & Tranel, 1989).

In this context, it is appropriate to consider how anosognosia may manifest in a neurological disease such as Huntington's disease (HD), and this is the focus of the current chapter. Although there are only a handful of empirical studies that have been aimed specifically at the topic of anosognosia and HD, the work is important and has indicated consistently that anosognosia can be a major component of HD, and can have treatment and management implications that are every bit as important as those that have been emphasized in more common conditions such as traumatic brain injury (e.g., see Prigatano, Chapter 12, this volume) and Alzheimer's disease (e.g., see Kaszniak & Edmonds, Chapter 11, this volume). The current chapter will begin with a review of the more recent literature (for a summary of the older literature, up to ca. 1990, the reader is referred to Prigatano & Schacter, 1991). This will be followed by a presentation of work from the University of Iowa, which has focused on anosognosia for cognitive, emotional, and functional abilities in patients with HD. The final section will consider some of the practical implications of the empirical findings for the diagnosis, treatment, and management of patients with HD (Helder et al., 2002).

A Review of the Literature

Huntington's disease is a devastating neurodegenerative disorder in which the affected individual progressively loses motor and cognitive abilities, and experiences psychiatric disturbance. Huntington's disease is an autosomal dominant genetic disorder with the onset of clinical symptoms typically beginning in the third or forth decade of life and unfolding over a long period of time (15 years or longer, on average). Although HD includes multiple symptoms, the clinical diagnosis of HD is made after the unequivocal presence of the movement disorder of HD in the context of a family history or genetic testing.

Given the catastrophic implications of HD, it is not surprising to see frequent references in the literature to the adaptive value of "denial" on the part of many HD patients (e.g., Hans & Gilmore, 1968; Jellife, 1908; Mendez, Adams, & Lewandowski, 1989). From this perspective, denial on the part of HD patients is seen as an understandable coping mechanism. Nonetheless, there has also been the notion that some component of denial and/or unawareness in HD could be neurological in nature, given that the disease affects the basal ganglia and related frontal lobe circuitry (e.g., Aylward et al., 1997; Gontkovsky, 1998; Peinemann et al., 2005; Shoulson, 1992), and that dysfunction in basal ganglia/frontal lobe circuitry has been associated with anosognosia (e.g., Cummings, 1993; Flashman, 2002; House & Hodges, 1988; McGlynn & Schacter, 1997).

Deckel and Morrison (1996) picked up on this idea in a study that investigated awareness of motoric, cognitive, and emotional disabilities in 19 patients with HD. The authors hypothesized that some component of denial in HD patients might represent anosognosia secondary to the degeneration of the basal ganglia and associated brain regions. To measure awareness, the authors utilized a brief set of rating scales comprising eight items (with 5-point ratings ranging from "very impaired" to "excellent") covering basic everyday abilities (walk, use hands and fingers), cognitive functions (talk, remember, concentrate, word finding), motor control (sit still), and emotional control. Anosognosia was operationalized by calculating a difference score between patient self-ratings and the average ratings of two staff raters (with greater discrepancies indicating more unawareness). The key finding was that in the HD group, the difference score was much higher ($M = 5.81$) than in a comparison group of 14 patients with various non-HD neurological conditions ($M = 1.25$). In other words, in the HD group, the raters rated the patients as much worse on the various abilities than the patients rated themselves. The authors also divided the HD group into patients with high anosognosia versus low anosognosia, and they found that the high subgroup had significantly worse performances on several neuropsychological tests, including the Wisconsin Card Sorting Test (WCST). The authors highlighted the WCST findings to argue for the notion that anosognosia in HD may reflect dysfunction in basal ganglia-frontal lobe circuitry (the study did not include any direct measure of neuroanatomical integrity).

Snowden, Craufurd, Griffiths, & Neary (1998) investigated awareness of involuntary movements in HD. The authors studied 40 HD patients, using a questionnaire that covered various aspects of physical symptoms in two main phenomenological categories, which the authors called *direct experience* (e.g., "Do you ever feel fidgety, as if your arms and legs are on the go?") and *consequences* (e.g., "Do you have difficulty doing up buttons?"). The patients' responses on this questionnaire were compared to objective measures of movement disorder derived from the Quantitated Neurologic Examination (QNE). The overall QNE score was correlated with the *consequences* component of the self-ratings (0.41), but interestingly, was *not* correlated with the *direct experience* component of the self-ratings (0.14). Even more striking was the lack of correlation between the Chorea Scale from the QNE and both the *consequences* self-ratings (–0.12) and *direct experience* self-ratings (0.06). Snowden et al., interpreted these findings to indicate that patients with HD have impaired subjective experience of chorea. They went on to suggest that a physiological mechanism for this impairment was likely (the nature of such a mechanism was not specified), since the patients were not generally denying or unaware of physical symptoms and did not have cognitive impairments (including defects on executive function tests) that would explain their impaired subjective experience reports. In short, the HD patients appeared to have accurate appreciation of the consequences of their motor dysfunction, but they lacked awareness of choreiform movements per se.

Similar results were reported by Vitale et al. (2001) in nine patients with HD. The authors had patients subjectively evaluate the presence of dyskinesias while performing specific motor tasks (e.g., gait, finger tapping), and then they compared these ratings to objective measures of dyskinesias. It was found that seven of the nine HD patients were completely unaware of their dyskinesias. Unawareness was significantly related to both disease severity and disease duration. The authors suggested that frontal lobe dysfunction might underlie the lack of awareness manifest in the HD patients.

Following a theme reiterated in earlier studies, whereby anosognosia has been attributed frequently to dysfunction in frontal lobe "executive" systems, Ho,

Robbins, and Barker (2006) conceptualized lack of insight within the context of "executive dysfunction" in patients with HD, and they studied the extent to which HD patients had impaired awareness of their executive impairments. The authors studied 75 HD patients and their caregivers, using the Dysexecutive Questionnaire (DEX) from the Behavioral Assessment of the Dysexecutive Syndrome battery of Wilson, Alderman, Burgess, Emslie, and Evans (1996). The DEX is a 20-item questionnaire (with 5-point Likert scales) that taps into changes in various aspects of executive functioning following brain disease, including emotional/personality changes, motivational changes, behavioral changes, and cognitive changes. The authors used an innovative strategy whereby they had HD patients rate themselves and their caregivers, and in addition, caregivers were asked to rate themselves and the HD patients. This approach allowed not only a means of determining whether HD patients had lack of insight into their own executive problems (by comparing the HD patients' ratings to those provided by their caregivers) but also a means of determining whether HD patients were able to rate executive behavior accurately per se (by comparing how HD patients rated their caregivers with how the caregivers rated themselves). Ho et al. (2006) reported a couple of important findings. The HD patients showed impaired awareness of their executive dysfunction, consistently rating themselves as having less change in the various areas tapped by the DEX than did caregivers. In fact, Ho et al., quantified this, and reported that HD patients underestimated the degree of their executive dysfunction by 26%. However, the HD patients did *not* have a general impairment in rating executive behavior in others, as they accurately rated their caregivers and produced ratings that corresponded well with those provided by the caregivers themselves. It was also shown that the caregivers' ratings of executive dysfunction in the HD patients were more highly correlated with objective measures of disease severity (from the UHDRS), suggesting that the caregivers were providing a more veridical picture of the HD patients' functional status than the HD patients themselves. The authors emphasized that the HD patients' lack of insight regarding dysexecutive behavior has important implications for patient management and rehabilitation.

Work from the University of Iowa

In a recent study from the University of Iowa Huntington's Disease Center of Excellence (Directors: Jane Paulsen, PhD, and Henry Paulson, MD, PhD; Hoth et al., 2007), we extended the work of previous investigators by examining awareness of a range of symptoms in HD, as well as some of the clinical correlates of impaired awareness. A discrepancy rating measure of awareness was utilized, similar to previous approaches to operationalize unawareness. Following the innovative strategy of Ho et al. (2006), we had 66 pairs of patients

Table 8.1 Patient and Collateral Demographic and Clinical Characteristics

Characteristic	Patients ($n = 66$)	Collaterals ($n = 66$)
Mean age (SD)	46.8 (10.0)	48.5 (10.7)
Mean education in years (SD)	14.5 (2.4)	14.6 (2.6)
Mean BDI-II total score (SD)	15.4 (11.1)	8.8 (8.2)
Mean duration of HD symptoms in years (SD)	7.1 (5.0)	NA
Mean UHDRS total functional capacity score (SD)	8.6 (3.1)	NA
Mean UHDRS independence scale (SD)	80.15 (12.25)	NA
Mean UHDRS motor total (SD)	37.8 (17.6)	NA
Sex		
Female (%)	27 (40.9%)	43 (66.2%)
Male (%)	39 (59.1%)	22 (33.8%)

BDI-II, Beck Depression Inventory-II; NA, not applicable or not collected in collaterals; UHDRS, Unified Huntington's Disease Rating Scale.

with HD and their collaterals (e.g., family members, friends, or caregivers) rate both the patient and the collateral on a range of symptoms from the Patient Competency Rating Scale (Prigatano et al., 1986) and additional motor items developed for our study (see Table 8.1 for demographic information about the sample). We examined discrepancies between ratings of both the patient and the collaterals' functioning across several psychometrically derived symptom domains (i.e., behavioral control, affective regulation, and activities of daily living). This permitted comparison of patients' ability to rate their own behavior and functioning versus their ability to rate the functioning of another person. An exploratory goal of the project was to examine the association between unawareness and cognitive functioning. A subset of 19 participants completed neuropsychological assessment measures so that we could examine relations between unawareness and overall dementia severity and executive functioning.

Based on previous work reviewed earlier, patients with HD were predicted to demonstrate unawareness of their symptoms as defined by higher self-ratings of their own competency compared to the ratings provided by their collaterals. Secondly, we predicted that patients would have unawareness across symptom domains, such that patients would rate themselves as more competent in all areas compared to collateral ratings. This hypothesis was motivated by previous findings that HD patients' level of unawareness did not differ for cognitive versus motor symptoms (McGlynn & Kaszniak, 1991), and that HD patients consistently underestimated dysfunction across different subscales on the Dysexecutive Questionnaire as reported by Ho et al. (2006). Thirdly, we anticipated that patients' awareness of their own level of functioning would be more disrupted than their ability to judge another individual's level of functioning consistent with Ho and colleagues' (2006) findings. Finally, we predicted that unawareness of symptoms would be significantly associated with greater dementia severity and poorer performance on measures of executive functioning.

Table 8.2 Patient and Collateral Ratings by Subscale

	Scale	Potential Range	Ratings by Patients		Ratings by Collaterals	
			Scale Mean	Mean Item Score	Scale Mean	Mean Item Score
Ratings of patients	Total	29–145	108.0 (21.8)	3.72	100.12 (21.8)	3.45
	Behavioral control	14–70	55.2 (10.7)	3.95	51.76 (10.2)	3.70
	Emotional control	8–40	27.1 (7.5)	3.38	24.3 (6.3)	3.04
	ADLs	7–35	25.7 (6.7)	3.67	24.1 (6.6)	3.44
Ratings of collaterals	Total	29–145	130.3 (19.2)	4.51	132.6 (8.7)	4.57
	Behavioral control	14–70	64.5 (9.0)	4.62	65.91 (1.2)	4.70
	Emotional control	8–40	33.7 (6.5)	4.23	33.0 (4.4)	4.12
	ADLs	7–35	32.1 (4.8)	4.60	33.9 (1.5)	4.85

ADLs, activities of daily living.

Patients with HD did overestimate their overall competency (including behavioral control, affective regulation, and activities of daily living) as compared to informants' ratings (see Table 8.2). Notably, patients' ratings of their functioning were not significantly associated with objective clinical measures (e.g., neurological exam and cognitive testing; see Table 8.3). In contrast, informants' ratings of the patients were associated with findings on neurological exam and cognitive testing (i.e., dementia severity, memory performance, and several measures of executive functioning). This provides further evidence that patients demonstrated impaired awareness of their actual functioning.

When the HD patients' awareness was examined by symptom domain, patients overestimated their competency in all areas (i.e., behavioral control, affective regulation, and activities of daily living). This is the first study to examine unawareness of affective control and self-care in HD and to compare the magnitude of unawareness across domains. Findings from this analysis support the hypothesized lack of differences in awareness across symptom domains and are consistent with the past literature finding no significant differences in HD patients' underestimation of their motor and cognitive symptoms (Caine & Shoulson, 1983) or across different subscales of the Dysexecutive Questionnaire (Ho et al., 2006).

An important contribution of our study was the comparison of patients' ability to rate their own behavior with their ability to rate the behavior of another person. This provided a test of whether patients' self-awareness was more impaired than their awareness of others' functioning. There was greater overall patient-collateral disagreement for ratings of the patients versus ratings of the collaterals across domains. The findings from our study are consistent with Ho and colleagues' (2006) observations and extend them by examining additional symptom domains (i.e., emotional control and activities of daily

Table 8.3 Intercorrelations between Patient and Collateral Ratings of the Patient and Clinical Measures

	Total Mean Item Score	
Variable	Patient Self-Ratings	Collateral Ratings of Patient
Patient age	.03	.21
Patient years of education	.03	.10
Patient BDI-II total	−.64***	−.20
Collateral age	.15	.15
Collateral years of education	.09	.03
Collateral BDI-II total	−.06	−.21
UHDRS neurological exam total	−.24	−.65**
UHDRS total functional capacity	.49***	.70***
DRS total score	.22	.62**
DRS attention	.08	.41
DRS initiation/perseveration	.18	.47*
DRS construction	.11	.24
DRS conceptualization	.09	−.03
DRS memory	.11	.59**
Verbal fluency	.07	.26
Stroop color/word	−.01	.22
Symbol digit	.23	.49*
IGT advantageous selections	.03	.29
WCST no. categories completed	.26	.32
WCST perseverative responses	−.31	−.55*
WCST failure to maintain set	.08	.12

$n = 66$ for demographic variables, BDI-II, and UHDRS total functional capacity; $n = 18$ for the WCST and the Stroop; $n = 19$ for the neurological exam and all other neuropsychological measures.
BDI-II, Beck Depression Inventory-II; DRS, Dementia Rating Scale; IGT, Iowa Gambling Task; UHDRS, Unified Huntington's Disease Rating Scale; WCST, Wisconsin Card Sorting Task.
*$p < .05$, **$p < .01$, ***$p < .001$.

living). Taken together, these findings allow the important conclusion that the defect in self-rating observed in HD patients cannot be explained simply as a general impairment in their ability to rate behavior.

Exploratory analysis of the association between patients' self-awareness and cognitive functioning provided some limited support for a relationship with dementia severity and executive functioning (see Table 8.4). Correlations between the awareness measures and global cognitive performance on the DRS were not statistically significant; however, relations were in the expected direction and the magnitude of the correlations was suggestive of a potential relationship. Furthermore, failure to maintain set on the Wisconsin Card Sorting Test (WCST) was associated with poorer patient self-awareness, consistent with a previous study that found a relationship between higher levels of anosognosia and WCST perseverative errors in HD patients (Deckel & Morrison, 1996). As mentioned above, reviews of the literature across different neurological and psychiatric disorders suggest that unawareness of deficits has often been

Table 8.4 Neuropsychological Task Performance and Intercorrelations with Patient-Collateral Discrepancy Scores

Measure	Neuropsychological Task Performance		Intercorrelations (r)	
	Mean Raw Score (SD)	Range	Patient-Collateral Mean Item Discrepancy	Patient-Collateral Absolute Value Mean Item Discrepancy
DRS total score	129.0 (7.3)	118–142	−.41	−.26
DRS attention	34.6 (1.3)	32–37	−.35	−.32
DRS initiation/ perseveration	30.5 (5.8)	19–37	−.30	−.20
DRS construction	5.8 (0.9)	2–6	−.14	−.33
DRS conceptualization	36.4 (2.6)	31–39	.14	.39
DRS memory	21.8 (2.3)	17–25	−.52*	−.51*
Verbal fluency total score	19.7 (10.8)	4–41	−.20	.01
Stroop color/word no. correct	29.1 (10.5)	11–53	−.26	−.07
Symbol digit	26.9 (10.3)	13–49	−.23	−.23
WCST no. categories completed	3.7 (2.2)	0–6	−.04	−.17
WCST perseverative responses	28.0 (20.0)	4–72	.24	.30
WCST failure to maintain set	1.4 (1.4)	0–4	−.05	.51*
IGT advantageous selections	54.4 (15.9)	25–84	−.27	−.42

$n = 18$ for the WCST and Stroop; $n = 19$ for all other tasks.
*$p < .05$.
DRS, Dementia Rating Scale; IGT, Iowa Gambling Task; WCST, Wisconsin Card Sorting Task.

associated with poor performance on cognitive measures of executive functioning, potentially implicating frontal systems as important neuroanatomical substrates of awareness (e.g., Flashman, 2002; McGlynn & Schacter, 1997).

Interestingly, there was also a significant correlation between patient unawareness and performance on the DRS memory subscale. The correlation suggests that more impaired memory abilities were associated with poorer self-awareness. Associations between poorer memory performance and unawareness have been documented in Alzheimer's disease (e.g., Starkstein et al., 1995; also see Kaszniak, Chapter 11, this volume), although findings regarding the role of memory impairment in awareness have been somewhat mixed (e.g., Auchus, Goldstein, Green, & Green, 1994; Lopez, Becker, Somsak, Dew, & DeKosky, 1994). The possibility that impaired updating of new memories may contribute to unawareness in HD could be examined in future studies including more comprehensive memory measures.

Our findings also address the possibility that differences in awareness may be associated with demographic or clinical variables. Patients who endorsed more depressive symptoms were more likely to report problems in other areas of behavior and functioning (see Table 8.3). This pattern of responding may reflect a depressive outlook on the world, leading more depressed patients to view themselves negatively, biasing their ability to accurately report about themselves. Another potential explanation is that depression negatively impacts patients' functioning. Post-hoc examination of the association between patients' symptoms of depression and awareness indicated that patients who were more depressed also underestimated their abilities compared to collaterals, suggesting that greater depression might be associated with less self-awareness ($r = -0.46$, $p < .001$). It is possible that among symptomatic individuals with HD, depression and impaired awareness are both associated with similar underlying aspects of disease (e.g., specific neurological dysfunction).

Patients' level of awareness was not associated with age, education, disease duration, or severity of motor signs on neurological exam in our sample. Thus, our study suggests that impaired awareness is not associated with general disease progression per se, at least not within the early to middle stages of HD. Instead, unawareness likely reflects a combination of emotional responses to disease and more specific neurological dysfunction. This idea is consistent with current definitions of awareness in the literature, suggesting that deficits in awareness result from neurological disease but may also occur in combination with psychological reactions to disease. This perspective reflects integrative models of unawareness that posit that it is possible for patients to acquire unawareness of specific impairments or more general unawareness of multiple impairments (e.g., Prigatano & Johnson, 2003).

Conclusion: Implications for Diagnosis, Treatment, and Management of Patients with Huntington's Disease

In closing, and picking up on the theme that "unawareness" or "denial of illness" may be manifestations of the combined effects of a neurobiological mechanism *and* a psychological mechanism, it is worth reiterating the message that anosognosia in HD is a very important part of the patient presentation, and something that has to be assessed accurately and then taken into account in patient treatment and rehabilitation. It goes without saying that patients who cannot or will not acknowledge their functional deficits are extremely challenging to treat, and this has long been recognized as a major obstacle to patient management and rehabilitation (e.g., Prigatano & Schacter, 1991). However, the challenge is not even that simple: there may very well be some psychologically adaptive value to denying or otherwise lacking insight into one's impairments, and approaches to management and rehabilitation have to remain cognizant of this side of the coin as well. One may do more harm than good, for example, by forcing too much attention to impairments and deficits. Also, it is important to conceptualize unawareness in HD within the more general context of illness perception, coping mechanisms, and patient well-being. For example, Helder et al. (2002)

have reported that illness perceptions and coping mechanisms in HD patients are significant predictors of patients' well-being. Specifically, illness perceptions characterized by a strong illness identity (such as embracing the inevitability of the HD course) were negatively correlated with patients' well-being. Coping mechanisms that Helder et al. (2002) found to be less useful included focusing on and venting emotions, behavioral disengagement, and mental disengagement; on the other hand, coping strategies that were directed at accepting the problems that HD brings about were significantly positively related to patients' well-being. The latter finding in particular has obvious implications for the consideration of anosognosia in HD.

Acknowledgments

Supported by NIDA R01 DA022549 and NINDS P01 NS19632 to D. Tranel, and NINDS RO1 NS040068, RO1 NS054893, the Huntington's Disease Society of America Center of Excellence Grant, and the CHDI Foundation to J. S. Paulsen. We would like to acknowledge collaboration with the National Research Roster for Huntington Disease Patients and Families (NINDS N01 NS32357).

References

Adair, J. C., Schwartz, R. L., & Barrett, A. M. (2003). Anosognosia. In K. M. Heilman & E. Valenstein (Eds.), *Clinical neuropsychology* (4th edition) (pp. 185–214). New York: Oxford University Press.

Anderson, S. W., & Tranel, D. (1989). Awareness of disease states following cerebral infarction, dementia, and head trauma: Standardized assessment. *The Clinical Neuropsychologist, 3*, 327–339.

Auchus, A. P., Goldstein, F. C., Green, J., & Green, R. C. (1994). Unawareness of cognitive impairments in Alzheimer's disease. *Neuropsychiatry, Neuropsychology, and Behavioral Neurology, 7*, 25–29.

Aylward, E. H., Li, Q., Stine, O. C., Ranen, N., Sherr, M., Barta, P. E., et al. (1997). Longitudinal change in basal ganglia volume in patients with Huntington's disease. *Neurology, 48*, 394–399.

Caine, E. D., & Shoulson, I. (1983). Psychiatric syndromes in Huntington's disease. *American Journal of Psychiatry, 140*, 728–733.

Cummings, J. L. (1993). Frontal-subcortical circuits and human behavior. *Archives of Neurology, 50*, 873–880.

Deckel, A. W., & Morrison, D. (1996). Evidence of a neurologically based "denial of illness" in patients with Huntington's disease. *Archives of Clinical Neuropsychology, 11*, 295–302.

Flashman, L. A. (2002). Disorders of awareness in neuropsychiatric syndromes: An update. *Current Psychiatry Reports, 4*, 346–353.

Gontkovsky, S. T. (1998). Huntington's disease: A neuropsychological overview. *The Journal of Cognitive Rehabilitation, 16*, 6–9.

Hans, M. B., & Gilmore, T. H. (1968). Social aspects of Huntington's chorea. *British Journal of Psychiatry, 114,* 93–98.

Helder, D. I., Kaptein, A. A., van Kempen, G. M. J., Weinman, J., van Houwelingen, H. C., & Roos, R. A. C. (2002). Living with Huntington's disease: Illness perceptions, coping mechanisms, and patients' well-being. *British Journal of Health Psychology, 7,* 449–462.

Ho, A. K., Robbins, A. O. G., & Barker, R. A. (2006). Huntington's disease patients have selective problems with insight. *Movement Disorders, 21,* 385–389.

Hoth, K. F., Paulsen, J. S., Moser, D. J., Tranel, D., Clark, L. A., & Bechara, A. (2007). Patients with Huntington's disease have impaired awareness of cognitive, emotional, and functional abilities. *Journal of Clinical and Experimental Neuropsychology, 29,* 365–376.

House, A., & Hodges, J. (1988). Persistent denial of handicap after infarction of the right basal ganglia: A case study. *Journal of Neurology, Neurosurgery, and Psychiatry, 51,* 112–115.

Jellife, S. E. (1908). A contribution to the history of Huntington's chorea: A preliminary report. *Neurographs, 1,* 117.

Lopez, O. L., Becker, J. T., Somsak, D., Dew, M. A., & DeKosky, S. T. (1994). Awareness of cognitive deficits and anosognosia in probable Alzheimer's disease. *European Neurology, 34,* 277–282.

McGlynn, S. M., & Kaszniak, A. W. (1991). Unawareness of deficits in dementia and schizophrenia. In G. P. Prigatano & D. L. Schacter (Eds.) *Awareness of Deficit after Brain Injury: Clinical and theoritical issues* (pp. 84–110). New York: Oxford University Press.

McGlynn, S. M., & Schacter, D. L. (1997). The neuropsychology of insight: Impaired awareness of deficits in a psychiatric context. *Psychiatric Annals, 27,* 806–811.

Mendez, N. F., Adams, N. L., & Lewandowski, K. S. (1989). Neurobehavioral changes associated with caudate lesions. *Neurology, 39,* 349–354.

Peinemann, A., Schuller, S., Pohl, C., Jahn, T., Weindl, A., & Kassubek, J. (2005). Executive dysfunction in early stages of Huntington's disease is associated with striatal and insular atrophy: A neuropsychological and voxel-based morphometric study. *Journal of the Neurological Sciences, 239,* 11–19.

Prigatano, G. P., Fordyce, D. J., Zeiner, H. K., Roueche, J. R., Pepping, M., & Case Wood, B. (Eds.) (1986). *Neuropsychological rehabilitation after brain injury.* Baltimore: The Johns Hopkins University Press.

Prigatano, G. P., & Johnson, S. A. (2003). The three vectors of consciousness and their disturbances after brain injury. *Neuropsychological Rehabilitation, 13,* 13–29.

Prigatano, G. P., & Schacter, D. L. (Eds.) (1991). *Awareness of deficits after brain injury: Clinical and theoretical issues.* New York: Oxford University Press.

Shoulson, I. (1992). Huntington's disease. In A. K. Asbury, G. M. McKhann, & W. J. McDonald (Eds.), *Diseases of the nervous system: Clinical neurobiology* (pp. 1159–1168). Philadelphia: W.B. Saunders Company.

Snowden, J. S., Craufurd, D., Griffiths, H. L., & Neary, D. (1998). Awareness of involuntary movements in Huntington's disease. *Archives of Neurology, 55,* 801–805.

Starkstein, S. E., Vazquez, S., Migliorelli, R., Teson, A., Sabe, L., & Leiguarda, R. (1995). A single-photon emission computed tomographic study of anosognosia in Alzheimer's disease. *Archives of Neurology, 52,* 415–420.

Vitale, C., Pellecchia, M. T., Grossi, D., Fragassi, N., Cuomo, T., Di Maio, L., & Barone, P. (2001). Unawareness of dyskinesias in Parkinson's and Huntington's diseases. *Neurological Science, 22*, 105–106.

Wilson, B. A., Alderman, N., Burgess, P. W., Emslie, H., & Evans, J. J. (1996). *Behavioural assessment of the dysexecutive syndrome (BADS)*. Bury St. Edmunds, England: Thames Valley Test.

9

Anosognosia and Parkinson's Disease

George P. Prigatano, Franziska Maier, and Richard S. Burns

Reports of anosognosia in persons with Parkinson's disease (PD) are relatively rare (McGlynn & Kaszniak, 1991). Yet clinicians can readily provide patient examples which suggest that some of these patients appear to have diminished awareness of their motor disorders and, at times, psychosocial consequences. For example, one patient reported: "My wife pointed out that I had difficulty swinging my left arm when walking. I never noticed this." Another PD patient with dysarthria was aware of his speech difficulties, but not the psychosocial consequences. When asked if there were any difficulties with people understanding him, he stated, "No," but he did admit people often ask him to repeat what he says.

Since PD is a progressive disorder, the prospective assessment of impaired self-awareness (ISA) of motor abnormalities in this patient group provides another "window of observation" as to the neurological and neuropsychological correlates of anosognosia. We have initiated a prospective study on anosognosia in PD patients, which will be reported in detail in the future (Maier et al., in preparation). In this chapter, we summarize information on the neurology and neuropsychology of PD that may have relevance to the study of anosognosia in this patient group. We also review selected preliminary findings and their theoretical implications.

Parkinson's Disease

Parkinson's disease is an age-related, neurodegenerative disease that is characterized by the development of bradykinesia, rigidity, resting tremor, a flexed posture, and postural instability. It is species specific, only occurring in humans. Parkinson's disease is the second most common neurodegenerative disorder with an estimated annual incidence and prevalence in individuals ≥65 years of age in the United States of 160/100,000 and 9.5/1,000, respectively (Hirtz et al., 2007). The number of individuals >50 years of age in Western Europe and the world's most populous countries with PD is expected to increase from an estimated 4.1 to 4.6 million in 2005 to 8.7 to 9.3 million in 2030 (Dorsey et al., 2007).

The clinical diagnosis of "probable Parkinson's disease" is based on the presence of bradykinesia and at least one of the other two cardinal features: rigidity and resting tremor. The diagnosis of "definite Parkinson's disease" is based on the clinical finding of one or more of the cardinal motor signs during life and the presence of the characteristic neuropathological changes on brain autopsy. Braak staging of the disease is based on the extent of the intraneuronal pathology using the distribution of α-synuclein immunoreactive Lewy bodies and Lewy neuritis as markers for progression of the disease (Braak et al., 2003). Stage 1 is characterized by pathological changes in the dorsal motor nucleus of the medulla and the anterior olfactory nucleus of the olfactory bulb. In stage 2, changes progress to involve the locus ceruleus of the pons. Only in stage 3 is the substantia nigra of the midbrain involved. By stage 4, pathological changes are found in the basal forebrain and entorhinal cortex, and by stage 5 in the association and prefrontal cortices. Stage 6 is characterized by diffuse involvement of the neocortex (Braak et al., 2003). It is in later stages of progression of the disease that brain regions known to be related to cognition are involved.

The classic neurochemical finding in PD is the deficiency of the neurotransmitter dopamine in the striatum (caudate nucleus and putamen) (Jellinger & Mizuno, 2003). This is attributed to the degeneration of the dopaminergic neurons in the substantia nigra compacta of the midbrain that project to the striatum and synapse on the population of GABA-ergic striatal output neurons that are critical to the function of basal ganglia motor circuits. The deficiency of dopamine in the striatum and impairment of neurotransmission in the nigrostriatal pathway is the basis of the use of replacement therapy with Levodopa, the natural precursor of dopamine, in PD.

The classic Alexander-DeLong model of basal ganglia circuits implies that the basal ganglia modulate cortical function via striato-thalamo-cortical circuits and the impairment of dopamine neurotransmission in the nigrostriatal pathway affects motor control by excessive thalamic inhibition of cortical function (Alexander, Crutcher, & DeLong, 1990; Lewis et al., 2007). A model of segregated reentrant loops and topographical organization has been proposed. According to this model, input to the basal ganglia from specific cortical areas terminates in specific territories within the basal ganglia, which are connected to specific regions of the thalamus, which in turn project to the original cortical region of activity. It has further been suggested that some neuropsychiatric conditions might arise from dysfunction within nonmotor loops of the basal ganglia circuits (DeLong & Wichmann, 2007).

It has been observed that the motor deficits in PD primarily affect internally guided rather than externally guided tasks (Lewis et al., 2007). Considering the question of the awareness of motor deficits by individuals with PD, it is a common clinical observation that patients are not aware of the reduction in arm swing on the affected side that occurs during walking. Also, some patients with involvement of their left, nondominant side seem not to be fully aware of the deficits in motor function that have taken place on that side of the body. An interesting clinical observation that contrasts the differences in conscious awareness of motor phenomena in Huntington's disease and PD is the occurrence of conversion of choreiform jerking movements to a purpose or semi-purposeful movements in Huntington's disease. Although the individual has no warning of the occurrence of a choreiform movement, the movements occur at a slow enough speed that patients with Huntington's disease may become aware of the movement and convert it into a gross purposeful movement. In the case of PD, chronic treatment with Levodopa frequently leads to the development of superimposed, extra, abnormal movements or peak-dose dyskinesia in the form of chorea. Patients with this type of chorea are generally not aware of the occurrence of the movements and do not convert the movements to semi-purposeful movements. This suggests a lack of recognition and/or awareness during the time span of the movements.

In addition to reported unawareness of motor abnormalities, there are reports of unawareness of naps in PD patients with excessive daytime sleepiness (Merino-Andrew, Arnulf, Konofal, Derenne, & Agid, 2003).

Clinical Classification of Severity of Parkinson's Disease

Like other disease states, various clinical stages of PD have been identified. The classification system by Hoehn and Yahr (1967) has been readily adopted by many. Using this classification system, Stage 1 refers to the clinical situation in which symptoms are only on one side of the body. In Stage 2, symptoms are on both sides of the body. Stage 3 is characterized further by balance difficulties. In Stage 4, assistance is required to walk and various motor symptoms are described as severe. In Stage 5, the patient is wheelchair bound.

A Unified Parkinson's Disease Rating Scale (UPDRS) has been developed to help clinicians and researchers describe various aspects of PD and to track the long-term changes associated with it (Stern & Hurtig, 1988). It evaluates the patient via interview and direct examination. Patients are classified along various dimensions, including "mentation, behavior, and mood," activities of daily living, motor functioning, and response to treatment. Various scores can be derived from this scale, including the relative presence of tremor and the severity of bradykinesia and motor rigidity.

The onset of PD is usually late in life and its progression is usually insidious. "Dementia is not an early feature of Parkinson's disease, but estimates of dementia later in the course vary from 15 to 40% or higher" (Blumenfeld, 2002, p. 713).

The Neuropsychology of Parkinson's Disease as It Relates to the Study of Anosognosia

Recently, Tröster and Fields (2008) reviewed the neuropsychological literature on nondemented PD patients. Citing the work of Lieberman (1998), they suggest that about 19% of nondemented PD patients have some form of cognitive impairment. Among these impairments, memory and "executive" dysfunction appear most common. Tröster and Fields (2008) also note that the disturbances in visuospatial problem solving are equally noteworthy in some PD patients. Under "executive function," Tröster and Fields (2008) list functions that involve planning, conceptualization, flexibility of thought, insight, judgment, and self-monitoring and regulation. While acknowledging these functional areas of potential susceptibility in PD, they conclude "...PD patients as a group do not have significant diminished awareness" (Seltzer, Vasterling, Mathias, & Brennan, 2001, p. 541). Disturbances of awareness secondary to any brain disorder, however, can range from subtle to severe and obvious. Certainly, in nondemented PD patients, frank anosognosia is often not present.

Starkstein et al. (1996) examined the neuropsychological and neuropsychiatric characteristics of patients with Alzheimer's disease (AD) and compared them to patients with PD and dementia. Their assessment battery included an anosognosia questionnaire. They noted that anosognosia was clearly more severe in persons with dementia of the Alzheimer's type. Parkinson's disease patients who were judged to be demented had relatively low scores of unawareness of disability.

Seltzer et al. (2001) compared 31 patients with probable AD with 32 patients who met criteria for PD who were not judged to be severely demented. The mean Mini-Mental State Examination (MMSE) score was 18.5 for patients with AD and 23.4 for patients with PD. All patients, however, were judged to be capable of completing study questionnaires. They employed the Patient Competency Rating Scale (PCRS), which was developed primarily for persons with traumatic brain injury (TBI) (Prigatano et al., 1986). It requires judgments about one's overall functional capacity in many areas, but it does not include items specific to the motor deficits associated with PD. To counteract this, the researchers did use nine items from the UPDRS to assess motor functioning. They concluded that in both patient groups there was a tendency for patients to rate their functional capacities higher than caregivers report, but the effect was clearly greater in the AD group. Seltzer et al. (2001) noted that for PD patients "...impaired awareness of self-care deficits and motor dysfunction ... was associated with poorer overall cognitive function..." (p. 126). They emphasized that "PD patients with comparatively intact function displayed relatively well-preserved awareness of their motor and self-care deficits" (p. 126).

Leritz, Loftis, Crucian, Friedman, and Bowers (2004) investigated impaired self-awareness (ISA) of functional difficulties in nondemented PD patients prior to them undergoing unilateral pallidotomy. Patients and caregivers rated the patient's performance on several items sampling motor and activities of daily living from the UPDRS. Generally speaking, PD patients did not show signs of ISA; however, on some items assessing activities of daily functioning, PD patients reported less impairment than their caregivers.

While impaired awareness of motor deficits is not anticipated in most PD patients who are nondemented, we have observed PD patients who are non-demented, yet seem unaware of certain abnormalities. They may be able to judge their overall functional capabilities compared to relatives' reports, and therefore do not show global anosognosia, yet still present with subtle signs of ISA for specific motor deficits when they occur.

Unawareness of Motor Abnormalities in Nondemented, Nondepressed Parkinson's Disease Patients

As noted above, the study of anosognosia in PD patients offers a unique opportunity. One can potentially observe the emergence of the phenomenon and track its neurological and neuropsychological correlates. The literature on anosognosia for hemiplegia suggests that right hemisphere dysfunction may have a special role to play (Cutting, 1978; also see Bottini et al., Chapter 2, this volume; Heilman & Harciarek, Chapter 5, this volume; Karnath & Baier, Chapter 3, this volume). Some authors suggest that the right frontal region may have an especially important role in realistic self-awareness (see Johnson & Ries, Chapter 18, this volume) and is specifically compromised in certain disease states (see Robertson, Chapter 15, this volume; Starkstein & Power, Chapter 10, this volume).

The literature on impaired self-awareness (ISA) in severe traumatic brain injury (TBI) suggests that bilateral cerebral dysfunction may underlie permanent ISA in this patient group (Prigatano, 1999). These two hypotheses can be tested in PD patients by studying the incidence and type of ISA in PD patients who begin by having only right-versus left-sided motor involvement (Stage 1 patients; Hoehn & Yahr, 1967) and then studying patients as they progress into bilateral motor impairments without significant balance difficulties (Stage 2). Moreover, if severity of motor impairment is related to ISA of abnormal motor movements, one would anticipate a greater incidence of anosognosia as patients move to Stages 3, 4, and 5. Finally, studying the level of cognitive impairment in relationship to the stage of motor illness would further help elucidate how cognitive impairment may or may not be related to anosognosia of motor abnormalities. We have initiated a study to track the development of anosognosia from a longitudinal perspective in PD patients (Maier et al., in preparation).

Assessing Anosognosia in Parkinson's Disease Patients

While there are different methods of assessing anosognosia, our research protocol first asks patients if they have any difficulty carrying out a variety of motor tasks. The motor tasks that are inquired about are as follows: rising from a chair, sitting, walking, finger tapping, conducting hand pronation/supination, and carrying out speech tasks. These judgments are compared to clinical ratings. After the patient is asked about potential difficulties in this area, a second test of awareness is conducted. The patient is asked to watch the examiner perform each of the motor tasks referenced above. The patient is then asked to carry out the same tasks that the examiner just performed. After the patient completes all of these tasks, the PD patient is again asked by the examiner whether he or she had any difficulties in carrying out these specific motor acts. The clinician thus notes if there is a disparity between what the patient reports and what is actually observed when carrying out the motor tasks. As a control, caregivers or spouses of the PD patients are asked to do the very same thing.

In addition to sampling "online" awareness of motor functions, PD patients are asked to complete the Parkinson's Disease Questionnaire-39 Items (PDQ-39). This is done to assess their overall view of their functional capacity in everyday life and how PD may have affected their functioning. The patient's caregiver also rates the patient on the PDQ-39. This allows for an additional assessment of awareness in PD patients, particularly as it relates to their functional limitations in their everyday life.

Our study protocol also requires PD patients to carry out a variety of neuropsychological tests, as well as a test of depression, to screen for dementia and/or depression. We are particularly interested in noting whether speed of finger tapping would be slower in PD patients who showed ISA versus non-ISA, since this one task has been shown to be sensitive to ISA in patients with severe TBI (Prigatano & Altman, 1990).

Preliminary Results

To date, we have studied 18 PD patients and their caregivers. Table 9.1 summarizes the demographic characteristics of the PD patients and their caregivers. Parkinson's disease patients tended to be male (13 out of 18), while caregivers tended to be female (5 out of 13). Parkinson's disease patients also had slightly lower MMSE scores, as would be anticipated. However, both PD patients and

Table 9.1 Demographic Data and Entry Criteria of Parkinson's Disease Patients and Caregivers

	PD Patients ($n = 18$)	Caregivers ($n = 18$)	Significance
Age (years)	58. 78 ± 9.39	52.17 ± 10.49	NS
Sex (male/female)	13/5	5/13	$p < .01$
Handedness (r/l/a)	16/1/1	14/3/1	NS
Education (years)	12.11 ± 4.18	10.94 ± 2.82	NS
BDI-II	10.28 ± 6.46	9.06 ± 5.18	NS
MMSE	28.50 ± 1.70	29.67 ± 0.77	$p < .05$

BDI-II, Beck Depression Inventory-II; MMSE, Mini-Mental State Examination; NS, not significant; PD, Parkinson's disease.

caregivers were functioning within the normal range. Also, the self-reported levels of depression on the Beck Depression Inventory-II was comparable between the PD patients and caregivers. Thus, the PD patients studied are nondemented and nondepressed.

Table 9.2 lists the number of PD patients enrolled in the study to date based on the Hoehn and Yahr stages. The table also documents which side of motor deficit was first observed when the patient was brought to medical attention.

On medications, the majority of patients were at Stage 2 (9 out of 18). Off medications, however, nine patients were at Stage 3. There was a preponderance of patients who have right-sided symptom onset, but motor indications of bilateral involvement were common. The progression of the PD in these patients was judged to be slow in 14 out of the 18 patients. It should also be emphasized that 11 out of the 18 patients were considered to have signs of bilateral motor involvement.

While the majority of PD patients were judged to show good awareness of basic motor and day-to-day functioning in everyday life (using the PDQ-39), specific inquiry as to whether they had reduced awareness of motor difficulties right after they carried out a series of motor tasks reveals different findings. Eight (8) out of the 18 patients (44%) had difficulty accurately reporting when abnormal movements occurred when they carried out a series of motor tasks.

Table 9.2 Number of Subjects Presently Enrolled in Study by Side of Motor Onset and Stage of Parkinson's Disease

Parkinson's Disease	Left-Sided Onset	Right-Sided Onset	Total
Unilateral: Hoehn & Yahr, Stage 1	2	5	7
Bilateral: Hoehn & Yahr, Stage 2	2	7	9
Bilateral: Hoehn & Yahr, Stage 3	1	1	2
Total	5	13	18

Table 9.3 Neuropsychological Test Performance of Nondemented Parkinson's Disease Patients Who Are Both "Aware" and "Unaware" of Motor Disturbances

Test	Aware (n = 10)	Unaware (n = 8)	p Value
WAIS-III Vocabulary T-scores	46.30 ± 7.80	47.75 ± 11.91	.759
WAIS-III Matrix Reasoning T-scores	51.30 ± 8.99	49.25 ± 11.30	.673
Finger Tapping Right Hand (raw score)	39.50 ± 11.13	31.13 ± 12.31	.149
Finger Tapping Left Hand (raw score)	43.00 ± 7.96	29.38 ± 11.58	.009
Finger Tapping Right Hand (age/gender adjusted T score)	38.60 ± 14.74	29.75 ± 17.47	.260
Finger Tapping Left Hand (age/gender adjusted T score)	47.50 ± 12.18	26.88 ± 13.75	.004

None of the caregivers demonstrated difficulties of this type. It appears, therefore, that there is a subgroup of PD patients who have limited awareness of motor difficulties when they occur. Parkinson's disease patients who showed this type of difficulty (i.e., unaware subgroup) tended to be older (63.88 years ± 8.71 years) compared to patients who appeared to be aware of motor abnormalities when they occur (mean age = 54.7 years ± 8.14 years, $p = .035$).

While the two groups of patients did not differ on overall level of intellectual functioning, speed of finger tapping in both hands appeared slower in the unaware group. Interestingly, the effect was more robust in the left hand (see Table 9.3).

On the UPDRS, unaware PD patients tended to show bilateral motor symptoms *while on medication*. Six out of 10 patients who were aware had signs of only unilateral motor involvement. In contrast, only 1 out of 7 patients that were unaware had unilateral motor difficulties ($p = .04$). Bilateral motor involvement was, therefore, much more common in PD patients who seem to be unaware of motor abnormalities right after they completed a series of motor tasks.

Implications of Preliminary Findings

Given the limited data presently available, little can be said about the incidence, potential causes, and correlates of ISA for motor abnormalities in nondemented, nondepressed PD patients. However, our preliminary findings suggest that this phenomenon may be more common in older patients who show bilateral motor involvement, but who are not cognitively compromised. This provides suggestive evidence that severity of PD and associated bilateral motor involvement may be related to anosognostic phenomena in PD patients. The role of the right, nondominant hemisphere in ISA for motor abnormalities in PD patients cannot be addressed until a more extensive data set is available. However, the present data reveals that left hand speed of finger tapping was reliably slower in the "unaware" PD patients compared to the "aware" PD patients. It should be emphasized again, however, that these patients show bilateral motor difficulties, and the left hand effect is in the presence of bilateral slow motor functioning.

Given the observations of Braak et al. (2003), degeneration of dopaminergic neurons in the midbrain, forebrain, and prefrontal cortex may play a role in this phenomenon. Stemmer, Segalowitz, Dywan, Panisset, and Melmed (2007) have suggested that error-related negativity (ERN) is "modulated by the midbrain dopaminergic system" (p. 1223). They report that PD patients have attenuated error negativity compared to normal, healthy controls. They also note that error negativity is diminished in early-stage nonmedicated PD patients and then in later stage, medicated PD patients. The implication is that disturbance of midbrain structures that particularly project to the frontal regions may be at the basis of ISA of motor deficits as they occur in some PD patients.

Another alternative is that a specific disturbance of the striatal thalamic cortical circuits may also underlie anosognostic phenomena in PD patients (Alexander et al., 1990). This hypothesis also needs to be further evaluated.

When previous researchers have attempted to investigate whether the side of onset of motor deficits relates to later cognitive impairments, the results have been mixed (Katzen, Levin, & Weiner, 2006; Tomer, Levin, & Weiner, 1993). We will investigate in future studies whether side of onset and the role of bilateral motor impairment in some way interact to produce a greater ISA in PD patients.

The study of anosognosia in PD patients does suggest that disturbance in the dopaminergic system may play an important role in ISA for motor impairments. Research on anosognosia in other patient groups often attempts to relate the disturbance to regional brain dysfunction, but not to specific neurotransmitter disturbances. The study of anosognosia in PD patients may, therefore, provide a new avenue of research that attempts to relate anosognosia to specific neurotransmitter disturbances, in addition to having certain regions of the brain compromised.

Conclusion

The prevailing literature on PD rightfully points out that frank anosognosia for motor deficits in nondemented PD patients is rare, if at all present. However, clinical experience has suggested that some nondemented, nondepressed PD patients may not be aware of motor abnormalities when they occur or shortly after they occur. Studying this group of PD patients over time may provide useful insights as to the mechanism underlying ISA of motor deficits in neurodegenerative disorders. The preliminary findings, based on a small sample, suggest that PD patients who are older and who show bilateral motor involvement tend to be the ones who do not detect abnormal motor movements when carrying out a series of simple motor tasks. These individuals, however, do not differ on estimates of intellectual ability, and therefore, cognitive impairment does not appear to be an explanatory concept.

The neurology of PD suggests that as the disease progresses, there is greater brainstem and possible frontal lobe involvement as a direct result of the dopaminergic disturbance underlying PD. Attenuation of error negativity measured by electroencephalographic recordings suggests that midbrain and frontal dysfunction may be at the basis of the failure to detect motor errors when they occur. Robertson's research (see Chapter 15, this volume) would be compatible with such an interpretation.

References

Alexander, G. E., Crutcher, M. D., & DeLong, M. R. (1990). Basal ganglia-thalamocortical circuits: Parallel substrate for motor, oculomotor, "prefrontal" and "limbic" functions. *Progressive Brain Research, 85*, 119–146.

Blumenfeld, H. (2002). *Neuroanatomy through clinical cases.* Sunderland, MA: Sinauer Associates, Inc.

Braak, H., Del Tredici, K., Rüb, U., de Vos, R.A., Jansen Steur, E. N., & Braak, E. (2003). Staging of brain pathology related to sporadic Parkinson's disease. *Neurobiology of Aging, 24*(2), 197–211.

Cutting, J. (1978). Study of anosognosia. *Journal of Neurology, Neurosurgery, and Psychiatry, 41,* 548–555.

DeLong, M. R., & Wichmann, T. (2007). Circuits and circuit disorders of the basal ganglia. *Archives of Neurology, 64,* 20–24.

Dorsey, E. R., Constantinescu, R., Thompson, J. P., Biglan, K. M., Holloway, R.G., Kieburtz, K., Marshall, F. J., Ravina, B. M., Schifitto, G., Siderowf, A., & Tanner, G. M. (2007). Projected number of people with Parkinson disease in the most populous nations, 2005 through 2030. *Neurology, 68*(5), 384–386.

Hirtz, D., Thurman, D. J., Gwinn-Hardy, K., Mohamed, M., Chaudhuri, A. R., & Zalutsky, R. (2007). How common are the "common" neurologic disorders. *Neurology, 68*(5), 326–337.

Hoehn, M. M., & Yahr, M. D. (1967). Parkinsonism: Onset, progression, and mortality. *Neurology, 12,* 427–442.

Jellinger, K. A., & Mizuno, Y. (2003). Parkinson's disease. In D.W. Dickson (Ed.) *Neurodegeneration: The molecular pathology of dementia and movement disorders* (pp. 159–187). Basel, Switzerland: ISN Neuropath Press.

Katzen, H. L., Levin, B. E., & Weiner, W. (2006). Side and type of motor symptom influence cognition in Parkinson's disease. *Movement Disorders, 21*(11), 1947–1953.

Leritz, E., Loftis, C., Crucian, G., Friedman, W., & Bowers, D. (2004). Self-awareness of deficits in Parkinson disease. *The Clinical Neuropsychologist, 18,* 352–361.

Lewis, M. M., Slagle, C. G., Smith, D. B., Truong, Y., Bai, P., McKeown, M., Milman, R., Belger, A., & Huang, X. (2007). Task specific influences of Parkinson's disease on the striato-thalamo-cortical and cerebello-thalamo-cortical motor circuits. *Neuroscience, 147*, 224–235.

Lieberman, A. (1998). Managing the neuropsychiatric symptoms of Parkinson's disease. *Neurology, 50*(Suppl. 6), S33–S38.

McGlynn, S. M., & Kaszniak, A. W. (1991). Unawareness of deficits in dementia and schizophrenia. In G. P. Prigatano & D. L. Schacter (Eds.), *Awareness of deficit after brain injury: Clinical and theoretical issues* (pp. 84–110). New York: Oxford University Press.

Merino-Andrew, J., Arnulf, I., Konofal, E., Derenne, J. P., & Agid, Y. (2003). Unawareness of naps in Parkinson's disease and in disorders with excessive daytime sleepiness. *Neurology, 60*, 1553–1554.

Prigatano, G. P. (1999). *Principles of neuropsychological rehabilitation.* New York: Oxford University Press.

Prigatano, G. P. & Altman, I. (1990). Impaired awareness of behavioral limitations after traumatic brain injury. *Archives of Physical Medicine and Rehabilitation, 71*, 1058–1064.

Prigatano, G. P., Fordyce, D. J., Zeiner, H. K., Roueche, J. R., Pepping, M., & Case Wood, B. (Eds.) (1986). *Neuropsychological rehabilitation after brain injury.* Baltimore: The Johns Hopkins University Press.

Seltzer, B., Vasterling, J. J., Mathias, C. W., & Brennan, A. (2001). Clinical and neuropsychological correlates of impaired awareness of deficits in Alzheimer disease and Parkinson disease: A comparative study. *Neuropsychiatry, Neuropsychology, and Behavioral Neurology, 14*(2), 122–129.

Starkstein, S. E., Sabe, L., Petracca, G., Chemerinski, E., Kuzis, G., Merello, M., & Leiguarda, R. (1996). Neuropsychological and psychiatric differences between Alzheimer's disease and Parkinson's disease with dementia. *Journal of Neurology, Neurosurgery, and Psychiatry, 61*, 381–387.

Stemmer, B., Segalowitz, S. J., Dywan, J., Panisset, M., & Melmed, C. (2007). The error negativity in nonmedicated and medicated patients with Parkinson's disease. *Clinical Neurophysiology, 118*, 1223–1229.

Stern, M. D., & Hurtig, H. I. (1988). *The comprehensive assessment of Parkinson's disease.* New York: PML Publications.

Tomer, R., Levin, B. E., & Weiner, W. J. (1993). Side of onset of motor symptoms influences cognition in Parkinson's disease. *Annals of Neurology, 34*(4), 579–584.

Tröster, A. I., & Fields, J. A. (2008). Parkinson's disease, progressive supranuclear palsy, corticobasal degeneration, and related disorders of the frontostriatal system. In J. Morgan & J. Ricker (Eds.), *Textbook of clinical neuropsychology* (pp. 536–577). New York: Taylor & Francis.

10

Anosognosia in Alzheimer's Disease: Neuroimaging Correlates

Sergio E. Starkstein and Brian D. Power

From an etymological perspective, anosognosia may be construed as the lack of knowledge or awareness of physical or mental disorders. Among patients with dementia, anosognosia was construed as the denial or lack of awareness of impairments in activities of daily living (ADL) and cognitive deficits. In this chapter, we will review those studies that examined neuroimaging correlates of anosognosia in dementia. Most studies have been carried out in patients with Alzheimer's disease (AD), although more recent studies have also included individuals with frontotemporal dementia (FTD) and mild cognitive impairment (MCI). Our review will include studies using a variety of imaging techniques, such as single-photon emission tomography (SPECT), positron emission tomography (PET), and functional magnetic resonance imaging (fMRI). Given the scant number of radiological studies on anosognosia in dementia, we will also review pertinent neuropathological studies.

Single-Photon Emission Tomography Studies of Anosognosia in Dementia

Reed, Jagust, and Coulter (1993) carried out the first study of anosognosia in dementia. They examined 20 patients with AD using SPECT and iodine 123-labeled N-isopropyl-p-iodoamphetamine. Anosognosia was diagnosed based on a relatively crude semi-structured interview, which classified patients into those with full awareness of cognitive impairment, "shallow" awareness (defined as the transient recognition of memory loss), and no awareness (defined as the denial of memory impairment in response to direct questions with regard to memory impairment). The main finding was that patients with either shallow or no awareness had significantly lower cerebral blood flow (CBF) involving the right dorsolateral frontal lobe as compared to patients with full awareness. One limitation of the study was that the diagnosis of poor or no awareness was carried out using an instrument of unknown reliability and validity. Patients had to rate the extent of their own memory problems, and awareness of deficits on other functional or behavioral domains was not assessed. Sample size was small ($n = 20$), and patients with or without anosognosia were not comparable on demographic and clinical variables that may impact SPECT findings (e.g., age, duration of illness, severity of cognitive impairment).

A second study was carried out by Starkstein and co-workers (1995) in a sample of 46 patients with AD. Anosognosia was diagnosed using the *Anosognosia Questionnaire-Dementia* (AQ-D), which consists of 30 questions that assess impairments on basic and instrumental ADL as well as behavioral changes (Starkstein, Sabe, Chemerinski, Jason, & Leiguarda, 1996). Answers range from no deficits to deficits always present, and higher scores indicate more severe impairments. The final score is the difference between caregiver's and patient's scores, so that positive scores indicate that the informant rated the patient as more impaired than the patient's own evaluation. The AQ-D demonstrated adequate reliability and validity (Starkstein et al., 1995). A cut-off score of 14 points for anosognosia was based on findings in an age-comparable healthy sample (Starkstein et al., 1995). Patients with anosognosia ($n = 12$) were matched for age, duration of illness, and Mini-Mental State Examination (MMSE) scores with patients with no anosognosia, and assessed with technetium Tc99m exametazime SPECT. There was a significant group by side interaction, with the anosognosia group showing a lower cerebral blood flow (CBF) in the right hemisphere as compared to the no anosognosia group (see Figure 10.1). There also was a significant group by side by region interaction: patients with anosognosia showed significantly lower CBF in frontal superior and inferior regions of the right hemisphere as compared to the group without anosognosia. One limitation of the study was that the diagnosis of anosognosia was based on cut-off scores on a severity rating scale rather than on valid diagnostic criteria for anosognosia.

Ott, Noto, and Fogel (1996) examined correlations between anosognosia and Tc99m-HMPAO-SPECT findings in a series of 40 patients with probable or possible AD (six patients had small infarctions, and three patients had primary progressive aphasia). Anosognosia was rated by a neurologist during an interview with the patient and a caregiver using the *Clinical Insight Rating Scale*, which assesses awareness of situation, memory deficits, functional deficits, and disease progression. Regions of interest (ROI) on the SPECT involved prefrontal, temporal, parietal, and lateral occipital regions, and measures consisted of counts per pixel normalized to average cerebellum count. There was a significant correlation between worse awareness and lower perfusion in inferior frontal, right posterior temporal and right occipital perfusion. However, a stepwise multivariate linear regression was

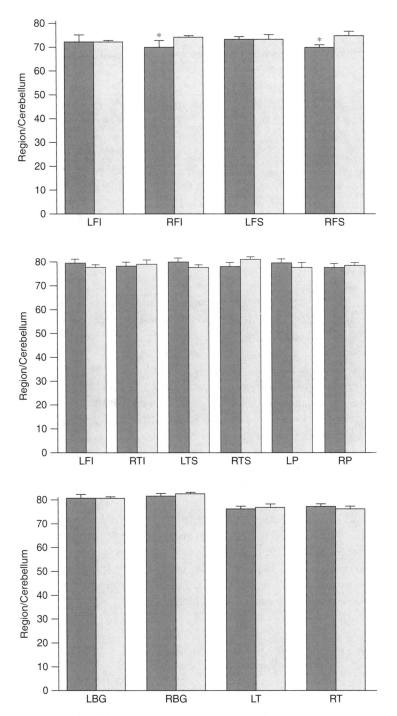

Figure 10.1 rCBF for different brain regions. Group × side interaction (F (1, 22) = 4.39, p < .05), group × side × region interaction (F (6, 132) = 2.82, p = .01. L = left, R = right, F = frontal, T = temporal, P = parietal, BG = basal ganglia, T = thalamus, I = inferior, S = superior.

significant for right occipital perfusion only. Based on these findings the authors suggested that AD patients with poor insight may have relatively more pathology in the left frontal and right temporo-occipital regions, or a disconnection of a transcortical frontotemporal circuit (Ott et al., 1996).

Mendez and Shapira (2005) examined with either PET or SPECT a series of 29 patients with FTD. Anosognosia was diagnosed based on the patients' responses to the insight question from the *Consortium to Establish a Registry in AD* (CERAD) instrument ("Tell me why you are here") and to three additional questions (whether the patient had an illness requiring medical attention, whether there was a behavioral change lately, and whether relatives or friends considered the patient to have an illness). The patients responses were graded as *(1)* awareness of a medical problem, *(2)* partial awareness, *(3)* no awareness of illness, but awareness of relatives' or friends' concerns, and *(4)* full unawareness. PET or SPECT images were visually inspected, and patients with right frontal hypometabolism had the greatest loss of insight.

Vogel and co-workers (Vogel, Hasselbalch, Gade, Ziebell, & Waldemar, 2005) examined the association between anosognosia and frontal CBF in a series of 36 patients with AD, 36 individuals with MCI, and 33 age-comparable healthy controls. Cerebral blood flow was measured with Tc99m-HMPAO SPECT. Anosognosia was assessed using two instruments: *(1) The Memory Questionnaire*, in which the patient and an informant are asked to rate the patient's memory ability currently as compared to 5 years before. The difference between the informant's and the patient's score is used as the measure of anosognosia; and *(2) The Anosognosia Rating Scale*, a categorical four-point scale rated by a clinical psychologist based on an overall impression after a neuropsychological assessment and an interview with the patient and an informant. Awareness is classified into full, shallow or no awareness, or denial of impairment. Image analysis was carried out on the orbitofrontal cortex, the middle frontal gyrus, and the inferior frontal gyrus. Thirty-eight percent of AD patients and 40% of MCI individuals had full insight, 24% and 48%, respectively, had shallow insight, and 24% and 12%, respectively, had no insight. There was a significant correlation between higher informant/patient discrepancies on The Memory Questionnaire and lower blood perfusion in right and left inferior frontal gyrus. On the other hand, the classification based on the Anosognosia Rating Scale produced no significant correlations with regional CBF.

Positron Emission Tomography Studies of Anosognosia in Dementia

Harwood and co-workers (2005) assessed the relationship between impaired insight into cognitive and functional deficits and brain metabolic changes using [18]-fluorodeoxyglucose ([18]FDG) PET in a study that included 41 patients with probable AD.

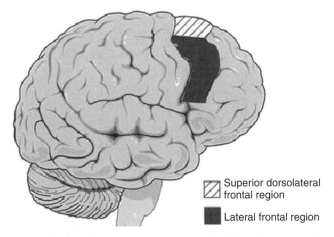

Superior dorsolateral
frontal region

Lateral frontal region

Figure 10.2 Brain drawing showing frontal regions significantly correlated with insight scores in AD.

Anosognosia was assessed with the Inaccurate Insight item of the *Neurobehavioral Rating Scale*. Briefly, the patient had to judge the extent of her or his own cognitive deficits and functional disability, and this information was compared to data obtained from an informant. Scores range from 0 (insight is well preserved; accurate appraisal of deficits and disability), to 6 (severe deficits of insight: the patient is unaware of her or his own deficits, and her or his plans entirely disregard cognitive limitations and may be dangerous). The main finding was that less insight was significantly correlated with hypometabolism involving the right lateral and superior dorsolateral frontal regions (see Figure 10.2). The main limitation of the study was that anosognosia was assessed based on answers to a single item on a generic rating scale for behavioral problems.

Salmon and co-workers (2006) used (^{18}FDG) PET to assess 209 patients with AD. Anosognosia was assessed with an experimental questionnaire that assessed 13 cognitive domains. This instrument provides a total score that corresponds to the caregiver evaluation of the patient's cognitive status, a total score as rated by the patient, and a discrepancy score (caregiver minus patient). The main finding was that after accounting for age, apathy, and severity of dementia, there still was a negative correlation between the discrepancy score and metabolic activity in the left and right temporoparietal cortex, bilateral inferior temporal cortex, and left inferior frontal sulcus (i.e., more severe anosognosia was associated with lower metabolic activity in those regions; see Figures 10.3 and 10.4). While these findings were consistent with previous reports of an association between ano-sognosia and hypometabolism in frontal and parietal association cortices, the authors were unable to replicate findings of more severe metabolic deficits in the

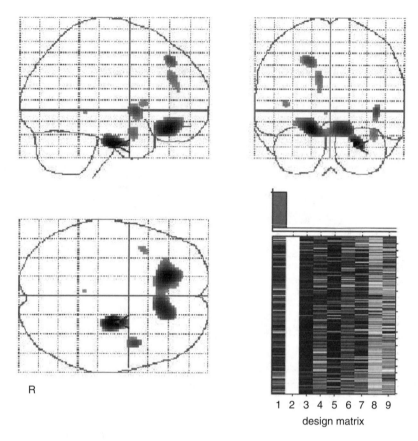

Figure 10.3 Relationship between brain metabolism in AD and self-cognitive assessment of patients. (From Salmon et al., 2006, reprinted with permission from John Wiley & Sons, Inc.: *Human Brain Mapping*, 27: 588–597.)

right as compared to the left hemisphere. They stressed the association between anosognosia and hypometabolism in right parahippocampal and orbitofrontal regions given the role of the latter in autobiographical memory, and they suggested that anosognosia could result from "a failure to retrieve episodes of memory problems" (Salmon et al., 2006). They further suggested that medial temporal dysfunction may impair a comparison mechanism between current information and personal knowledge of cognitive abilities. Based on the hypothesis that orbitofrontal dysfunction may result in failure to suppress irrelevant memories and to select appropriate information, the authors suggested that anosognosia may also result from reduced inhibition of proactive interference of remote experiences and from deficits "to update associations between impaired cognitive capacities and their decreased qualitative value" (Salmon et al., 2006). A final suggestion was that the association between anosognosia and metabolic deficits in the temporoparietal junction and superior frontal sulcus

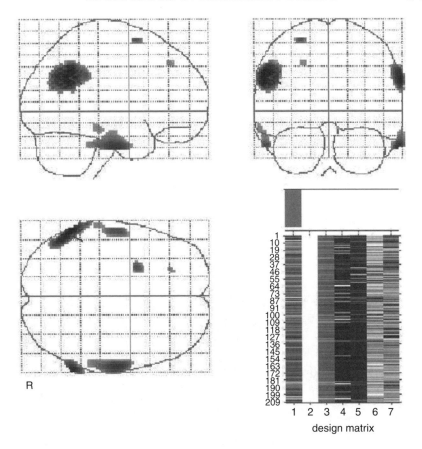

Figure 10.4 Relationship between brain metabolism in AD and the discrepancy (carer minus patient) score. (From Salmon et al., 2006, reprinted with permission from John Wiley & Sons, Inc.: *Human Brain Mapping*, 27: 588–597.)

may reflect "impairment of self-referential processes." Based on empirical findings and theoretical interpretations, the authors suggested two different neural substrates for anosognosia: *(1)* the impairment on self-assessment of cognitive impairment may involve the orbitofrontal cortex and may be related to disturbed judgment processes, *(2)* the increased caregiver minus patient discrepancy may be related to temporo-parietal changes and may result from disturbed comparative judgments required during "perspective taking."

Ruby and co-workers (2007) recruited 21 patients with FTD to examine associations between awareness about personality traits and behavior in social and emotional circumstances and brain metabolic activity as assessed with [18]FDG-PET. Anosognosia was assessed with two questionnaires: (1) The *"behavior prediction"* questionnaire includes questions describing life events likely to trigger an emotional reaction, and participants indicate how they would react to the event by choosing one out of three potential reactions (this was referred to as the "first-person perspective condition"). Participants were also asked how their respective informants (usually their partners) would react ("third-person perspective condition"); (2) The *"personality assessment"* consisted of a series of adjectives describing personality traits, and participants had to score how accurately each adjective described their own and their partner's personality. There were no significant correlations between discrepancy scores on the personality questionnaire and regional brain metabolic activity. On the other hand, there were significant correlations between more severe unawareness of one's own social behavior and decreased metabolic activity in the temporal poles (see Figure 10.5). Given the role of the left temporal cortex on memory and emotional processing, the authors suggested that anosognosia for social disability in the frontal variant of FTD may result from "deficits affecting autobiographical information involving the self in socioemotional interaction" (Ruby et al., 2007). More specifically, they proposed that anosognosia may result from a

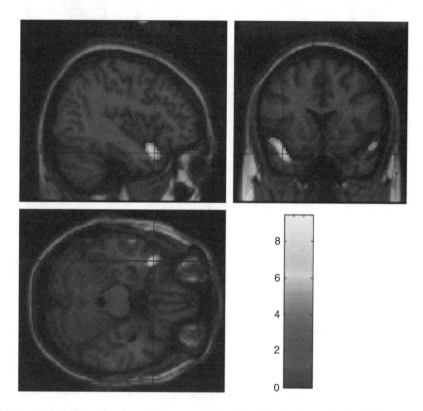

Figure 10.5 Left temporal activation correlates with the score for social disability among patients with FTD. (From Ruby et al., 2007, reprinted with permission from the Massachusetts Institute of Technology: *Journal of Cognitive Neuroscience*, 19: 671–683.)

mismatch between current behavior and impaired processing of personal and emotional events in memory.

Functional Magnetic Resonance Imaging Studies of Anosognosia in Dementia

Ries and co-workers (2007) examined the neural correlates of anosognosia in MCI using fMRI. The authors conceptualized anosognosia as a continuum of awareness deficits ranging from mild to severely impaired. Based on studies showing that the medial prefrontal cortex and the anterior cingulate cortex are activated by tasks that require appraisal of self-relevant information, Ries and co-workers (2007) hypothesized that dysfunction of the medial prefrontal cortex could account for anosognosia in MCI. Anosognosia was assessed based on the discrepancy score (informant rating minus patient rating) on the *Informant Questionnaire on Cognitive Decline in the Elderly* (IQCODE; Jorm, 2004). The study included 16 patients with MCI and 16 healthy elderly controls. None of the patients with MCI had evidence of decline in activities of daily living. The fMRI technique consisted of a self-appraisal task and a baseline semantic condition. The self-appraisal condition consisted of the presentation of adjectives (e.g., calm, creative) and participants had to decide whether each presented word would apply to their personality. The main result was a significant negative correlation between IQCODE differential scores and activation on medial prefrontal and posterior cingulate regions during the self-appraisal task (i.e., the lower the discrepancy the higher the activation). This correlation remained unchanged after adjusting for the severity of memory deficits. The authors concluded that dysfunction of "cortical midline structures" are linked to anosognosia for cognitive deficits in MCI. One methodological limitation is that due to the relatively small sample size, the correlation analysis was restricted to a small number of a priori selected brain regions. Another limitation is that individuals with MCI had lower IQCODE scores than controls. Given that IQCODE mostly assesses deficits in daily life activities, it is possible that some MCI individuals may have had early dementia.

In a more recent study, Ruby and co-workers (2008) examined the hypothesis that anosognosia for behavioral and personality changes in AD is related to deficits in memory and "perspective taking." The study included 14 individuals with mild AD and 17 elderly controls. Participants were asked to make personality assessments concerning themselves and their closest caregiver, based on their own ("first-person perspective") or their caregiver's perspective ("third-person perspective"). All participants were assessed with fMRI and regions of interest were selected a priori based on their association with specific cognitive functions (personality trait assessment, perspective taking, autobiographical and semantic memory). When AD patients assessed their own personality there was a significant

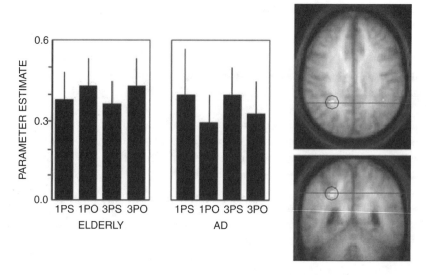

Figure 10.6 Activation clusters in the intra-parietal sulcus in the AD group as compared to elderly controls. 1PS = first person perspective on self, 1PO = first person perspective on other, 3PS = third person perspective on self, 3PO = third person perspective on other. (From Ruby et al., 2008, reprinted with permission from Elsevier, *Neurobiology of Aging*, 30: 1637–51.) (See Color Plate 10.6)

bilateral activation of the intraparietal sulcus, as compared to greater activation of the ventromedial prefrontal cortex for elderly controls on the same task (Figure 10.6). The authors considered that this result is congruent with the involvement of the intraparietal sulci in "self-processing," whereas the stronger frontal activation in their elderly controls as compared to the AD subjects is consistent with the use of "more reflective, recollective and evaluative processes."

When the AD patients had to take a third-person perspective (regardless of whether their own or their caregiver's personality was being assessed), there was greater activation of the posterior dorsomedial prefrontal cortex and the lateral orbitofrontal cortex. These activations were stronger than the ones observed in elderly controls, although they were similar to activations in a group of young volunteers. Of note, self-awareness scores for the AD group were not significantly different than in controls. The authors interpreted that the more efficient knowledge of elderly controls of their own and their relatives' personality could explain a diminished need of inferential and reasoning activities, and therefore a lesser need of frontal activation as compared to the AD group. The authors also hypothesized that deficits in "perspective taking" may be related to impairments in processing a mismatch between "self and other perspective of self abilities." Due to deficits on episodic memory and impairments to "correctly represent others' reaction and mind," Patients with AD may fail to assess their own personality and may depend on others to make the mismatch explicit.

Third-person perspective deficits may also account for poor awareness of personality changes referring to social emotion. The authors admitted that several confounding variables, such as the magnitude of brain atrophy and hemodynamic changes in AD, were not accounted for and that the increased activations in AD could be affected by these factors.

Neuropathological Studies of Anosognosia in Dementia

Marshall and co-workers (2004) examined the neuropathological correlates of anosognosia among 41 individuals with neuropathologically verified AD. Based on information obtained during a clinical interview and formal neuropsychological testing, patients were divided into four categories: *(1)* spontaneous complaint, *(2)* agrees when questioned, *(3)* unaware, and *(4)* denies but appears aware. Patients in one of the first two categories were included in the "aware" group ($n = 23$), while patients in one of the last two categories ($n = 18$) were included in the "no aware" group. Neuropathological analysis consisted in counting senile plaques as well as neurofibrillary tangles bilaterally in the superior and middle frontal gyrus, superior temporal lobe, prosubiculum, and entorhinal cortex. The main finding was that patients with no awareness had a greater number of senile plaques in the right prosubiculum as compared to patients with awareness, and this finding remained significant after groups were matched for the severity of cognitive deficit. No other significant between-group difference was found on the other brain regions examined.

Summary of Neuroimaging Results

Given the heterogeneity of methods used to diagnose anosognosia, the variety of neuroimaging techniques (e.g., SPECT studies using different radioactive markers and cameras, PET, and fMRI studies using different activation paradigms), the variety of patients assessed (e.g., MCI, mild and/or moderate AD, FTD), the relatively small number of neuroimaging studies, and differences in statistical analysis (e.g., calculating differences between patients with or without anosognosia, or calculating correlations between neuroimaging findings and severity of anosognosia), discrepant findings are certainly expected. Nevertheless, the fact that 6 of the 11 studies reviewed above showed a significant association between anosognosia and perfusion or metabolic changes in the right frontal lobe represents a rather robust finding. This association comprises studies that used either SPECT or PET, and patients with either AD or FTD. These studies focused on the whole frontal lobe, "superior" and "inferior" frontal regions, or the "dorsolateral" frontal region, but without more detailed regional analysis. Other studies demonstrated an association between anosognosia and temporal lobe dysfunction. One of these studies also found concomitant inferior frontal changes (Ruby et al., 2008), another showed bilateral temporo-parietal changes (Salmon et al., 2006), and a third was a neuropathological study which found a significant association between more pathology in a restricted region of the temporal lobe and more severe anosognosia (Marshall et al., 2004).

A summary of fMRI findings is more difficult to convey. These studies used original and innovative paradigms that may clarify, in a sophisticated fashion, the human mechanisms of insight. On the other hand, the relationship between the activation paradigms and the clinical construct of anosognosia is of unclear validity. The activation of the intraparietal sulcus during the self-appraisal of personality traits, and the activation of the prefrontal and orbitofrontal cortices during third-person appraisals may not be comparable with the results produced by the more straightforward approach to measure anosognosia used in PET and SPECT studies.

Methodological Limitations

Methodological limitations of neuroimaging studies in dementia may be subsumed into three groups: *(1)* the methodology used to assess and diagnose anosognosia, *(2)* the neuroimaging methods, and *(3)* sampling methods.

Most studies reviewed above defined anosognosia as the discrepancy between caregiver and patient ratings of deficits on activities of daily living. Thus, positive scores indicate that the caregiver rated the patient as more impaired than the patient's own evaluation (i.e. the patient was less aware of her or his functional deficits). One of the main limitations of this method is that the caregiver's score becomes the de facto gold standard, and caregivers may potentially misjudge the extent of the patients' deficits. The second limitation is that the subtraction method may minimize discrepancies among patients with early dementia and less functional impairments. Several studies classified patients into different levels of awareness using a semi-structured interview with unknown reliability and validity, short scales with good reliability but unknown validity, or single items from generic assessments, supplemented by additional ad-hoc questions. Other studies required patients to estimate their current memory ability as compared to 5 years before, and anosognosia was calculated as the discrepancy between the caregivers' and patients' estimations. One of the limitations of this method is that it depends at least partially on the patients' memory performance, which may have an important impact on the overall estimation of anosognosia.

Recent studies using fMRI activation estimated anosognosia based on conceptually complex paradigms, such as asking patients to characterize their own personality attributes, as well as the potential behavior of patients in theoretical emotional and social contexts. These mental exercises had to be carried out from a "first-person perspective" (the way patients see themselves) or a "third-person perspective" (the patients' estimations on how their personality and behaviors may be regarded by their respective caregivers). While novel and provocative, these methods have yet to be established as valid markers of anosognosia in dementia (a critical analysis of these methods exceeds this review). A final methodological problem is found in studies that use estimations of deficits on activities of daily living (such as the IQCODE) to assess anosognosia among individuals with MCI, which, by definition, are supposed to have intact functioning. This suggests that some MCI studies may have included some patients with early dementia.

Methodological limitations also apply to the different neuroimaging techniques. As briefly mentioned above, SPECT studies used different radioactive markers, cameras with different definition, and different methods to identify ROIs. Positron emission tomography studies used different thresholds of significance and different statistical techniques (group comparisons or correlations). Functional magnetic resonance imaging studies are interesting new additions to the study of anosognosia in dementia, but whether the paradigms being used are valid measures of anosognosia remains to be established.

Finally, the studies reviewed above included heterogeneous samples, ranging from patients meeting criteria for mild or moderate AD, to those with FTD or MCI. Nevertheless, rather than a limitation, sampling differences may be considered a strength, given that demonstrating similar neuroimaging correlates of anosognosia in different populations may actually reinforce the relevance of the structural–clinical association.

Mechanism of Anosognosia: Evidence from Neuroimaging

Neuroimaging studies of anosognosia led to the proposal of different mechanisms for this condition. Studies by Reed, Mendez, Vogel, and Starkstein suggested that anosognosia may result from deficits of self-monitoring or response-inhibition secondary to right frontal dysfunction. Nevertheless, the concepts of "self-monitoring" or "response-inhibition" have not been clarified in these studies. For instance, it is unclear in what consists the "self-monitoring" process that allows an individual to be aware of her or his own capacities. Some authors suggested that deficits of self-monitoring in dementia may result from executive dysfunction, but most studies could not find a significant association between executive dysfunction and anosognosia in AD.

Harwood and co-workers (2005) reported right frontal dysfunction among AD patients with anosognosia and/or delusions and suggested that poor insight may facilitate the production of delusions "via impaired simulation and reality-checking mechanisms." Other authors based their theory on the premise that anosognosia may result from deficits of self-assessment of cognitive abilities, as well as autobiographical and episodic memory deficits. Salmon and co-workers (2006) associated impaired self-evaluation (i.e. updating qualitative judgments associated with cognitive deficits) with orbitofrontal hypometabolism, and deficits comparing current information with cognitive and personal knowledge with medial temporal hypometabolism. They also considered that the significant correlation between discrepancy scores (i.e. caregiver minus patient) and temporo-polar hypometabolism reflects deficits of "self-referential process and perspective taking." In other words, anosognosia in dementia was proposed to be secondary to deficits to remember episodes of memory problems and to deficits with personal factual knowledge. A "ventral limbic complex" (comprising the hippocampus and orbitofrontal cortex) was considered to play an important role in mediating conceptual information of personal significance. Salmon and co-workers (2006) further suggested that the hippocampus may work as a "comparator" whose dysfunction may impair matching current information with self-knowledge of cognitive capacities. Anosognosia was also considered to result from deficits to inhibit "proactive inference of remote experiences," and to associate current cognitive deficits with their decreased "quality value." Based on suggestions that the temporo-parietal region may mediate self-referential processes and perspective taking, Salmon and co-workers construed their finding of a significant correlation between increased discrepancy scores and temporo-parietal hypometabolism as underlying deficits in personal and "third-person" self-knowledge. Taken together, these PET findings were interpreted as showing that anosognosia may result from orbitofrontal dysfunction and concomitant deficits in "present reality" monitoring with a negative impact on judgment and decision making, as well as temporo-parietal dysfunction and concomitant deficits in "self versus other comparative judgment" and "impaired ability to see oneself with a third-person perspective." These novel and provocative hypotheses based on sophisticated activation paradigms raise, however, a number of methodological and conceptual issues. For instance, the meaning of assessing oneself with a "third-person perspective" is unclear. This may simply be the knowledge patients have about what their respective caregivers believe about themselves. An impaired ability to see oneself through a third-person perspective does not necessarily mean the patient has a specific deficit in "perspective taking." This impairment could result from a host of other factors, such as refusing to accept the point of view of the caregiver due to behavioral changes in the patient (e.g., irritability, increased stubbornness), ambiguities in the caregiver's opinion (e.g., occasionally refusing to confront the patient with her or his limitations), and divergent contextual information from different sources. In some cases, deficits of "perspective taking" could be a manifestation rather than the cause of anosognosia. Deficits of "present reality monitoring" are neither necessary nor sufficient to produce anosognosia, given that some patients deny or minimize their functional deficits irrespective of the context in which they are, or may fully acknowledge their limitations but explain them away as secondary to non-illness-related causes.

Based on their finding of a significant association between decreased metabolic activity in the left temporal pole and anosognosia for behavioral change in social situations (but not for personality changes), Ruby and co-workers (2007) proposed independent mechanisms for subtypes of anosognosia among patients with FTD. Anosognosia for behavioral change in social and emotional contexts was explained as secondary to a role for the temporal poles to retrieve personality-relevant and time-specific memories "involving the self in socio-emotional interactions" (Ruby et al., 2007). Temporal lobe dysfunction may lead to deficits to remember personal behaviors in social contexts, which may result in a "self-representation that does not match the current behaviour" (Ruby et al., 2007). On the other hand, the authors proposed that contextual feedback may allow FTD patients to sense the potential mismatch between self-representation and actual behavior. They suggested that impaired third-person perspective may contribute to build an impaired self-representation in social situations, preventing the proper adjustment of self-representation and contextual feedback. In the authors' words "perspective taking ability is necessary for building a self-representation that agrees with the individual's current behaviour." Anosognosia for social disabilities was construed as related to impaired processing of social/emotional autobiographical information, leading to "an inability to remember the self as it behaves in social situations," while perspective taking disability may prevent FTD from correcting self-representations based on contextual information.

While theoretically appealing and building on previous findings, this theory has several limitations. The concept of "matching" self-representations with current behaviors is not clearly explained, and it is unclear how this matching may occur (e.g., how a "self-representation" is selected to be matched with a putative "social behavior," what are the criteria for a "correct" matching, what are the neural structures engaged in judging the result of the matching process). Some methodological issues should be noted as well. In some studies activations are considered to indicate that the activated region subserves (appropriately) a given cognitive function so that reduced activations are considered abnormal, while in other studies diminished activations are considered to represent a decreased need of resources, and therefore, to reflect better functioning.

On the basis that memory deficits are not sufficient to produce anosognosia, Ruby and co-workers (2008) suggested that anosognosia may result from a faulty processing of a mismatch between "self and other perspectives on self abilities" secondary to deficits in perspective taking. The authors further hypothesized that when AD patients' avowals of personality traits contradict their current behavior, it is only external information that may correct this mismatch. But in case the external information cannot be correctly "represented," there will be no awareness of mismatch. The authors suggested that patients may be unable to rely on episodic memory for correct awareness, and therefore, they depend on "online representation of other's mind about themselves to sense a mismatch and correct the self-representation." The authors suggested that the significant association between prefrontal activation and impaired third-person perspective taking may indicate "recruitment of inferring and monitoring more than memory processes." Anosognosia for personality changes was suggested to result from judgments based on nonupdated biographical knowledge and deficits using a third-person perspective for correcting self-evaluation. These hypotheses raise conceptual issues that are similar to the ones already described. It is unclear how external information is "represented," and what the criteria for a "correct" representation are. A discussion of the concept of "self-personality assessment" is beyond the scope of the present chapter, but it should not be reduced to the relatively simple paradigms used in activation studies.

Finally, the neuropathological finding of an association between prosubiculum changes and anosognosia was suggested to depend on reciprocal connections between this structure and the amygdala. The authors suggested this circuit may mediate "information regarding emotional valence supporting awareness." The connections between the prosubiculum and the anterior cingulate were considered to be relevant to error detection, self-reflection, and self-awareness. As with the studies reviewed above, the concept of self-reflection or how error detection works will need further elaboration.

Conclusions

While anosognosia is a frequent finding in AD and other dementias, neuroimaging studies on this interesting and clinically relevant phenomenon are still few. Given the heterogeneity in sampling (with studies including patients with AD, FTD, or MCI), different imaging techniques (SPECT, PET, and fMRI), and methods to assess anosognosia (ranging from nonstandardized clinical interviews to well-validated scales), it is relevant that most studies showed a significant association between anosognosia and right frontal abnormalities. Recent activation studies using fMRI techniques and sophisticated paradigms that assess awareness of personality and behavioral changes showed activations in frontal and parietal regions. These findings suggest that anosognosia in AD may result from defective self-representations and third-person perspective, but further study of these complex psychological constructs and their relationship with brain dysfunction are needed.

References

Harwood, D. G., Sultzer, D. L., Feil, D., Monserratt, L., Freedman, E., & Mandelkern, M. A. (2005). Frontal lobe hypometabolism and impaired insight in Alzheimer disease. *American Journal of Geriatric Psychiatry, 13*(11), 934–941.

Jorm, A. F. (2004). The Informant Questionnaire on cognitive decline in the elderly (IQCODE): A review. *International Psychogeriatrics, 16*(3), 275–293.

Marshall, G. A., Kaufer, D. I., Lopez, O. L., Rao, G. R., Hamilton, R. L., & DeKosky, S. T. (2004). Right prosubiculum amyloid plaque density correlates with anosognosia in Alzheimer's disease. *Journal of Neurology, Neurosurgery & Psychiatry, 75*(10), 1396–1400.

Mendez, M. F., & Shapira, J. S. (2005). Loss of insight and functional neuroimaging in frontotemporal dementia. *Journal of Neuropsychiatry & Clinical Neurosciences, 17*(3), 413–416.

Ott, B. R., Noto, R. B., & Fogel, B. S. (1996). Apathy and loss of insight in Alzheimer's disease: A SPECT imaging study. *Journal of Neuropsychiatry & Clinical Neurosciences, 8*(1), 41–46.

Reed, B. R., Jagust, W. J., & Coulter, L. (1993). Anosognosia in Alzheimer's disease: Relationships to depression, cognitive function, and cerebral perfusion. *Journal of Clinical & Experimental Neuropsychology, 15*(2), 231–244.

Ries, M. L., Jabbar, B. M., Schmitz, T. W., Trivedi, M. A., Gleason, C. E., Carlsson, C. M., et al. (2007). Anosognosia in mild cognitive impairment: Relationship to activation of cortical midline structures involved in self-appraisal. *Journal of the International Neuropsychological Society, 13*(3), 450–461.

Ruby, P., Collette, F., D'Argembau, A., Peters, F., Degueldre, C., Balteau, E., et al. (2008). Perspective taking to assess self-personality: What's modified in Alzheimer's disease? *Neurobiology of Aging, 30*(10), 1637–1651.

Ruby, P., Schmidt, C., Hogge, M., D'Argembeau, A., Collette, F., & Salmon, E. (2007). Social mind representation: Where does it fail in frontotemporal dementia? *Journal of Cognitive Neuroscience, 19*(4), 671–683.

Salmon, E., Perani, D., Herholz, K., Marique, P., Kalbe, E., Holthoff, V., et al. (2006). Neural correlates of anosognosia for cognitive impairment in Alzheimer's disease. *Human Brain Mapping, 27*(7), 588–597.

Starkstein, S. E., Sabe, L., Chemerinski, E., Jason, L., & Leiguarda, R. (1996). Two domains of anosognosia in Alzheimer's disease. *Journal of Neurology, Neurosurgery & Psychiatry, 61*(5), 485–490.

Starkstein, S. E., Vazquez, S., Migliorelli, R., Teson, A., Sabe, L., & Leiguarda, R. (1995). A single-photon emission computed tomographic study of anosognosia in Alzheimer's disease. *Archives of Neurology, 52*(4), 415–420.

Vogel, A., Hasselbalch, S. G., Gade, A., Ziebell, M., & Waldemar, G. (2005). Cognitive and functional neuroimaging correlate for anosognosia in mild cognitive impairment and Alzheimer's disease. *International Journal of Geriatric Psychiatry, 20*(3), 238–246.

11

Anosognosia and Alzheimer's Disease: Behavioral Studies

Alfred W. Kaszniak and Emily C. Edmonds

Babinski (1914) first coined the term *anosognosia* in reference to the curious behavior of several patients who suffered left-sided paralysis due to right-hemisphere cerebral damage. These patients seemed to be unaware of their paralysis and never complained about their impairment. Since Babinski's description, a large number of reports have been published that confirm the frequent occurrence of the syndrome and extend use of the term *anosognosia* to include similar unawareness of deficit phenomena in patients suffering from a variety of neurological impairments (for reviews, see McGlynn & Schacter, 1989; Prigatano & Schacter, 1991a, 1991b; Vuilleumier, 2000). Within the present chapter, we use the terms *anosognosia* and *impaired awareness* of deficit synonymously, although it is recognized that these and other terms (e.g., *denial of deficit, impaired self-awareness of deficit, loss or lack of insight*) used within the relevant literature can reflect differing connotations and theoretical commitments (for discussion, see Markova, Clare, Wang, Romero, & Kenny, 2005).

Alzheimer's disease (AD) is the most common neurological illness causing the syndrome of dementia, characterized by progressive impairment of memory and other cognitive functions (Bondi, Salmon, & Kaszniak, 2009; Cummings & Benson, 1992; Kaszniak, 1986, 2002). Alzheimer's disease is a neurodegenerative disorder with neuropathological features of neuron loss, neuritic plaques, and neurofibrillary tangles that are most prominent in the mediotemporal, posterior temporal, parietal, and frontal brain regions (Braak & Braak, 1991; DeKosky & Scheff, 1990; Hyman, Van Hoesen, Damasio, & Barnes, 1984). Persons with AD show significant memory impairment early in the course of their dementia, along with somewhat milder attention and executive function deficits. These and other cognitive functions become increasingly impaired with disease progression (Kaszniak, Wilson, Fox, & Stebbins, 1986). The nature and progression of these cognitive impairments appear to correspond with the pattern of observed neuropathological changes (see Bondi et al., 2009). Clinical observations have suggested anosognosia to be a relatively frequent feature of AD (McGlynn & Schacter, 1989). Although variation in methods used to identify anosognosia, and in dementia severity of patient samples that have been studied, prevents confident determination of anosognosia prevalence in AD (Clare, 2004), it has been estimated that anywhere from approximately 20% (Migliorelli et al., 1995) to as many as 81% of AD patients (Reed, Jagust, & Coulter, 1993) show impaired awareness of their deficits. Research on anosognosia in AD has clear practical relevance. It has been proposed that anosognosia may pose a challenge to early identification and diagnosis, and a threat to treatment compliance (Cosentino & Stern, 2005). Anosognosia may also increase injury risk for AD patients (e.g., Cotrell & Wild, 1999; Kaszniak, Keyl, & Albert, 1991; Pachana & Petriwskyj, 2006; Starkstein, Jorge, Mizahi, Adrian, & Robinson, 2007), and it has been found to be associated with increased caregiver burden (DeBettignies, Mahurin, & Pirozzolo, 1990; Seltzer, Vasterling, Yoder, & Thompson, 1997).

Several reviews of research on anosognosia in AD have been published (e.g., Agnew & Morris, 1998; Clare, 2004; Cosintino & Stern, 2005; Kaszniak, 2003; Kaszniak & Zak, 1996; Markova et al., 2005; McGlynn & Kaszniak, 1991a; Moulin, 2002; Ownsworth, Clare, & Morris, 2006). Most of these reviews comment upon the inconsistency, across studies, regarding whether anosognosia is present in AD, and if present, whether it is correlated with other patient characteristics and behaviors. In the present chapter, we draw from and update these reviews, with a particular emphasis on how different approaches to assessing the presence, degree, and nature of agnosognosia in AD constrain conclusions that may be drawn. Studies concerned with neuroimaging correlates of anosognosia in AD are excluded, since these are discussed by Starkstein and Power (see Chapter 10, this volume). The chapter begins with a brief discussion of motivational versus nonmotivational factors in apparent anosognosia, followed by sections describing clinician observations and clinical rating studies, and interpretations permitted by differing research methods. We then discuss a neuropsychological model of the heterogeneity of anosognosia in AD, followed by an examination of the methods and results of empirical research employing experimental procedures designed to explore the nature of anosognosia in this illness. The chapter closes with a summary emphasizing theoretical and practical implications.

Motivational versus Nonmotivational Aspects of Anosognosia in Alzheimer's Disease

There has been debate concerning the question of whether anosognosia, in various neurological disorders, is due primarily to motivational or nonmotivational factors. Motivated unawareness of deficit (also termed "defensive denial";

see Markova et al., 2005; McGlynn & Schacter, 1989) accounts of anosognosia posit an "ego-protective" blocking of symptoms or deficits from conscious awareness, via psychodynamic defense mechanisms. Weinstein and Kahn (1955), the most influential advocates of this view, held that "The effect of the brain damage is to provide the milieu of altered function in which the patient may deny *anything* that he feels is wrong with him. Some motivation to deny illness and incapacity exists in everyone and the level of brain function determines the particular perceptual-symbolic organization, or language, in which it is expressed" (p. 123). Focusing primarily upon anosognosia for hemiplegia, Ramachandran (1995) points out that a psychodynamic interpretation fails to account for two important aspects of anosognosic syndromes. First, anosognosia appears to be associated with damage to particular brain structures (e.g., in anosognosia for hemiplegia, inferoparietal cortex, frontal lobes, and subcortical structures connecting to these cortical regions, with greater incidence of unawareness seen in right- than in left-hemisphere damage) and is not generally observed when peripheral, spinal, lower brain stem, or cortical primary sensory or motor areas alone are affected (McGlynn & Schacter, 1989). Second, unawareness is often domain specific. For example, a patient may deny an obvious hemiplegia but simultaneously admit to other disabling or distressing symptoms. Further, an occasional patient with upper and lower extremity hemiplegia may admit that his or her leg is paralyzed but insist that his or her arm is not (Ramachandran, 1995). Similar arguments can be made regarding anosognosia in AD. Research concerned with neuropsychological (see below) and neuroimaging (see Starkstein & Power, Chapter 10, this volume) correlates have frequently shown that anosognosia in AD is associated with measures assumed to reflect dysfunction of particular brain regions, and not consistently with overall level of dementia severity or length of disease progression. In addition, there is some evidence, albeit controversial (as discussed more fully below), that awareness varies across the different cognitive, behavioral, and functional impairments/changes in AD, even when these might appear to be equally disabling or potentially distressing (e.g., Green, Goldstein, Sirockman, & Green, 1993; Kaszniak & Christenson, 1996; Kotler-Cope & Camp, 1995; Vasterling, Seltzer, Foss, & Vanderbrook, 1995).

Thus, motivated unawareness does not appear to be a sufficient explanation for anosognosia in AD. However, the possible influence of motivated or defensive denial, in combination with neurologic/neuropsychologic variables, must be given consideration, and accepted or rejected on relevant empirical grounds, in the study of anosognosic phenomena in any patient group (Markova et al., 2005; Weinstein, 1991). Ownsworth et al. (2006) have proposed an integrated biopsychosocial framework for understanding awareness disorders in AD, which includes neurocognitive factors (e.g., frontal cerebral damage and executive system dysfunction), psychological factors (premorbid personality characteristics, defensive reactions, reliance on pre-illness ways of thinking and reacting), and socio-environmental context (e.g., perception of whether the individual stands to gain or lose from disclosing problems in the specific assessment context; availability of relevant information or opportunities to recognize changes in functioning; cultural values; whether selected assessment tasks have provided an opportunity for the display of awareness of deficit). Although focusing primarily upon research that implicitly or explicitly assumes a neuropsychological model of anosognosia in AD, whenever motivational factors and/or context are specifically addressed in research reports, they are given consideration in the following review.

Clinical Observations and Clinician Rating Scales for Anosognosia in Alzheimer's Disease

Clinical accounts of anosognosia in AD began appearing in the early 1980s (e.g., Gustafson & Nilsson, 1982). Reference to impaired awareness of memory and other cognitive deficits can also be found in clinical descriptions of other dementing illness (for reviews, see McGlynn & Kaszniak, 1991a; Pannu & Kaszniak, 2005). These include vascular dementia (most often associated with multiple and bilaterally distributed small cerebral infarctions), frontotemporal dementia, including Pick's disease (a relatively rare neurodegenerative disorder that presents with impaired impulse control, poor social judgment, and cognitive deficit, and typically involves severe atrophy of frontal and temporal cortices), Huntington's disease (an autosomal dominant genetic neurodegenerative disorder marked by motor, cognitive, and emotional impairments, which are associated with prominent caudate nucleus atrophy and frontal lobe changes), and cognitive impairment associated with human immunodeficiency virus (HIV) infection.

Published clinician rating studies of anosognosia in AD have been based upon patient record review (Auchus, Goldstein, Green, & Green, 1994), unstructured interview (e.g., Verhey, Rozendaal, Ponds, & Jolles, 1993), and structured interview (e.g., Sevush & Leve, 1993). These clinician rating studies have disagreed in their conclusions regarding whether anosognosia occurs early (Frederiks, 1985) or late (Schneck, Reisberg, & Ferris, 1982; Sevush & Leve, 1993) in the course of a progressive dementia. As noted in the review by Kaszniak and Zak (1996), some clinical observation reports have supported an association between anosognosia for cognitive deficits and greater dementia severity in AD (e.g., Migliorelli et al., 1995; Sevush & Leve, 1993; Starkstein, Sabe, Chemerinski, Jason, & Leiguarda, 1996; Verhey et al., 1993), while other reports have not (e.g., Auchus et al., 1994; Reed et al., 1993). It has also been noted that some patients in the advanced stages of AD may verbalize acknowledgment of their impairments (Mayhew, Acton, Yauk, & Hopkins, 2001). Clinical rating studies of anosognosia in AD have similarly come to varying conclusions regarding association with the specific severity of memory impairment (Auchus et al., 1994; Reed et al., 1993; Starkstein et al., 1995; Weinstein, Friedland, & Wagner, 1994). There is some evidence, from clinician rating studies, for the proportion of AD patients rated as showing unawareness of deficit to increase over time. McDaniel and colleagues (1995) reported a 33.1% increase over 2 years, and Weinstein et al. (1994) reported an 8.2 % increase over 2 to 3 years. However, as pointed out by Clare and Wilson (2006), these percentages also suggest that the majority of AD patients in these reports did not show significant change in unawareness of deficit over the follow-up interval.

Clinical rating studies have thus not found a consistent relationship between anosognosia in AD and length of illness, dementia severity, or memory impairment severity. Given that there is evidence for an association between impaired self-awareness of memory functioning (as indexed by experimental metamemory tasks) and focal frontal lobe damage (Janowsky, Shimamura, & Squire, 1989; Pannu, Kaszniak, & Rapcsak, 2005; Schnyer et al., 2004), clinical rating studies have examined the possibility of an association between anosognosia in AD and measures thought to reflect frontal lobe functioning. Clinical observation of differing dementia diagnoses have encouraged such investigation. Persons with frontotemporal dementia have been described as unaware of the marked changes in their social behavior and personality that are observed by family members and other informants (Gregory & Hodges, 1996). Some clinical observers (e.g., Gustafson & Nilsson, 1982) have suggested that anosognosia occurs earlier in the course of Picks disease than in AD. Both of these illnesses are typically associated with evidence of frontal lobe pathology, but frontal pathology is more severe in the early stages of Pick's disease than AD (for review, see Bondi et al., 2009). Studies examining the correlates of clinically rated anosognosia in AD have supported an association with neuropsychological measures thought related to frontal lobe dysfunction. Loebel, Dager, Berg, and Hyde (1990) found a positive correlation between decreased fluency of speech (generative naming test, which has been found to be associated with left or bilateral frontal cortex damage; e.g., Janowsky, Shimamura, Kritchevsky, & Squire, 1989) and clinical ratings of impaired awareness of memory deficit in persons with AD. Lopez, Becker, Somsak, Dew, and DeKosky (1994) found their clinical classification of impaired awareness in a large sample of persons with probable AD to be associated with both lower mental status test performance and specific impairment on measures of executive functions (e.g., choice reaction time, behavioral set-shifting) that have been associated with frontal lobe damage (for review of relevant evidence, see Duke & Kaszniak, 2000). Possibly reflecting the difficult behavioral disturbances that may accompany frontal dysfunction in AD (Johnson, Brun, & Head, 2007), clinical ratings of anosognosia have been found to be related to self-report measures of increased caregiver burden (Seltzer et al., 1997). Despite this convergence of evidence relating clinical ratings of anosognosia in AD to frontal lobe dysfunction, it should be noted that Clare, Wilson, Carter, Roth, and Hodges (2004) found no association between a clinical rating scale evaluating awareness of memory deficit in AD and performance on several neuropsychological executive function tests.

Weinstein et al. (1994) reported that among the 41 persons with AD whom they interviewed, 7 claimed that their memory was good but admitted to difficulty in finding words, several others denied memory impairment but admitted to reading difficulties, and 12 denied all cognitive deficits. Weinstein and colleagues (1994) argue that denial of particular impairments among their AD patients was related to premorbid personality traits (conscientiousness, a strong work ethic, high expectations for oneself, and the view that illness is a sign of weakness). Similarly, Cotrell and Lein (1993), based on interviews with AD patient caregivers, concluded that denial of difficulties in AD is linked to pre-morbid coping styles. Problems in evaluating such motivated unawareness inter-pretations of clinical interview reports include a relative lack of specificity regarding how and under what conditions the clinical interviews were obtained. Adding to the difficulty in evaluating such reports are the possibilities that some patients who do not describe themselves as impaired may be aware of deficits but choose not to disclose them within a particular context (Ownsworth et al., 2006), while other patients may describe awareness of deficits and yet show poor recognition of these deficits during related task performance and fail to employ compensatory strategies (Giovanetti, Libon, & Hart, 2002). Alternative interpretations and theoretical models for understanding apparent anosognosia domain specificity in AD are discussed below.

Clinician ratings of anosognosia in AD, particularly when based on struc-tured interview, may have advantages over other assessment methods (such as those described below), when comprehension deficits may limit the validity of patient responses to printed questionnaires or other verbal tasks (Sevush & Leve, 1993). As noted by Kaszniak and Zak (1996), clinical observations and ratings also remain important for generating empirically testable hypotheses, but they allow for only limited and tentative conclusions concerning both the correlates and nature of anosognosia in AD. Methods employed in making clinical obser-vations, such as clinical rating scales and patients' responses to interview ques-tions have sometimes been unstructured (e.g., Reed et al., 1993; Verhey et al., 1993) and the types of rating scales or questionnaires are variable across reports, limiting the ability to compare across studies. Clinical observation reports have sometimes involved clinician ratings that use nominal (i.e., aware or unaware; Auchus et al., 1994; Loebel et al., 1990) or limited-range ordinal scale levels of measurement (e.g., three-point scales used by Sevush & Leve, 1993 and Weinstein et al., 1994; the four-point Anosognosia Rating Scale developed by Reed et al., 1993). This limits rating scale reliability and the statistical power available for either comparing patient groups or for correlation with other variables. It also appears to be the case that few persons with dementia are completely unaware of their memory deficits. Most mildly to moderately impaired AD patients appear to rate their memory as not being as good as their spouse's, but rate themselves as less impaired than they are rated by their spouses or than their task performance would indicate (e.g., McGlynn & Kaszniak, 1991b). Dementia patients thus typically exhibit *underawareness* or underappreciation of the severity and extent of their deficits. As argued by Kaszniak and Zak (1996), nominal or ordinal scale clinical ratings of impaired awareness of deficit that use relatively few rating categories may be unable to capture more subtle degrees of underawareness. Other authors (Clare & Wilson, 2006; McDaniel et al., 1995; Verhey et al., 1993) have also criticized clinician ratings of deficit unawareness for being excessively global and insufficiently reliable.

Finally, clinician ratings do not allow for detailed examination of questions regarding the *nature* of anosognosia. These questions include whether apparent anosognosia represents inaccurate self-efficacy beliefs (see Hertzog & Dixon, 1994), perhaps reflecting a failure to update stored representations concerning the self, poor self-monitoring of memory and other cognitive functions, impaired cognitive estimation ability, or some combination of these or other factors. Systematic patient–informant questionnaire discrepancy approaches, and experimental metacognitive measures, which employ explicit operational definitions and quantification of deficit awareness, do appear capable of addressing such questions. The following section examines the questions regarding the nature of anosognosia in AD that appear to be addressable by particular research methodologies, followed by sections that review the procedures and results of research employing these methods.

Questions Regarding the Nature of Anosognosia in Alzheimer's Disease

Several reviewers (e.g., Clare, 2004; Cosentino & Stern, 2005; Kaszniak & Zak, 1996; Moulin, 2002) have pointed out that conclusions concerning the presence, degree, and nature of apparent anosognosia are substantially dependent upon the research methods employed. In addition to possible variability between different measures in reliability, and in sensitivity and specificity for detecting unawareness of deficit, it also appears that different methods provide information relevant to different theoretical constructs concerning metacognition (a term referring to our personal "knowledge about how we perceive, remember, think, and act"; Metcalfe & Shimamura, 1994, p. xi) and the nature of anosognosia. Since Hart (1965) introduced the feeling-of-knowing (or recall-judgment-recognition) research paradigm, metacognition research on normal adults has focused predominantly upon metamemory (that aspect of metacognition specifically concerned with one's own memory functioning). Over the past 25 years, an increasing number of studies have utilized both questionnaire and performance-referenced experimental metamemory tasks in an effort to understand the nature of impaired awareness of memory deficits in several different neurological disorders, including AD (for review, see Pannu & Kaszniak, 2005).

Investigators with an interest in exploring the nature of anosognosia in AD from a metacognitive perspective have typically used one or more of the following methodologies: *(1)* examination of questionnaire discrepancies between patient self-ratings and informants' (typically family caregivers) ratings of patient impairment/disability, and *(2)* patient performance on various experimental metacognitive tasks (e.g., feeling-of-knowing judgments, judgments of learning, ease-of-learning judgments, recall readiness tasks, global task performance predictions and postdictions, retrospective confidence judgments; see below for task descriptions). Following the framework proposed by Hertzog and Dixon (1994), metacognitive research can be categorized into three general groups of constructs that have been examined: *(1)* knowledge about how memory and other cognitive processes function and the utility of different strategies in task performance; *(2)* self-monitoring of memory and other cognitive process, defined as awareness of the current state of one's own memory or other cognitive systems; and *(3)* self-referent beliefs about memory or other cognitive functions (memory/cognition self-efficacy beliefs). It has been argued (Kaszniak & Zak, 1996) that studies using patient–informant question-naire discrepancy measures of anosognosia in AD have provided information relevant primarily to questions concerning the construct of memory/cognition self-efficacy beliefs. In contrast, studies that have used various performance-referenced experimental metacognitive tasks have provided information that can be interpreted as relevant to questions about "online" memory/cognition self-monitoring, as well as memory/cognition self-efficacy beliefs and knowledge about the functioning of memory and other cognitive processes. The rationale for this argument is provided within the review of specific relevant studies in the sections that follow.

Neuropsychological Theoretic Models of the Nature of Anosognosia in Alzheimer's Disease

Agnew and Morris (1998) were the first to propose a specific metacognitive/neuropsychological model concerning the nature of anosognosia in AD, drawing from and expanding upon the more general neuropsychological model of anosognosia put forward by McGlynn and Schacter (1989). As illustrated in Figure 11.1, Agnew and Morris (1998) theorize that incoming information about an incident of memory failure enters episodic memory, from which it is sent on to a conscious awareness system (CAS; Schacter, 1990), theorized to be dependent upon the parietal lobes, allowing the incident to be consciously

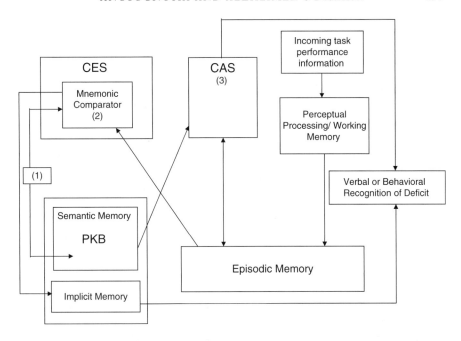

Figure 11.1 Agnew and Morris model of anosognosia in Alzheimer's disease. (Adapted and modified from Agnew & Morris, 1989; Ansell & Bucks, 2006. Modified by permission from Elsevier Publishers: *Neuropsychologia, 44*, 1095–1102, Copyright, 2006.) CAS, conscious awareness system; CES, central executive system; PKB, personal knowledge base. Numbers indicate theorized location of dysfunction, relating to differing types of anosognosia in Alzheimer's disease: 1, mnemonic anosognosia; 2, executive anosognosia; 3, primary anosognosia.

experienced. The information from the incident is simultaneously sent to a "mnemonic comparator" (an aspect of the central executive system [CES] thought to be largely dependent upon frontal brain structures/processes) and compared to a semantic "personal knowledge base" (PKB), in which are stored representations of one's own memory ability in relation to that of others. When a mismatch is detected by the mnemonic comparator, the PKB is then updated, through inputs from episodic to semantic memory, and this updated information from the PKB is directed back into the CAS, allowing for an awareness of deficit. Focusing upon the apparent heterogeneity of anosognosia in AD, Agnew and Morris (1998) apply this model to describe three different types of anosognosia: *Mnemonic anosognosia* is posited to reflect a dysfunction in the path between the mnemonic comparator of the CES and semantic memory of the PKB. Individuals with this type of anosognosia might demonstrate short-term knowledge of a memory failure immediately upon completing a task, but this knowledge would not effectively update the PKB. These individuals would thus have no enduring awareness of their memory impairment, although they might exhibit emotional or behavioral responses suggesting implicit (nonconscious) knowledge of their deficit (pathways between the mnemonic comparator and implicit memory assumed to be intact). *Executive anosognosia* is theorized to reflect a dysfunctional mnemonic comparator. In this case, the episode of memory failure is registered in short-term memory but is never compared with representations in the PKB. Thus, neither explicit awareness of impairment nor behavioral/emotional reactions reflecting implicit knowledge of deficits would be observed (since the PKB is not updated, no new information is sent to either the CAS or implicit knowledge systems). *Primary anosognosia* is proposed to reflect an impaired CAS, with resultant lack of conscious awareness of the functioning of all cognitive domains, including memory, even though the comparator of the CES may detect the failure and register this in implicit memory. According to this model, AD patients with primary anosognosia would not be expected to show domain-specific unawareness of deficit, since the entire CAS is held to be impaired. However, implicit knowledge of deficits might lead to behavioral/emotional reactions, such as social withdrawal, when confronted by tasks at which the individual is impaired.

In addition to these theorized sources of heterogeneity in anosognosia among AD patients, it has been proposed that consideration should be given to whether depression exists as a comorbid condition. Depression occurs more frequently in AD than in nondemented individuals of similar age (Wragg & Jeste, 1989), and it could influence patients' reports of deficit (e.g., those with depression being more likely to acknowledge their deficits). There is evidence that, in healthy individuals, self-report of poor memory functioning is more related to negative affect than to actual memory performance (e.g., Larrabee & Levin, 1986; Seidenberg, Taylor, & Haltiner, 1994). Agnew and Morris (1998) also acknowledge the appeal of a hypothesis that depression is a psychological reaction to awareness of cognitive loss, which then decreases as awareness of deficit becomes impaired with progression of AD. However, they note that empirical evidence supporting an association between depression and awareness of deficits in AD (across studies utilizing a variety of methods for assessing awareness of deficit and for assessing depression) has been equivocal. Some studies have reported depression to be more prevalent in mild as opposed to more severely demented AD patients while others have not (for review of relevant studies, see Agnew & Morris, 1998; Clare, 2004).

Patient–Informant Questionnaire Discrepancy Studies of Anosognosia in Alzheimer's Disease

Several studies have employed the patient–informant questionnaire discrepancy method first described by Reisberg and colleagues (1985) in their study of AD patients, and they have shown that AD patients generally estimate their memory, self-care, and activities of daily living abilities as being less impaired than these areas of functioning are rated by informants, most typically relatives who are caregivers for the patient (Anderson & Tranel, 1989; Clare & Wilson, 2006; Correa, Graves, & Costa, 1996; DeBettignies et al., 1990; Duke, Seltzer, Seltzer, & Vasterling, 2002; Feher, Mahurin, Inbody, Crook, & Pirozzolo, 1991; Freidenberg, Huber, & Dreskin, 1990; Kaszniak, DiTraglia, & Trosset, 1993; Mangone et al., 1991; McGlone et al., 1990; Migliorelli et al., 1995; Ott, Noto, & Fogel, 1996; Salmon et al., 2008; Seltzer, Vasterling, Hale, & Khurana, 1995; Starkstein et al., 1996; Vasterling et al., 1995).

McGlynn and Kaszniak (1991b) introduced a new variation to the questionnaire discrepancy method, having persons with AD and their relatives rate both their own and their relative's memory difficulties (i.e., patients rated themselves and their spouses; spouses rated themselves and the patient) in response to questions regarding various memory tasks of everyday life (e.g., remembering what you just said a few minutes ago, remembering where you put things). The AD group rated their own memory difficulties as greater than those of their spouses but also as significantly less severe than relatives rated the patients' problems. This discrepancy increased with greater degrees of patient's cognitive impairment as assessed by the Mini-Mental State Examination (MMSE; Folstein, Folstein, & McHugh, 1975). However, no significant differences were found between the patients' and relatives' ratings of the relatives' daily memory difficulties. The authors note that their data were not consistent with any general impairment in cognitive estimation as accounting for the apparent anosognosia of the AD group. If this had been the case, the authors argue, there would be errors expected in patients' estimations of both their own and their caregivers' problems. McGlynn and Kaszniak (1991b) conclude that their results are consistent with a breakdown of metacognitive processes with progression of disease in AD, "... resulting in patients' failure to update knowledge about their *own* cognitive performance" (p. 187). McGlynn and Kaszniak (1991b) also conclude that the impaired awareness appears to be restricted to evaluations regarding the self, since AD patients were generally accurate when making judgments about their relatives' memory functioning. A problem for this interpretation, however, is the possibility that patients' questionnaire responses regarding the daily difficulties of both themselves and their spouses are based upon episodic and semantic knowledge about both self and other that has not been updated, due to the patients' memory impairment (i.e., mnemonic anosognosia within the Agnew & Morris, 1998 model). Since the AD patients have presumably deteriorated in their functioning, while their spouses have not, patient questionnaire responses based upon nonupdated information would thus appear to be accurate in regard to their spouses' functioning, though inaccurate for themselves. The data of McGlynn and Kaszniak (1991b) thus may not adequately address the question of whether the apparent underestimation of deficit demonstrated by their AD groups is specific to evaluation of self and not other.

Several studies have examined patient–informant questionnaire discrepancy scores in relationship to various other patient characteristics. Studies assessing the relationship of discrepancy magnitude and severity of dementia (utilizing a variety of measures) or duration of illness have produced conflicting results. Several reports support a modest relationship between the magnitude of discrepancy and increasing severity of dementia (Anderson & Tranel, 1989; Duke et al., 2002; Feher et al., 1991; Mangone et al., 1991; McGlynn & Kaszniak, 1991b; Migliorelli et al., 1995; Ott, Noto, & Fogel, 1996; Reisberg et al., 1985; Seltzer, Vasterling, Hale, & Khurana, 1995; Starkstein et al., 1996; Vasterling et al., 1995; Verhey, Rozendaal, Ponds, & Jolles, 1993; Wagner, Spangenberg, Bachman, & O'Connell, 1997). However, other investigators report an absence of significant correlation between patient–informant discrepancy and measures of dementia severity (Clare & Wilson, 2006; Correa et al., 1996; DeBettignies, Mahurin, & Pirozzolo, 1990; Feher, Larrabee, Sudilovsky, & Crook, 1994; Green et al., 1993; Kotler-Cope & Camp, 1995; Michon, Deweer, Pillon, Agid, & Dubois, 1994). Similar variability exists among reports of the relationship between questionnaire discrepancy measures of anosognosia and severity of memory impairment, with some studies supporting a relationship (Feher et al., 1991; Migliorelli et al., 1995) and other studies not (Derouesné et al., 1999; Vogel, Hasselbalch, Gade, Ziebell, & Waldemar, 2005). Some of the variability in studies examining relationships between questionnaire discrepancy measures of anosognosia and memory could be related to the nature of the memory tests used in the particular study. Gallo and colleagues (2007) provide evidence suggesting that measures of anosognosia and memory are more likely to correlate in AD patient groups when memory tests require the effortful retrieval of nondistinctive information. There is also some variability in the results of studies that have evaluated longitudinal changes in AD patient–informant discrepancy measures, with follow-up intervals ranging from 1 to 2 years. Four longitudinal studies have reported significant increases in patient–caregiver questionnaire discrepancies (Derouesné et al., 1999; Kaszniak & Christenson, 1995, 1996; Starkstein et al., 1997; Vasterling, Seltzer, & Watrous, 1997), while another study (Clare & Wilson, 2006) found small, nonsignificant increases in mean discrepancy scores. Overall, such variability in study results suggests that neither dementia severity nor progression over time is able to reliably account for patient–informant discrepancy indices of anosognosia in AD.

Consistent with the results of clinical observation studies reviewed above, more recent research has suggested that the patient characteristic more closely associated with questionnaire discrepancy measures of deficit unawareness in AD may be degree of frontal-lobe dysfunction, rather than general dementia severity. Salmon and colleagues (2008), examining patient–caregiver discrepancy on questions covering several cognitive domains, found evidence of underawareness of deficits in a large group of AD patients but also found their AD group to demonstrate greater awareness than a group of frontotemporal patients of similar overall dementia severity. In a group of mildly to moderately demented persons with AD, Michon et al. (1994) found the magnitude of discrepancy between patients' self-ratings and family members' ratings of these patients on a memory-functioning questionnaire to be highly correlated with patient performance on neuropsychological tasks thought to be sensitive to frontal lobe functioning (e.g., Wisconsin Card Sorting Task, Verbal Fluency), but not with performance on general mental status, memory, or linguistic tasks. Kashiwa et al. (2005) reported a similar relationship between a patient–informant discrepancy measure of anosognosia in AD and the color-word conflict portion of the Stroop Task (a measure that has also been found to be related to frontal functioning; see Stuss, 2007). Not all studies, however, have found a relationship between AD patient–informant questionnaire discrepancy and neuropsychological measures assumed to be related to frontal lobe functioning. For example, Vogel et al. (2005) found their discrepancy measure to be unrelated to performance on several neuropsychological measures of executive functioning (although it was related to a SPECT measure of regional cerebral blood flow in the right inferior frontal gyrus and to a Frontal Behavioral Inventory score). The apparent dissociation between neuropsychological and neuroimaging or behavioral indices of frontal functioning, in relation to a patient–informant discrepancy measure of deficit awareness, may reflect the fact that so-called executive functioning tasks are "...complex and multifactorial, and individuals can fail for many reasons..." (Stuss, 2007, p. 294), and/or that certain measures of executive cognitive function may not be sensitive to frontal dysfunction in those regions (e.g., ventromedial) that may be most important in subserving metacognitive processes (Stuss, Rosenbaum, Malcolm, Christiana, & Keenan, 2005). Other evidence of an association between functional neuroimaging indices of frontal dysfunction in AD and questionnaire discrepancy measures of deficit awareness are reviewed by Starkstein and Power (see Chapter 10, this volume).

Several investigators have also used discrepancy scores to examine whether unawareness is limited to memory or extends to other cognitive and emotional impairments or symptoms. Kaszniak et al. (1993) examined 19 persons with mildly to moderately severe AD, using a questionnaire (modified from the Gilewski, Zelinski & Schaie [1990] Memory Functioning Questionnaire) to assess patient–caregiver discrepancies in ratings of the frequency and seriousness of patients' memory failures, problems in other areas of cognitive functioning, and emotional problems, such as depression, anxiety, or anger. Compared to their caregiver's assessments, AD patients significantly underestimated both the frequency and seriousness of their difficulties with memory, language, praxis, and attention. Patients and their caregivers, however, were in close agreement that the patients made little use of mnemonic aids in their daily lives. Kaszniak and colleagues (1993) interpreted this observation as inconsistent with a defensive denial explanation, since patients who are defensively denying their difficulties might be expected to utilize mnemonic aids despite minimization of their frequency and seriousness of forgetting. Patients and caregivers in the

Kaszniak et al. (1993) study also were in agreement about the frequency and seriousness of patients' emotional difficulties, which were minimal in their sample of AD patients. Vasterling et al. (1995) reported that patient–caregiver discrepancy for a group of mildly to moderately demented persons with AD was largest for ratings of memory and self-care ability, moderate for ratings of anxiety and irritability, and least for ratings of depression and general health status. Similarly, Kotler-Cope and Camp (1995), in a study of a small number of more severely demented persons with AD, found large patient–caregiver discrepancies for questionnaire ratings of memory and other cognitive impairments, but not for ratings of agitation, depression, or need for routine. Green et al. (1993) also compared awareness of memory deficits with awareness of other aspects of impaired cognition and disturbed behavior. Their group of mildly impaired AD patients rated themselves as significantly more able than they were rated by their family members. Discrepancies were largest for ratings of recent memory and everyday activity abilities, were smaller for attention, and were minimal for memory of events from the distant past (remote memory).

Thus, questionnaire discrepancy measures might appear to provide some evidence for selectivity of unawareness, since patients were in closer agreement with their spouses on their ratings of some, but not other deficits. This would have theoretical implications regarding the nature of anosognosia in AD, since domain specificity of unawareness of deficits would weigh against an interpretation that AD patients can be described as having *primary anosognosia*, as defined by the Agnew and Morris (1998) model. It remains possible, however, that this apparent selectivity in deficit awareness is a measurement artifact. Overall, the largest discrepancies appear to occur for those domains of functioning where informants rated the patients as most impaired. As noted by Kaszniak and Zak (1996) and by Clare (2004), it is thus unclear whether discrepancy score differences across domains of functioning reflect domain-specific anosognosia or are an artifact of differences in degree of impairment. Cognitive and behavioral domains for which there are closer patient–spouse agreement in rating deficits (e.g., remote memory, depression, agitation) may be those for which the particular AD patient sample being studied shows little impairment or abnormality. Consistent with this possibility, Kaszniak and colleagues (1993) found that patients and caregivers were highly discrepant in ratings of the patients' memory for recent events, but in agreement regarding memory for events in the remote past. Although remote memory becomes impaired with disease progression in AD, older memories generally tend to be more accessible than recent ones (Kopelman, 1989). Similarly, inspection of the Vasterling et al. (1995) data suggests that the magnitude of patient–caregiver disagreement in this study was proportional to the caregivers' ratings of severity of patient impairment. Thus, in some domains there may be little "deficit" of which the patient could be said to be aware, and self-ratings of normal functioning in these domains would necessarily be in close agreement with caregiver ratings.

A limitation for interpretation and integration of patient–informant questionnaire discrepancy research is that the specific questionnaires vary from one study to another and generally have unknown psychometric properties. However, recent research has emphasized establishing the reliability and validity of questionnaires, including the Anosognosia Questionnaire for Dementia (Migliorelli et al., 1995; Sato et al., 2007), the Memory Awareness Rating Scale (Clare, Wilson, Carter, Roth, & Hodges, 2002), the Memory Awareness Rating Scale—Adjusted (Hardy, Oyebode, & Clare, 2006), the Dementia Quality of Life Scale (Ready, Ott, & Grace, 2006), the Everyday Memory Questionnaire (Efklides et al., 2002; Sunderland, Harris, & Baddeley, 1983), and the Apathy inventory (Robert et al., 2002). This should assist in reducing some of the unsystematic variance related to methodological factors in future questionnaire discrepancy studies of anosognosia in AD. Another potential weakness of the questionnaire method is the dependence on the subjective judgment of the informant, whose responses may be biased by a number of factors, including the nature of their relationship with the patient and their potential motivation to make the patient look more or less impaired (Cosentino & Stern, 2005). Nevertheless, structured questionnaires offer a simple and convenient method of measuring patients' level of awareness, which may be particularly valuable in clinical settings when administering the kinds of tasks described below is not feasible.

Alzheimer's Disease Patient Questionnaire Self-Report versus Memory Test Performance

A small number of studies have been published in which investigators have examined discrepancies between AD patient questionnaire self-report and performance on objective memory tests (Anderson & Tranel, 1989; Dalla Barba, Parlato, Iavarone, & Boller, 1995; Feehan, Knight, & Partridge, 1993; Wagner, Spangenberg, Bachman, & O'Connell, 1997). Although providing evidence consistent with anosognosia in varying proportions of the AD patients participating in each study, this research method poses interpretation difficulties. As noted by Clare (2004), concern can be raised about whether questionnaire scores are equivalent in levels of measurement to scores obtained on various memory tests. It is thus unclear how comparisons between these two types of measures should be made. Clare (2004) also points out that the questionnaires employed in these studies often inquire about everyday memory tasks, while the memory tests (e.g., list recall, paired-associate learning) may involve tasks that are less familiar. Fortunately, other research is available in which AD patients are asked to make predictions about their performance on the same memory tasks (following initial task familiarization) on which the memory performance is assessed.

Accuracy of Alzheimer's Disease Patients' Performance Predictions on Specific Cognitive Tasks

Schacter, McLachlan, Moscovitch, and Tulving (1986) (more fully described in Schacter, 1991) asked three groups of memory-disordered patients (due to AD, head injury, and ruptured anterior communicating artery aneurysms, respectively) to study two 20-item categorized lists and then to predict the number of items they would be able to recall without cueing. Schacter and colleagues found that those with head injury or ruptured anterior communicating artery aneurysms were nearly as accurate in their performance predictions as their matched controls. However, the AD group consistently overpredicted their performance, even though the severity of memory deficit was fairly equivalent between the groups. This suggested that the apparent unawareness of memory deficit in persons with AD could not be accounted for by simply assuming that patients are unable to remember that they have a deficit. Schacter (1991) concluded that the inability of persons with AD to accurately predict their recall performance is consistent with unawareness of deficit. Unfortunately, alternative explanations of performance prediction inaccuracy, such as nonspecific problems in cognitive estimation, poor task comprehension, or response bias, cannot be ruled out on the basis of the data of the Schacter et al. (1986) study alone. In an attempt to address these possible alternative explanations, McGlynn and Kaszniak (1991b) designed a performance prediction experiment in which persons with AD were asked to make predictions about their own and their family caregiver's performance on various memory tasks (e.g., immediate and delayed word list recall, immediate and delayed picture recall, verbal recognition memory). Similarly, the family members predicted both their own and the patient's performance on these same tasks. Overall, the persons with AD overestimated their own performance on the memory tasks, but were more accurate when predicting their relatives' performance. Relatives were generally accurate in predicting both their own and their patient's performance. It was also found that the patients were as sensitive as their relatives in predictions regarding expected effects of retention interval and the different demands of recall versus recognition memory tasks. That is, both the patients and their family members predicted that they would perform better in recognition than in free recall tasks, and predicted that they would remember less at delayed than in immediate recall testing. Thus, the AD group in this study showed no evidence of deterioration in general knowledge about how memory processes work. McGlynn and Kaszniak (1991b) interpreted their results as reflecting a breakdown in the ability to self-monitor memory in AD, rather than any more general difficulty in cognitive estimation (which would have affected predictions for both self and relatives' performance) or disrupted knowledge about how memory works.

Another study (Moulin, Perfect, & Jones, 2000b) investigated whether memory performance prediction accuracy improves as a function of task exposure. In this study, AD patients were instructed to make predictions regarding their ability to remember words from a list, both prior to and after list encoding. The prediction accuracy data showed the AD patients to overestimate their recall performance. However, the AD patients made a significant improvement with respect to their postdictions after study, suggesting that they retain some ability to monitor memory. Ansell and Bucks (2006) similarly reported that their AD patient group, although showing performance prediction evidence of underawareness of their memory deficits prior to a word-recall task, improved in estimation accuracy following the recall task performance and largely retained this improvement after a 20-minute delay. The authors interpret their findings as providing partial support for a mnemonic anosognosia in AD, as posited by Agnew and Morris (1998). Although the Agnew and Morris model would have predicted that awareness of deficit following the delay period should have returned to pre-task-performance levels (due to a hypothetical inability of the AD patients to update their personal knowledge base), the authors suggest that this might have been observed with a longer delay or a change to a different environment where the testing situation would not cue them about their memory impairments.

It should be noted that an improvement in prediction accuracy following task performance has not always been observed in performance prediction studies. Barrett, Eslinger, Ballentine, and Heilman (2005) had their AD patients make self-assessment ratings, using Likert scales (marking each of 10 vertical lines) to indicate estimates of their abilities in the domains of memory, attention, generative behavior (ability to generate words and movements), confrontation naming, visuospatial skill, limb praxis, mood, and uncorrected visual acuity, both prior to and after performance on standardized neuropsychological tests assessing these same domains. Relative to controls, the AD group initially overestimated their visuospatial skill, but on post-testing overestimated their memory performance. The control group underestimated their attention at pre-testing, and overestimated their limb praxis and vision performance at post-testing. The authors suggest that pre-testing ability estimates may be related to self-semantics (i.e., abstract knowledge about oneself), while post-testing ability estimates may be more closely related to arousal/vigilance and online monitoring ability. They also propose that the AD group's overprediction for only some domains, with different domains overpredicted pre- versus post-testing, is inconsistent with a global deficit in judgment. Given the wide differences in measurement scales across the various neuropsychological tests used to assess performance in this study, it is difficult to evaluate these proposals.

Souchay, Isingrini, Pillon, and Gill (2003) used a performance prediction-postdiction accuracy approach in a study comparing AD patients and a small number of patients with frontotemporal dementia (FTD). Accuracy predictions were made both before and after participants studied a list of 20 cue-target pairs. Results showed both the AD and FTD groups to overpredict their subsequent recall performance, and for after-study predictions, the FTD group was more inaccurate than the AD group. Examination of covariance with several different neuropsychological tests indicated that performance prediction accuracy was primarily related to a composite of memory tests for the AD group, and to a composite of executive function tests for the FTD group.

As noted by Trosset and Kaszniak (1996), an interpretive difficulty for the method originally described by McGlynn and Kaszniak (1991b) involves the procedure they used for calculating patients' performance prediction accuracy scores. These scores were computed by subtracting the relative's accuracy ratio (relative's predicted ÷ relative's actual performance) from the patient's accuracy ratio (patient's predicted ÷ patient's actual performance), and an analogous procedure was used for calculating caregiver performance prediction accuracy. McGlynn and Kaszniak (1991b) selected this approach as a way to allow for evaluation of whether patients are less accurate in predicting their own than in predicting their relative's performance, while also adjusting for any tendency to overpredict one's own performance in comparison to the performances of others. However, the problem for this approach is that the comparison of two accuracy scores by subtraction is incompatible with the measurement of accuracy by division because the interpretation of the difference depends on the actual values of the ratios being compared. Thus, the difference of 1.0 between the ratios 1.5 and 0.5 is clearly not equivalent to the difference of 1.0 between the ratios 6.0 and 5.0. A more natural comparison is obtained by computing the quotient of the patient and relative accuracy ratios. Trosset and Kaszniak (1996) therefore proposed a comparative prediction accuracy measure (i.e., a ratio of ratios) and showed that this approach provides a single index of deficit unawareness that exceeds unity only when the patient exaggerates self-prediction relative to other prediction more than the caregiver does.

Kaszniak and Christenson (1995, 1996) replicated the general performance prediction methodology of the McGlynn and Kaszniak (1991b) study, utilizing the comparative prediction accuracy measure of Trosset and Kaszniak (1996) and adding longitudinal observations (retesting at 1 year). A group of mildly to moderately demented persons with AD and their caregivers made predictions concerning each other's performance on various memory tasks. Comparative prediction accuracy scores supported an interpretation that the AD group was, on average, impaired in their awareness of deficits, with their performance overprediction not being explainable as reflecting any general patient or caregiver response bias. Impaired awareness, by this measure, was not significantly correlated with clinician, patient, or family caregiver ratings of patients' or caregivers' depression-related symptoms. The longitudinal reassessment data showed the comparative prediction accuracy measures to remain relatively constant over a 1-year interval. Thus, patients' overprediction of their performance did not increase from baseline to follow-up, arguing against unawareness being related to either length of illness or increasing dementia severity, since the patients' actual performance did deteriorate over the year interval. This also seems to suggest that persons with AD are actually able to make some adjustments in their self-assessment of memory functioning as their memory deficit increases, but they remain consistently underaware of the severity of their memory impairment. Kaszniak and Christenson (1995, 1996), however, obtained somewhat conflicting results when they examined longitudinal data in their memory functioning questionnaire discrepancy data. They found the discrepancy between patient and family caregiver ratings of patients' frequency of forgetting to significantly increase over the 1-year interval. The persons with AD rated their frequency of forgetting similarly at the baseline and follow-up assessment points, whereas caregivers rated the patients' forgetting as significantly more frequent at the 1-year, compared to the baseline assessment. Thus, the questionnaire discrepancy data would seem to argue against the suggestion from the performance prediction data that persons with AD are able to somewhat adjust their self-assessment of memory functioning. The disagreement in conclusions from these two types of data may reflect the different cognitive processes involved in deficit awareness between the methods. Kaszniak and Zak (1996) proposed that the patient–informant questionnaire discrepancy method depends primarily upon an individual's generalized self-efficacy beliefs regarding his or her abilities, whereas performance prediction appears to involve both generalized self-efficacy beliefs and online self-monitoring. If the AD patients in the Kaszniak and Christenson (1995, 1996) longitudinal study had predominantly mnemonic anosognosia (in the Agnew & Morris, 1998 terminology), then it might be expected that they would fail to adequately update their personal knowledge base, and thus show greater discrepancy from their caregivers in memory difficulty questionnaire ratings from baseline to the 1-year reassessment. However, if most of these same patients had relatively intact online self-monitoring ability (i.e., did not have executive anosognosia in Agnew & Morris, 1998 terms), then the feedback provided by the actual tasks (demonstrated to the patients before their administration) might be expected to result in the patients being able to somewhat adjust their performance predictions at the 1-year reassessment, according to the increased severity of their objective memory impairment.

The study reported by Duke et al. (2002) provides data consistent with this interpretation of the differences in results for longitudinal patient–informant questionnaire discrepancy versus performance prediction approaches. Duke and colleagues (2002) used both questionnaire discrepancy and performance prediction-postdiction methods with a group of mostly mildly impaired AD patients and their spouse caregivers. Both groups predicted/postdicted their own and their spouses' performance on both a delayed-recall list learning test (predictions/postdictions for recall at each of three learning trials and after a 20-minute delay) and a verbal fluency (generative animal naming) test. Performance predictions occurred immediately prior to each task performance, and postdictions involved participants' estimation of their performance immediately following completion of each trial/task. Postdictions were added to the typical performance prediction method, in accord with the argument that post-dictions more clearly involve online self-monitoring. It has been proposed (Kaszniak & Zak, 1996) that performance predictions may involve contributions of both online self-monitoring and generalized self-efficacy beliefs, while questionnaire discrepancy data may primarily reflect self-efficacy beliefs. In contrast, postdictions, particularly when obtained immediately after task performance, would appear to provide a clearer reflection of cognitive self-monitoring (e.g., operation of the mnemonic comparator component of central executive systems posited by Agnew & Morris, 1998). Kaszniak and Zak (1996) also recognized a possibility that the relative accuracy shown by AD patients when predicting their relatives' memory task performance (and in giving questionnaire ratings of their caregiver's memory difficulties) could be based upon recall of their caregiver's abilities as they were several years ago (i.e., prior to the beginning of the patient's own memory deterioration and subsequently not updated). The persons with AD in performance prediction and questionnaire discrepancy studies may thus have failed to update their personal knowledge base concerning current cognitive abilities of others, as well as of self. Given the probability that their caregivers' memory functioning was not deteriorating, this (rather than a specific deficit in *self*-monitoring) could account for patients overpredicting their own performance, while appearing to accurately predict their caregivers' performance. Kaszniak and Zak (1996) proposed that this possibility could be evaluated by future studies in which patients are asked to predict the memory task performance or rate the daily memory difficulties of other persons with memory impairment with whom they have become recently familiar. Duke et al. (2002) attempted such an evaluation by including a condition in their study in which AD patient–caregiver questionnaire discrepancy and learning/memory task prediction/postdiction data were obtained for participant estimations regarding a previously unfamiliar memory-disordered patient observed on videotape.

Duke and colleagues' (2002) questionnaire discrepancy data showed their AD patients to have underestimated their difficulties in daily cognitive, self-care, and social tasks. The performance prediction-postdiction data was analyzed using the comparative performance prediction-postdiction accuracy (CPA) index of Trosset and Kaszniak (1996), in addition to secondary analyses of independent ratio scores for each prediction and postdiction. The secondary analyses were designed to further evaluate whether the CPA results could be best explained by underawareness of deficit by the AD patients or by underestimation of self-performance by caregivers (a possibility not resolvable by examination of the CPA ratio of ratios alone). These analyses demonstrated that the AD patients overpredicted their own verbal learning/memory performance prior to the first list-learning trial. The extent of overestimation decreased for their learning trial postdictions (post-trial estimates), indicating some preservation of memory self-monitoring capacity (see Oyebode, Telling, Hardy, & Austin,

2007, for similar evidence of improved accuracy from memory task prediction to postdiction). However, after a 20-minute delay the AD patients in the Duke et al., study again overpredicted their memory performance, suggesting that they were unable to effect any longer-term updating of their personal knowledge base of self-efficacy beliefs, based on their poor memory task performance. Both patients and their spouse caregivers accurately estimated caregiver verbal learning/ memory performances, and they showed similar general tendencies to predict increasing levels of learning with repeated exposure of the word list, and some decrease of memory for the words after a 20-minute distraction-filled delay. The AD patients also made fairly accurate predictions and postdictions concerning their own and their caregivers' verbal fluency task performance (which was objectively impaired for the AD group). For analysis of the patient and caregiver predictions and postdictions regarding the previously unfamiliar patient whom they viewed being interviewed on videotape, Duke and colleagues used a modification of the Trosset and Kaszniak (1996) comparative performance prediction/postdiction accuracy (CPA) index (utilizing published normative data based upon comparably mildly memory-impaired AD patients as proxies for the learning/memory task performance of the unfamiliar videotaped patient). It was found that both the AD patients and their caregivers overestimated performances of this patient.

Duke and colleagues (2002) interpreted their data as supporting the following conclusions: *(1)* Mildly impaired AD patients and their nondemented spouse caregivers have similar general knowledge concerning how memory functions (i.e., adjusting the predictions according to immediate versus delayed recall conditions and the expectation of increased recall over repeated learning trials); *(2)* These same AD patients appear underaware of their own memory and other cognitive deficits, as reflected in questionnaire discrepancy and memory performance prediction results; *(3)* This underawareness of deficit may vary across different cognitive domains (i.e., accurate prediction for their verbal fluency performance, but overprediction of their memory performance); *(4)* Mildly impaired AD patients appear to retain some capacity to monitor their own memory performances in an online fashion (i.e., reduction in extent of overestimation when making postdictions compared to predictions; also similar number of attempts at self-correcting recall performances for the AD patients and their caregivers). However, this self-monitoring does not appear to result in effective and longer-lasting updating of memory self-efficacy beliefs in their personal knowledge base; *(5)* Since both the AD patients and their caregivers overpredicted the performance of the previously unfamiliar patient viewed on videotape, the question of whether the AD patients have a specific impairment in *self*-awareness of their deficits, rather than a more global impairment in awareness, remains unresolved.

In light of the observed patterns in their data, Duke et al. (2002) suggest that the generally mildly impaired AD patients in their study show evidence for what

Agnew and Morris (1998) termed *mnemonic anosognosia*. The apparent preserved capacity of their AD patients for online self-monitoring would argue against the presence of executive anosognosia, although Duke and colleagues (2002) acknowledge that, given the relatively mild dementia syndromes shown by most of their patients, evidence for executive anosognosia could manifest with further dementia progression in their sample. This expectation is based upon evidence showing online memory self-monitoring abilities to be associated with frontal lobe (particularly right ventromedial) functioning, and the evidence for increasing frontal neuropathology seen with AD disease progression (Braak & Braak, 1991).

By combining both patient–informant questionnaire discrepancy and performance prediction approaches, McGlynn and Kaszniak (1991b), Kaszniak and Christenson (1995, 1996), and Duke et al. (2002) obtained both convergent and divergent evidence regarding impaired awareness of memory deficit in AD (see also Correa et al., 1996). Although both approaches provide evidence for impaired awareness of deficit in AD, they do not provide results that are highly correlated with each other. Indeed, the computed correlation between the questionnaire and performance prediction measures (at baseline) indicated approximately 13% shared variance in the Kaszniak and Christenson (1995, 1996) study, and only 3% shared variance in the Duke et al. (2002) study. To some extent, these weak correlations between methods may reflect differences in skills being assessed (e.g., the questionnaire discrepancy measure focusing upon general self-care skills, and the performance prediction task upon memory in the Duke et al., 2002 study). Some support for the contribution of different skill assessment to the low correlation between measures of awareness of deficit comes from the AD longitudinal study of Clare and Wilson (2006). Using analogous (i.e., focusing upon the same skill domains) patient–caregiver questionnaire discrepancy and performance postdiction scales, they found little difference between the two types of measures in the pattern of change over a 1-year retest interval. Caution, however, must be exercised in interpreting the Clare and Wilson (2006) data, given the limited sample size (12 AD patients), and the fact that only nonsignificant trends toward change over time were seen in either measurement scale. Limited correlation between questionnaire discrepancy and performance prediction/postdiction measures may also reflect the different metacognitive process involved in these different awareness of deficit measures. As discussed by Kaszniak and Zak (1996) and by Duke et al. (2002), questionnaire discrepancy measures may primarily reflect generalized self-efficacy beliefs about cognitive and self-care abilities, while performance prediction, and especially postdiction, measures may reflect both self-efficacy beliefs and online self-monitoring. From this perspective, studies of anosognosia in AD that utilize these two different methods suggest that, at least for relatively mildly impaired AD patients, there is a failure to update their personal knowledge base (i.e., mnemonic anosognosia), but that memory self-monitoring capacity may remain relatively more intact (i.e., a lack of evidence for executive anosognosia). Further, the evidence for some preservation of self-monitoring ability and the data from performance-prediction studies (e.g., Duke et al., 2002; Kaszniak & Christenson, 1995, 1996) that provide evidence (albeit not conclusive) for domain specificity suggest that the AD patients in the samples studied cannot be fairly characterized as showing what Agnew and Morris (1998) term *primary anosognosia.*

Studies Using Other Metamemory Tasks to Explore Anosognosia in Alzheimer's Disease

In addition to memory performance prediction/postdiction, there are several other metamemory tasks that have been used to explore the nature of anosognosia in AD. These tasks include feeling-of-knowing judgments, retrospective confidence judgments, judgments of learning, and recall readiness judgments. More extensive descriptions of these tasks, and results from studies that have employed them with healthy individuals, across the age range, can be found in Dunlosky and Metcalfe (2009).

Metamemory Task Procedures

The *feeling-of-knowing* (FOK) task requires the participant to attempt recall of a previously presented item, and if it is not currently recallable, to specify whether the answer will be remembered at a later time (Hart, 1965; Nelson & Narens, 1990). Two hypotheses have been proposed to account for the cognitive processes by which FOK judgments are made. The cue familiarity hypothesis posits that a cue present at the time of the FOK judgment is processed for familiarity versus novelty (Metcalfe, Schwartz, & Joaquim, 1993). The sense of familiarity or novelty is hypothesized to be accessed by control processes that then affect the FOK judgment. A second hypothesis is the accessibility account, stating that that FOK judgments are based on all information that is present at the time the judgment is made (e.g., letters or sounds associated with the to-be-retrieved word), including but not limited to cue familiarity (Koriat, 1993). The two FOK hypotheses are not incompatible and empirical studies of healthy adults support both views (see Koriat & Levy-Sadot, 2001).

Feeling-of-knowing judgment studies of AD patients have used either tasks assessing semantic memory/general knowledge or episodic memory tasks in which the new information is learned during a study phase. A typical episodic task requires subjects to learn new sentences and then reproduce the last word of the sentence at test. If subjects fail to recall the word, they then make an FOK judgment, reporting their confidence that they will correctly recognize the word at a later time. The accuracy of FOK judgments are evaluated by one or more of three different statistical indices of concordance between the ratings of confidence and the actual recognition memory performance. These indices are: *(1)* the Goodman-Kruskal gamma coefficient (see Nelson, 1984), a symmetric index of association based on a ratio of the difference between concordant and discordant item confidence-recognition pairs divided by the sum of concordant plus discordant pairs (eliminating from the computation any tied pairs). The gamma coefficient has been taken to be a measure of monitoring resolution (i.e., the extent to which the person is able to distinguish between known and unknown items); *(2)* the less frequently used Somers' *d* (Somers, 1962), an asymmetric statistic (although able to be rendered symmetric by an averaging procedure) that is identical to the gamma coefficient, except that it includes tied pairs in the denominator of the gamma equation; and *(3)* the Hamann index, measuring correspondence of confidence judgments and objective recognition performance, which although argued to be a better measure than gamma (Schraw, 1995), has been found to be highly related to gamma in empirical study comparisons (e.g., Schnyer et al., 2004; Souchay, Isingrini, & Espagnet, 2000). Panuu and Kaszniak (2005) provide a more expanded discussion of these indices and the steps involved in their computation.

Retrospective confidence judgments are made regarding a recently retrieved item from memory. In typical experiments, these judgments are made following a recall or recognition attempt, but preceding an FOK judgment. For example, in a semantic memory/general knowledge task, participants might be asked to recall an item of general knowledge. If some information is recalled, the individual is asked to make a retrospective confidence judgment regarding whether he or she thinks that his or her response is correct. If the individual does not provide an answer, he or she is asked to make an FOK judgment regarding subsequent recall or recognition of the correct answer. Retrospective confidence and FOK are different types of judgments in that the former is an assessment that follows retrieval and the latter a prospective judgment regarding future recall or recognition. These two types of judgments may also depend on somewhat different brain regions. Schnyer et al. (2004) provide structural neuroimaging evidence, for a group of patients with frontal lobe focal damage, that the ventromedial (particularly right) prefrontal cortex may be critical for accurate FOK judgments. The lateral prefrontal cortex, which has been postulated to be involved in retrieval monitoring effort (Henson, Rugg, & Shallice, 2000), may be the critical region involved in accurate retrospective confidence judgments (Pannu et al., 2005).

In *judgments of learning* (JOLs), predictions are made about participants' ability to later remember items that are currently available for study (Nelson & Narens, 1990). In a typical JOL task, an individual item (e.g., word) is studied for a limited time, and the likelihood of later word recall is rated. As with FOK judgments, JOL accuracy is measured (using similar statistical indices) by comparison of the JOLs to objective recall performance. Judgments of learning can be made either immediately following the learning session or following a delay. Studies of healthy adult participants have found that delayed JOLs tend to be more accurate than immediate JOLs (Nelson & Dunlosky, 1991). One explanation for this could be that participants monitor working memory during an immediate judgment, and this information may not be available to retrieve at a later time. Delayed JOLs, however, may be based upon information from long-term memory and therefore tend to be more accurate reflections of what the participant will be able to recall.

Recall readiness experiments require subjects to study stimuli (e.g., words) and declare when they feel they have studied the stimulus sufficiently to subsequently recall it. Thus, for a self-paced word list, each subsequent word is presented only when the participant indicates that the previous word has been adequately studied for future recall. Following the recall readiness trial, the participant is asked to recall the studied words, and the accuracy of the prior recall readiness judgments is determined (e.g., through indices of relationship between self-determined study time and recall accuracy).

Study Results

Pappas et al. (1992) reported on FOK experiments for both previously acquired general knowledge and for newly learned information, studying a group of 12 moderately demented persons with AD and 12 age-matched control participants. Pappas and colleagues (1992) obtained FOK judgments for subsequent recognition of information not initially recalled and also had participants rate their confidence (on a six-point scale) that each of their initial recall responses was correct (retrospective confidence judgment). The accuracy of retrospective confidence judgments regarding correctness of initial recall attempts was indexed by the gamma coefficient, computed in a manner analogous to that described for FOK judgments. Pappas and colleagues (1992) found that their AD patients were as accurate as the control group in their confidence ratings for correctness of initial recall responses, for both general knowledge (semantic) and recently presented (episodic) memory items, despite profoundly impaired recall of information from both semantic and episodic memory. However, the patients showed impaired FOK accuracy for long-term knowledge, in that they were significantly less accurate than controls at predicting the likelihood that they would subsequently recognize correct answers to knowledge questions which they had been unable to initially recall (although their accuracy did exceed chance). Unfortunately, for the new information (episodic memory) task, neither the persons with AD nor the healthy age-matched control groups showed sufficient variation in FOK judgments to calculate gamma. Pappas et al. (1992) posit that this may reflect the absence of repeated items in their procedure, possibly reducing the range of memory strength, and hence the range of FOK judgments. Thus, although providing some support for impaired memory self-monitoring in their AD sample, the finding of apparently unimpaired accuracy in retrospective confidence ratings for recall attempts suggests that these different metamemory measures are dissociable in AD. Similar to what the present authors proposed above for the different results of memory performance prediction and postdiction accuracy, the dissociation between retrospective confidence and FOK indices observed by Pappas and colleagues (1992) may reflect a differential contribution of online monitoring in these two tasks. That is, retrospective confidence ratings may primarily reflect online memory monitoring, while FOK judgments may involve some combination of online monitoring and self-efficacy beliefs from the individual's personal knowledge base. As noted above, these two types of metamemory judgment tasks may also depend upon different frontal cortical regions.

Conflicting results were reported by Bäckman and Lipinska (1993), who studied mildly demented AD patients and normal older adults, in FOK judgments for a general knowledge test. On both tests of recall and recognition, no significant group differences in FOK accuracy were found. As expected, the AD group recalled and recognized less general knowledge information than the healthy older adult group. In a follow-up study, the datedness of general knowledge questions was varied (Lipinska & Bäckman, 1993). The authors hypothesized that AD patients would show better monitoring for older material than newer material. However, the patient group and the control group again did not differ in their metamemory judgments, regardless of the datedness of the material. Based on the results of these two studies, the authors conclude that monitoring is relatively intact during the early stages of AD. It remains unclear why the general knowledge FOK accuracy results of Pappas et al. (1992) and of Bäckman and Lipinska (1993) differ.

More consistent conclusions have been reached by investigators who studied FOK accuracy for episodic memory in AD. As already noted, Pappas et al. (1992) attempted to examine FOK accuracy for episodic memory, but there was insufficient variation in FOK judgments to calculate gamma. Duke and Kaszniak (2001) found episodic memory (sentence completion learning/memory task) FOK judgments to be less accurate in a group of mildly to moderately impaired AD patients compared to their spouse caregiver controls. Feeling-of-knowing accuracy was unrelated to severity of memory impairment in this study. Souchay, Isingrini, and Gil (2002) employed an episodic memory task to examine FOK accuracy in mildly impaired AD patients compared to healthy age-matched control participants. The participants studied 20 cue-target word pairs, and results showed FOK accuracy (measured by both gamma correlations and the Hamann index) to be significantly worse for the AD group than for a healthy control group. Examination of partial correlations between the FOK accuracy measures (both by gamma and Hamann indices) and composite scores from a battery of neuropsychological tests indicated that FOK accuracy was more related to memory than executive function neuropsychological measures.

Research examining retrospective confidence accuracy in AD has produced conflicting results. Duke and Kaszniak (2001) examined retrospective confidence for an episodic sentence completion learning/memory task and found their AD group to be less accurate in these judgments than their spouse caregiver control group. However, Moulin, James, Perfect, and Jones (2003), using a forced-choice recognition paradigm, found AD patients to be as accurate as controls in assigning retrospective confidence ratings to their recognition performance.

Moulin (2002) has argued that episodic FOK accuracy measures are confounded by the generally poor accuracy (and hence floor effects) of AD patients on the memory task. In order to examine memory monitoring at encoding without this confound, they analyzed JOL prediction ratings that patients made during encoding and determined how sensitive their predictions were, based on normative data indicating the difficulty of each item, with the assumption that items considered to be more difficult relative to other items should be rated as less likely to be recalled. Indeed, they found that the AD patients made appropriate judgments at encoding, suggesting that memory monitoring was intact despite their poor accuracy on the memory test (Moulin, Perfect, & Jones, 2000c). However, in another study, Moulin, Perfect, and Jones (2000a) found that AD patients, unlike age-matched controls, did not adjust their JOLs over repeated presentations of a word list, although the AD patients did show faster recall readiness over repetitions. The authors suggest that this difference in results from their two purported measures of memory monitoring sensitivity may reflect JOLs being explicit (i.e., conscious) judgments, while recall readiness time is an implicit measure.

Given the discrepant conclusions in the literature regarding whether memory monitoring abilities are intact in AD patients, it is clear that future studies are needed, particularly ones which integrate multiple different methodologies in order to provide a clearer picture of the metacognitive abilities of AD patients.

Summary, Conclusions, and Practical Implications

In summary, the large majority of studies reviewed in the present chapter provide support for the conclusion that anosognosia is common in AD. Despite the variety of research methods that have been used, results of available studies do allow for several general conclusions. Anosognosia in AD does not appear to be accounted for by general impairment in questionnaire/task comprehension or cognitive estimation. Relevant results suggest that, at least for more mildly impaired AD patients, there is no impairment in knowledge regarding how memory operates (e.g., that memory performance is better immediately following learning than after a delay). Several studies provide support for the hypothesis that anosognosia in AD reflects, at least in part, a failure to update memory/cognitive self-efficacy beliefs (an aspect of the individual's hypothetical personal knowledge base). However, the question of whether there is also an impairment of online self-monitoring has not been convincingly resolved. Thus, the majority of relevant research results would appear to support the presence of mnemonic anosognosia in AD, using Agnew and Morris' (1998) terminology. However, additional research will be needed to more fully compare different methods of assessing awareness of deficits, particularly contrasting those approaches that appear to reflect theoretically distinct constructs (e.g., memory self-monitoring versus the updating of memory self-efficacy beliefs/personal knowledge).

There is variation in reported findings regarding the relationship between unawareness of deficits and the overall severity of dementia or the specific severity of memory impairment. Although not entirely consistent across studies, there is somewhat better support for a hypothesized relationship between executive functioning, thought to largely reflect frontal lobe functioning, and anosognosia in AD. Several investigators have found depressive symptoms in AD to be associated with the degree of impaired awareness, while others have not.

As described above, some of the variability in the results of research designed to explore the nature of metacognitive deficits in AD may reflect differences in tasks used to measure awareness of deficits. One relevant difference may involve the type of mental representations that are monitored in metamemory judgment tasks. Some tasks involve semantic memory monitoring, such as FOK for general knowledge, while others, such as FOK for newly learned words or sentences involve episodic memory monitoring. Episodic memory tasks may be more difficult because they make greater cognitive demands than semantic memory tasks and may also pose greater monitoring difficulty. Those FOK studies that used an episodic memory task have more consistently shown differences in metamemory accuracy between AD patients and healthy control subjects, while FOK studies that used a semantic memory task have provided conflicting results. Another relevant task difference may involve whether judgments about task performance are made prior to or after task performance. Several, although not all, studies indicate that judgment accuracy improves following, as compared to before task performance for AD patients. A third relevant task difference appears to be whether memory monitoring accuracy or sensitivity is assessed. Several, though not all, studies support the presence of impaired FOK and JOL accuracy in AD, while other studies show that monitoring sensitivity to such memory-relevant variables as learning list repetition appears preserved.

Evidence suggestive of some domain specificity of impaired deficit awareness in AD, across different areas of cognitive and emotional functioning, has been reported. However, because of methodological limitations in available studies, further exploration of possible dissociations of impaired deficit awareness in AD patients is needed. Such research will need to simultaneously investigate unawareness of deficits across different cognitive and functional domains for which patients show similar severity of impairment. The increased use of longitudinal designs may elucidate how awareness of deficits and its correlates change over time in the progressive dementia of AD. Since premorbid patient characteristics may be related to anosognosia, prospective studies (e.g., of individuals at increased risk for AD, due to genetic or associated illness factors) are also needed to address this issue and explore the earliest changes in awareness of deficits in AD.

A greater understanding of the processes and mechanisms of anosognosia in AD may have important clinical and practical implications for patients and their families, particularly for the development and use of dementia management/ rehabilitation interventions. Although research in this area is currently sparse, at least two studies have examined the role of anosognosia in treatment outcome. Koltai, Welsh-Bohmer, and Schmechel (2001) identified patients' awareness of their deficits as a potential moderator in the perceived outcome of a Memory and Coping Program (MCP) intervention that enrolled 24 patients with mild to moderate dementia. The MCP is a multicomponent approach that addresses both cognitive and affective functioning. Specifically, it aims to improve memory functioning by teaching strategies such as spaced retrieval, verbal elaboration, repetition, face-name recall strategies, and the use of external aides. The MCP also targets emotional distress by teaching adaptive coping strategies and communication skills. Results of the Koltai et al. (2001) study revealed that patients' awareness of their deficits (retrospectively rated by therapists) was significantly related to perceived level of improvement following the intervention. Those rated as showing greater awareness of deficits reported benefiting more than patients with less rated awareness of their impairments, as well as more than patients in a no-treatment control group. The relationship between deficit awareness and outcome was not straightforward, however, as caregivers perceived more improvement in the intervention group relative to the control group regardless of patients' insight status. A major limitation of this study is that awareness of deficit was not formally assessed prior to the intervention, but was based on post hoc therapist ratings using a dichotomous variable (i.e., "insight" or "no insight").

This limitation was addressed in a later study by Clare et al. (2004), who reported the first study examining the role of awareness in cognitive rehabilitation using a prospective design. Twelve patients diagnosed with early-stage probable AD were characterized using the Memory Awareness Rating Scale, assessing the discrepancy between patient and informant reports of memory difficulties as well as the discrepancy between patient prediction and actual performance on cognitive tasks, yielding a mean discrepancy score. A negative correlation was found between mean discrepancy scores and outcome on an intervention that sought to retrain patients in face-name associations for acquaintances and public figures. Interestingly, this relationship remained robust after controlling for variance associated with dementia severity, as measured by the MMSE.

The findings of these two studies offer initial encouraging support for the hypothesis that anosognosia hinders treatment gain in AD patients, at least for those types of interventions employed in these studies. Future research should address different types of cognitive rehabilitation programs, particularly those that target behaviors relevant to the everyday lives of patients and their caregivers, such as activities of daily living and reduction of dangerous behaviors. Cotrell and Wild (1999) reported that unawareness of deficits was associated with failure of AD patients to restrict driving activity, and a more recent study by Starkstein et al. (2007) reported a threefold increase of dangerous behaviors (assessed by patient and caregiver questionnaire) in AD patients with questionnaire discrepancy evidence of anosognosia. These findings highlight the need for developing practical applications based on an understanding of anosognosia in AD.

Another potential avenue for future research would be to develop ways in which awareness could be increased in patients with AD, perhaps by capitalizing on those cognitive functions that are preserved. There is some evidence that patients' awareness of their memory functioning improves after sufficient exposure to the specific memory task (e.g., Moulin et al., 2000a) and that such gains are maintained after a short delay (Ansell & Bucks, 2006). Clare, Roth, and Pratt (2005) have argued that awareness in dementia is a multidimensional construct that may be affected by a number of psychological and social factors, some of which could be targeted for intervention. For example, Clare et al. (2005) have shown that particular kinds of coping styles appear to be related to a higher level of explicit awareness in patients with dementia. These findings are encouraging from the perspective of potentially developing interventions that could increase awareness of deficit in patients with AD by targeting cognitive, psychological, and/or social aspects of the disease (e.g., Watkins, Cheston, Jones, & Gilliard, 2006). Successfully increasing the awareness of patients with AD and helping them to appreciate the severity of their cognitive deficits and the consequences of these deficits in everyday life could potentially serve to reduce dangerous behaviors, facilitate greater independence, and improve quality of life for patients and caregivers alike.

Acknowledgments

Preparation of this chapter was supported by an Alzheimer's Disease Core Center grant (#P30 AG019610, Eric Reiman, M.D., Principal Investigator) from the U.S. National Institute on Aging/National Institutes of Health, and State of Arizona funding for the Arizona Alzheimer's Consortium.

References

Auchus, A. P., Goldstein, F. C., Green, J., & Green, R. C. (1994). Unawareness of cognitive impairments in Alzheimer's disease. *Neuropsychiatry, Neuropsychology, and Behavioral Neurology, 7*, 25–29.

Agnew, S. K., & Morris, R. G. (1998). The heterogeneity of anosognosia for memory impairment in Alzheimer's disease: A review of the literature and a proposed model. *Aging & Mental Health, 2*, 7–19.

Anderson, S. W., & Tranel, D. (1989). Awareness of disease states following cerebral infarction, dementia, and head trauma: Standardized assessment. *The Clinical Neuropsychologist, 3,* 327–339.

Ansell, E. L., & Bucks, R. S. (2006). Mnemonic anosognosia in Alzheimer's disease: A test of Agnew and Morris (1998). *Neuropsychologia, 44,* 1095–1102.

Babinski, J. (1914). Contribution a l'etude des troubles mentaux dans l'hemiplegie organique cerebral (Anosognosie). [Contribution to the study of mental disturbance in organic cerebral hemiplegia. (Anosognosia).] *Revue Neurologique, 27,* 845–848.

Bäckman, L., & Lipinska, B. (1993). Monitoring of general knowledge: Evidence for preservation in early Alzheimer's disease. *Neuropsychologia, 31,* 335–345.

Barrett, A. M., Eslinger, P. J., Ballentine, N. H., & Heilman, K. M. (2005). Unawareness of cognitive deficit (cognitive anosognosia) in probable AD and control subjects. *Neurology, 64,* 693–699.

Bondi, M., Salmon, D., & Kaszniak, A. W. (2009). The neuropsychology of dementia. In I. Grant, & K.Adams (Eds.), *Neuropsychological assessment of neuropsychiatric and neuromedical disorders* (3rd edition, pp.159-198). New York: Oxford University Press.

Braak, H., & Braak, E. (1991). Neuropathological staging of Alzheimer-related changes. *Acta Neuropathologica.* 82, 239–259.

Clare, L. (2004). Awareness in early-stage Alzheimer's disease: A review of methods and evidence. *British Journal of Clinical Psychology, 43,* 177–196.

Clare, L., Roth, I., & Pratt, R. (2005). Perceptions of change over time in early-stage Alzheimer's disease. *Dementia: The International Journal of Social Research and Practice, 4,* 487–520.

Clare, L., & Wilson, B. A. (2006). Longitudinal assessment of awareness in early-stage Alzheimer's disease using comparable questionnaire-based and performance-based measures: A prospective one-year follow-up study. *Aging & Mental Health, 10,* 156–165.

Clare, L., Wilson, B. A., Carter, G., Roth, I., & Hodges, J. (2002). Assessing awareness in early stage Alzheimer's disease: Development and piloting of the Memory Awareness Rating Scale. *Neuropsychological Rehabilitation, 12,* 341–362.

Clare, L., Wilson, B. A., Carter, G., Roth, I., & Hodges, J. R. (2004). Awareness in early-stage Alzheimer's disease: Relationship to outcome of cognitive rehabilitation. *Journal of Clinical and Experimental Neuropsychology, 26,* 215–226.

Correa, D. D., Graves, R. E., & Costa, L. (1996). Awareness of memory deficit in Alzheimer's disease patients and memory-impaired older adults. *Aging, Neuropsychology, and Cognition, 3,* 215–228.

Cosentino, S., & Stern, Y. (2005). Metacognitive theory and assessment in dementia: Do we recognize our areas of weakness? *Journal of the International Neuropsychological Society, 11,* 910–919.

Cotrell, V., & Lein, L. (1993). Awareness and denial in the Alzheimer's disease victim. *Journal of Gerontological Social Work, 19,* 115–132.

Cotrell, V., & Wild, K. (1999). Longitudinal study of self-imposed driving restrictions and deficit awareness in patients with Alzheimer disease. *Alzheimer Disease and Associated Disorders, 13,* 151–156.

Cummings, J. L., & Benson, D. F. (1992). *Dementia: A clinical approach* (2nd edition). Boston: Butterworth-Heinemann.

Dalla Barba, G., Parlato, V., Iavarone, A., & Boler, F. (1995). Anosognosia, intrusions and "frontal" functions in Alzheimer's disease and depression. *Neuropsychologia, 33*, 247–259.

DeBettignies, V. H., Mahurin, R. K., & Pirozzolo, F. J. (1990). Insight for impairment in independent living skills in Alzheimer's disease and multi-infarct dementia. *Journal of Clinical and Experimental Neuropsychology, 12*, 355–363.

DeKosky, S. T., & Scheff, S. W. (1990). Synapse loss in frontal cortex biopsies in Alzheimer's disease: Correlation with cognitive severity. *Annals of Neurology, 27*, 457–464.

Derouesné, C., Thibault, S., Lagha-Pierucci, S., Baudouin-Madec, V., Ancri, D., & Lacomblez, L. (1999). Decreased awareness of cognitive deficits in patients with mild dementia of the Alzheimer type. *International Journal of Geriatric Psychiatry, 14*, 1019–1030.

Duke, L., & Kaszniak, A. W. (2001). Impaired self-monitoring of episodic memory in Alzheimer's disease. *Journal of the International Neuropsychological Society, 7*, 125.

Duke, L. M., & Kaszniak, A. W. (2000). Executive control functions in degenerative dementias: A comparative review. *Neuropsychology Review, 10*, 75–99.

Duke, L. M., Seltzer, B., Seltzer, J. E., & Vasterling, J. J. (2002). Cognitive components of deficit awareness in Alzheimer's disease. *Neuropsychology, 16*, 359–369.

Dunlosky, J., & Metcalfe, J. (2009). *Metacognition.* Los Angeles, CA: Sage.

Efklides, A., Yiultsi, E., Kangellidou, T., Kounti, F., Dina, F., & Tsolaki, M. (2002). Wechsler Memory Scale, Rivermead Behavioral Memory Test, and Everyday Memory Questionnaire in healthy adults and Alzheimer patients. *European Journal of Psychological Assessment, 18*, 63–77.

Feehan, M., Knight, R. G., & Partridge, F. M. (1993). Cognitive complaint and test performance in elderly patients suffering depression or dementia. *International Journal of Geriatric Psychiatry, 6*, 287–293.

Feher, E. P., Larrabee, G. J., Sudilovsky, A., & Crook, T. H. (1994). Memory self-report in Alzheimer's disease and age-associated memory impairment. *Journal of Geriatric Psychiatry and Neurology, 7*, 58–65.

Feher, E. P., Mahurin, R. K., Inbody, S. B., Crook, T. H., & Pirozzolo, F. (1991). Anosognosia in Alzheimer's disease. *Neuropsychiatry, Neuropsychology, and Behavioral Neurology, 4*, 136–146.

Folstein, M.F., Folstein, S.E., & McHugh, P. R. (1975). "Mini-mental state." *Journal of Psychiatric Research, 12*, 189–198.

Frederiks, J. A. M. (1985). The neurology of aging and dementia. In J. A. M. Frederiks (Ed.), *Handbook of clinical neurology* (Vol. 2, pp. 199–219). Amsterdam: Elsevier.

Freidenberg, D. L., Huber, S. J., & Dreskin, M. (1990). Loss of insight in Alzheimer's disease. *Neurology, 40*(Suppl. 1): 240 (Abstract).

Gallo, D. A., Chen, M. J., Wiseman, A. L., Schacter, D. L., & Budson, A. E. (2007). Retrieval monitoring and anosognosia in Alzheimer's disease. *Neuropsychology, 21*, 559–568.

Gilewski, M. J., Zelinski, E. M., & Schaie, K. W. (1990). The Memory Functioning Questionnaire for assessment of memory complaints in adulthood and old age. *Psychology and Aging, 5*, 482–490.

Giovannetti, T., Libon, D. J., & Hart, T. (2002). Awareness of naturalistic action errors in dementia. *Journal of the International Neuropsychological Society, 8,* 633–644.

Green, J., Goldstein, F. C., Sirockman, B. E., & Green, R. C. (1993). Variable awareness of deficits in Alzheimer's disease. *Neuropsychiatry, Neuropsychology, and Behavioral Neurology, 6,* 159–165.

Gregory, C. A., & Hodges, J. R. (1996). Frontotemporal dementia: Use of consensus criteria and prevalence of psychiatric features. *Neuropsychiatry, Neuropsychology and Behavioral Neurology, 9,* 145–153.

Gustafson, L., & Nilsson, L. (1982). Differential diagnosis of presenile dementia on clinical grounds. *Acta Psychiatrica Scandinavica, 65,* 194–209.

Hardy, R. M., Oyebode, J. R., & Clare, L. (2006). Measuring awareness in people with mild to moderate Alzheimer's disease: Development of the Memory Awareness Rating Scale—adjusted. *Neuropsychological Rehabilitation, 16,* 178–193.

Hart, J. T. (1965). Memory and the feeling-of-knowing experience. *Journal of Educational Psychology, 56,* 208–216.

Henson, R. N., Rugg, M. D., & Shallice, T. (2000). Confidence in recognition memory for words: Dissociating right prefrontal roles in episodic memory. *Journal of Cognitive Neuroscience, 12,* 913–923.

Hertzog, C., & Dixon, R. A. (1994). Metacognitive development in adulthood and old age. In J. Metcalfe & A. P. Shimamura (Eds.), *Metacognition: Knowing about knowing* (pp. 227–251). Cambridge, MA: MIT Press.

Hyman, B. T., Van Hoesen, G. W., Damasio, A., & Barnes, C. (1984). Alzheimer's disease: Cell-specific pathology isolates the hippocampal formation. *Science, 225,* 1168–1170.

Janowsky, J. S., Shimamura, A. P., Kritchevsky, M., & Squire, L. R. (1989). Cognitive impairment following frontal lobe damage and its relevance to human amnesia. *Behavioral Neuroscience, 103,* 548–560.

Janowsky, J. S., Shimamura, A. P., & Squire, L. R. (1989). Memory and metamemory: Comparisons between patients with frontal lobe lesions and amnesic patients. *Psychobiology, 17,* 3–11.

Johnson, J. K., Brun, A., & Head, E. (2007). Frontal variant of Alzheimer's disease. In B. L. Miller & J. L. Cummings (Eds.), *The human frontal lobes: Functions and disorders* (2nd edition, pp. 429–444). New York: Guilford Press.

Kashiwa, Y., Kitabayashi, Y., Narumoto, J., Nakamura, K., Ueda, H., & Fukui, K. (2005). Anosognosia in Alzheimer's disease: Association with patient characteristics, psychiatric symptoms and cognitive deficits. *Psychiatry and Clinical Neurosciences, 59,* 697–704.

Kaszniak, A. W. (1986). The neuropsychology of dementia. In I. Grant & K. M. Adams (Eds.), *Neuropsychological assessment of neuropsychiatric disorders* (pp. 172–220). New York: Oxford University Press.

Kaszniak, A. W. (2002). Dementia. In V. S. Ramachandran (Ed.), *Encyclopedia of the human brain* (pp. 89–100). San Diego, CA: Elsevier Science.

Kaszniak, A. W. (2003). Anosognosia. In L. Nadel (Ed.), *Encyclopedia of cognitive science* (pp. 160–163). London: Macmillan.

Kaszniak, A. W., & Christenson, G. D. (1995). One-year longitudinal changes in the metamemory impairment of Alzheimer's disease. *Journal of the International Neuropsychological Society, 1*, 145.

Kaszniak, A. W., & Christenson, G. D. (1996). Self-awareness of deficit in patients with Alzheimer's disease. In S. R. Hameroff, A. W. Kaszniak, & A. C. Scott (eds.), *Toward a science of consciousness: The first Tucson discussions and debates* (pp. 227–242). Cambridge, MA: MIT Press.

Kaszniak, A. W., DiTraglia, G., & Trosset, M. W. (1993). Self-awareness of cognitive deficit in patients with probable Alzheimer's disease. *The Journal of Clinical and Experimental Neuropsychology, 15*, 30 (Abstract).

Kaszniak, A. W., Keyl, P., & Albert, M. (1991). Dementia and the older driver. *Human Factors, 33*, 527–537.

Kaszniak, A. W., Wilson, R. S., Fox, J. H., & Stebbins, G. T. (1986). Cognitive assessment in Alzheimer's disease: Cross-sectional and longitudinal perspectives. *Canadian Journal of Neurological Sciences, 13*, 420–423.

Kaszniak, A. W., & Zak, M. G. (1996). On the neuropsychology of metamemory: Contributions from the study of amnesia and dementia. *Learning and Individual Differences, 8*, 355–381.

Koltai, D. C., Welsh-Bohmer, K. A., & Schmechel, D. E. (2001). Influence of anosognosia on treatment outcome among dementia patients. *Neuropsychological Rehabilitation, 11*, 455–475.

Kopelman, M. D. (1989). Remote and autobiographical memory, temporal cortex memory and frontal atrophy in Korsakoff and Alzheimer patients. *Neuropsychologia, 27*, 437–460.

Koriat, A. (1993). How do we know that we know? The accessibility model of the feeling-of-knowing. *Psychological Review, 100*, 609–639.

Koriat, A., and Levy-Sadot, R. (2001). The combined contributions of the cue-familiarity and accessibility heuristics to feelings of knowing. *Journal of Experimental Psychology: Learning, Memory, and Cognition, 27*, 34–53.

Kotler-Cope, S., & Camp, C. J. (1995). Anosognosia in Alzheimer disease. *Alzheimer Disease and Associated Disorders, 9*, 52–56.

Larrabee, G. J., & Levin, H. S. (1986). Memory self-ratings and objective test performance in a normal elderly sample. *Journal of Clinical and Experimental Neuropsychology, 8*, 275–284.

Lipinska, B., & Bäckman, L. (1993). Monitoring of general knowledge: Evidence for preservation in early Alzheimer's disease. *Neuropsychologia, 31*, 335–345.

Loebel, J. P., Dager, S. R., Berg, G., & Hyde, T. S. (1990). Fluency of speech and self-awareness of memory deficit in Alzheimer's disease. *International Journal of Geriatric Psychiatry, 5*, 41–45.

Lopez, O. L., Becker, J. T., Somsak, D., Dew, M. A., & DeKosky, S. T. (1994). Awareness of cognitive deficits and anosognosia in probable Alzheimer's disease. *European Neurology, 34*, 277–282.

Mangone, C. A., Hier, D. B., Gorelick, P. B., Ganellen, R. J., Langenberg, P., Boarman, R., & Dollear, W. C. (1991). Impaired insight in Alzheimer's disease. *Journal of Geriatric Psychiatry and Neurology, 4*, 189–193.

Markova, I. S., Clare, L., Wang, M., Romero, B., & Kenny, G. (2005). Awareness in dementia: Conceptual issues. *Aging & Mental Health, 9*, 386–393.

Mayhew, P., Acton, G. J., Yauk, S., & Hopkins, B. A. (2001). Communication from individuals with advanced DAT: Can it provide clues to their sense of awareness and well-being? *Geriatric Nursing, 22*, 106–110.

McDaniel, K. D., Edland, S. D., Heyman, A., & The Cerad Clinical Investigators (1995). Relationship between level of insight and severity of dementia in Alzheimer's disease. *Alzheimer Disease and Associated Disorders, 9*, 101–104.

McGlone, J., Gupta, S., Humphrey, D., Oppenheimer, S., Mirsen, T., & Evans, D. R. (1990). Screening for early dementia using memory complaints from patients and relatives. *Archives of Neurology, 47*, 1189–1193.

McGlynn, S. M., & Kaszniak, A. W. (1991a). Unawareness of deficits in dementia and schizophrenia. In G. P. Prigatano & D. L. Schacter (Eds.), *Awareness of deficit after brain injury: Clinical and theoretical issues* (pp. 84–110). New York: Oxford University Press.

McGlynn, S. M., & Kaszniak, A. W. (1991b). When metacognition fails: Impaired awareness of deficit in Alzheimer's disease. *Journal of Cognitive Neuroscience, 3*, 183–189.

McGlynn, S. M., & Schacter, D. L. (1989). Unawareness of deficits in neuropsychological syndromes. *Journal of Clinical and Experimental Neuropsychology, 11*, 143–205.

Metcalfe, J., Schwartz, B. L., & Joaquim, S. G. (1993). The cue-familiarity heuristic in metacognition. *Journal of Experimental Psychology: Learning, Memory, and Cognition, 19*, 851–864.

Metcalfe, J. & Shimamura, A. P. (Eds.) (1994). *Metacognition: Knowing about knowing.* Cambridge, MA: MIT Press.

Michon, A., Deweer, B., Pillon, B., Agid, Y., & Dubois, B. (1994). Relation of anosognosia to frontal lobe dysfunction in Alzheimer's disease. *Journal of Neurology, Neurosurgery, and Psychiatry, 57*, 805–809.

Migliorelli, R., Teson, A., Sabe, L., Petracca, G., Petracchi, M., Leiguarda, R., & Starkstein, S. E. (1995). Anosognosia in Alzheimer's disease: A study of associated factors. *The Journal of Neuropsychiatry and Clinical Neurosciences, 7*, 338–344.

Moulin, C. (2002). Sense and sensitivity: Metacognition in Alzheimer's disease. In T. Perfect (Ed.), *Applied metacognition* (pp. 197–223). West Nyack, NY: Cambridge University Press.

Moulin, C., James, N., Perfect, T., & Jones, R. (2003). Knowing what you cannot recognize: Further evidence for intact metacognition in Alzheimer's disease. *Aging, Neuropsychology, and Cognition, 10*, 74–82.

Moulin, C. J. A., Perfect, T. J., & Jones, R. W. (2000a). The effects of repetition on allocation of study time and judgements of learning in Alzheimer's disease. *Neuropsychologia, 38*, 750–758.

Moulin, C. J. A., Perfect, T. J., & Jones, R. W. (2000b). Global predictions of memory in Alzheimer's disease: Evidence for preserved metamemory monitoring. *Aging, Neuropsychology, and Cognition, 7*, 230–244.

Moulin, C. J. A., Perfect, T. J., & Jones, R. W. (2000c). Evidence for intact memory monitoring in Alzheimer's disease: Metamemory sensitivity at encoding. *Neuropsychologia, 38*, 1242–1250.

Nelson, T. O. (1984). A comparison of current measures of the accuracy of feeling-of-knowing. *Psychological Bulletin, 95,* 109–133.

Nelson, T. O. & Dunlosky, J. (1991). When peoples' judgments of learning (JOLs) are extremely accurate at predicting subsequent recall: The "Delayed-JOL Effect." *Psychological Science, 2,* 267–270.

Nelson, T. O., & Narens, L. (1990). Metamemory: A theoretical framework and new findings. In G. Bower (Ed.), *The psychology of learning and motivation* (Vol. 26, pp. 125–322). New York: Academic Press.

Ott, B. R., Noto, R. B., & Fogel, B. S. (1996). Apathy and loss of insight in Alzheimer's disease: A SPECT imaging study. *The Journal of Neuropsychiatry and Clinical Neurosciences, 8,* 41–46.

Ownsworth, T., Clare, L., & Morris, R. (2006). An integrated biopsychosocial approach to understanding awareness deficits in Alzheimer's disease and brain injury. *Neuropsychological Rehabilitation, 16,* 415–438.

Oyebode, J. R., Telling, A. L., Hardy, R. M., & Austin, J. (2007). Awareness of memory functioning in early Alzheimer's disease; Lessons from a comparison with healthy older people and young adults. *Aging & Mental Health, 11,* 761–767.

Pachana, N. A., & Petriwskyj, A. M. (2006). Assessment of insight and self-awareness in older drivers. *Clinical Gerontologist, 30,* 23–38.

Pannu, J. K., & Kaszniak, A. W. (2005). Metamemory experiments in neurological populations: A review. *Neuropsychology Review, 15,* 105–130.

Pannu, J. K., Kaszniak, A. W., & Rapcsak, S. Z. (2005). Metamemory for faces following frontal lobe damage. *Journal of the International Neuropsychological Society, 11,* 668–676.

Pappas, B. A., Sunderland, T., Weingartner, H. M., Vitiello, B., Martinson, H., & Putnam, K. (1992). Alzheimer's disease and feeling-of-knowing for knowledge and episodic memory. *Journal of Gerontology, 47,* P159–P164.

Prigatano, G. P. & Schacter, D. L. (Eds.) (1991a). *Awareness of deficit after brain injury: Clinical and theoretical issues.* New York: Oxford University Press.

Prigatano, G. P. & Schacter, D. L. (1991b). Introduction. In G. P. Prigatano & D. L. Schacter (Eds.), *Awareness of deficit after brain injury: Clinical and theoretical issues* (pp. 3–16). New York: Oxford University Press.

Ramachandran, V. S. (1995). Anosognosia in parietal lobe syndrome. *Consciousness and Cognition, 4,* 22–51.

Ready, R. E., Ott, B. R., & Grace, J. (2006). Insight and cognitive impairment: Effects on quality-of-life reports from mild cognitive impairment and Alzheimer's disease patients. *American Journal of Alzheimer's Disease and Other Dementias, 21,* 242–248.

Reed, B. R., Jagust, W. J., & Coulter, L. (1993). Anosognosia in Alzheimer's disease: Relationship to depression, cognitive function, and cerebral perfusion. *The Journal of Clinical and Experimental Neuropsychology, 15,* 231–244.

Reisberg, B., Gordon, B., McCarthy, M., Ferris, S. H., & deLeon, M. J. (1985). Insight and denial accompanying progressive cognitive decline in normal aging and Alzheimer's disease. In B. Stanley (Ed.), *Geriatric psychiatry: Clinical, ethical, and legal issues* (pp. 19–39). Washington, DC: American Psychiatric Press.

Robert, P. H., Clairet, S., Benoit, M., Koutaich, J., Bertogliati, C., Tible, O., Caci, H., Borg, M., Brocker, P., & Bedoucha, P. (2002). The apathy inventory: Assessment of apathy and awareness in Alzheimer's disease, Parkinson's disease and mild cognitive impairment. *International Journal of Geriatric Psychiatry, 17*, 1099–1105.

Salmon, E., Perani, D., Collette, F., Feyers, D., Kalbe, E., Holthoff, V., Sorbi, S., & Herholz, K. (2008). Comparison of unawareness in frontotemporal dementia and Alzheimer's disease. *Journal of Neurology, Neurosurgery, and Psychiatry, 79*, 176–179.

Sato, J., Nakaaki, S., Murata, Y., Shinagawa, Y., Matusi, T., Hongo, J., Tatsumi, J., Akechi, T., & Furukawa, T. A. (2007). Two dimensions of anosognosia in patients with Alzheimer's disease: Reliablity and validity of the Japanese version of the anosognosia questionnaire for dementia (AQ-D). *Psychiatry and Clinical Neurosciences, 61*, 672–677.

Schacter, D. L. (1990). Toward a cognitive neuropsychology of awareness: Implicit knowledge and anosognosia. *Journal of Clinical and Experimental Neuropsychology, 12*, 155–178.

Schacter, D. L. (1991). Unawareness of deficit and unawareness of knowledge in patients with memory disorder. In G. P. Prigatano & D. L. Schacter (Eds.), *Awareness of deficit after brain injury: Clinical and theoretical issues* (pp. 127–151). New York: Oxford University Press.

Schacter, D. L., McLachlan, D. R., Moscovitch, M., & Tulving, E. (1986). Monitoring of recall performance by memory-disordered patients. *The Journal of Clinical and Experimental Neuropsychology, 8*, 130.

Schneck, M. K., Reisberg, B., & Ferris, S. H. (1982). An overview of current concepts of Alzheimer's disease. *American Journal of Psychiatry, 139*, 165–173.

Schnyer, D. M., Verfaellie, M., Alexander, M. P., LaFleche, G., Nicholls, L., & Kaszniak, A. W. (2004). A role for right medial prefrontal cortex in accurate feeling of knowing judgments: Evidence from patients with lesions to frontal cortex. *Neuropsychologia, 42*, 957–966.

Schraw, G. (1995). Measures of feeling-of-knowing accuracy: A new look at an old problem. *Applied Cognitive Psychology, 9*, 321–332.

Seidenberg, M., Taylor, M. A., & Haltiner, A. (1994). Personality and self-report of cognitive functioning. *Archives of Clinical Neuropsychology, 9*, 353–361.

Seltzer, B., Vasterling, J. J., Hale, M. A., & Khurana, R. (1995). Unawareness of memory deficit in Alzheimer's disease: Relation to mood and other disease variables. *Neuropsychiatry, Neuropsychology, and Behavioral Neurology, 8*, 176–181.

Seltzer, B., Vasterling, J. J., Yoder, J., & Thompson, K. (1997). Awareness of deficit in Alzheimer's disease: Relation to caregiver burden. *Gerontologist, 37*, 20–24.

Sevush, S., & Leve, N. (1993). Denial of memory deficit in Alzheimer's disease. *American Journal of Psychiatry, 150*, 748–751.

Somers, R. H. (1962). A new asymmetric measure of association for ordinal variables. *American Sociological Review, 27*, 799–811.

Souchay, C., Isingrini, M., & Espagnet. (2000). Aging, episodic memory feeling-of-knowing, and frontal functioning. *Neuropsychology, 14*, 299–309.

Souchay, C., Isingrini, M., & Gil, R. (2002). Alzheimer's disease and feeling-of-knowing in episodic memory. *Neuropsychologia, 40*, 2386–2396.

Souchay, C., Isingrini, M., Pillon, B., & Gill, R. (2003). Metamemory accuracy in Alzheimer's disease and frontotemporal lobe dementia. *Neurocase, 9*, 482–492.

Starkstein, S. E., Chemerinski, E., Sabe, L., Kuzis, G., Petracca, G., Teson, A., & Leiguarda, R., (1997). Prospective longitudinal study of depression and anosognosia in Alzheimer's disease. *British Journal of Psychiatry, 171,* 47–52.

Starkstein, S. E., Jorge, R., Mizahi, R., Adrian, J., & Robinson, R. G. (2007). Insight and danger in Alzheimer's disease. *European Journal of Neurology, 14,* 455–460.

Starkstein, S. E., Sabe, L., Chemerinski, E., Jason, L., & Leiguarda, R. (1996). Two domains of anosognosia in Alzheimer's disease. *Journal of Neurology, Neurosurgery, and Psychiatry, 61,* 485–490.

Starkstein, S. E., Vazquez, S., Migliorelli, R., Teson, A., Sabe, L., & Leiguarda, R. (1995). A single-photon emission computed tomographic study of anosognosia in Alzheimer's disease. *Archives of Neurology, 52,* 415–420.

Stuss, D. T. (2007). New approaches to prefrontal lobe testing. In B.L. Miller & J.L. Cummings (Eds.), *The human frontal lobes: Functions and disorders* (2nd edition, pp. 292–305). New York: Guilford Press.

Stuss, D. T., Rosenbaum, R. S., Malcolm, S., Christiana, W., & Keenan, J. P. (2005). The frontal lobes and self-awareness. In T. E. Feinberg & J. P. Keenan (Eds.), *The lost self: Pathologies of the brain and identity* (pp. 50–64). New York: Oxford University Press.

Sunderland, A., Harris, J. E., & Baddeley, A. D. (1983). Do laboratory tests predict everyday memory? *Journal of Verbal Learning and Verbal Behavior, 22,* 341–357.

Trosset, M. W., & Kaszniak, A. W. (1996). Measures of deficit unawareness for predicted performance experiments. *Journal of the International Neuropsychological Society, 2,* 315–322.

Vasterling, J. J., Seltzer, B., Foss, J. W., & Vanderbrook, V. (1995). Unawareness of deficit in Alzheimer's disease: Domain-specific differences and disease correlates. *Neuropsychiatry, Neuropsychology, and Behavioral Neurology, 8,* 26–32.

Vasterling, J. J., Seltzer, B., & Watrous, W. E. (1997). Longitudinal assessment of deficit unawareness in Alzheimer's disease. *Neuropsychiatry, Neuropsychology, & Behavioral Neurology, 10,* 197–202.

Verhey, F. R., Rozendaal, N., Ponds, R. W., & Jolles, J. (1993). Dementia, awareness and depression. *International Journal of Geriatric Psychiatry, 8,* 851–856.

Vogel, A., Hasselbalch, S. G, Gade, A., Ziebell, M., & Waldemar, G. (2005). Cognitive and functional neuroimaging correlates for anosognosia in mild cognitive impairment and Alzheimer's disease. *International Journal of Geriatric Psychiatry, 20,* 238–246.

Vuilleumier, P. (2000). Anosognosia: The neurology of beliefs and uncertainties. *Cortex, 40,* 9–17.

Wagner, M. T., Spangenberg, K. B., Bachman, D. L., & O'Connell, P. (1997). Unawareness of cognitive deficit in Alzheimer disease and related dementias. *Alzheimer Disease and Related Disorders, 11,* 125–131.

Watkins, R., Cheston, R., Jones, K, & Gilliard, J. (2006). "Coming out" with Alzheimer's disease: Changes in awareness during a psychotherapy group for people with dementia. *Aging & Mental Health, 10,* 166–176.

Weinstein, E. A. (1991). Anosognosia and denial of illness. In G. P. Prigatano & D. L. Schacter (Eds.), *Awareness of deficit after brain injury: Clinical and theoretical issues* (pp. 240–257). New York: Oxford University Press.

Weinstein, E. A., Friedland, R. P., & Wagner, E. E. (1994). Denial/unawareness of impairment and symbolic behavior in Alzheimer's disease. *Neuropsychiatry, Neuropsychology, and Behavioral Neurology, 7*, 176–184.

Weinstein, E. A., & Kahn, R. L. (1955). *Denial of illness: Symbolic and physiological aspects.* Springfield, IL: Charles C. Thomas.

Wragg, R., & Jeste, D. (1989). Overview of depression and psychosis in Alzheimer's disease. *American Journal of Psychiatry, 146*, 577–587.

12

Anosognosia after Traumatic Brain Injury

George P. Prigatano

The hallmark of traumatic brain injury (TBI) is a loss or disruption of consciousness followed by a period of "confusion," or post-traumatic amnesia (PTA; Russell, 1971). Depending on the length of unresponsiveness or coma and the duration of PTA, severe neurocognitive and neurobehavioral problems may be observed (Dikmen, Machamer, Winn, & Temkin, 1995; Levin et al., 1990). These include disorders of memory, processing speed, attention, language, and abstract or analytic reasoning abilities. Patients often report less tolerance for frustration and being more irritable (Prigatano, 1999). Family members may report that patients are socially inappropriate and appear unaware of their cognitive and behavioral limitations (Oddy, Coughlan, Tyerman, & Jenkins, 1985).

Early reports of the neurocognitive consequences of TBI alluded to disturbances in self-awareness following moderate to severe TBI (Meyer, 1904). However, it was the efforts at intensive neuropsychological rehabilitation that clearly revealed that a portion of these patients show residual impairments in self-awareness several months and even years post-TBI (Prigatano et al., 1986). Residual disturbances in self-awareness have been shown to impact both the process and outcome of neurorehabilitation (Prigatano, 2008). The mechanisms responsible for this lack of awareness of one's residual cognitive and/or behavioral/personality disturbances remain debated. In this chapter, I will present a partial review of the literature on disturbances of self-awareness, or anosognosia, associated with TBI.

A Brief Historical Review of Observations on Impaired Self-Awareness after Traumatic Brain Injury

Adolf Meyer (1904) provided an early attempt to relate specific neuropathological findings to changes in cognition and personality after TBI. While not using the terms *anosognosia* or *impaired self-awareness* (ISA), he provided clinical vignettes of patients that suggested a lack of awareness of functional limitations. For example, he described dramatic personality changes in a 38-year-old mill operator who was struck on the head by a 45-pound weight. He described the patient as less efficient at work, but the patient attributed these inefficiencies to co-workers who "put things in his way" (p. 378).

Several years later, Paul Schilder (1934) described the "confusion" patients demonstrate when regaining consciousness following TBI, and he gave examples of apparent "denial" phenomena. For instance, he described a 46-year-old man who was found unconscious in the street. When the patient regained conscious-ness, he had obvious memory difficulties and was disoriented. Schilder (1934) noted that the patient at one point stated: "I really don't think anything is the matter with my leg" (p. 160). Schilder noted, however, that the left leg of the patient had to be amputated. His contradictory statements about himself were explained on the basis of disorientation and severe memory impairment.

Schilder (1934) went on to note that the "two fundamental symptoms" after severe head injury are "the clouding of consciousness with confusion" and memory disturbance. He also noted that "it is astonishing how little the patients are concerned about their head injuries" (p. 165). This lack of concern (or anosodiaphoria) is often observed in neurological patients who are unaware of a hemiparetic limb following stroke (Bisiach & Geminiani, 1991). Using more contemporary terminology, we could describe these TBI patients as showing a disruption in their self-awareness of residual cognitive, personality, or sensori-motor losses following moderate to severe brain injuries (Prigatano, 1991).

Goldstein (1952), the father of neuropsychological rehabilitation, attributed the diminished self-awareness of deficit after TBI to a "protective mechanism" aimed at helping the patient avoid a "catastrophic condition—of anxiety" (p. 257). Goldstein noted that the whole thrust of adaptation is for the organism to avoid any condition that would put it in a state of panic, and therefore it may well keep out of awareness any experience that would be threatening to its ability to survive. This type of explanation argues that for biological and/or psychological reasons, the patient remains "unaware" as a method of coping.

An alternative explanation is that unawareness of deficit, or frank anosog-nosia, is not a method of coping, but a failure of the brain to integrate (and perhaps remember) important experiences that allow for conscious perception of a disturbed function. Critchley (1953) quoting from a paper by Nielsen (1938) made the following observations: the patient "denied that the paralyzed arm was hers. When it was demonstrated that the hand was attached by way of the arm to her own body, she replied: 'but my eyes and my feelings don't agree, and I must believe my feelings. I know they look like mine, but I can feel that they are not, and I cannot believe my eyes'" (Nielsen as quoted in Critchley, 1953, p. 236). This patient's description of her subjective experience may provide important clues as to the nature of anosognosia in TBI patients.

Problems in Studying Anosognosia or Impaired Self-Awareness after Traumatic Brain Injury

While clinicians frequently observe phenomena that suggest a person with moderate to severe TBI may have limited or impaired self-awareness of certain neurocognitive and behavioral disturbances, there are numerous difficulties in systematically studying ISA after TBI. Persons with TBI who show ISA may vary greatly as to their pre-morbid and post-morbid neuropsychological and psychiatric functioning. Seldom if ever is ISA seen in isolation of other significant neurocognitive and neuropsychiatric disturbances (Prigatano & Maier, 2008). The correlational findings reported in the literature are, therefore, interesting but seldom explanatory in nature.

Present measurement techniques are limited when assessing a person's subjective experience. Answers obtained from questionnaires or structured interviews may not reveal the underlying nature or phenomenological experience of ISA. Questionnaire data always measures ISA indirectly. Comparing the patient's self-report on questionnaires to family members' reports (Prigatano & Altman, 1990) or professional judgments (Prigatano, Ogano, & Amakusa, 1997) is helpful, but it is vulnerable to methodological error, including response bias (Bach & David, 2006).

The type of question asked of the patient can also produce varying results and misleading findings. Post-acute TBI patients with a history of severe injuries are not generally globally unaware of their difficulties. They typically have specific areas in which they have reduced awareness and early research suggested that those areas center around problems with emotional control and social interactions (Prigatano, Altman, & O'Brien, 1990). Using questionnaires that ask about general health-related difficulties, but do not focus on specific areas of potential difficulty that would reflect ISA are likely to produce either negative findings or unclear findings, despite the robust statistics that may be employed in a given study (e.g., Pagulauan, Temkin, Machamer, & Dimken, 2007).

A further complication is that some patients who appear unaware may actually be in a state of denial (Weinstein & Kahn, 1955). These patients seem to have knowledge of their difficulties but may be overwhelmed by their limitations (Prigatano & Klonoff, 1997). Seldom do researchers systematically assess patient statements to detect possible methods of coping versus a lack of awareness of disturbance in functional capacity. This failure has led to numerous misunderstandings, particularly the notion that depression is a natural consequence of improved self-awareness.

It is true that patients who become aware of deficits can be initially distressed by their knowledge of functional limitations. Whether awareness of their deficits in and of itself produces depression may vary from individual to individual and change over the course of time. Many severely impaired patients with TBI are genuinely confused over the feedback they obtain from others concerning their inappropriate social behaviors (Prigatano, 1991). With a better understanding of their difficulties, they are seldom depressed and are often grateful to have a reduction in their cognitive perplexity (some research has supported this clinical observation: Malec & Moessner, 2000; Ownsworth & Clare, 2006). There is no doubt, however, that prolonged failure in social interactions will likely lead to depression. Patients who have neurobehavioral problems frequently have long-term difficulties with social interaction; therefore, one could misinterpret the role of ISA in mediating these two phenomena (Bach & David, 2006).

What can be said with some clinical confidence is that ISA changes with time and most notably is more pronounced during the acute stages of TBI. Second, severity of TBI and location of brain lesions appear to play an important role in the extent and the type of ISA that is observed. Finally, premorbid and post-morbid personality (and cultural factors) may influence how deficits or impairments are interpreted by the patient, the family, and their doctor. Developing innovative methods of assessing these potential complex interactions will help us better understand the true nature of anosognosia after TBI.

Disturbances of Self-Awareness of Deficits after Traumatic Brain Injury: Time and Severity Interactions

At the moment of impact, persons who suffer a TBI either lose consciousness or very briefly are "confused" about what just happened to them. In cases of mild TBI (i.e., Glasgow Coma Scale [GCS] scores of 13 to 15; Jennett & Teasdale, 1981), the period of both retrograde and anterograde amnesia (the latter term is often referred to as PTA) is brief—lasting from a few seconds to no more than 20 minutes (Bigler, 2005). Typically these individuals quickly become aware of disturbances in balance, memory, and concentration, as well as a variety of sensory disturbances, including sensitivity to light and noise. Some may have severe headache and vomit. Understandably, these individuals are frightened and distressed over their symptoms. As they improve in their neurological and neuropsychological functioning, the distress level abates and usually within 30 to 90 days post trauma, these individuals feel much better. If anything, they are aware of changes in their functional capacities that are not easily assessed by existing neurological and neuropsychological methods.

When asked to rate their functional capabilities on measures such as the Patient Competency Rating Scale (PCRS; Prigatano et al., 1986), they report either similar levels of functioning as their family members perceive, or at times, higher levels of difficulty (particularly in such areas as memory) than what relatives report about them. Research by Leathem, Murphy, and Flett (1998) supports this clinical observation. Malec, Testa, Rush, Brown, and Moessner

(2007), using another scale to measure ISA, came to a similar conclusion (i.e., patients with mild TBI do not demonstrate ISA).

The clinical picture is entirely different in cases of severe TBI (admitting GCS scores between 3 and 8) where there is a prolonged loss of consciousness (i.e., greater than 24 hours) or an extended period of PTA (in excess of 2 to 3 weeks). The patients often do not have any recollection of what happened to them, are convinced that they do not need to be in the hospital, and may report no cognitive impairments. During their hospital stays, they may literally "walk and talk" and give elaborate explanations (often confabulatory in nature) as to why they are in the hospital. During this time they demonstrate severe memory impairment. For example, one patient who was an aspiring actor indicated that he was not in a hospital but rather on a movie set depicting a MASH scene in which he was an actor. The individuals appearing as doctors and nurses were also actors on the movie set. Progressively, this patient did accept that he had suffered injuries, but during his hospital stay and immediately post discharge, reported no significant neuropsychological disturbances. Physical disturbances, on the other hand, are typically acknowledged within weeks and months following severe TBI (Sherer et al., 1998a).

Patients who suffered severe TBI were seen in a holistic neuropsychological rehabilitation program in which they were treated 6 hours a day, 5 days a week for 6 months (Prigatano et al., 1984; Prigatano et al., 1986). Most of these patients were in excess of 1 to 2 years post trauma and had already undergone traditional inpatient neurorehabilitation. In working with these patients, it became evident that many of these individuals were not aware of their neuropsychological impairments and/or the extent of those impairments (Prigatano et al., 1984).

Early studies showed that in this population of patients their ISA was not "global" several months post injury, but a proportion (estimated between 30% and 40%) did not subjectively experience significant cognitive impairments and particularly were noted to not accurately perceive their socially inappropriate behavior or their difficulties handling emotionally charged situations. In contrast, their family members were acutely aware of difficulties in these areas (Prigatano et al., 1990). These basic observations were later replicated (Prigatano, 1996) and confirmed by other researchers (Fischer, Trexler, & Gauggel, 2004; O'Keefe, Dockree, Moloney, Carton, & Robertson, 2007).

Patients with moderate TBI (i.e., GCS scores between 9 and 12) tend to be aware of their neurological and neuropsychological disturbances once PTA abates, but their picture is more complicated when they suffer frontal lesions to the brain. Some of these patients could be described as having "moderately severe" TBI and a portion of these patients do, in fact, demonstrate ISA. As a group they have not been thoroughly studied and are often combined with patients who have suffered severe TBI (e.g., Dirette & Plaisier, 2007) for research purposes. Not unexpectedly, combining these groups often results in findings that are more difficult to interpret.

Clinical observations suggest that patients with severe TBI may show improvement in their ISA over time (i.e., as they move into the post-acute or chronic phases typically 1 year or longer post TBI), but still demonstrate ISA if properly examined. For example, Hoofien, Gilboa, Vakil, and Barak (2004) reported that approximately 27% of their TBI patients showed evidence of ISA 13.8 years ($SD = 5.8$) post injury. It is often a mistake, therefore, to assume that as PTA resolves in persons with severe TBI that their altered self-awareness returns to "normal." On the surface many patients appear to have adequate insight or awareness of their difficulties, but under certain examining conditions, subtle but important impairments of self-awareness may exist.

Lesion Location and Impaired Self-Awareness after Severe Traumatic Brain Injury

Neuroradiographic findings associated with moderate to severe TBI secondary to acceleration/deceleration forces frequently reveal hemorrhagic contusions and/or hematomas in the prefrontal and anterior temporal regions of the brain (Gentry, 2002). Lesions can occur, however, anywhere in the brain. Bilateral and asymmetrical lesions are common and may include the brain stem and cerebellum. Pathological findings further demonstrate diffuse neuronal loss and white matter degeneration (Bigler, 2005).

It is not uncommon, given the nature of the neuropathology of severe TBI, to find individual cases in which bilateral prefrontal hemorrhagic contusions are present in patients who make socially inappropriate comments and who are not aware of them (e.g., Anderson, Damasio, Tranel, & Damasio, 2000; Prigatano, 1991). However, ISA in patients with severe TBI can also exist for memory deficits, as well as other cognitive and behavioral disturbances. It is not surprising that two neuroimaging studies that have attempted to relate ISA to lesion location reveal multiple site lesions and a greater number of lesions in TBI patients with ISA, compared to TBI patients who do not show ISA (Prigatano & Altman, 1990; Sherer, Hart, Whyte, Nick, & Yablon, 2005). These findings do not tell us how different types of anosognosia or ISA relate to different neurocircuit disturbances in different regions of the brain. They do emphasize, however, that severity of TBI is an important predictor of ISA.

Schmitz, Rowley, Kawahara, and Johnson (2006) employed functional MRI techniques to address two interacting questions concerning ISA in TBI patients. First, when TBI patients are asked to reflect on their personal traits and abilities, do they show a pattern of brain activation similar to those found in normal adults (Johnson et al., 2002)? Second, using a linear regression analysis, what areas of the brain activate when TBI patients show more accurate self-awareness? Their results suggest that TBI patients and controls showed similar patterns of brain activation when engaged in a self-reflection task (i.e., activation of medial prefrontal cortex, retrosplenial cortex, left parahippocampal gyrus, and thalamus). Interestingly, TBI patients showed greater activation (i.e., increased signal change) when conducting the self-evaluation task in the anterior cingulate, precuneus, and the right temporal pole, compared to controls. These researchers also found that increased activation of the right anterior dorsal prefrontal cortex (PFC) was associated with more accurate self-insight in the TBI population. The implication, of course, is that damage to this region might be especially important in persistent ISA after severe TBI.

Impaired Awareness of a Neurological or Neuropsychological Impairment versus Its Functional Implications

Crosson et al. (1989) brought attention to an issue in the study of ISA after TBI. A person may have awareness that a function is impaired (i.e., deemed "intellectual awareness") but may not be aware of its functional implications as it is happening (i.e., "emergent awareness") or when it might occur in the future (i.e., "anticipatory awareness"). Thus, separating ISA for a deficit versus its functional implications may be important in some cases. This idea has not found much empirical support (O'Keefe et al., 2007).

Against this background, there are two interesting published case reports about anosognosia for neurological dysfunction after TBI that deserve special attention.

Anton's Syndrome in a Patient with Post-Traumatic Optic Neuropathy and Bifrontal Contusions

McDaniel and McDaniel (1991) provided a detailed case study of a woman who suffered right optic nerve damage secondary to a suicide attempt. The patient denied any visual loss during her first 11 days post trauma. The patient also suffered bilateral frontal contusions and demonstrated several behavioral signs of frontal systems dysfunction (i.e., marked disinhibition, impulsiveness, and disorganized behavioral responses). Like many patients during PTA, she denied she was in the hospital and reported no difficulties with her legs, even though they were in casts and her left leg was in traction. They described her as globally anosognostic with confabulation. With time, her "frontal lobe" functions improved and she no longer "denied" her visual loss, but like many patients she explained any residual visual problems that were demonstrated to her secondary to external factors (i.e., the lighting was poor in the room). This version of Anton's syndrome (i.e., a loss of vision with no conscious acknowledgement of that loss) may be due to disturbances of frontal lobe function involved in self-monitoring and the capacity for self-insight (McDaniel and

McDaniel, 1991). The disorder was attributed to a pattern of frontal lobe dysfunction in the context of a dense PTA.

Chronic Anosognosia for Hemiplegia after Severe Traumatic Brain Injury

Cocchini, Beschin, and Della Sala (2002) present a case of a 27-year-old male who suffered a severe TBI. Neuroimaging of the brain showed both cortical and subcortical lesions. He reportedly had bilateral frontal lobe lesions, but mainly in the left hemisphere. He was noted to have a right frontal parietal, a left temporal lobe, and right internal capsule lesion. One year post trauma he still demonstrated left extrapersonal neglect, anosognosia for left hemiplegia, and a profound memory disturbance of which he was unaware. He had dense retrograde amnesia, as well as anterograde amnesia. He showed substantial difficulties with visuospatial problem solving. Furthermore, it was noted that he had a hemianopsia and demonstrated extinction to double stimulation of tactile and auditory stimuli.

When his visuospatial neglect was ultimately demonstrated to him, he explained his failure on the basis of his not really concentrating. These researchers pointed out that he reportedly " . . . correctly analyzed information from the social environment and was able to comply with social rules, sometimes making whimsical, socially-appropriate comments" (p. 2032).

When the experimenters were able to briefly demonstrate that he could not use his limbs when testing Heilman's (1991) feed-forward theory of anosognosia for hemiplegia, the patient was able to momentarily be aware of his failure. They reported him saying: "Oh dear me, it's not moving." Reportedly "he was so upset that the experiment had to be halted" (p. 2032). However, they noted that he quickly forgot the event and returned to his state of unawareness. While the investigators did not attribute his anosognosia for hemiplegia solely on the basis of his dense amnesia, they drew the following conclusions:

> N.S. (the patient) was unaware because of his personal neglect coupled with sensory feedback mis-routing, which prevented him from detecting his motor impairment. When he overcame these problems he became fully aware of his hemiplegia. Yet he could not retain this information and update his premorbid beliefs about himself. The result was that the new information decayed after a few minutes and N.S. was once again unaware of his motor deficits, referring to himself through the accrued schema of a healthy person." (p. 2032)

This very thoughtful and theoretically relevant case study has several important observations that should be kept in mind when understanding anosognosia in TBI patients. First, bilateral frontal lobe lesions were present with several other cortical and subcortical lesions noted. Second, anosognosia for hemiplegia is associated with other significant neuropsychological disturbances (in this case, severe neglect and dense amnesia). Third, frank anosognosia persisted when retrograde and anterograde amnesia persisted (in many ways the patient was still in a period of post-traumatic amnesia). Fourth, the internal conscious representation of sensory (bodily feelings) input was deprived, and when this was overcome the patient was momentarily aware with an associated catastrophic reaction, as described years ago by Goldstein (1952). These facts should be kept in mind when attempting to understand ISA for neuropsychological disturbances in TBI patients after PTA ends (i.e., the resolution of significant retrograde or anterograde amnesia).

Impaired Self-Awareness after the Period of Post-Traumatic Amnesia Resolves in Patients with Severe Traumatic Brain Injury

Impaired Self-Awareness for Socially Inappropriate Behavior

After the resolution of PTA, patients with a history of severe TBI can demonstrate ISA for any neuropsychological dysfunction. Perhaps the most common area, however, is a failure to experience difficulties in social interaction and appropriate control of emotional responses. For example, one young man who suffered severe TBI and who showed bilateral frontal contusions on computed tomography was observed interacting with a young woman in a hospital cafeteria. Like many young males, he was eager to have a girlfriend. On this particular occasion he was waiting in line in the hospital cafeteria when he caught the eye of an attractive young physical therapist. The patient desperately wanted to talk to the therapist, but she was obviously not interested. As the physical therapist moved up in line to obtain her food, the patient began to smile at her in somewhat of a childish manner. The therapist, not interested, turned her head away to avoid eye contact. The patient did not pick up on this subtle cue, but continued to walk close to the physical therapist, attempting to engage her in communication. At one point, the patient said to the therapist that she had pretty hair. The therapist acknowledged this, but again looked the other way, giving a clear social signal that she was not interested in further dialogue.

As they walked up further in the line, the patient became bolder, making a comment that her hair was exceptionally pretty and long. Again, the therapist recognized this and turned the other way. Her facial expression became sterner. The patient did not appear to pick up on this cue.

Finally, the patient became somewhat desperate to engage the physical therapist in conversation and made the comment that her hair was so long that he wondered where "she got it." At this point the young woman, frustrated with this man's behavior, abruptly stated, "I grew it out of my head." At that, the patient simply responded, "Oh." He sensed that something may have gone wrong, but he was unaware that he had missed several social cues.

I had an opportunity to talk to the patient about this during a group psychotherapy session, which followed the lunch break. When I brought my observations to his attention, the patient's response was, "You psychologists look for problems everywhere." He did not recognize that what he had said or done was uncomfortable for the woman. We agreed that we would have one of the staff members contact the physical therapist to see if in fact she was upset. The patient agreed that if he was told via our staff occupational therapist that the physical therapist was upset, he would accept it as accurate feedback. When that feedback was given to him, his response was one of mild confusion. He simply did not know or understand what he had done wrong.

This type of scenario can be observed over and over again in clinical settings. Prigatano, Altman, and O'Brien (1990) documented that post-acute patients with severe TBI underestimate problems of social interaction and emotional control, but do not demonstrate global unawareness for other areas of functioning (such as the degree of physical independence). These findings have been replicated (Fischer et al., 2004; O'Keefe et al., 2007; Prigatano, 1996) and are compatible with Oddy et al.'s (1985) initial observations of these patients.

Impaired Self-Awareness for Memory Disturbances

Memory complaints are common after severe traumatic brain injury. It is not uncommon, however, to observe that these patients often underestimate the degree of memory impairment compared to relatives' reports. In order to further explore whether this lack of awareness of memory impairment is psychologically motivated or if it reflects a true disturbance of impaired aware-ness, the following took place in our early rehabilitation program. A 35-year-old woman suffered a severe TBI with associated cerebral and brainstem involvement and demonstrated a dense amnesia. She was extensively asked about her memory difficulties. When questioned, she would frequently insist that her memory was "fine." When several memory failures were brought to her attention, she would explain her behavior as falling within the realm of normal or indicating that whatever memory failures took place, they were inconsequential.

In the context of individual psychotherapy sessions, the patient was progres-sively confronted over her poor memory, and evidence was provided to support the severity of her difficulties. When more and more pressure was put on her to face her memory impairment, she would become emotionally upset. She reported being upset that others were misinterpreting her failures in memory. Clinically, she appeared to be unaware of her difficulties rather than denying their existence.

Hoofien et al. (2004) reported that approximately one-third of patients studied 13 years post severe TBI underreported their memory difficulties. This study, which was conducted in Israel, provides partial cultural cross-validation of this phenomenon.

Impaired Self-Awareness for Slow Processing Speed

It is well established that processing speed difficulties are common in both adults (Dikmen et al., 1995) and children (Prigatano, Gray, & Gale, 2008) after severe TBI. Some patients who show severe processing deficits may not report processing speed difficulties or may minimize them. A 24-year-old male who suffered severe TBI was seen 2-1/2 years post trauma. His neuroimaging findings are presented in Figure 12.1.

The patient was a trained mechanic and had lost six jobs in 2 years following his injury. When asked why it was difficult for him to maintain employment, his response was: "I don't know." He seemed honestly perplexed as to why he had lost so many jobs in such a short period of time. His wife reported, however, that employers stated that he simply was too slow to meet job expectations. When this information was presented to him, he did not seem to challenge it, but appeared "neutral" in his response. He reported that he did not perceive any significant difficulties with speed of information processing.

His neuropsychological test scores showed a probable reduction in overall intelligence (Verbal IQ = 81; Performance IQ = 79) and severe difficulties in processing speed and memory. Despite repeated attempts to help him accept the reality that he was slow in processing information, he was unable to achieve this insight without extensive neuropsychological rehabilitation. Reviewing his neuropsychological test performance had very little impact on his awareness of his difficulties.

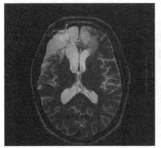 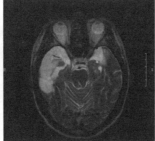 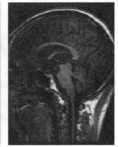

Figure 12.1 Post acute MRI of the brain showing encephalomalacia and enlarged ventricles following severe TBI in a 24-year-old male.

Despite the frequency of processing speed deficits after severe TBI, no studies were found that specifically demonstrate a lack of awareness of this dysfunction after TBI.

Prolonged Impaired Self-Awareness and Paranoid Ideation after Severe Traumatic Brain Injury

While not commonly reported, long-term follow-up of patients with severe TBI and persistent ISA suggest that some may go on to develop frank paranoid ideations of psychotic proportions (Prigatano, 1988). For example, a 26-year-old male had suffered a severe TBI (admitting GCS score = 6). When seen approximately 1 year post injury, he insisted that he was able to return back to work without any limitations. His level of neuropsychological impairment, however, was severe and clearly precluded him from returning back to work. At that time, the patient was asked to complete the PCRS. If an individual reports on the 30 items on the PCRS that they can complete each item "with ease," their total score would be 150/150 points. At that time this patient rated himself 143/150 points. However, his mother rated him 85/150 points. The disparity indicates that his mother recognized her son had significantly more limitations than what the patient was reporting.

The patient returned 13 years later. At this time he was floridly psychotic. He was easily upset and showed angry outbursts. He insisted that he was "not crazy." He also insisted that he could go back to work, but people were keeping him from work in order to control him. At that time he had a Verbal IQ of 84 with a Performance IQ of 64. On the PCRS, his total score was now 138/150 points. The only thing he admitted differently now was problems in driving a car due to visual difficulties. His mother's ratings were 84/150, showing high stability over the 13 years. Unfortunately, this patient was not successfully treated through any form of pharmacological intervention or psychotherapy. Unresolved or untreated anosognosia after severe TBI may result in paranoid ideation for some TBI patients.

Consequences and/or Correlations of Impaired Self-Awareness after Severe Traumatic Brain Injury

Numerous studies have been conducted on the relationship of ISA after brain injury and a variety of behavioral and outcome measures. Bach and David (2006) noted that patients with poor self-awareness are more likely to be described as having significant behavioral abnormalities. Trahan, Pépin, and Hopps (2006) have reported that poor self-awareness in TBI patients was related to poor treatment compliance during the early stages of rehabilitation. Schönberger, Humle, and Teasdale (2006a) reported that patients' level of self-awareness appeared to be related to their capacity to form a working alliance with their rehabilitation therapists. This latter variable has repeatedly been shown to relate to productivity status after neuropsychological rehabilitation (Prigatano et al., 1994; Schönberger et al., 2006b).

Sherer et al. (1998b), Sherer et al. (2003), and Malec, Buffington, Moessner, and Degiorgio (2000) have linked poor self-awareness to failure to obtain gainful employment after rehabilitation. Whether this relationship reflects the severity of brain injury per se or the specific role of ISA remains to be demonstrated. However, Sherer et al. (1998b) demonstrated that even after severity of TBI was statistically controlled, ISA independently predicted gainful employment.

Other studies have linked ISA to changes in personality (Ownsworth, McFarland, & Young, 2002) and have specifically studied it in relationship to the emergence of depression (Malec et al., 2007). Whether improved ISA automatically leads to depression remains a matter of debate. It is clear, however, that disturbances in self-awareness are often associated with substantial neurocognitive and behavioral problems, which result in a restriction in a patient's life. Years of restricted independent living is, of course, fruitful grounds for a variety of behavioral problems, as well as the presence of depression.

Related to this observation is that poor self-awareness after TBI is correlated with elevated distress levels in family members (Prigatano, Borgaro, Baker, & Wethe, 2005). Collectively these studies highlight the negative impact of ISA on psychosocial functioning for both the patient and the family.

Premorbid Personality, Cultural Factors, and Impaired Self-Awareness

Does the patient's premorbid personality and/or cultural factors influence how they report their symptoms and consequently impact estimates of ISA? Weinstein and Kahn (1955) argued that premorbid personality factors play an important role. Their argument was that the underlying brain disorder would result in specific disabilities but that it could not explain the mechanism of denial per se. The later insightful work of Bisiach, Vallar, Perani, Papagno, and Berti (1986) challenged this notion, arguing that it was the underlying brain disorder that in fact was responsible for impairment in self-awareness.

Yet it has become progressively clear that cultural factors may influence how individuals actually describe their disabilities, and this has to be taken into consideration when measuring ISA. Prigatano and Leathem (1993) noted that Maori New Zealanders who suffered TBI reported less behavioral competency than non-Maori TBI patients. Only the non-Maori TBI patient's responses on the PCRS replicated the previous findings reported in American TBI patients (Prigatano, Altman, & O'Brien, 1990). One explanation for these findings included the idea that Maori TBI patients may report themselves as less competent to researchers who are white and non-Maori (i.e., the Pakeha). It was recommended that future studies employ researchers with the same cultural and language background as the participants to obtain information on ISA.

In a subsequent study, Prigatano, Ogano, and Amakusa (1997) had Japanese therapists ask Japanese family members of individuals who suffered TBI and/or stroke about impaired awareness. They found that in that culture, wives of elderly Japanese men who had suffered brain injury were much less likely to report that their husband had any disability, whether in the psychosocial realm or the physical realm. Again, when using relative reports, one must understand how their comments do or do not coincide with the local cultural mores, as this could influence how ISA is recorded and measured.

These observations suggest that cultural factors must be considered when obtaining any information regarding ISA that involves significant others' reports concerning a brain-dysfunctional person. The choice of questions and how they are asked could also influence the clinician's opinion about whether the individual demonstrates ISA.

The more complicated question of whether premorbid personality actually influences the expression of ISA remains debated. Weinstein and Kahn (1955) argued that individuals who are obsessive-compulsive in nature and have to dominate social situations are much more likely to deny any disability. Weinstein and Kahn (1955) also argued that the choice of words that patients use to describe their lack of awareness often betrays that they have some implicit knowledge of their impairment. Ramachandran (1994) has also argued that under the right circumstances (for example, using caloric stimulation) one can reveal that a patient who shows apparent anosognosia for hemiplegia may in fact have awareness of his/her deficit. This area of inquiry continues to be important, but it has received very little attention in the scientific community.

Impaired Self-Awareness before and after Neurorehabilitation

Ranseen, Bohaska, and Schmitt (1990) had TBI patients complete the PCRS within the first week of an inpatient rehabilitation program, and then again at the time of discharge. During this early phase of rehabilitation, they noted: "Virtually all of the patients viewed themselves as having greater competencies and fewer deficits than viewed by the staff member who was closely working with the patient. Unfortunately, there was little to suggest that over the course of approximately one month of intensive inpatient rehabilitation . . . there was any notable change in this discrepancy" (p. 33). Schönberger, Humle, and Teasdale (2006a) more recently came to the same conclusion in studying patients in Denmark who underwent a holistic neuropsychological rehabilitation program several months post injury. Ownsworth, Fleming, Desbois, Strong, and Kuipers (2006) also noted after utilizing an intensive behavioral modification program to help a TBI patient become more vigilant of errors, error detection improved but the patient's awareness of his limitations did not seem to improve.

Malec and Moessner (2000), studying a mixed group of patients (74% of them having suffered a TBI), report improved ISA for some patients after attending a brain injury rehabilitation program modeled after the work of Ben-Yishay and Prigatano (1990). Improved ISA was correlated with goal attainment following rehabilitation.

Ownsworth and McFarland (2004) attempted to measure ISA and "personality-related denial" via the Marlow-Crowne Social Desirability Scale (M-CSDS). They also used the Symptom Expectancy Checklist (SEC) as a measure of "coping-related denial." Measures were obtained before and after a 16-week group rehabilitation program aimed at improving awareness and coping skills after an "acquired brain injury." Patients were described as "clinically improved" versus "not improved." The authors report that persons with high levels of defensiveness were less likely to improve.

In a follow-up study, Ownsworth et al. (2007) argued that there are "awareness typologies" that do relate to psychosocial outcome after various forms of acquired brain injury (TBI included). They identified four groups. Their groups included those with poor self-awareness, good self-awareness, high "defensiveness," as well as high "symptom-reporting." They note that patients with acquired brain injury who have poor self-awareness and high symptom-reporting typically show the worst outcomes compared to those with good self-awareness and high defensiveness.

These observations suggest that some patients with TBI who are defensive and who are given feedback regarding their performance may, in fact, improve with the passage of time. The same could be said for TBI patients who are perplexed by feedback secondary to their poor awareness. These findings parallel previous observations made by Prigatano and Klonoff (1997).

It remains to be demonstrated whether intensive neuropsychological rehabilitation programs can improve self-awareness after TBI or reduce denial of disability (DD). In many instances, the patient's self-awareness does not seem to improve, but there are differences of opinion regarding this observation. Holistic neuropsychological rehabilitation programs should therefore make every effort to determine under what conditions ISA and/or DD may or may not improve.

Impaired Self-Awareness in Children with Traumatic Brain Injury

Jacobs (1993) noted that children with severe TBI appear to have limited knowledge about their injuries and many seem to have poor awareness of residual neuropsychological disturbances. Beardmore, Tate, and Liddle (1999) empirically replicated a portion of Jacobs' observations. They studied children between the ages of 9 and 16 who had a history of severe TBI. They noted that these children had very poor understanding of what a TBI is and how it may impact their behavior. They go on to report, however, that children spontaneously report fewer problems in their day-to-day functioning compared to parents' reports (something commonly clinically observed). Using a checklist procedure, they note that these children are able to endorse a larger number of problems than when asked open-ended questions. Using a discrepancy index score (similar to what has been used with adults; see Prigatano, Altman, & O'Brien, 1990), they note that these children with TBI tend to minimize their deficits. Areas most reflective of a disagreement between their view and their parents' view were centered on motor disturbances, planning difficulties, and fatigue.

Beardmore et al. (1999) also noted that a brief (one-session) training experience did increase the child's level of knowledge about TBI, but had no impact on improving their self-awareness. While their sample size was relatively small ($n = 21$), they judged that less than 20% of the children that they studied had adequate knowledge about their personal deficits. They make the interesting observation that as school-age children grow into adolescence, the underlying problem of ISA may become more obvious. This is often seen in clinical practice, but it has not been empirically studied and demonstrated with group data.

In studying children and their awareness of their deficits, several challenges exist. It is important to ask questions at a level that is compatible with the child's vocabulary level and conceptual capacities. Also the questions have to be asked in multiple ways in order to obtain a consistent picture as to whether the child really has a lack of awareness. George P. Prigatano (in preparation) has developed a self-report questionnaire, Children's Daily Functioning Scale (CDFS), that asks children to make simple "yes" or "no" responses to statements about their daily functioning (e.g., I remember to brush my teeth at night without my parents having to remind me). Their parents also complete the questionnaire. Preliminary data suggest that children's responses become more concordant with the parents' responses as they move from ages 6 to 12. Children and adolescents with severe TBI often show significant difficulties with social interaction and integration. Preliminary data on these children suggest that poor social integration may be associated with impaired self-awareness, as reflected by low concordance between their self-reports and their parents' self-reports concerning their daily functioning.

Multiple Brain Lesions, Overlapping Neuropsychological Disturbances, and Impaired Self-Awareness after Severe Traumatic Brain Injury: Some Theoretical Considerations

Given the complex neuropathology commonly observed in persons with severe TBI (Gentry, 2002; Jennett & Teasdale, 1981), it would seem improbable that this patient group could meaningfully be studied from a neuroscience perspective in order to reveal the nature of anosognosia in general, and the mechanisms responsible for anosognosia in this particular patient population. While the problems are indeed formidable, studying this patient group has one distinct advantage. Patients can be studied from the time they are rendered unconscious through the period of regaining consciousness, and during and after the time that PTA resolves. These states represent a continuum of consciousness and provide multiple opportunities to study variables that may interact with one another and later correlate with the type and degree of ISA seen in the post-acute and chronic phases after TBI.

Posner, Saper, Schiff, and Plum (2007) define consciousness as "the state of full awareness of the self and one's relationship to the environment" (p. 5). They go on to say, "consciousness has two major components: content and arousal. The *content* of consciousness represents the sum of all functions mediated at the cerebral cortex level, including both cognitive and affective responses" (p. 5). The arousal component is the behavioral manifestations associated with the sleep-wake cycle. This latter dimension is known to be highly dependent on "a specific set of brainstem and diencephalic pathways" (p. 5) (see Figure 12.2).

It is highly probable that anosognosia after TBI represents a complex interaction of neural network abnormalities that occur at the level of the cerebral cortex and the brain stem. In fact, this must be the case, since patients who demonstrate persistent anosognosia or ISA are known to have sleep disturbances, slowed information processing, decreased memory capacity, and reduced problem-solving and planning abilities. These overlapping neuropsychological problems are almost always seen in patients who have ISA and suggest by their presence that multiple neural network circuits are either directly or indirectly negatively affected when this syndrome occurs.

It is curious, however, that no single neuropsychological disturbance (as measured by existing tests) seems to predict the extent or type of ISA observed after TBI (e.g., Anderson & Tranel, 1989; Prigatano & Altman, 1990). This observation led to the proposition that ISA after TBI is not a purely cognitive function (Prigatano, 1991, 1999). It appears to represent some form of disintegration of the normal bond between thinking and feeling that "pushes consciousness into existence in the first place" (see Prigatano, 1999).

More than one clinician (i.e., Bisiach & Geminiani, 1991; Cutting, 1978; Nielsen, 1938) has noted that anosognostic patients after stroke often show a

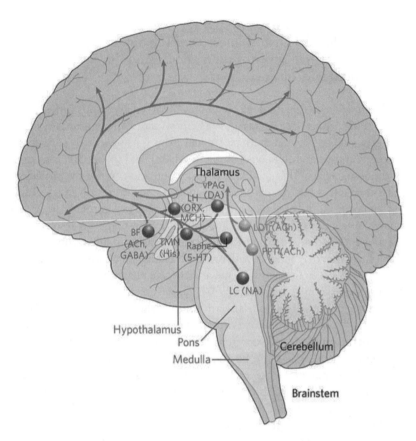

Figure 12.2 A summary diagram of the ascending arousal system. The cholinergic system, shown in yellow, provides the main input to the relay and reticular nuclei of the thalamus from the upper brainstem. This inhibits the reticular nucleus and activates the thalamic relay nuclei, putting them into transmission mode for relaying sensory information to the cerebral cortex. The cortex is activated simultaneously by a series of direct inputs, shown in red. These include monoaminergic inputs from the upper brainstem and posterior hypothalamus, such as noradrenaline (NA) from the locus coeruleus (LC), serotonin (5-HT) from the dorsal and median raphe nuclei, dopamine (DA) from the ventral periaqueduetal gray matter (vPAG), and histamine (His) from the tuberomammillary nucleus (TMN); petidergic inputs from the hypothalamus such as orexin (ORX) and melanin-concentrating hormone (MCH) both from the lateral hypothalamus (LH); and both cholinergic (ACH) and gamma-aminobulyric acid (GABA)-ergic inputs from the basal forebrain (BF). Activation of the brainstem yellow pathway in the absence of the red pathways occurs during rapid eye movement (REM) sleep, resulting in the cortex entering a dreaming state. LDT, laterodorsal tegmental nuclei; PPT, pedunculopontine. (From Saper, CB, Scammell, TE, Lu J. Hypothalamic regulation of sleep and circadian rhythms. *Nature* 437: 1257–1263, 2005. Reprinted with permission from Macmillan Publishers LTD) (See Color Plate 12.2)

"flatness of affect" or an indifference over their neurological deficits. The importance of these affective disturbances in conjunction with the apparent lack of insight has never been integrated into any comprehensive theory of anosognosia.

In an effort to understand the relationship between these findings, a theoretical model of consciousness is needed. Prigatano and Johnson (2003), building on a review paper by Zeman (2001), suggest that there are actually three "vectors of consciousness" that can be described and that are observed in day-to-day life before and after brain injury. The first vector of consciousness has to do with the sleep-wake cycle and is responsible for what Posner et al. (2007) refer to as the arousal dimension of consciousness. The brain circuits and neurochemistry involved in this first vector of consciousness are illustrated in Figure 12.2. Disturbance of this vector initially produces a loss of consciousness and may contribute to prolonged coma. It is suggested that as the patients emerge from coma, they still may be in a state of hypoarousal secondary to disturbances of this first vector of consciousness.

Zeman (2001) had reviewed studies that attempted to measure metabolic changes associated with dreaming. During REM sleep, there appears to be increase in blood flow in the rostral brain stem, thalamus, and limbic regions. At the same time there is a decrease in blood flow in the prefrontal regions of the cortex, as well as in the posterior cingulate and in regions of the parietal cortex.

During dreaming, the individual does not know what is real. Prigatano and Johnson (2003) suggest that for humans to know what is "real," the first vector of consciousness must be functional. Damage to this vector may well produce a disturbance in the perception of reality, even during the waking state. It may contribute to the development of psychosis when prolonged anosognosia exists in TBI patients for several years. Frontal-basal systems dysfunction are commonly seen when Vector 1 is compromised.

The second vector of consciousness represents that aspect of consciousness that has traditionally been associated with anosognosia. It is the vector of consciousness that allows for a phenomenological state to exist, in which the individual can identify himself/herself as "me" in the "here and now." It is the basis of the experiential or subjective realities that an individual is able to enjoy (or suffer through). It has been argued that heteromodal cortical regions are crucial for this vector of consciousness to emerge (Prigatano, 1991). It has also been argued that depending on the regions of heteromodal damage, different syndromes of impaired awareness may be observed after TBI or other brain disorders (Prigatano, 1999).

This model proposes that the heteromodal cortex integrates inputs from the primary sensorimotor cortex and the limbic belt in order to combine external and internal realities to produce the phenomenological or subjective state, which, by its nature, has both thinking and feeling components (for a more complete description of this model, see Prigatano, 1999). Bilateral cerebral dysfunction is necessary to produce permanent complete syndromes of ISA. As the patient recovers and/or certain regions of the lesioned and nonlesioned hemispheres begin to function normally (Perani, Vallar, Paulesu, Alberoni, & Fasio, 1993), then partial awareness may develop. This is the case for most patients who have severe TBI. They have partial or limited awareness without showing a frank anosognostic syndrome, although there are exceptions, such as the case documented by Cocchini et al. (2002). In instances where there is a partial syndrome of impaired self-awareness, one can use both defensive and nondefensive methods of coping. It is at this juncture that denial of disability and ISA are frequently confused.

A third vector of consciousness has to do with the conscious awareness of another's mental state. More recently this has been referred to as a "theory of mind" capacity. Bibby and McDonald (2005) have studied theory of mind capacities in persons with TBI. They raise the interesting question of whether poor performance on theory of mind tasks in patients with severe TBI is simply a function of poor abstract reasoning and problem-solving skills, or whether in fact it does suggest some unique difficulty in making inferences which are important in social interactions. Their findings produced mixed results. Perhaps not unexpectedly, patients with severe TBI perform more poorly (compared to controls) on a variety of cognitive tasks irrespective of whether they specifically attempted to assess theory of mind capabilities. They did note, however, that patients with severe TBI had difficulties with some tasks reportedly sampling theory of mind that could not be accounted for on the basis of their overall inference ability. This study provides indirect support that a third level of ISA may exist in some TBI patients.

Returning to Clinical Realities

The patient previously described (his neuroimaging findings were presented in Figure 12.1) highlights the complexity of what is clinically observed. While this patient had unequivocal processing speed difficulties for which he was unaware, he also had impairments of memory, of which he appeared not to be fully aware. He had obvious difficulties with abstract reasoning and problem solving. His wife noted that he was less socially sensitive to her than he had been in the past (perhaps a theory of mind problem?). While he denied fatigue, his wife indicated that he was much more fatigued than what he frequently reported. He appeared to have diminished awareness of his actual physiological arousal state.

Utilizing the model proposed by Prigatano and Johnson (2003), one can superimpose on this patient's neuroimaging studies how the three vectors of consciousness might be theoretically affected by his brain lesions (see Figure 12.3). While admittedly a crude and oversimplified picture, Figure 12.3 attempts to demonstrate that lesions in the frontal and temporal areas would

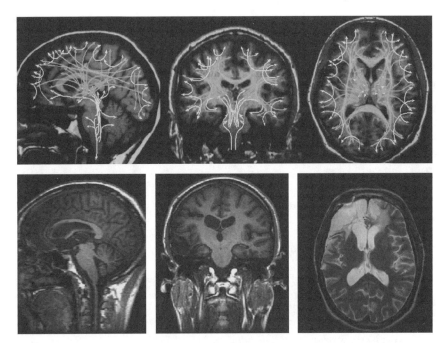

Figure 12.3 Top part of the figure is an over-simplified and theoretical representation of how three vectors of consciousness may be distributed in an overlapping fashion in the adult brain. Bottom part of the figure represents encephalomalacia associated with severe TBI. It is presented for comparison purposes to see how different vectors of consciousness may be differentially affected depending on the brain regions that are affected following severe TBI. (See Color Plate 12.3)

affect Vector 1 level of consciousness as well as Vector 2 and Vector 3. Depending on the bilateral nature and the extensiveness of the lesions, all aspects of consciousness potentially could be affected. This may help explain why this individual patient had minimal awareness of multiple areas of dysfunction, ranging from the more physical (i.e., fatigue or arousal level) to the more psychosocial (i.e., insensitivity to social cues from his wife).

Summary

In this chapter I have attempted to summarize several studies on ISA associated with moderately severe to severe TBI. I note that disturbances of self-awareness after moderately severe to severe TBI have actually been reported by investigators since the turn of the last century, even though it was not recognized as a problem of anosognosia or ISA. Over the years, several empirical findings have been reported. These findings, however, have not led to a single theory explaining the phenomenon.

Impaired self-awareness can occur for a variety of neuropsychological and neurological disturbances, both during the period of post-traumatic amnesia and after it resolves. It has been progressively recognized that ISA changes with the passage of time, often giving different impressions regarding its etiology. Patients who have ISA after severe TBI may have complete versus partial knowledge of their deficits. Patients with partial knowledge may use denial as a method of coping while others do not. The information in this chapter suggests, however, that anosognosia is a part of a complex series of disturbances of human consciousness that occur as a result of severe TBI, even after the patient emerges from coma and PTA.

References

Anderson, S. W., Damasio, H., Tranel, D., & Damasio, A. R. (2000). Long-term sequelae of prefrontal cortex damage acquired in early childhood. *Developmental Neuropsychology, 18*, 281–296.

Anderson, S. W., & Tranel, D. (1989). Awareness of disease states following cerebral infarction, dementia, and head trauma: standardized assessment. *The Clinical Neuropsychologist, 3*, 327–339.

Bach, L. F., & David, A. S. (2006). Self-awareness after acquired and traumatic brain injury. *Neuropsychological Rehabilitation, 16*, 397–414.

Beardmore, S., Tate, R., & Liddle, B. (1999). Does information and feedback improve children's knowledge and awareness of deficits after traumatic brain injury? *Neuropsychological Rehabilitation, 9*, 45–62.

Ben-Yishay, Y., & Prigatano, G. P. (1990). Cognitive remediation. In E. Griffith, M. Rosenthal, M. R. Bond, & J. D. Miller (Eds.), *Rehabilitation of the adult and child with traumatic brain injury* (pp. 393–409). Philadelphia: F.W. Davis Company.

Bibby, H., & McDonald, S. (2005). Theory of mind after traumatic brain injury. *Neuropsychologia, 43*, 99–114.

Bigler, E. D. (2005). Structural imaging. In J. M. Silver, T. W. McAllister, & S. C. Yudofsky (Eds.), *Textbook of traumatic brain injury*. Washington, D.C.: American Psychiatric Publishing, Inc.

Bisiach, E., & Geminiani, G. (1991). Anosognosia related to hemiplegia and hemianopia. In G. P. Prigatano & R. L. Schacter (Eds.), *Awareness of deficit after brain injury: Clinical and theoretical issues* (pp. 17–39). New York: Oxford University Press.

Bisiach, E., Vallar, G., Perani, D., Papagno, & Berti, A. (1986). Unawareness of disease following lesions of the right hemisphere: Anosognosia for hemiplegia and anosognosia for hemianopia. *Neuropsychologia, 24*, 471–482.

Cocchini, G., Beschin, N., & Della Sala, S (2002). Chronic anosognosia: A case report and theoretical account. *Neuropsychologia, 40*, 2030–2038.

Critchley, M. (1953). *The parietal lobes*. New York: Hafner.

Crosson, B., Barco, P. P., Velozo, C. A., Bolesta, M. M., Cooper, P. V., Werts, D., & Brobeck, T. C. (1989). Awareness and compensation in postacute head injury rehabilitation. *Journal of Head Trauma and Rehabilitation, 4*, 46–54.

Cutting, J. (1978). Study of anosognosia. *Journal of Neurology and Neurosurgery Psychiatry, 41*, 548–555.

Dikmen, S. S., Machamer, J. E., Winn, H. R., & Temkin, N. R. (1995). Neuropsychological outcome at 1-year post head injury. *Neuropsychology, 9*, 80–90.

Dirette, D. K., & Plaisier, B. R. (2007). The development of self-awareness of deficits from 1 week to 1 year after traumatic brain injury: Preliminary findings. *Brain Injury, 21*, 1131–1136.

Fischer, S., Trexler, L.E., & Gauggel, S. (2004). Awareness of activity limitations and prediction of performance in patients with brain injuries and orthopedic disorders. *Journal of the International Neuropsychological Society, 10*, 190–199.

Gentry, L. R. (2002). Head trauma. In S. W. Atlas (Ed.), *Magnetic resonance imaging of the brain and spine* (3rd edition, Vol. II, pp.1059–1098). Philadelphia: Lippincott, Williams, and Wilkins.

Goldstein, K. (1952). The effect of brain damage on the personality. *Psychiatry, 15*, 245–260.

Heilman, K. M. (1991). Anosognosia: Possible neuropsychological mechanisms. In G. P. Prigatano & D. L. Schacter (Eds.), *Awareness of deficit after brain injury: Clinical and theoretical issues* (pp. 53–62). New York: Oxford University Press.

Hoofien, D., Gilboa, A., Vakil, E., & Barak, O. (2004). Unawareness of cognitive deficits and daily functioning among persons with traumatic brain injuries. *Journal of Clinical and Experimental Neuropsychology, 26*, 278–290.

Jacobs, M. P. (1993). Limited understanding of deficit in children with brain dysfunction. *Neuropsychological Rehabilitation, 3*, 341–365.

Jennett, B., & Teasdale, G. (1981). *Management of head injuries*. Philadelphia: F. A. Davis.

Johnson, S. C., Baxter, L. C., Wilder, L. S., Pipe, J. G., Heiserman, J. E., & Prigatano, G. P. (2002). Neural substrates of self-reflective thought. *Brain, 125*, 1808–1814.

Leathem, J. M., Murphy, L. J., & Flett, R. A. (1998). Self- and informant-ratings on the Patient Competency Rating Scale in patients with traumatic brain injury. *Journal of Clinical and Experimental Neuropsychology, 20*, 694–705.

Levin, H. S., Gary, H. E., Eisenberg, H. M., Ruff, R. M., Barth, J. T., Kreutzer, J. S., High, W. M., Portman, S., Foulkes, M. A., Jame, J. A., Marmarou, A., & Marshall, L. F. (1990). Neurobehavioral outcome 1 year after severe head injury: Experience of the Traumatic Coma Data Bank. *Journal of Neurosurgery, 73*, 699–709.

Malec, J. F., Buffington, A. L. H., Moessner, A. M., & Degiorgio, L. (2000). A medical/vocational case coordination system for persons with brain injury: An evaluation of employment outcomes. *Archives of Physical Medicine and Rehabilitation, 81*, 1007–1015.

Malec, J. F., & Moessner, A. M. (2000). Self-awareness, distress, and postacute rehabilitation outcome. *Rehabilitation Psychology, 45*, 227–241.

Malec, J. F., Testa, J. A., Rush, B. K., Brown, A. W., & Moessner, A. M. (2007). Self-assessment of impairment, impaired self-awareness, and depression after traumatic brain injury. *Journal of Head Trauma and Rehabilitation, 22*, 156–166.

McDaniel, K. D., & McDaniel, L. D. (1991). Anton's Syndrome in a patient with posttraumatic optic neuropathy and bifrontal contusions. *Archives of Neurology, 48*, 101–105.

Meyer, A. (1904). The anatomical facts and clinical varieties of traumatic insanity. *American Journal of Insanity, 60*, 373–441.

Nielsen, J. M. (1938). Disturbances of the body scheme: Their physiological mechanism. *Bulletin of the Los Angeles Neurological Society, 3*, 127–135.

Oddy, M., Coughlan, T., Tyerman, A., & Jenkins, D. (1985). Social adjustment after closed head injury: A further follow-up seven years after injury. *Journal of Neurology, Neurosurgery, and Psychiatry, 48*, 564–568.

O'Keefe, F., Dockree, P., Moloney, P., Carton, S., & Robertson, I. H. (2007). Awareness of deficits in traumatic brain injury: A multidimensional approach to assessing metacognitive knowledge and online-awareness. *Journal of the International Neuropsychological Society, 13*, 38–49.

Ownsworth, T., & Clare, L. (2006). The association between awareness deficits and rehabilitation outcome following acquired brain injury. *Clinical Psychology Review, 26*, 783–795.

Ownsworth, T., Fleming, J., Desbois, J., Strong, J., & Kuipers, P. (2006). A metacognitive contextual intervention to enhance error awareness and functional outcome following traumatic brain injury: A single-case experimental design. *Journal of the International Neuropsychological Society, 12*, 54–63.

Ownsworth, T., Fleming, J., Strong, J., Radel, M., Chan, W., & Clare, L. (2007). Awareness typologies, long-term emotional adjustment and psychosocial outcomes following acquired brain injury. *Neuropsychological Rehabilitation, 17*, 129–150.

Ownsworth, T., & McFarland, K. (2004). Investigation of psychological and neuropsychological factors associated with clinical outcome following a group rehabilitation programme. *Neuropsychological Rehabilitation, 14*, 535–562.

Ownsworth, T. L., McFarland, K., & Young, R. M. (2002). The investigation of factors underlying deficits in self-awareness and self-regulation. *Brain Injury, 16*, 291–309.

Pagulayan, K. F., Temkin, N. R., Machamer, J. E., & Dikmen, S. S. (2007). The measurement and magnitude of awareness difficulties after traumatic brain injury: A longitudinal study. *Journal of the International Neuropsychological Society, 13*, 561–570.

Perani, D. Vallar, G., Paulesu, E., Alberoni, M., & Fazio, F. (1993). Left and right hemisphere contribution to recovery from neglect after right hemisphere damage—an[18F] FDG PET study of two cases. *Neuropsychologia, 31*, 115–125.

Posner, J. B., Saper, C. B., Schiff, N. D., & Plum, F. (Eds.). (2007). *Plum and Posner's diagnosis of stupor and coma* (4th edition). New York: Oxford University Press.

Prigatano, G. P. (1988). Anosognosia, delusions, and altered self-awareness after brain injury: A historical perspective. *BNI Quarterly, 4*, 40–48.

Prigatano, G. P. (1991). Disturbances of self-awareness of deficit after traumatic brain injury. In G. P. Prigatano & D. L. Schacter (Eds.), *Awareness of deficit after brain injury: Clinical and theoretical issues* (pp. 111–126). New York: Oxford University Press.

Prigatano, G. P. (1996). Behavioral limitations TBI patients tend to underestimate: A replication and extension to patients with lateralized cerebral dysfunction. *The Clinical Neuropsychologist, 10*, 191–201.

Prigatano, G. P. (1999). *Principles of neuropsychological rehabilitation*. New York: Oxford University Press.

Prigatano, G. P. (2008). Anosognosia and the process and outcome of neurorehabilitation. In D. T. Stuss, G. Winocur, and I. H. Robertson (Eds.), *Cognitive neurorehabilitation: Evidence and application* (2nd edition, pp. 218–231). Cambridge,
England: Cambridge University Press.

Prigatano, G. P., & Altman, I. M. (1990). Impaired awareness of behavioral limitations
after traumatic brain injury. *Archives of Physical Medicine and Rehabilitation, 71*,
1058– 1064.

Prigatano, G. P., Altman, I. M., & O'Brien, K. P. (1990). Behavioral limitations that
traumatic brain injured patients tend to underestimate. *The Clinical
Neuropsychologist, 4*, 163–176.

Prigatano, G. P., Borgaro, S. R., Baker, J., & Wethe, J. (2005). Awareness and distress
after traumatic brain injury: A relative's perspective. *Journal of Head Trauma
Rehabilitation, 20*, 359–367.

Prigatano, G. P., Fordyce, D. J., Zeiner, H. K., Roueche, J. R., Pepping, M., & Wood, B.
(1984). Neuropsychological rehabilitation after closed head injury in young adults.
Journal of Neurology, Neurosurgery and Psychiatry, 47, 505–513.

Prigatano, G. P., Fordyce, D. J., Zeiner, H. K., Roueche, J. R., Pepping, M., & Wood, B. C.
(1986). *Neuropsychological rehabilitation after brain injury*. Baltimore: Johns
Hopkins University Press.

Prigatano, G. P., Gray, J. A., & Gale, S. D. (2008). Individual case analysis of processing
speed difficulties in children with and without traumatic brain injury. *The Clinical
Neuropsychologist, 22*, 603–619.

Prigatano, G. P., & Johnson, S. C. (2003). The three vectors of consciousness and
their disturbances after brain injury. *Neuropsychological Rehabilitation, 13*,
13–29.

Prigatano, G. P., & Klonoff, P. S. (1997). A clinician's rating scale for evaluating impaired
self-awareness and denial of disability after brain injury. *The Clinical
Neuropsychologist, 11*, 1–12.

Prigatano, G. P., & Leathem, J. M. (1993). Awareness of behavioral limitations after
traumatic brain injury: A cross-cultural study of New Zealand Maoris and Non-
Maoris. *The Clinical Neuropsychologist, 7*, 123–135.

Prigatano, G. P., & Maier, F. (2008). Neuropsychiatric, psychiatric, and behavioral
disorders associated with traumatic brain injury. In I. Grant and K. Adams (Eds.),
Neuropsychological assessment of neuropsychiatric disorders (3rd edition,
pp. 618–631). New York: Oxford University Press.

Prigatano, G. P., Ogano, M., & Amakusa, B. (1997). A cross-cultural study on impaired
self-awareness in Japanese patients with brain dysfunction. *Neuropsychiatry,
Neuropsychology, and Behavioral Neurology, 10*, 135–143.

Ramachandron, V. S. (1994). Phantom limbs, neglect syndromes, repressed memories,
and Freudian Psychology. *International Review of Neurobiology, 37*, 291–372.

Ranseen, J. D., Bohaska, L. A., & Schmitt, F. A. (1990). An investigation of anosognosia
following traumatic head injury. *International Journal of Clinical Neuropsychology,
12*, 29–35.

Russell, W. R. (1971). *The traumatic amnesias*. London: Oxford University Press.

Schilder, P. (1934). Psychic disturbances after head injuries. *American Journal of
Psychiatry, 91*, 155–188.

Schmitz, T. W., Rowley, H. A., Kawahara, T. N., & Johnson, S. C. (2006). Neural correlates of self-evaluative accuracy after traumatic brain injury. *Neuropsychologia, 44,* 762–773.

Schönberger, M., Humle, F., & Teasdale, T. W. (2006a). The development of the therapeutic working alliance, patients' awareness and their compliance during the process of brain injury rehabilitation. *Brain Injury, 20,* 445–454.

Schönberger, M., Humle, F., & Teasdale, T. W. (2006b). Subjective outcome of brain injury rehabilitation in relation to the therapeutic working alliance, client compliance and awareness. *Brain Injury, 20,* 1271–1282.

Sherer, M., Bergloff, P., Levin, E., High Jr., W. M., Oden, K. E., & Nick, T. G. (1998b). Impaired awareness and employment outcome after traumatic brain injury. *Journal of Head Trauma and Rehabilitation, 13,* 52–61.

Sherer, M., Boake, C., Levin, E., Silver, B. V., Ringholz, G., & High Jr., W. M. (1998a). Characteristics of impaired awareness after traumatic brain injury. *Journal of the International Neuropsychological Society, 4,* 380–387.

Sherer, M., Hart, T., Nick, T. G., Whyte, J., Thompson, R. N., & Yablon, S. A. (2003). Early impaired self-awareness after traumatic brain injury. *Archives of Physical Medicine and Rehabilitation, 84,* 168–176.

Sherer, M., Hart, T., Whyte, J., Nick, T. G., & Yablon, S. A. (2005). Neuroanatomical basis of impaired self awareness after traumatic brain injury: Findings from early computed tomography. *Journal of Head Trauma Rehabilitation, 20,* 287–300.

Trahan, E., Pépin, M., & Hopps, S. (2006). Impaired awareness of deficits and treatment adherence among people with traumatic brain injury or spinal cord injury. *Journal of Head Trauma and Rehabilitation, 21,* 226–235.

Weinstein, E. A., & Kahn, R. L. (1955). *Denial of illness: Symbolic and physiological aspects.* Springfield, IL: Charles C. Thomas.

Zeman, A. (2001). Invited review: Consciousness. *Brain, 124,* 1263–1289.

13

Anosognosia in Schizophrenia and Other Neuropsychiatric Disorders: Similarities and Differences

James Gilleen, Kathryn Greenwood, and Anthony S. David

In the past 20 years we have seen a renaissance of interest in awareness in clinical psychiatry. Like much psychiatric research, this interest began with schizophrenia and psychosis but soon spread through the whole of the discipline. Lack of illness awareness is a prevalent feature in people with schizophrenia (Mohamed, Fleming, Penn, & Spaulding, 1999), with approximately 60% of schizophrenia patients believing they do not have a mental disorder (Amador et al., 1994; Keshavan, Rabinowitz, DeSmedt, Harvey, & Schooler, 2004). Nevertheless, it is only in this relatively recent past that awareness has been more thoroughly examined through empirical research rather than just clinical observation, and in that time our conceptualization and understanding of awareness have evolved considerably. Awareness into schizophrenia and related disorders, or *insight*—to use the term favored by psychiatrists—is a topic for entire volumes and cannot really be done justice in a single chapter (see Amador & David, 2004; Markova, 2005; Osatuke, Ciesla, Kaschow, Zisook, & Mohamed, 2008). However, what we will attempt is an overview of the main conceptual issues and empirical findings in relation to awareness of illness in schizophrenia with emphasis on the commonalities and differences between psychiatric and neurological disorders, ending with new data directly comparing awareness of deficits in such disorders.

Terminology

The terms "anosognosia," "insight," "lack of awareness," and even "denial" are often used synonymously, yet they differ taxonomically with respect to the historical context and mental diagnoses to which they refer. Anosognosia, referred to throughout this volume, is generally used to convey lack of awareness of encapsulated functions seen after brain injury, such as hemiplegia. In contrast, "insight" and "lack of awareness" are typically used to describe the phenomenon in psychiatric disorders, such as schizophrenia, where the awareness in question refers to that of being ill and the capacity to judge the content of symptoms, such as delusions and hallucinations, as not being real. These terms, therefore, each refer to "awareness" per se, but the nature and form of awareness differ in scope, as does the *"object"*(s) to which they refer (see Markova, 2005). This is crucial since awareness of an objective, obvious deficit such as hemiplegia would seem to be different in kind from that of an objectively verifiable but invisible deficit such as amnesia, which is different again from a subjective experience such as an hallucination.

A critical operational difference between anosognosia in brain injury and dementia and "awareness" or "insight" in schizophrenia is that the latter may be conceptualized as pertaining to a *secondary judgment* (e.g., the *interpretation* and *attribution* given to the phenomenology of auditory hallucinations), whereas the former could be conceptualized as a lack of conscious *access to the information* (at one of several points). This distinction might map onto a broad information processing model: anosognosia follows dysfunction in perceptual and attentional systems while lack of awareness or insight is attributed to higher-level processing failures from memory to judgement and reasoning. However, this scheme is incomplete and unsatisfactory, being founded entirely on deficits. Cognitive neuropsychiatry (Bentall, 1995; David, 1993, 1995) provides a more nuanced approach that encompasses, in addition to deficits, biases (i.e., the weighting of certain bits of information over others) and leaves room for social and interpersonal processes, too (Gigante & Castel, 2004; Johnson & Orrell, 1996; Saravanan, Jacob, Prince, Bhugra, & David, 2004; Smith, Barzman, & Pristach, 1997). From this it follows that there is the need to contrast stated awareness with behavioral awareness, publicly avowed over privately held, and self versus other deception (Cooke, Peters, Kuipers, & Kumari, 2005; Subotnik et al., 2005).

One attempt to get a handle on this complexity within the schizophrenia field has been to dissect insight into different components or *dimensions* of awareness, which may, to some degree, be independent (e.g., Amador et al., 1991, 1993; David, 1990; David, Buchanan, Reed, & Almeida, 1992). David (1990) proposed three dimensions: recognition of having a mental illness, compliance with treatment, and the ability to label unusual events as pathological. Amador et al. (1993) splits insight into five components: the first two relate to (un) awareness of having a mental disorder in general and the symptoms in particular, and the others to the effects of medication, of consequences of illness and of specific symptoms, and the final component is the attribution of symptoms to illness. Popular measures of insight include the Schedule for the Assessment of Insight–Expanded version (SAI-E; Kemp & David, 1997; Sanz, Constable,

Table 13.1 Common Measures of Insight or Illness Awareness

Self-report scales
  Insight Scale (IS; Birchwood et al., 1994)
Clinician ratings
  Single items
   Item G12 of the Positive and Negative Syndrome Scale (PANSS) (Kay et al., 1987)
   Present State Examination (PSE item 104; Wing et al., 1974)
  Full scales
   Schedule for the Assessment of Insight (expanded) (SAI-E; David & Kemp, 1997)
   Insight and Treatment Attitudes Questionnaire (ITAQ; McEvoy et al., 1989)
   Scale for the Assessment of Unawareness of Mental Disorder (SUMD; structured
    interview; Amador et al., 1993)
Informant ratings
  Patient Competency Rating Scale (PCRS: Prigatano & Fordyce, 1986)
  Dysexecutive quesionnaire (DEX: Burgess et al., 1998)
Discrepancy ratings
  Informant vs. Patient: PCRS, DEX
  Prediction vs. Postdiction Memory Awareness Rating Scale (MARS; Clare et al., 2002)
  Objective score vs. Patient rating (MARS; Clare et al., 2002)

Lopez-Ibor, Kemp, & David, 1998); the semi-structured interview: Scale to Assess Unawareness of Mental Disorder (SUMD; Amador et al., 1993); the simple clinician rated: Insight and Treatment Attitudes Questionnaire (ITAQ; McEvoy et al., 1989); and the Birchwood self-report Insight Scale (IS; Birchwood et al., 1994). All these scales have reasonably good intercorrelation (Sanz et al., 1998) (see Tables 13.1 and 13.4). Many authors have used a single item from general psychopathology schedules, and others, particularly in the dementia and brain injury fields, have made use of patient–caregiver discrepancy questionnaires (see Kaszniak & Edmonds, Chapter 11, this volume).

Models

Theories seeking to explain awareness in neuropsychiatric conditions broadly fall into three categories. Lack of awareness is conceptualized as a direct manifestation of psychiatric symptomatology (or a symptom in itself), a function of general or specific neuropsychological (e.g., executive) impairment, or a motivated response to a mental disorder to preserve self-esteem and protect against low mood. Bearing in mind the above caveats, we will concentrate in this chapter on the cognitive and neuropsychological aspects of insight in schizophrenia.

Awareness and Symptomatology

Before the early nineteenth century it would have been seen as a logical contradiction in terms to talk of "insight" into psychiatric symptoms such as delusions, yet at around this time, early French "alienists" began to acknowledge the concept of "partial" insanity, where "madness" could be accompanied by lucidity indicating that some aspects of mental function could be "deranged" while others were preserved (Berrios & Markova, 2004; Markova, 2005). It seems intuitive that awareness would be associated with severity of psychopathology, such that increased severity of delusions and hallucinations would necessarily by their very nature leave sufferers unaware that their experiences were not real. However, the literature suggests a more complex picture (Cuesta & Peralta, 1994; David et al., 1995; Flashman, McAllister, Andreasen, & Saykin, 2000; Lysaker & Bell, 1994; McEvoy, Schooler, Friedman, Steingard, & Allen, 1993; McEvoy et al., 1996; McGlashan & Carpenter, 1981). Several studies have shown a relationship between awareness and global psychopathology (David et al., 1992; Fennig et al., 1996; Kemp & Lambert, 1995; Keshavan et al., 2004; Rossell, Coakes, Shapleske, Woodruff, & David, 2003; Takai, Uematsu, Ueki, Sone, & Kaiya, 1992; Young, Davila, & Scher, 1993; Young et al., 1998), while others have found associations only with positive symptoms (Almeida, Levy, Howard, & David, 1996; Carroll et al., 1999; Kim, Sakamoto, Kamo, Sakamura, & Miyaoka, 1997; Lysaker, Bell, Bryson, & Kaplan, 1998; McCabe, Quayle, Beirne, & Duane, 2002; Olfson, Marcus, Wilk, & West, 2006; Schwartz, 1998) or only negative symptoms (Collins, Remington, Coulter, & Birkett, 1997; Cuesta, Peralta, & Zarzuela, 2000; Laroi et al., 2000; MacPherson, Jerrom, & Hughes, 1996) or positive and negative symptoms (e.g., Mintz, Addington, & Addington, 2004). Other studies find awareness to be associated with specific symptoms such as "formal thought disorder" (Baier et al., 2000; Smith, Hull, Israel, & Willson, 2000); "degree of grandiosity" (Heinrichs, Cohen, & Carpenter, 1985); or with degree of "unusual thought content" (equivalent to delusions) as measured by the Brief Psychiatric Rating Scale (Keshavan et al., 2004; Overall & Gorham, 1962). Still others have found specific symptoms correlated with specific subdimensions of awareness. For example, Sevy, Nathanson, Visweswaraiah, & Amador (2004) found lack of awareness of the illness and its social consequences was only correlated with the positive symptom dimension from the Positive and Negative Syndrome Scale (PANSS; Kay, Fiszbein, & Opler, 1987).

In an effort to clarify the relationship of awareness and psychopathology, Mintz, Dobson, and Romney (2003) conducted a meta-analysis of 40 relevant studies and found small negative associations between awareness and global, positive, and negative symptoms accounting for 7.2%, 6.3%, and 5.2% of the variance in awareness, respectively. This would strongly suggest that symptomatology plays only a small part in the degree of awareness displayed by schizophrenia patients. Some studies have reported improvements in patients' awareness over time, which seem to be relatively independent of improvements in psychopathology over the same time (Cuesta et al., 2000; Fennig et al., 1996; Jorgensen, 1995; McEvoy et al., 1989; Michalakeas et al., 1994), which further complicates the overall picture (Markova, 2005). McEvoy et al. (1989), for example, reported that clinical improvement in 52 schizophrenia patients was not consistently accompanied by improvement in awareness, with 40% showing no substantial change in awareness during hospitalization. Finally, in a large longitudinal study based on a cohort who had enrolled in a pharmacological trial, almost half of the 614 patients were rated as having impaired insight on the PANSS (Gharabawi, Lasser, Bossie, Zhu, & Amador, 2006). This correlated with global symptom score severity and as insight improved so did global symptoms over 1 year. Taken together, it must be concluded that insight is related to psychopathology—as one increases, the other tends to decrease. Nevertheless, the association is weak cross-sectionally and variable longitudin-ally. There would, therefore, appear to be a strong prima facie case for regarding awareness as more than "just psychopathology" (David, 2004) and certainly worth studying in its own right.

It is also of interest to consider how the syndrome of schizophrenia may differ in comparison to other disorders with respect to the level of awareness that patients hold. Several studies have shown that schizophrenia patients present with less awareness than patients with other diagnoses such as bipolar disorder and major depressive disorder (Fennig et al., 1996; Michalakeas et al., 1994); and schizo-affective disorder and mood disorder with and without psychosis (Amador et al., 1994; but see Ghaemi & Rosenquist, 2004; Varga, Magnusson, Flekkoy, David, & Opjordsmoen, 2007); or similar levels of awareness as bipolar patients but less awareness than patients with unipolar affective disorder (Pini, Cassano, Dell'Osso, & Amador, 2001; Weiler, Fleisher, & Arthur-Campbell, 2000). However, others have found no significant differences between different patient groups (Arduini et al., 2003; Cuesta et al., 2000; David et al., 1992; David et al., 1995; Smith et al., 2000).

The Contribution of Clinical and Demographic Factors

There is little consistency across studies regarding reliable sociodemographic predictors of awareness in schizophrenia (see Markova, 2005). For example, age and gender do not appear to be associated with level of awareness. Nor does awareness appear to be related to level of education (Amador et al., 1993). Studies which report positive findings have occasionally done so in opposite directions, for example, duration of illness and awareness (Marks, Fastenau, Lysaker, & Bond, 2000; Pyne, Bean, & Sullivan, 2001). Age has been found to associate with awareness in only a few studies (Amador et al., 1993; Kim et al., 1997; Lysaker et al., 1998; Weiler et al., 2000) while four studies report that white patients were rated as having significantly more awareness than those from minority ethnic groups (Johnson & Orrell, 1996), patients of African-Caribbean origin (Goldberg, Green-Paden, Lehman, & Gold, 2001; Rathod, Kingdon, Smith, & Turkington, 2005), and patients born outside the United Kingdom (White, Bebbington, Pearson, Johnson, & Ellis, 2000). This may potentially be attributed to the blurring of delusional themes and culturally appropriate beliefs. For example, references to black magic/voodoo are more likely to be considered delusional than those pertaining to Christian beliefs (but see Saravanan et al., 2004, 2007 for discussion).

Initial studies on variables, including course, age at onset, and number of hospitalizations, have each been shown to have low to moderate correlations with various awareness dimensions as assessed by the SUMD (Amador et al., 1993), yet awareness may also improve with greater number of previous hospital admissions (Amador et al., 1993; Ghaemi, Hebben, Stoll, & Pope, 1996; Peralta & Cuesta, 1994; Takai et al., 1992). A meta-analysis reported that age of onset of the disorder moderated the relationship between awareness and symptom clusters (Mintz et al., 2003), such that acute patient status was found to act as a moderator variable between awareness and positive symptoms; acutely ill patients were least aware. There is, however, little evidence of increased awareness being associated with any specific medication (Burton, 2006), although Pallanti, Quercioli, and Pazzagli (1999) reported increased awareness was associated with clozapine administration.

Awareness and Neurocognition

Intelligence and Awareness

Several studies have established a relationship between intelligence (IQ) and awareness in schizophrenia (David et al., 1992, 1995, reviewed in David, 1999; Donohoe, Corvin, & Robertson, 2005; Fennig et al., 1996; Jones, Guth, Lewis, & Murray, 1994; Koren et al., 2004; Lysaker, Bell, Milstein, Bryson, & Beam-Goulet, 1994; Lysaker & Bell, 1994; Lysaker, Clements, Plascak-Hallberg, Knipscheer, & Wright, 2002; Marks et al., 2000; Smith et al., 2000; Startup, 1996; Young et al., 1993, 1998). This would appear to be problematic for any overarching theory of unawareness for specific focal deficits (e.g., the unawareness that Anton's patient *Ursula M* had for her blindness but not her word finding difficulties; David, Owen, & Forstl, 1993; Laroi, Barr, & Keefe, 2004). Other studies, however, do not find a relationship between awareness and IQ (Almeida et al., 1996; Carroll et al., 1999; Cuesta & Peralta, 1994; Dickerson, Boronow, Ringel, & Parente, 1997; Donohoe, Donnell, Owens, & O'Callaghan, 2004; Drake & Lewis, 2003; Freudenreich, Deckersbach, & Goff, 2004; Ghaemi et al., 1996; Goldberg et al., 2001; Kemp & David, 1996; Kim, Jayathilake, & Meltzer, 2003; Laroi et al., 2000; Lysaker et al., 1998; Lysaker et al., 2002; Marks et al., 2000; McCabe et al., 2002; McEvoy et al., 1993, 1996; Nakano, Terao, Iwata, Hasako, & Nakamura, 2004; Rossell et al., 2003; Sanz et al., 1998; Takai et al., 1992).

Confirming an unequivocal relationship between intelligence and awareness has, therefore, proved to be difficult and some studies have suggested that unawareness may be related to educational background more than intelligence. Macpherson et al. (1996), for example, reported that one of the two main factors that contributed to level of awareness in 64 people with schizophrenia was length of education. There is a possible confound, however, in that level of education will be affected by earlier or more severe onset of schizophrenia. Yet education about illness has also been shown to significantly improve awareness (Macpherson et al., 1996). Despite this, lack of awareness does not appear to be related to *knowledge* about mental illness. Startup (1997) showed that both high- and low-awareness patients were able to identify case vignettes as descriptions of mental illness, but they simply failed to associate the symptoms to themselves (see also Milton Rockeach's classic *Three Christs of Ypsilanti* [1964]), suggesting awareness is not a function of knowledge of psychopathology and may be independent of educational background. Greater awareness has also been linked to having more "common sense" (McEvoy et al., 1996) or real-world knowledge.

Executive Function

As early as 1934, future doyen of U.K. psychiatry Aubrey Lewis asserted that poor awareness of illness was rooted in neuropsychological dysfunction (Lewis, 1934). Indeed, a neuropsychological theory of awareness would offer a parsimonious explanation for both loss of awareness in psychosis and loss of awareness as seen in anosognosia. Studies in schizophrenia have made a great deal of the association between awareness and performance on "frontal-lobe" tasks such as the Wisconsin Card Sorting Test (WCST). The WCST is the most commonly used test of executive/frontal lobe functioning in awareness studies, despite lacking cognitive specificity (Donohoe & Robertson, 2003) and clarity over the functional components it measures. The WCST is generally thought to be a measure of set-shifting ability, where impairment has been hypothesized to be analogous to patients' inability to shift from a previously established "set" (that of being well) to a more accurate, postmorbid "set" (of being ill) (e.g., see Laroi et al., 2000; Lysaker & Bell, 1994). Drake and Lewis (2003) explain that set-shifting may be analogous to the ability to "hold an abstract representation related to an actual situation, but different from it, at the same time as the more obvious immediate representation. . .maintaining an objective appraisal of the [psychotic] experience" (p. 166).

Young et al. (1993) reported that the WCST "categories achieved" and "perseverative errors" scores could significantly discriminate between subjects with high and low awareness. In contrast, other studies have reported no association between any WCST score and SUMD awareness scores (Arduini et al., 2003) or SAI-E awareness scores (Collins et al., 1997). Cooke et al. (2005) examined 29 studies that included a measure of WCST performance and awareness and found that 11 studies reported no association between any WCST measure and awareness; 9 studies found all WCST measures taken correlated with awareness; and 9 found some but not all WCST measures correlated with awareness. All findings were in the anticipated direction, with lower awareness being associated with poorer WCST performance. In total, 12 of the 29 studies reported a correlation between "perseverative errors" and awareness; and 9 between "sets achieved" and awareness. It has been suggested that cognitive perserveration may underlie patients "perseverating in denial of illness despite evidence to the contrary" (Lysaker & Bell, 1994), but the evidence remains contradictory (Morgan & David, 2004). The most comprehensive, quantitative review of work in this area is a meta-analysis by Aleman, Agrawal, Morgan, and David (2006), which suggests that WCST performance has more in common with awareness than other measures such as IQ or memory. In this meta-analysis 13 studies created a pooled effect size of $r = .23$ (Aleman et al., 2006). As the WCST is a task largely free of language skills, it has been suggested that awareness may have closer links to nonverbal cognitive abilities (Morgan & David, 2004).

Studies investigating awareness also commonly administer a test of verbal fluency in which patients are given 1 minute in which to say as many words as possible that begin with each of the letters "F," "A," and "S." This test, a measure of word generation, self-monitoring, and perseveration is again thought to be a test of "executive" functioning; however, Morgan and David (2004) reported that very few studies find a positive association between verbal fluency and awareness, although an exception is provided by Simon, Berger, Giacomini, Ferrero, and Mohr (2006). Yet other studies have furnished evidence to doubt the supposed "strong link" between executive functions and awareness. Freudenreich et al. (2004), for example, found no association between awareness in a group of 122 patients and any neuropsychological variable, including WCST, leading the authors to conclude that lack of awareness may be a non-reducible symptom of schizophrenia. Goodman, Knoll, Isakov, and Silver (2005) also reported no association between awareness and "frontal" tests, including abstraction and set shifting, as did Cuesta et al. (2006) using both a cross-sectional and longitudinal design. Despite these exceptions, the majority of studies indicate that executive functions are, to some degree, involved in determining level of awareness but clearly there are other important factors to take into account.

Awareness and Other Neuropsychological Tests

Aside from executive tests, poor awareness in schizophrenia has also variously been found to be associated with poor digit span performance (Upthegrove, Oyebode, George, & Haque, 2002); letter-number sequencing (Marks et al., 2000), block design (Laroi et al., 2000), right-left orientation (McEvoy et al., 1996), and poor finger-tapping speed (see Morgan & David, 2004, for review; Prigatano, 1999). Impaired temporal lobe functioning (in conjunction with impaired performance on tasks assumed to reflect prefrontal cortex function) has also been implicated and may indicate that lack of awareness is mediated by a broad range of cognitive dysfunction (Keshavan et al., 2004). Specific cognitive components are not immediately discernible from the tests listed above, such that findings of poor performance on these tasks do not indicate a clear causal mechanism for lack of awareness.

Several studies have reported correlations between awareness and memory. Goodman et al. (2005) reported greater verbal memory to be associated with better awareness, whereas, somewhat counter-intuitively, Cuesta and Peralta (1994) found lower awareness correlated with *better* verbal and visual memory performance. Yet other studies found no association between awareness and visual and verbal memory (Almeida et al., 1996; Lysaker et al., 1998; McEvoy et al., 1993), nor awareness and short-term and working memory (Aleman, de Haan, & Kahn, 2002). Donohoe et al. (2005) investigated awareness and specific dissociable executive components (working memory, inhibition, set-shifting, and attention), and found the low-awareness group performed worse than the high-awareness group on a working memory test only (see also Mutsatsa, Joyce, Hutton, & Barnes, 2006). The meta-analysis by Aleman et al. (2006) confirmed an association between memory and awareness in schizophrenia but not psychosis, with the effect size less than that of executive tasks.

Awareness and the Right Hemisphere

Lack of awareness has also been linked to right hemisphere/parietal dysfunction, or impairment independent of executive function impairments (e.g., Berti et al., 2005; Laroi et al., 2004). Interestingly, both unawareness of unilateral space as seen in unilateral neglect cases (see Karnath, Berger, Kuker, & Rorden, 2004) and delusions (the definitive "psychiatric" state of unawareness) in brain injury populations (see Fleminger, Strong, & Ashton, 1996) are seen almost exclusively following right hemisphere damage, suggesting a strong role of right hemisphere structures in awareness per se. Furthermore, patients with visuospatial neglect and patients with schizophrenia have recently been shown to demonstrate the reciprocal pattern of biases in spatial and motor task performance, which may reflect common pathways of parietal dysfunction (Cavezian et al., 2007). Despite this, proxy tests of (right and left) parietal functioning have largely failed to show associations with measures of awareness (Morgan & David, 2004; for an exception, see McEvoy et al., 1996), yet neuroimaging studies have also implicated right hemisphere functioning with self-awareness.

Neuroimaging

As interest in awareness has blossomed, so has the use of MRI as an investigative tool. The findings to date suggest an association between poor insight and reduced total brain volume (Flashman et al., 2000; McEvoy et al., 2006), frontal lobe atrophy (Laroi et al., 2000), reduced frontal lobe volume (Flashman et al., 2001; Sapara et al., 2007), reduced cingulate gyrus and temporal lobe grey matter volume (Sapara et al., 2007), and ventricular enlargement (Takai et al., 1992). There is, however, some inconsistency in these findings and much study variation in the location of brain-insight correlates and in some instances a failure to identify any brain abnormalities associated with poor insight (Bassitt, Neto, de Castro, & Busatto, 2007). (Table 13.2 summarizes brain structure-insight findings.)

One explanation for this inconsistency could be the use of different image analysis techniques, such as region of interest measurements or voxel-based methods of analysis. In some studies a single insight assessment item has been used (David et al., 1995; Ha et al., 2004) while in others, insight schedules were employed (Rossell et al., 2003). Shad et al. (2006) investigated SUMD scores and

Table 13.2 Summary of Structural Neuroimaging Studies in Relation to Insight and Psychosis

Authors	Patients	Main Findings (Association with Insight and Brain Volume*)	Insight Measure
Morgan (2002 and in prep)	First episode psychosis ($n = 82$)	↓ Posterior cingulate and right precuneus/ cuneus grey density	SAI-E
Sapara et al. (2007)	Sz, chronic, OPs ($n = 28$)	↓ Prefrontal grey	SAI-E
McEvoy et al. (2006)	Sz ($n = 251$)	↓ Total grey/white/ whole brain	ITAQ
Bassitt et al. (2007)	Sz ($n = 50$)	No assoc. with prefrontal grey/ white vols	SUMD
Ha et al. (2004)	Sz OPs ($n = 35$)	↓ Grey L post / R ant. cingulate and bilateral inf temporal	PANSS
Rossell et al. (2003)	Sz (males) ($n = 78$)	No assoc. whole brain, white / grey vols	SAI-E
Laroi et al. (2000)	Schizophrenic ($n = 20$)	Frontal lobe atrophy and ↓ insight (CT)	SUMD
Flashman et al. (2000)	Sz spectrum ($n = 30$)	↓ Whole brain vol. poor insight	SUMD
David (1995)	Mixed psychosis ($n = 128$)	No assoc. with ventricular vol. (CT)	PANSS
Takai et al. (1992)	Sz, chronic ($n = 22$)	Ventricular enlargement	PANSS

* Magnetic resonance imaging (MRI) unless otherwise stated.

CT, computed tomography; ITAQ, Insight and Treatment Attitudes Questionnaire; Ops, outpatient; PANSS, Positive and Negative Symptoms of Schizophrenia Scale; SAI-E, Schedule for the Assessment of Insight (expanded); SUMD, Scale for the assessment of Unawareness of Mental Disorder; Sz: schizophrenia patients.

brain volume in 14 patients with schizophrenia and found lower awareness of current symptoms to be associated with lower right dorsolateral prefrontal cortex volume, while misattribution of current symptoms was associated with higher right medial orbitofrontal cortex (OFC) volume. Morgan et al. (2002; 2007; and in preparation) used voxel-based methods in a large sample of first-episode psychosis patients and found deficits particularly with respect to attribution of symptoms in cingulate cortex, perhaps related to the midline cerebral system for self-processing (see Johnson & Reis, Chapter 18, this volume). In addition there were right posterior grey matter deficits—reminiscent of regions implicated in neurological cases of anosognosia of hemiplegia and neglect (Berti et al., 2005). Damage to any of these putative systems could potentially account for impaired self-awareness.

Metacognition and Awareness

More recently, research has suggested that a direct relationship between awareness and cognitive function may be overly simplistic, and that metacognition, the reflective capacity for *thinking about one's thinking*, may be a more appropriate measure for inquiry. This is because metacognition reflects one's self-monitoring and the ensuing regulation of one's performance, and as such may mediate between basic-level cognitive deficits and the observed clinical phenomena of poor awareness (Koren et al., 2004). It follows that the capacity to make judgements on performance (metacognition), and not performance itself, is directly of interest. Thus, Koren and colleagues (2004) administered the standard WCST but in addition asked various "metacognitive" questions about their performance. Awareness into illness had higher correlations with metacognitive indices derived from confidence ratings and "volunteered sorts" (whether subjects wanted a trial to contribute to their final score) than with the conventional scores from the WCST. Although metacognition is also strongly correlated with frontal lobe structure and integrity (Pannu & Kaszniak, 2005), Koren et al., conclude that metacognitive capacity may better predict level of awareness, as measured by the SUMD, than standard neuropsychological tests. Lysaker et al. (2005) also report good awareness to be associated with greater metacognition in relation to one's own thinking in the context of purposeful problem solving.

In a different manner, Beck, Baruch, Balter, Steer, and Warman (2004), in developing the self-completed Beck Cognitive Insight Scale, have sought to investigate metacognition in terms of self-reflectivity and self-certainty. In the original study, the total "cognitive insight" score was significantly associated with greater awareness of having a mental disorder, as assessed by the SUMD. Greater self-reflectivity was associated with greater awareness of having delusions; and changes in score were associated with changes in positive and negative symptoms. If patients are unable to distance themselves from the phenomenon of illness, and have impaired ability to evaluate their "aberrant perceptions," they will be compelled to believe their experiences are real (Beck et al., 2004). Thus, self-reflection and its opposite, self-certainty, may reveal an important cognitive foundation of unawareness.

Finally, research on Theory of Mind (ToM), or the ability to infer the thoughts and feelings of other persons, has entered the insight field. People with schizophrenia are generally impaired on ToM tasks (Sprong, Schothorst, Vos, Hox, & van Engeland, 2007). It has been proposed that insight depends on the ability to take the perspective of another person in order to evaluate that person's own situation and so may share common processing abilities. A few studies have investigated the relationship between the two but with mixed results (Bora, Sehitoglu, Aslier, Atabay, & Veznedaroglu, 2007; Langdon & Ward, 2009; Pousa et al., 2008a, 2008b) perhaps because so far the distinction between self and other appraisal has not been incorporated into extant paradigms.

Psychological Coping

Rather than a purely cognitive basis for awareness, Startup (1996) postulated that awareness may instead be a product of an interaction of cognitive functioning and psychological coping style. Patients with poor neuropsychological function will necessarily have poor awareness, while those patients with good neuropsychological function may either retain good awareness or alternatively have the capacity to subsequently recruit denial strategies to cope with their deficits. Indeed, Startup (1996) revealed a curvilinear relationship between neuropsychological performance (IQ) and awareness, suggesting this may indeed be the case. At the very least, such a relationship must speak to additional factors being implicated in awareness.

This idea has been supported by Lysaker, Lancaster, Davis, and Clements (2003), who found that a subgroup of 66 patients with schizophrenia exhibited a profile of "high executive functioning–low awareness" scores who endorsed a significantly greater preference for denial as a coping strategy than the "poor awareness–poor executive function" group. These findings serve to highlight the role of multiple etiological factors in level of awareness, where psychological styles may act secondary to neuropsychological functioning in determining awareness. Inconsistencies elsewhere between awareness and cognition may in fact be due to a potential nonlinear relationship (Aleman et al., 2006), so coping strategies cannot be ruled out as an etiologically significant factor in denial of illness (Mintz et al., 2003).

Mood

One of the more reliable findings in the literature is the positive correlation between awareness and depression or dysthymia (and between elevated mood and lack of awareness; Ghaemi & Rosenquist, 2004), which has been shown across different patient groups (Clare, 2004b; Markova, 2005; see Tranel, Paulsen, & Hoth, Chapter 8, this volume). Although findings are variable, many studies have reported that increased awareness in schizophrenia is associated with greater depressive symptoms (Carroll et al., 1999; Iqbal, Birchwood, Chadwick, & Trower, 2000; Moore, Cassidy, Carr, & O'Callaghan, 1999; Mutsatsa et al., 2006; Pyne et al., 2001; Schwartz, 2001; Smith et al., 1998, 2000; White et al., 2000), including the meta-analysis by Mintz et al. (2003). In this way, low awareness of symptoms and illness is conceptualized as a form of denial, in order to maintain self-esteem and preclude the psychological consequences of acknowledging one has a mental illness. This in turn preserves mood. Whether this process is "conscious" (self-motivated) or "unconscious" (automatic) is, however, rarely addressed in research, and certainly difficult to measure empirically (although, as mentioned, see Lysaker et al., 2003; Startup, 1996).

A critical question is to address the causal direction of the relationship between awareness and depression. Does a depressive mood ensue from awareness of illness, or does a depressive mood foster a more self-critical attitude? Iqbal et al. (2000) interviewed patients five times over 1 year and found increases in awareness did not predate worsening mood; they tended to change together. This, however, does not rule out the possibility that awareness and depressive symptoms could be more temporally entwined, such that changes in one factor may cause immediate/reactionary reciprocal changes in the other. Smith et al. (2000), however, separated high- and low-depression schizophrenia patients at baseline and measured awareness at a 6-month follow-up. The high-depression group was associated with increases in awareness at follow-up, while the low-depression group was associated with worsening awareness at follow-up, suggesting mood may be a causal force in determining level of awareness, rather than vice versa. The framework of "depressive realism" goes a long way to explain this (see Ghaemi, 2007). On the other hand, Rathod et al. (2005) reports that patients undergoing CBT intervention to improve awareness became depressed subsequent to gaining awareness (Kemp, Kirov, Everitt, Hayward, & David, 1998). Of course, depressive symptomatology in nonpsychiatric populations is often associated with more accurate self-appraisal (Pyszczynski & Greenberg, 1987), but again the causal direction of the relationship is unclear.

There has been concern that attempts to improve insight in schizophrenia may lead to increased thoughts of self-harm and even suicide. Several studies have now shown that the association between insight and self-harm is complex (Schwartz & Smith, 2004; Schwartz-Stav, Apter, & Zalsman, 2006). A longitudinal analysis of a large medication trial showed that, while at baseline, low mood, insight, and suicidal thoughts were associated; as insight improved, suicidal thoughts diminished (Bourgeois et al., 2004). Furthermore, the impact of lack of insight on outcome in schizophrenia, especially as mediated via noncompliance is potentially grave. Hence, any concern that improving insight might have a negative impact on outcome—for example, through an increase in self-harm—is far outweighed by the association between poor insight and suicide (Hawton, Sutton, Haw, Sinclair, & Deeks, 2005).

There are other paradoxical findings with respect to broader social outcomes such as quality of life and insight. If we take subjective assessments of quality of life to be valid and this is by no means uncomplicated (see Whitty et al., 2004), a number of people have shown better insight correlates with poorer quality of life (Hasson-Ohayon, Kravetz, Roe, David, & Weiser, 2006). This appears to be related to the emotional distress in some people, caused or attributed to greater awareness of their predicament, or on the other hand, that an attitude of denial of illness frees people from the constraints of illness behavior and the limitation on their horizons their illness induces. However, all these associations are complex and may be mediated through low mood (see Karow & Pajonk, 2006) and coping style (Cooke et al., 2007). For example, Kaiser, Snyder, Corcoran, and Drake (2006) found a curvilinear relationship between insight and satisfaction with social support, that is, both low and high insight tended to go together with greater satisfaction.

Insight in Relation to Clinical Outcome

One of the best validations for clinical concepts, particularly in schizophrenia, is that they offer useful predictive value in relation to outcome. A number of prospective studies have been carried out in relation to insight (see David, 2004 for a review; Lincoln, Lullmann, & Rief, 2007). In brief, these studies tend to show that good insight, when first assessed, predicts better outcome. The strength of the association is hard to quantify and previously identified predictors of outcome such as premorbid adjustment and other social factors and more recently, cognitive impairment, are probably far more important. Furthermore, as noted above, the story is not so simple in that there have been suggestions that good insight might relate to less favorably judged quality of life and with suicidal thoughts and tendencies. Drake et al. (2007) reported on a first-episode nonaffective psychosis cohort from England. Data on relapse over a period of 18 months were available on 236 patients. Just over half of the patients relapsed in the follow-up period with a third of the sample being readmitted to the hospital. The authors showed that those scoring highest for insight on the Birchwood Insight Scale (Birchwood et al., 1994) had a 34% reduction in risk for re-admission and 39% reduction in risk for relapse compared to those with no insight. Several other longitudinal studies bear on this issue. Saeedi, Addington, and Addington (2007) reported on 278 patients admitted to a Canadian early psychosis service. The group was dichotomized on the basis of the PANSS insight score into those with good or poor insight, the latter defined as a score of $\geq 4/7$, which applied to 110 patients of the sample. Over 3 years there was a tendency to improve in most of this cohort in the first year but those with persistently poor insight had persistently more symptoms and cognitive impairment. A study by Ceskova et al., (2007) also showed a general tendency in first-episode schizophrenia patients to improve on insight, although those who failed to show remission at 1 year had poorer insight scores. Insight at baseline did not predict remission, but those patients whose insight improved relatively early on in treatment had the better outcome.

Overall, the many studies that have looked at the relationship between length of history or number of previous admissions and insight scores have not led to any firm conclusions. This is perhaps because over time two opposite forces are at play. On the one hand, patients with poor insight suffer more relapses, perhaps related to poor treatment compliance. On the other hand, another group of patients successively develops insight through learning from experience, becomes less defensive (Thompson, McGorry, & Harrigan, 2001), and at the very least, becomes more adept at using medical terms (Markova, 2005). Hence, these two effects tend to cancel themselves out. The current vogue for early diagnosis of psychosis, and services aimed at its detection, has added a new twist to this story. Studies in patients with the operationally defined "At-Risk Mental State," that is, symptoms of psychosis short of reaching full diagnostic criteria, have been found to show significant deficits in insight. Lappin et al. (2007) reported however that such individuals had higher insight scores than those with an established first episode of psychosis, although these were help-seeking individuals. This must be set against other studies, for example, Thompson et al. (2001), which showed a significant difference between patients in their first episode and multi-episode patients, with the latter group having more insight. Again these discrepancies are probably explained by the different influences of learning from experience versus circumstances of the initial presentation. Indeed, a person with symptoms but without a firm diagnosis of schizophrenia can hardly be expected to have a clear view that his or her problems are due to illness when the treating clinicians may be just as unsure.

Interim Summary

Awareness or insight in schizophrenia and allied disorders is an important clinical variable. The relationship between poor awareness and neuropsychological impairments are wide ranging and fit no particular explanatory pattern (David & Kemp, 1997; Koren et al., 2004; McGlynn & Schacter, 1997), although on balance executive deficits seem slightly more to blame (Aleman et al., 2006). As suggested explicitly or implicitly by several authors, there may be different pathways to unawareness. It may be that other nonexecutive factors such as psychological style and metacognition play a key role in determining level of awareness, although these may perhaps be secondary to neuropsychological functioning. If awareness is multiply determined by defensive mechanisms or cognitive impairment, then with a large enough sample, one might expect to see clusters of patients whose awareness show distinct patterns of associations, as indeed reported by Lysaker et al. (2003). Note that of 40 studies reviewed by Morgan and David (2004) only 7 studies had samples greater than 90; and 6 of these reported awareness to be associated with some measure of cognition, whereas only 21 of the remaining 33 smaller studies reported a positive finding.

Direct Comparison of Insight or Awareness in Patients with Schizophrenia, Alzheimer's Disease, and Brain Injury

Most studies of awareness investigate a single patient population. Is there a case for comparing different patient groups on the same measures (see Banks & Weintraub, 2009; O'Keeffe et al., 2007)? Such comparisons may reveal more about the nature of awareness per se, as well as allow us to observe how awareness may differ in these different groups where pathology is a known factor. By contrasting different patient groups, it may elucidate the mechanisms that subserve awareness, or alternatively it may reveal that patients from different clinical groups show lack of awareness for different reasons.

Just as patients with schizophrenia have, in addition to their core symptoms, cognitive impairments and behavioral and social deficits, patients with Alzheimer's disease and brain injury may have a range of psychopathologies into which they may or may not have varying degrees of awareness. Comparison within- as well as between-groups may have important theoretical implications. For example, if patient groups with widely divergent pathologies (e.g., Alzheimer and schizophrenia patients) both have memory deficits, then we can ask whether the same factors associated with awareness of these are consistent across the groups (see e.g., Kircher, Koch, Stottmeister, & Durst, 2007; Medalia & Lim, 2004, Flashman, Roth, McAllister, Pendergrass, Garlinghouse, & Saykin, 2007 for awareness of cognitive deficits in schizophrenia). If the answer is broadly affirmative, it suggests that a common cognitive structure of awareness pertains and this in turn can prompt overarching cognitive models which need not be overly concerned with diagnosis. Furthermore, if say, awareness of psychopathology is relatively independent of awareness into cognitive deficits (the correlation was nonsignificant in one recent study (Medalia et al., 2004)—regardless of diagnosis—it points to modularity in awareness. Modularity of "awarenesses" is perhaps the most likely pattern from the neurological literature (McGlynn & Schacter, 1989) but has seldom been tested using broad domains such as psychopathology and behavioral problems (alongside neuropsychological impairments). Where it has, as in the large pan-European brain injury study (Teasdale et al., 1997), considerable within-diagnosis hetero-geneity was found. Similarly, in the dementia field, different levels of awareness have been noted by contrasting behavior with cognition (Vasterling, Seltzer, Foss, & Vanderbrook, 1995; Vasterling, Seltzer, & Watrous, 1997) and as demonstrated in the original edition of this volume, between awareness of motor disorders such as involuntary movements and cognitive impairment in Huntington's disease (McGlynn & Kaszniak, 1991). Again, this latter combina-tion has been examined in patients with schizophrenia and tardive dyskinesia; insight into psychopathology seemingly dissociates from insight into dyskinesia (Arango, Adami, Sherr, Thaker, & Carpenter, 1999).

We recently conducted a study (in press) in which we compared different aspects of awareness in three different neuropsychiatric populations: schizo-phrenia, brain injury, and probable Alzheimer's disease (Table 13.3). The former were mostly subacute, chronic, and treated outpatients plus some inpati-ents at the Maudsley Hospital, London, while the Alzheimer group were locally dwelling subjects identified as part of a larger cohort study. The brain injury patients were a heterogeneous group with a mixture of traumatic, hypoxic, and vascular etiologies and with behavioral problems. We were keen to address, among other things, to what extent awareness in the same domain differed between neuropsychiatric patient groups and whether differences could be mea-sured using standard scales such as the Patient Competency Rating Scale (PCRS; Prigatano & Fordyce, 1986), which is applicable to all three patients groups. As the PCRS breaks down into subfactors of functioning, this also enabled us to investigate whether there may be, as has been proposed, a hierarchy of awareness, either within the schizophrenia group, or even common across all groups. Several authors drawn mostly from the brain injury literature (Prigatano & Altman, 1990; Sherer et al., 2003) have reported that awareness is greater for "low-level"

Table 13.3 Demographic and Insight Data on Clinical Groups

Variable Mean (SD)	Schizophrenia $n = 31$	Brain Injury $n = 26$	Alzheimer $n = 27$
Age, years	38.3 (10.4)	40.0 (12.1)	82.4 (4.3)
Sex, m/f	16/15	22/4	14/13
Premorbid IQ, (NART)	102.3 (12.8)	102.2 (13.8)	109.1 (12.8)
SAI-E	11.2 (7.15)	15.4 (5.7)	7.0 (6.4)
SUMD awareness of mental illness	3.37 (1.6)	1.92 (1.43)	4.04 (1.4)
PCRS (plus ToM items)	1.17 (range: −64 to 42)	−33.7 (range: −92 to 13)	−54.7 (range: −96 to −5)

IQ, intelligence quotient; NART, National Adult Reading Test; PCRS, Patient Competency Rating Scale; SAI-E, Schedule for the Assessment of Insight (expanded);

SD, standard deviation; SUMD, Scale for the Assessment of Unawareness of Mental Disorder; ToM, theory of mind.

functioning such as motor functioning and peripheral senses, but lower for "higher-level" functioning such as cognition (Teasdale et al., 1997).

Naturally, the patients were not matched on factors such as age and length of history. We contend that for the purposes of making inferences about the pattern of awareness deficits in different pathological groups and contrasting profiles of awareness within groups, this is not critical. The groups were, however, comparable in terms of estimated premorbid IQ. All were rated on the SAI-E, SUMD (it was found that the awareness of mental illness was the most useful item from the scale; many Alzheimer patients were on no medication), and a modified version of the PCRS.

Patient Competency Rating Scale

Patients were asked to rate themselves on an adjusted 37-item version (Bach et al., 2006) of the Patient Competency Rating Scale (PCRS) rating scale (Prigatano & Fordyce, 1986), which measures problems with activities of daily living (ADL) and interpersonal, cognitive, and emotional problems. The PCRS was originally a 30-item self-report questionnaire, developed by Prigatano, Fordyce and Roueche (see Prigatano et al., 1986; Fordyce & Roueche, 1986), that asks patients and family members to make independent judgments about the perceived degree of competency the patient shows on various behavioral, cognitive, and emotional tasks such as the ability to take care of his or her finances or stay involved in activities when tired or bored. More recently, Bach and David (2006) extended the original PCRS to include a ToM dimension that incorporates an additional seven questions, which ask the respondent, for example, "How much of a problem do I have: being tactful/ understanding jokes/understanding what others are thinking, etc.?" Responses are made on a 5-point Likert scale. Some authors have used (0) "can't do" to (4) "can do with ease" (Fordyce & Roueche, 1986). Other authors have used a 5-point rating scale from (1) "can't do" to (5) "can do with ease." This results in different total scores that have been published in the literature. In our research, we used a 0 to 4-point scoring system. Therefore, the extended PCRS is scored out of a maximum of 148. Informants complete an analogous version of the questionnaire. Informant-rated scores are subtracted from the patient-rated scores to produce discrepancy scores, which can range from −148 to +148, where 0 represents informant–patient agreement; the greater the discrepancy, the greater the unawareness. Negative scores reflect an overestimation of functioning by the patient. Using the standard version of the PCRS, Prigatano and Altman (1990) reported test-retest reliability coefficients of .97 for patients and .92 for caregivers. Other studies have reported test-retest reliability in a similar range (Fleming et al., 1996; Sherer et al., 2003). Leathem, Murphy, and Flett (1998), in following from Heilbronner, Roueche, Everson, and Epler (1989), identified a four-factor solution to the PCRS, consisting of problems with ADLs, and interpersonal, cognitive, and emotional problems. In order to investigate whether awareness may dissociate between domains of impairment, mean scores for the five factors (i.e., plus ToM) were calculated and used in the analysis.

The validity of the discrepancy index to measure insight and awareness may be questioned since it assumes that the informant is the "gold standard." Informants may overestimate deficits (e.g., because of their own frustration or inability to cope) or underestimate them (e.g., because they are hidden, or because the informant wishes to protect the person they care for). Correlation with clinician ratings may be poor (see Clare, 2004a, 2004b). Nevertheless, the methodology has been found to be generally valuable and consistently shows underestimation of deficits by patients in relation to informal caregivers.

Results of Within-Group Contrasts (Schizophrenia)

In contrast to patients within the schizophrenia group showing very good awareness of behavioral problems, they were mostly lacking awareness of being mentally ill, of having symptoms, and attributing those symptoms to mental illness. Figure 13.1 shows the variation in distribution of awareness scores across the different dimensions within the SUMD. Generally speaking, as a group, patients were moderately aware of the need for medication (SUMD-meds; mean = 2.46 out of 5, SD = 1.52), moderately unaware of the presence of symptoms (mean = 3.48, SD = 1.49), and moderately unable to correctly attribute them to mental illness (mean = 3.85, SD = 1.15), although there was large variation in scores. These different dimensions of awareness intercorrelated in the order of $r = 0.4$ to 0.7, which suggests both common variance and independence and is similar to that shown previously (e.g., David et al., 1992). SAI-E total scores also reflected low to moderate, but variable levels of awareness, with low to moderate awareness of illness, attitudes toward medication, and ability to relabel symptoms as pathological. Informants rated the average patient attitude to medication as "passive acceptance," which correlated, at best, modestly with other awareness scores. Thus, despite low to moderate awareness, patients accepted their medication. SAI-E and SUMD total scores correlated very highly, in the region of $r = -0.8$ to -0.9, as did the respective "attribution" subfactors from both scales (NB. the SUMD measures *un*-awareness: higher score = lower insight; see Table 13.4).

That patients with schizophrenia as a group are aware of behavioral problems but lack awareness of mental illness demonstrates that awareness can fractionate both *between* (e.g., mental illness compared to behavioral deficits) and *within* domain (e.g., awareness of the need for medication compared to awareness of symptoms).

First of all, within just the schizophrenia patients, there were significant differences between PCRS subfactors, for example, patients modestly underestimated their ADL and emotional problems, which were significantly different

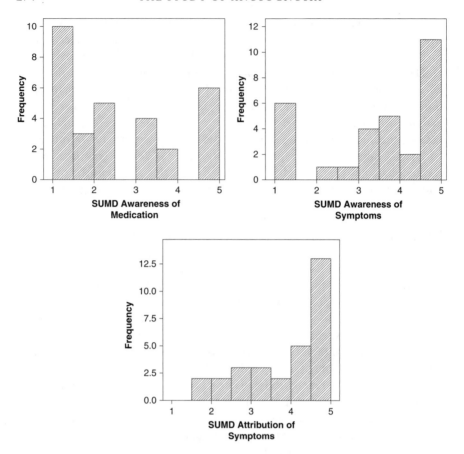

Figure 13.1 Frequency distribution of awareness scores across the different dimensions of the Scale to Assess Unawareness of Mental Disorder (SUMD) in schizophrenia patients. Higher scores reflect lower awareness.

to the modest *overestimation* of cognitive, ToM, and interpersonal problems (p's < 0.05). Despite this, scores on each of these factors correlated positively in the order of .3 to .7, suggesting that lack of awareness in one dimension is generally associated with lack of awareness in another—it is just that the *level* of awareness differs between dimensions.

There was also a great deal of variation in the scores, as revealed in Figure 13.2, which shows selected patient "profiles" of awareness across the PCRS factors. Patients 5 and 6, for example, have similar levels of unawareness of interpersonal functioning yet the former is greatly unaware of cognitive problems, while the latter is very aware of cognitive problems. Patients 6 and 7 show similar levels of awareness of emotional problems yet differ greatly on awareness of problems of ToM. Patients 4 and 5 show similar unawareness of

Table 13.4 Intercorrelation of Awareness Measures in Schizophrenia Patients

	SUMD				Total	Illness	Compliance	Relabeling
	Medication	Awareness	Attribution	Total				
SUMD Mental Awareness	.58**	.43*	.62**	.74**	−.82**	−.84**	−.42*	−.77**
SUMD-Medication		.52**	.63**	.88**	−.81**	−.50**	−.57**	−.68**
−Awareness			.69**	.75**	−.62**	−.45*	−.24	−.80**
−Attribution				.84**	−.87**	−.68**	−.46*	−.91**
SUMD Total					−.83**	−.66**	−.47**	−.85**
SAI-Total						.92**	.72**	.90**
SAI-Illness							.29	.69**
SAI-Compliance								.44*
SAI-Relabeling								

All correlations are Pearson correlations, except those involving SUMD awareness of mental illness measures, which are Spearman correlations, as they are not "normally" distributed.

** Correlation is significant at the .01 level (2-tailed).

* Correlation is significant at the .05 level (2-tailed).

SAI, Schedule for the Assessment of Insight; SUMD, Scale for the Assessment of Unawareness of Mental Disorder.

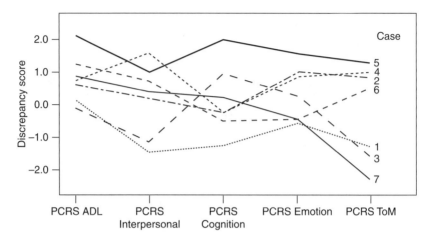

Figure 13.2 Differential patterns of awareness of functional deficits measured on the Patient Competency Rating Scale (PCRS) in seven selected schizophrenia patients. Each line represents the "profile" of one patient. Higher scores reflect greater unawareness. Zero reflects patient–informant concordance.

ToM problems, yet patient 5 is much less aware of problems of ADL than patient 4. Of interest is that between any two factors there are two patients which can be used to demonstrate a double dissociation, which would indicate that awareness of deficits on each factor is, at least to some extent, independent.

Between-Group Contrasts

Across the groups, patient- and informant-ratings of behavioral problems, as measured by the total PCRS score, were highly discrepant in the brain-injury and Alzheimer's disease groups (see Figure 13.3), but this was much less so in the schizophrenia group, and suggests that patients exhibit different levels of unawareness of behavioral deficits. Importantly, ratings made by either patients or informants in any patient group were not grossly at ceiling or floor, but varied somewhat, suggesting that these scales provided sensitivity in measuring behavioral impairment, and in turn, awareness.

It was also of interest to see on what dimensions awareness between domains may differ, and whether there is an extant hierarchy of awareness. Comparison of subfactor scores between groups can also reveal whether there are different "profiles" of awareness in different patient groups. From Figure 13.4 it can be seen that both the brain injury and Alzheimer groups rated *themselves* as having good to very good behavioral functioning (in the region of 3.5 points out of 4). The two groups differed in that the informants in the Alzheimer group rated these patients as having much greater impairments, especially in terms of cognition.

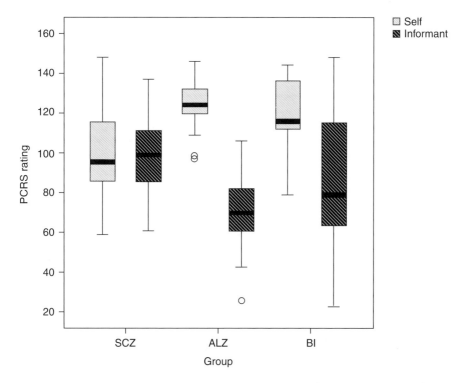

Figure 13.3 Box plot showing the mean total Patient Competency Rating Scale (PCRS) self- and informant ratings (possible range is 0 to 148) for each of the three groups. Higher ratings reflect greater rated functioning. Error bars at 1 SE. ALZ, Alzheimer patients; BI, brain injury patients; SCZ, schizophrenia patients. Circles represent scores from individual outliers.

Comparatively, the schizophrenia group rated themselves as lower functioning, but their ratings were concordant with the informants view across all subdomains, which reflect good awareness of behavioral problems. The lower panel shows that this results in lowest awareness for the Alzheimer group, and greatest awareness for the schizophrenia group, but also that there is no consistent profile across patients, failing to support the notion of a hierarchy of awareness.

It was also observed that PCRS discrepancy scores correlated moderately in the expected direction with clinician-rated insight for the Alzheimer and brain injury groups singly and combined but not the schizophrenia group alone (see Table 13.5). This might be taken to suggest that impaired awareness of behavioral and social competencies is governed by similar processes in these "organic" groups but in chronic schizophrenia a relatively intact system monitors behavioral competencies. This system is in turn separate from the one or more which monitors abnormal experiences, beliefs, and the need for treatment. The association of more awareness and lower mood, as indexed by the BDI, seemed to pertain to all groups.

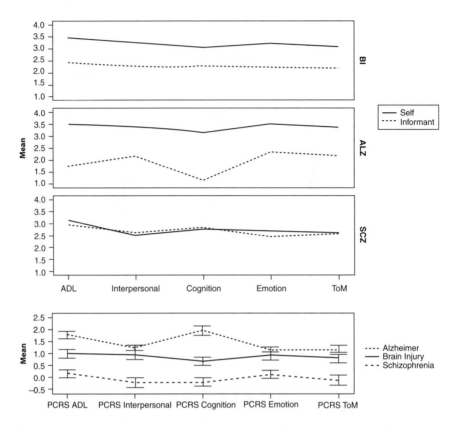

Figure 13.4 Graphs showing mean Patient Competency Rating Scale (PCRS) self and informant subfactor scores paneled according to patient group. Positive scores reflect greater rated functioning, where a score of "4" is perfect functioning. The lower panel shows the resultant PCRS discrepancy scores for the three groups. ADL, activities of daily living; ALZ, Alzheimer patients; BI, brain injury patients; SCZ, schizophrenia patients; ToM, theory of mind.

Table 13.5 Correlation Coefficients for the Modified PCRS-Discrepancy Scores, Depression and Insight Measures: Schizophrenia Patients Alone and Combined with Brain Injury and Alzheimer Patients

PCRS+ToM	Beck Depression Inventory	SAI-E	SUMD
Schizophrenia group ($n = 31$)	0.341	.009	.019
Whole group ($n = 86$)	0.546**	0.319*	−.271*

PCRS, Patient Competency Rating Scale; SAI-E, Schedule for the Assessment of Insight (expanded); SUMD, Scale for the Assessment of Unawareness of Mental Disorder; ToM, theory of mind.

Summary and Conclusions

In summary, insight or awareness in schizophrenia may be multiply determined, although broadly speaking, there is converging evidence for key etiological factors, such as executive function and positive psychopathology, with mood playing a mediating role. Insight is an important indicator of prognosis and outcome. Some of these associations are complex and nonlinear, for example, insight and subjective quality of life, with cognitive ability and denial showing statistical interactions.

These conclusions are based largely on the published literature plus our own recent findings presented above; however, there are several inconsistencies. There are many possible reasons for this, such as the use of different awareness scales, different batteries of neuropsychological tests, and heterogeneous patient groups. Another potential source of heterogeneity is the application of common rating tools to very different patient groups as described above. This last methodology is relatively novel and open to criticism, so the findings must be regarded as preliminary. However, the approach does raise interesting questions.

It has also been demonstrated by our work and that of others that awareness may be dissected within and also between domains of functioning. That is to say, it may fractionate. In the data we present here, patients with chronic schizophrenia show good awareness of their functional and behavioral problems compared to brain injury and Alzheimer's disease patients despite being mostly unaware of their mental illness or being unable to attribute their symptoms to mental illness. In turn, these dimensions are largely independent from compliance with medication. Pooling the neuropsychiatric patients together showed that overall awareness as measured by the PCRS discrepancy correlated inversely with symptom severity and positively with mood (worse symptoms, worse awareness; lower mood, better awareness). These results are generally in favor of modularity of awareness with a degree of consistency regardless of diagnosis. We propose, tentatively, that the pattern is consistent with there being a common cognitive architecture for awareness of psychopathologies which may be disrupted following varied neurophysiological and neuroanatomical dysfunction. This would go against focal localization of such an architecture, but instead it points to a somewhat distributed or multiple, function-specific system(s). However, such a system or systems appear to rely on general support systems—such as executive processing—and may be modulated by generalized factors such as mood.

Acknowledgments

James Gilleen was supported by an MRC PhD studentship. We are grateful to Professor Simon Lovestone for facilitating access to his Alzheimer cohort; Laura

Bach helped with recruitment of brain injury patients. We are grateful to all the patients and caregivers who generously took part in our studies.

References

Aleman, A., Agrawal, N., Morgan, K. D., & David, A. S. (2006). Insight in psychosis and neuropsychological function: Meta-analysis. *British Journal of Psychiatry, 189*, 204–212.

Aleman, A., de Haan, E. H., & Kahn, R. S. (2002). Insight and neurocognitive function in schizophrenia. *Journal of Neuropsychiatry and Clinical Neurosciences, 14*, 241–242.

Almeida, O. P., Levy, R., Howard, R. J., & David, A. S. (1996). Insight and paranoid disorders in late life (late paraphrenia). *International Journal of Geriatric Psychiatry, 11*, 653–658.

Amador, X. F., & David, A. S., (Eds.) (2004). *Insight and psychosis: Awareness of illness in schizophrenia and related disorders* (2nd edition). Oxford, England: Oxford University Press.

Amador, X. F., Flaum, M., Andreasen, N. C., Strauss, D. H., Yale, S. A., Clark, S. C., & Gorman, J. M. (1994). Awareness of illness in schizophrenia and schizoaffective and mood disorders. *Archives of General Psychiatry, 51*, 826–836.

Amador, X. F., Strauss, D. H., Yale, S. A., Flaum, M. M., Endicott, J., & Gorman, J. M. (1993). Assessment of insight in psychosis. *American Journal of Psychiatry, 150*, 873–879.

Amador, X. F., Strauss, D. H., Yale, S. A., & Gorman, J. M. (1991). Awareness of illness in schizophrenia. *Schizophrenia Bulletin, 17*, 113–132.

Arango, C., Adami, H., Sherr, J. D., Thaker, G. K., & Carpenter, W. T. (1999). Relationship of awareness of dyskinesia in schizophrenia to insight into mental illness. *American Journal of Psychiatry, 156*, 1097–1099.

Arduini, L., Kalyvoka, A., Stratta, P., Rinaldi, O., Daneluzzo, E., & Rossi, A. (2003). Insight and neuropsychological function in patients with schizophrenia and bipolar disorder with psychotic features. *Canadian Journal of Psychiatry, 48*, 338–341.

Babinski, J. (1914). Contributions à l'étude des troubles mentaux dans l'hémiplégie organique cérébrale (anososngosie). *Revue Neurologique, 27*, 845–848.

Bach, L. J., & David, A. S. (2006). Self-awareness after acquired and traumatic brain injury. *Neuropsychological Rehabilitation, 16*, 397–414.

Baier, M., DeShay, E., Owens, K., Robinson, M., Lasar, K., Peterson, K., & Bland, R. S. (2000). The relationship between insight and clinical factors for persons with schizo-phrenia. *Archives of Psychiatric Nursing, 14*, 259–265.

Banks, S.J., & Weintraub, S. (2009). Generalized and symptom-specific insight in beha-vioral variant frontotemporal dementia and primary progressive aphasia. *Journal of Neuropsychiatry and Clinical Neuroscience, 21*, 299–306.

Bassitt, D. P., Neto, M. R. L., de Castro, C. C., & Busatto, G. F. (2007). Insight and regional brain volumes in schizophrenia. *European Archives of Psychiatry and Clinical Neuroscience, 257*, 58–62.

Beck, A. T., Baruch, E., Balter, J. M., Steer, R. A., & Warman, D. M. (2004). A new instrument for measuring insight: The Beck Cognitive Insight Scale. *Schizophrenia Research, 68,* 319–329.

Bentall, R. P. (1995). Brains, biases, deficits, and disorders. *British Journal of Psychiatry, 167,* 152–158.

Berrios, G. E., & Markovà, I. S. (2004). Insight in the psychoses: A conceptual history. In X. F. Amador, & A. S. David (Eds.), *Insight and psychosis: Awareness of illness in schizophrenia and related disorders* (2nd edition, pp. 31–50). Oxford, England: Oxford University Press.

Berti, A., Bottini, G., Gandola, M., Pia, L., Smania, N., Stracciari, A., Castiglioni, I., Vallar, G., & Paulesu, E. (2005). Shared cortical anatomy for motor awareness and motor control. *Science, 309,* 488–491.

Birchwood, M., Smith, J., Drury, V., Healy, J., Macmillan, F., & Slade, M. (1994). A self-report Insight Scale for psychosis: Reliability, validity and sensitivity to change. *Acta Psychiatrica Scandinavica, 89,* 62–67.

Bora, E., Sehitoglu, G., Aslier, M., Atabay, I., & Veznedaroglu, B. (2007). Theory of mind and unawareness of illness in schizophrenia: Is poor insight a mentalizing deficit? *European Archives of Psychiatry & Clinical Neuroscience, 257,* 104–111.

Bourgeois, M., Swendsen, J., Young, F., Amador, X., Pini, S., Cassano, G. B., Lindenmayer, J.-P., Hsu, C., Alphs, L., Meltzer, H. Y., & The InterSePT Study Group. (2004). Awareness of disorder and suicide risk in the treatment of schizophrenia: Results of the International Suicide Prevention Trial. *American Journal of Psychiatry, 161,* 1494–1496.

Burgess, P. W., Alderman, N., Evans, J., Emslie, H., & Wilson, B. A. (1998). The ecological validity of tests of executive function. *Journal of the International Neuropsychological Society, 4,* 547–558.

Burton, S. (2006). Symptom domains of schizophrenia: The role of atypical antipsychotic agents. *Journal of Psychopharmacology, 20*(6) (Suppl.), 2–19.

Carroll, A., Fattah, S., Clyde, Z., Coffey, I., Owens, D. G., & Johnstone, E. C. (1999). Correlates of insight and insight change in schizophrenia. *Schizophrenia Research, 35,* 247–253.

Cavezian, C., Rossetti, Y., Danckert, J., d'Amato, T., Dalery, J., & Saoud, M. (2007). Exaggerated leftward bias in the mental number line of patients with schizophrenia. *Brain and Cognition, 63,* 85–90.

Clare, L. (2004a). The construction of awareness in early-stage Alzheimer's disease: A review of concepts and models. *British Journal of Clinical Psychology, 43,* 155–175.

Clare, L. (2004b). Awareness in early-stage Alzheimer's disease: A review of methods and evidence. *British Journal of Clinical Psychology, 43,* 177–196.

Clare, L., Wilson, B. A., Carter, G., Roth, I., & Hodges, J. R. (2002). Assessing awareness in early-stage Alzheimer's disease: Development and piloting of the Memory Awareness Rating Scale. *Neuropsychological Rehabilitation, 12,* 341–362.

Collins, A. A., Remington, G. J., Coulter, K., & Birkett, K. (1997). Insight, neurocognitive function and symptom clusters in chronic schizophrenia. *Schizophrenia Research, 27,* 37–44.

Cooke, M., Peters, E., Fannon, D., Anilkumar, A. P., Aasen, I., Kuipers, E., & Kumari, V. (2007). Insight, distress and coping styles in schizophrenia. *Schizophrenia Research, 94*, 12–22.

Cooke, M. A., Peters, E. R., Kuipers, E., & Kumari, V. (2005). Disease, deficit or denial? Models of poor insight in psychosis. *Acta Psychiatrica Scandinavica, 112*, 4–17.

Cuesta, M. J., & Peralta, V. (1994). Lack of insight in schizophrenia. *Schizophrenia Bulletin, 20*, 359–366.

Cuesta, M. J., Peralta, V., & Zarzuela, A. (2000). Reappraising insight in psychosis. Multi-scale longitudinal study. *British Journal of Psychiatry, 177*, 233–240.

Cuesta, M. J., Peralta, V., Zarzuela, A., & Zandio, M. (2006). Insight dimensions and cognitive function in psychosis: A longitudinal study. *BMC Psychiatry, 6*, 26.

Ceskova, E., Prikryl, R., Kasparek, T., & Kucerova, H. (2007). Insight in first episode schizophrenia. *International Journal of Psychiatry in Clinical Practice, 12*, 36–40.

David, A. (1995). The future of diagnosis: Commentary on: "Cognitive Neuropsychiatry and the PC model of the mind." *British Journal of Psychiatry, 167*, 155–157.

David, A., Buchanan, A., Reed, A., & Almeida, O. (1992). The assessment of insight in psychosis. *The British Journal of Psychiatry, 161*, 599–602.

David, A., & Kemp, R. (1997). Five perspectives on the phenomenon of insight in psychosis. *Psychiatric Annals, 27*, 791–797.

David, A., van Os, J., Jones, P., Harvey, I., Foerster, A., & Fahy, T. (1995). Insight and psychotic illness. Cross-sectional and longitudinal associations. *British Journal of Psychiatry, 167*, 621–628.

David, A. S. (1990). Insight and psychosis. *British Journal of Psychiatry, 156*, 798–808.

David, A. S. (1993). Cognitive neuropsychiatry? *Psychological Medicine, 23*, 1–5.

David, A. S. (1999). "To see ourselves as others see us." Aubrey Lewis's insight. *British Journal of Psychiatry, 174*, 210–216.

David, A. S. (2004). The clinical importance of insight. In X. F. Amador, & A. S. David (Eds.), *Insight and psychosis: Awareness of illness in schizophrenia and related disorders* (pp. 359–390). Oxford, England: Oxford University Press.

David, A. S., Owen, A. M., & Forstl, H. (1993). An annotated summary and translation of "On self-awareness of focal brain diseases by the patient in cortical blindness and cortical deafness" by Gabriel Anton. *Cognitive Neuropsychology, 10*, 263–272.

Dickerson, F. B., Boronow, J. J., Ringel, N., & Parente, F. (1997). Lack of insight among outpatients with schizophrenia. *Psychiatric Services, 48*, 195–199.

Donohoe, G., Corvin, A., & Robertson, I. H. (2005). Are the cognitive deficits associated with impaired insight in schizophrenia specific to executive task performance? *Journal of Nervous and Mental Disease, 193*, 803–808.

Donohoe, G., Donnell, C. O., Owens, N., & O'Callaghan, E. (2004). Evidence that health attributions and symptom severity predict insight in schizophrenia. *Journal of Nervous and Mental Disease, 192*, 635–637.

Donohoe, G., & Robertson, I. H. (2003). Can specific deficits in executive functioning explain the negative symptoms of schizophrenia? A review. *Neurocase, 9*, 97–108.

Drake, R. J., & Lewis, S. W. (2003). Insight and neurocognition in schizophrenia. *Schizophrenia Research, 62*, 165–173.

Drake, R. J., Pickles, A., Bentall, R. P., Kinderman, P., Haddock, G., Tarrier, N., & Lewis, S. W. (2004). The evolution of insight, paranoia and depression during early schizophrenia. *Psychological Medicine, 34,* 285–292.

Drake, R.J., Dunn, G., Tarrier, N., Bentall, R.P., Haddock, G., & Lewis, S.W. (2007). Insight as a predictor of the outcome of first episode non-affective psychosis in a prospective cohort study in England. *Journal of Clinical Psychiatry, 68,* 81–6.

Fennig, S., Everett, E., Bromet, E. J., Jandorf, L., Fennig, S. R., Tanenberg-Karant, M., & Craig, T. J. (1996). Insight in first-admission psychotic patients. *Schizophrenia Research, 22,* 257–263.

Flashman, L. A., McAllister, T. W., Andreasen, N. C., & Saykin, A. J. (2000). Smaller brain size associated with unawareness of illness in patients with schizophrenia. *American Journal of Psychiatry, 157,* 1167–1169.

Flashman, L. A., McAllister, T. W., Johnson, S. C., Rick, J. H., Green, R. L., & Saykin, A. J. (2001). Specific frontal lobe subregions correlated with unawareness of illness in schizophrenia: A preliminary study. *Journal of Neuropsychiatry and Clinical Neurosciences, 13,* 255–257.

Flashman, L. A., Roth, R. M., McAllister, T. W., Pendergrass, J. C., Garlinghouse, M. A., & Saykin, A. J. (2007). Dissociation of awareness of different components of illness in schizophrenia. *Journal of Neuropsychiatry and Clinical Neurosciences, 19,* 221–222.

Fleming, J. M., Strong, J., & Ashton, R. (1996). Self-awareness of deficits in adults with traumatic brain injury: How best to measure? *Brain Injury, 10,* 1–15.

Fordyce, D. J., & Roueche, J. R. (1986). Changes in perspectives of disability among patients, staff, and relatives during rehabilitation of brain injury. *Rehabilitation Psychology, 31,* 217–229.

Freudenreich, O., Deckersbach, T., & Goff, D. C. (2004). Insight into current symptoms of schizophrenia. Association with frontal cortical function and affect. *Acta Psychiatrica Scandinavica, 110,* 14–20.

Ghaemi, S. N. (2007). Feeling and time: The phenomenology of mood disorders, depressive realism, and existential psychotherapy. *Schizophrenia Bulletin, 33,* 122–130.

Ghaemi, S. N., Hebben, N., Stoll, A. L., & Pope, H. G., Jr. (1996). Neuropsychological aspects of lack of insight in bipolar disorder: A preliminary report. *Psychiatry Research, 65,* 113–120.

Ghaemi, S. N., & Rosenquist, K. J. (2004). Is insight in mania state-dependent? A meta-analysis. *Journal of Nervous & Mental Disease, 192,* 771–775.

Gharabawi, G. M., Lasser, R. A., Bossie, C. A., Zhu, Y., & Amador, X. (2006). Insight and its relationship to clinical outcomes in patients with schizophrenia or schizoaffective disorder receiving long-acting risperidone. *International Clinical Psychopharmacology, 21,* 233–240.

Gigante, A. D., & Castel, S. (2004). Insight into schizophrenia: A comparative study between patients and family members. *Sao Paulo Medical Journal, 122,* 246–251.

Goldberg, R. W., Green-Paden, L. D., Lehman, A. F., & Gold, J. M. (2001). Correlates of insight in serious mental illness. *Journal of Nervous and Mental Disease, 189,* 137–145.

Goodman, C., Knoll, G., Isakov, V., & Silver, H. (2005). Insight into illness in schizophrenia. *Comprehensive Psychiatry, 46,* 284–290.

Ha, T., Youn, T., Ha, K., Rho, K., Lee, J., Kim, I., Kim, S., & Kwon, J. (2004). Grey matter abnormalities in paranoid schizophrenia and their clinical correlations. *Psychiatry Research: Neuroimaging, 132,* 251–260.

Hasson-Ohayon, I., Kravetz, S., Roe, D., David, A. S., & Weiser, M. (2006). Insight into psychosis and quality of life. *Comprehensive Psychiatry, 47,* 265–269.

Hawton, K., Sutton, L., Haw, C., Sinclair, J., & Deeks, J. J. (2005). Schizophrenia and suicide: Systematic review of risk factors. *British Journal of Psychiatry, 187,* 9–20.

Heilbronner, R. L., Roueche, J. R., Everson, S. A., & Epler, L. (1989). Comparing patient perspectives of disability and treatment effects with quality of participation in a post-acute brain injury rehabilitation programme. *Brain Injury, 3,* 387–395.

Heinrichs, D. W., Cohen, B. P., & Carpenter, W. T., Jr. (1985). Early insight and the management of schizophrenic decompensation. *Journal of Nervous and Mental Disease, 173,* 133–138.

Iqbal, Z., Birchwood, M., Chadwick, P., & Trower, P. (2000). Cognitive approach to depression and suicidal thinking in psychosis. 2. Testing the validity of a social ranking model. *British Journal of Psychiatry, 177,* 522–528.

Johnson, S., & Orrell, M. (1996). Insight, psychosis and ethnicity: A case-note study. *Psychological Medicine, 26,* 1081–1084.

Jones, P. B., Guth, C., Lewis, S. W., & Murray, R. M. (1994). Low intelligence and poor educational achievement precede early onset schizophrenic psychosis. In A. S. David, & J. Cutting (Eds.), *The neuropsychology of schizophrenia* (pp. 131–144). London: Lawrence Erlbaum Associates.

Jorgensen, P. (1995). Recovery and insight in schizophrenia. *Acta Psychiatrica Scandinavica, 92,* 436–440.

Kaiser, S. L., Snyder, J. A., Corcoran, R., & Drake, R. J. (2006). The relationships among insight, social support, and depression in psychosis. *Journal of Nervous & Mental Disease, 194,* 905–908.

Karnath, H. O., Berger, M. F., Kuker, W., & Rorden, C. (2004). The anatomy of spatial neglect based on voxelwise statistical analysis: A study of 140 patients. *Cerebral Cortex, 14,* 1164–1172.

Karow, A., & Pajonk, F. G. (2006). Insight and quality of life in schizophrenia: Recent findings and treatment implications. *Current Opinion in Psychiatry, 19,* 637–641.

Kay, S. R., Fiszbein, A., & Opler, L. A. (1987). The Positive and Negative Syndrome Scale (PANSS) for schizophrenia. *Schizophrenia Bulletin, 13,* 261–276.

Kemp, R., & David, A. (1996). Psychological predictors of insight and compliance in psychotic patients. *British Journal of Psychiatry, 169,* 444–450.

Kemp, R., & David, A. S. (1997). Insight and compliance. In B. Blackwell (Ed.), *Treatment compliance and the therapeutic alliance* (pp. 61–86). Amsterdam: Harwood Academic Publishers.

Kemp, R., Kirov, G., Everitt, B., Hayward, P., & David, A. (1998). Randomised controlled trial of compliance therapy: 18 month follow-up. *British Journal of Psychiatry, 172,* 413–419.

Kemp, R. A., & Lambert, T. J. (1995). Insight in schizophrenia and its relationship to psychopathology. *Schizophrenia Research, 18,* 21–28.

Keshavan, M. S., Rabinowitz, J., DeSmedt, G., Harvey, P. D., & Schooler, N. (2004). Correlates of insight in first episode psychosis. *Schizophrenia Research, 70,* 187–194.

Kim, C. H., Jayathilake, K., & Meltzer, H. Y. (2003). Hopelessness, neurocognitive function, and insight in schizophrenia: Relationship to suicidal behavior. *Schizophrenia Research, 60*, 71–80.

Kim, Y., Sakamoto, K., Kamo, T., Sakamura, Y., & Miyaoka, H. (1997). Insight and clinical correlates in schizophrenia. *Comprehensive Psychiatry, 38*, 117–123.

Kircher, T. T. J., Koch, K., Stottmeister, F., & Durst, V. (2007). Metacognition and reflexivity in patients with schizophrenia. *Psychopathology, 40*, 254–260.

Koren, D., Seidman, L. J., Poyurovsky, M., Goldsmith, M., Viksman, P., Zichel, S., & Klein, E. (2004). The neuropsychological basis of insight in first-episode schizophrenia: A pilot metacognitive study. *Schizophrenia Research, 70*, 195–202.

Langdon, R., & Ward, P. (2009). Taking the perspective of the other contributes to awareness of illness in schizophrenia. *Schizophrenia Bulletin, 35*, 1003–1011.

Lappin, J. M., Morgan, K. D., Valmaggia, L. R., Broome, M. R., Woolley, J. B., Johns, L. C., Tabraham, P., Bramon, E., & McGuire, P. K. (2007). Insight in individuals with an at risk mental state. *Schizophrenia Research, 90*, 238–244.

Laroi, F., Fannemel, M., Ronneberg, U., Flekkoy, K., Opjordsmoen, S., Dullerud, R., & Haakonsen, M. (2000). Unawareness of illness in chronic schizophrenia and its relationship to structural brain measures and neuropsychological tests. *Psychiatry Research, 100*, 49–58.

Larøi, F., Barr, W. B., & Keefe, R. S. E. (2004). The neuropsychology of insight in psychiatric and neurological disorders. In X. F. Amador, & A. S. David (Eds.), *Insight and psychosis: Awareness of illness in schizophrenia and related disorders* (pp. 119–156). Oxford, England: Oxford University Press.

Leathem, J. M., Murphy, L. J., & Flett, R. A. (1998). Self- and informant-ratings on the patient competency rating scale in patients with traumatic brain injury. *Journal of Clinical and Experimental Neuropsychology, 20*, 694–705.

Lewis, A. (1934). The psychopathology of insight. *British Journal of Medical Psychology, 14*, 332–348.

Lincoln, T. M., Lullmann, E., & Rief, W. (2007). Correlates and long-term consequences of poor insight in patients with schizophrenia. A systematic review. *Schizophrenia Bulletin, 33*, 1324–1342.

Lysaker, P., & Bell, M. (1994). Insight and cognitive impairment in schizophrenia. Performance on repeated administrations of the Wisconsin Card Sorting Test. *The Journal of Nervous and Mental Disease, 182*, 656–660.

Lysaker, P. H., Bell, M. D., Bryson, G., & Kaplan, E. (1998). Neurocognitive function and insight in schizophrenia: Support for an association with impairments in executive function but not with impairments in global function. *Acta Psychiatrica Scandinavica, 97*, 297–301.

Lysaker, P. H., Bell, M., Milstein, R., Bryson, G., & Beam-Goulet, J. (1994). Insight and psychosocial treatment compliance in schizophrenia. *Psychiatry, 57*, 307–315.

Lysaker, P. H., Carcione, A., Dimaggio, G., Johannesen, J. K., Nicolo, G., Procacci, M., & Semerari, A. (2005). Metacognition amidst narratives of self and illness in schizophrenia: Associations with neurocognition, symptoms, insight and quality of life. *Acta Psychiatrica Scandinavica, 112*, 64–71.

Lysaker, P. H., Clements, C. A., Plascak-Hallberg, C. D., Knipscheer, S. J., & Wright, D. E. (2002). Insight and personal narratives of illness in schizophrenia. *Psychiatry, 65,* 197–206.

Lysaker, P. H., Lancaster, R. S., Davis, L. W., & Clements, C. A. (2003). Patterns of neurocognitive deficits and unawareness of illness in schizophrenia. *Journal of Nervous and Mental Disease, 191,* 38–44.

Macpherson, R., Jerrom, B., & Hughes, A. (1996). Relationship between insight, educational background and cognition in schizophrenia. *The British Journal of Psychiatry, 168,* 718–722.

Markova, I. S. (2005). *Insight in psychiatry.* Cambridge, England: Cambridge University Press.

Marks, K. A., Fastenau, P. S., Lysaker, P. H., & Bond, G. R. (2000). Self-Appraisal of Illness Questionnaire (SAIQ): Relationship to researcher-rated insight and neuropsychological function in schizophrenia. *Schizophrenia Research, 45,* 203–211.

McCabe, R., Quayle, E., Beirne, A. D., & Duane, M. M. (2002). Insight, global neuropsychological functioning, and symptomatology in chronic schizophrenia. *Journal of Nervous and Mental Disease, 190,* 519–525.

McEvoy, J. P., Apperson, L. J., Appelbaum, P. S., Ortlip, P., Brecosky, J., Hammill, K., Geller, J. L., & Roth, L. (1989). Insight in schizophrenia. Its relationship to acute psychopathology. *Journal of Nervous and Mental Disease, 177,* 43–47.

McEvoy, J. P., Hartman, M., Gottlieb, D., Godwin, S., Apperson, L. J., & Wilson, W. (1996). Common sense, insight, and neuropsychological test performance in schizophrenia patients. *Schizophrenia Bulletin, 22,* 635–641.

McEvoy, J. P., Johnson, J., Perkins, D., Lieberman, J. A., Hamer, R. M., Keefe, R. S., Tohen, M., Glick, I. D., & Sharma, T. (2006). Insight in first-episode psychosis. *Psychological Medicine, 36,* 1385–1393.

McEvoy, J. P., Schooler, N. R., Friedman, E., Steingard, S., & Allen, M. (1993). Use of psychopathology vignettes by patients with schizophrenia or schizoaffective disorder and by mental health professionals to judge patients' insight. *American Journal of Psychiatry, 150,* 1649–1653.

McGlashan, T. H., & Carpenter Jr, W. T. (1981). Does attitude toward psychosis relate to outcome? *American Journal of Psychiatry, 138,* 797–801.

McGlynn, S. M., & Schacter, D. L. (1989). Unawareness of deficits in neuropsychological syndromes. *Journal of Clinical and Experimental Neuropsychology, 11,* 143–205.

McGlynn, S. M., & Kaszniak, A. W. (1991). Unawareness of deficits in dementia and schizophrenia. In G. P. Prigatano & D. L. Schacter (Eds.) *Awareness of Deficit after Brain Injury: Clinical and theoritical issues* (pp. 84–110). New York: Oxford University Press.

McGlynn, S. M., & Schacter, D. L. (1997). The neuropsychology of insight: Impaired awareness of deficits in a psychiatric context. *Psychiatric Annals, 27,* 806–811.

McGlynn, S. M., Schacter, D. L., & Glisky, E. L. (1989). Unawareness of deficits in organic amnesia. *Journal of Clinical and Experimental Neuropsychology, 11,* 50.

Medalia, A., & Lim, R. W. (2004). Self-awareness of cognitive functioning in schizophrenia. *Schizophrenia Research, 71,* 331–338.

Michalakeas, A., Skoutas, C., Charalambous, A., Peristeris, A., Marinos, V., Keramari, E., & Theologou, A. (1994). Insight in schizophrenia and mood disorders and its relation to psychopathology. *Acta Psychiatrica Scandinavica, 90*, 46–49.

Mintz, A. R., Addington, J., & Addington, D. (2004). Insight in early psychosis: A 1-year follow-up. *Schizophrenia Research, 67*, 213–217.

Mintz, A. R., Dobson, K. S., & Romney, D. M. (2003). Insight in schizophrenia: A meta-analysis. *Schizophrenia Research, 61*, 75–88.

Mohamed, S., Fleming, S., Penn, D. L., & Spaulding, W. (1999). Insight in schizophrenia: Its relationship to measures of executive functions. *Journal of Nervous and Mental Disease, 187*, 525–531.

Moore, O., Cassidy, E., Carr, A., & O'Callaghan, E. (1999). Unawareness of illness and its relationship with depression and self-deception in schizophrenia. *European Psychiatry, 14*, 264–269.

Morgan, K. D., & David, A. S. (2004). Neuropsychological studies of insight in patients with psychotic disorders. In X. F. Amador, & A. S. David (Eds.), *Insight and psychosis: Awareness of illness in schizophrenia and related disorders* (pp. 275–298). Oxford, England: Oxford University Press.

Morgan, K. D., Dazzan, P., Orr, K. G., Hutchinson, G., Chitnis, X., Sucking, J., Lythgoe, D., Pollock, S.-J., Rossell, S., Shapleske, J., Fearon, P., Morgan, C., David, A., McGuire, P. K., Jones, P. B., Leff, J., & Murray, R. M. (2007). Grey matter abnormalities in first-episode schizophrenia and affective psychosis. *British Journal of Psychiatry, 191* (Suppl. 51), s111–116.

Morgan, K. D., Dazzan, P., & Suckling, J. (2002). Neuroanatomical correlates of poor insight: The AESOP first-onset psychosis study. *Schizophrenia Research, 53*, 101–102.

Mutsatsa, S. H., Joyce, E. M., Hutton, S. B., & Barnes, T. R. (2006). Relationship between insight, cognitive function, social function and symptomatology in schizophrenia: The West London first episode study. *European Archives of Psychiatry & Clinical Neuroscience, 256*, 356–363.

Nakano, H., Terao, T., Iwata, N., Hasako, R., & Nakamura, J. (2004). Symptomatological and cognitive predictors of insight in chronic schizophrenia. *Psychiatry Research, 127*, 65–72.

O'Keeffe, F. M., Murray, B., Coen, R. F., Dockree, P. M., Bellgrove, M. A., Garavan, H., Lynch, T., & Robertson, I. H. (2007). Loss of insight in frontotemporal dementia, corticobasal degeneration and progressive supranuclear palsy. *Brain, 130*, 753–764.

Olfson, M., Marcus, S. C., Wilk, J., & West, J. C. (2006). Awareness of illness and nonadherence to antipsychotic medications among persons with schizophrenia. *Psychiatric Services, 57*, 205–211.

Osatuke, K., Ciesla, J., Kasckow, J. W., Zisook, S., & Mohamed, S. (2008). Insight in schizophrenia: A review of etiological models and supporting research. *Comprehensive Psychiatry, 49*, 70–77.

Overall, J. E., & Gorham, D. (1962). The Brief Psychiatric Rating Scale. *Psychological Reports, 10*, 799–812.

Pallanti, S., Quercioli, L., & Pazzagli, A. (1999). Effects of clozapine on awareness of illness and cognition in schizophrenia. *Psychiatry Research, 86*, 239–249.

Pannu, J. K., & Kaszniak, A. W. (2005). Metamemory experiments in neurological populations: A review. *Neuropsychology Review, 15*, 105–130.

Peralta, V., & Cuesta, M. (1994). Lack of insight: Its status within schizophrenic psychopathology. *Biological Psychiatry, 36*, 559–561.

Pini, S., Cassano, G. B., Dell'Osso, L., & Amador, X. F. (2001). Insight into illness in schizophrenia, schizoaffective disorder, and mood disorders with psychotic features. *American Journal of Psychiatry, 158*, 122–125.

Pousa, E., Duno, R., Blas Navarro, J., Ruiz, A. I., Obiols, J. E., & David, A. S. (2008a). Exploratory study of the association between insight and Theory of Mind (ToM) in stable schizophrenia patients. *Cognitive Neuropsychiatry, 13*, 210–232.

Pousa, E., Duñó, R., Brebion, G., David, A. S., Ruiz, A. I., & Obiols J. E. (2008b). Theory of mind deficits in chronic schizophrenia: Evidence for state dependence. *Psychiatry Research, 158*, 1–10.

Prigatano, G. P. (1999). Impaired awareness, finger tapping, and rehabilitation outcome after brain injury. *Rehabilitation Psychology, 44*, 145–159.

Prigatano, G. P., & Altman, I. M. (1990). Impaired awareness of behavioral limitations after traumatic brain injury. *Archives of Physical & Medical Rehabilitation, 71*, 1058–1064.

Prigatano, G. P., & Fordyce, D. J. (1986). Cognitive dysfunction and psychosocial adjustment after brain injury. In *Neuropsychological rehabilitation after brain injury* (pp. 96–118). Baltimore: The John Hopkins University Press.

Pyne, J. M., Bean, D., & Sullivan, G. (2001). Characteristics of patients with schizophrenia who do not believe they are mentally ill. *Journal of Nervous and Mental Disease, 189*, 146–153.

Pyszczynski, T., & Greenberg, J. (1987). Self-regulatory perseveration and the depressive self-focusing style: A self-awareness theory of reactive depression. *Psychological Bulletin, 102*, 122–138.

Rathod, S., Kingdon, D., Smith, P., & Turkington, D. (2005). Insight into schizophrenia: the effects of cognitive behavioural therapy on the components of insight and association with sociodemographics—data on a previously published randomised controlled trial. *Schizophrenia Research, 74*, 211–219.

Rockeach, M. (1964). *The Three Christs of Ypsilanti*. New York: Knopf.

Rossell, S. L., Coakes, J., Shapleske, J., Woodruff, P. W., & David, A. S. (2003). Insight: Its relationship with cognitive function, brain volume and symptoms in schizophrenia. *Psychological Medicine, 33*, 111–119.

Saeedi, H., Addington, J., & Addington, D. (2007). The association of insight with psychotic symptoms, depression, and cognition in early psychosis: A 3-year follow-up. *Schizophrenia Research, 89*, 123–128.

Sanz, M., Constable, G., Lopez-Ibor, I., Kemp, R., & David, A. S. (1998). A comparative study of insight scales and their relationship to psychopathological and clinical variables. *Psychological Medicine, 28*, 437–446.

Sapara, A., Cooke, M., Fannon, D., Francis, A., Buchanan, R. W., Anilkumar, A. P. P., Barkataki, I., Aasen I., Kuipers E., & Kumari V. (2007). Prefrontal cortex and insight in schizophrenia: A volumetric MRI study. *Schizophrenia Research, 89*, 22–34.

Saravanan B., Jacob K. S., Johnson S., Prince M., Bhugra D., & David A. S. (2007). Assessing insight in schizophrenia: East meets West. *British Journal of Psychiatry, 190*, 243–247.

Saravanan, B., Jacob, K. S., Prince, M., Bhugra, D., & David, A. S. (2004). Culture and insight revisited. *British Journal of Psychiatry, 184,* 107–109.

Schwartz, R. C. (1998). Symptomatology and insight in schizophrenia. *Psychological Reports, 82,* 227–233.

Schwartz, R. C. (2001). Self-awareness in schizophrenia: Its relationship to depressive symptomatology and broad psychiatric impairments. *Journal of Nervous and Mental Disease, 189,* 401–403.

Schwartz, R. C., & Smith, S. D. (2004). Suicidality and psychosis: The predictive potential of symptomatology and insight into illness. *Journal of Psychiatric Research, 38,* 185–191.

Schwartz-Stav, O., Apter, A., & Zalsman, G. (2006). Depression, suicidal behaviour and insight in adolescents with schizophrenia. *European Child & Adolescent Psychiatry, 15,* 352–359.

Sevy, S., Nathanson, K., Visweswaraiah, H., & Amador, X. (2004). The relationship between insight and symptoms in schizophrenia. *Comprehensive Psychiatry, 45,* 16–19.

Shad, M. U., Muddasani, S., & Keshavan, M. S. (2006). Prefrontal subregions and dimensions of insight in first-episode schizophrenia—A pilot study. *Psychiatry Research, 146,* 35–42.

Sherer, M., Hart, T., Nick, T. G., Whyte, J., Thompson, R. N., & Yablon, S. A. (2003). Early impaired self-awareness after traumatic brain injury. *Archives of Physical Medicine and Rehabilitation, 84,* 168–176.

Simon, A. E., Berger, G. E., Giacomini, V., Ferrero, F., & Mohr, S. (2006). Insight, symptoms and executive functions in schizophrenia. *Cognitive Neuropsychiatry, 11,* 437–451.

Smith, C. M., Barzman, D., & Pristach, C. A. (1997). Effect of patient and family insight on compliance of schizophrenic patients. *Journal of Clinical Pharmacology, 37,* 147–154.

Smith, T. E., Hull, J. W., Israel, L. M., & Willson, D. F. (2000). Insight, symptoms, and neurocognition in schizophrenia and schizoaffective disorder. *Schizophrenia Bulletin, 26,* 193–200.

Smith, T. E., Hull, J. W., & Santos, L. (1998). The relationship between symptoms and insight in schizophrenia: A longitudinal perspective. *Schizophrenia Research, 33,* 63–67.

Sprong, M., Schothorst, P., Vos, E., Hox, J., & van Engeland, H. (2007). Theory of mind in schizophrenia: Meta-analysis. *British Journal of Psychiatry, 191,* 5–13.

Startup, M. (1996). Insight and cognitive deficits in schizophrenia: Evidence for a curvilinear relationship. *Psychological Medicine, 26,* 1277–1281.

Startup, M. (1997). Awareness of own and others' schizophrenic illness. *Schizophrenia Research, 26,* 203–211.

Subotnik, K. L., Nuechterlein, K. H., Irzhevsky, V., Kitchen, C. M., Woo, S. M., & Mintz, J. (2005). Is unawareness of psychotic disorder a neurocognitive or psychological defensiveness problem? *Schizophrenia Research, 75,* 147–157.

Takai, A., Uematsu, M., Ueki, H., Sone, H., & Kaiya, H. (1992). Insight and its related factors in chronic schizophrenic patients: a preliminary study. *European Journal of Psychiatry, 6,* 159–170.

Teasdale, T. W., Christensen, A. L., Willmes, K., Deloche, G., Braga, L., Stachowiak, F., Vendrell, J. M., Castro-Caldas, A., Laaksonen, R. K., & Leclercq, M. (1997). Subjective experience in brain injured patients and their close relatives: A European Brain Injury Questionnaire study. *Brain Injury, 11,* 543–564.

Thompson, K. N., McGorry, P. D., & Harrigan, S. M. (2001). Reduced awareness of illness in first-episode psychosis. *Comprehensive Psychiatry, 42,* 498–503.

Upthegrove, R., Oyebode, F., George, M., & Haque, M. S. (2002). Insight, social knowledge and working memory in schizophrenia. *Psychopathology, 35,* 341–346.

Varga, M., Magnusson, A., Flekkoy, K., David, A. S., & Opjordsmoen, S. (2007). Clinical and neuropsychological correlates of insight in schizophrenia and bipolar I disorder: Does diagnosis matter? *Comprehensive Psychiatry, 28,* 583–591.

Vasterling, J. J., Seltzer, B., Foss, J. W., & Vanderbrook, V. (1995). Unawareness of deficit in Alzheimer's disease. Domain-specific differences and disease correlates. *Neuropsychiatry, Neuropsychology, and Behavioral Neurology, 8,* 26–32.

Vasterling, J. J., Seltzer, B., & Watrous, W. E. (1997). Longitudinal assessment of deficit unawareness in Alzheimer's disease. *Neuropsychiatry, Neuropsychology, and Behavioral Neurology, 10,* 197–202.

Weiler, M. A., Fleisher, M. H., & Arthur-Campbell, D. (2000). Insight and symptom change in schizophrenia and other disorders. *Schizophrenia Research, 45,* 29–36.

White, R., Bebbington, P., Pearson, J., Johnson, S., & Ellis, D. (2000). The social context of insight in schizophrenia. *Social Psychiatry and Psychiatric Epidemiology, 35,* 500–507.

Whitty, P., Browne, S., Clarke, M., McTigue, O., Waddington, J., Kinsella, T., Larkin, C., & O'Callaghan, E. (2004). Systematic comparison of subjective and objective measures of quality of life at 4-year follow-up subsequent to a first episode of psychosis. *Journal of Nervous & Mental Disease, 192,* 805–809.

Wing, J. K., Cooper, J. E., & Sartorius, N. (1974). *Measurement and classification of psychiatric symptoms: An instruction manual for the PSE and CATEGO program.* New York: Cambridge University Press.

Young, D. A., Davila, R., & Scher, H. (1993). Unawareness of illness and neuropsychological performance in chronic schizophrenia. *Schizophrenia Research, 10,* 117–124.

Young, D. A., Zakzanis, K. K., Bailey, C., Davila, R., Griese, J., Sartory, G., & Thom, A. (1998). Further parameters of insight and neuropsychological deficit in schizophrenia and other chronic mental disease. *Journal of Nervous and Mental Disease, 186,* 44–50.

IV

Anosognosia and Specific Cognitive and Affective Disturbances

14

Anosognosia and Personality Change in Neurodegenerative Disease

Katherine P. Rankin

Investigation into the phenomenon of anosognosia over the past few decades has primarily focused on its most striking elements, including the failure to recognize obvious deficits in cognitive and physical functioning. However, loss of the ability to accurately characterize one's own personality and social behavior is an important corollary to this body of research, particularly in the context of brain injury and disease. Despite often drastic changes in personality following traumatic brain injury or the onset of a neurodegenerative condition, patients often will demonstrate, and even explicitly report, a completely inaccurate and often falsely positive sense of their social persona. Clinically, this dimension of anosognosia can impair patients' ability to successfully navigate their social environment, particularly when they are asked by a supervisor or loved one to change their behavior, but refuse because their flaws are invisible to them.

One feature that makes this domain of anosognosia particularly difficult to investigate is the fact that, unlike body awareness or the ability to recognize errors in speech or memory, otherwise healthy adults can demonstrate widely divergent degrees of social self-awareness. In fact, evaluation apprehension theory has demonstrated that lower levels of social self-monitoring and a certain imperviousness to negative social feedback can actually be adaptive (Uziel, 2007), and may be selected for in high-conflict social and occupational settings such as law enforcement or business (Miller, 2008). When it is observed in neurologic patients who were previously considered to be sensitive to social feedback, however, or when these patients are unable to change their minds about their own behavior in the face of overwhelming evidence contradicting their self-concept, this inaccurate self-perception enters the realm of anosognosia, and probably emerges directly from an organic etiology. These same unfortunate patients can shed light on both normal and pathological processes underlying the self-perception of behavior and personality.

This chapter will examine the mechanisms and possible neuroanatomic correlates of anosognosia for personality change, specifically focusing on this phenomenon in patients with neurodegenerative disease. Interpersonal, social elements of personality will be the primary focus, largely because more private or intrapsychic elements of personality are less observable in neurodegenerative disease patients. First, cognitive processes underlying the derivation of social self-awareness in nonpatient samples will be described, with attention to predicted neuroanatomic substrates. Second, the clinical phenomenon of acute loss of social self-awareness in neurodegenerative disease will be reviewed in the context of these normal cognitive processes. Finally, two novel experiments will be described that investigate the causal pathways involved in social self-monitoring deficits in dementia patients and healthy older adults.

Sources of Self-Knowledge about Personality and Social Behavior

Theoretically, derivation of an accurate concept of one's social persona is achieved through a complex series of cognitive steps, based on processing information from personal observations or from others' social feedback.

Self-Knowledge Derived from Personal Observation

1. Introspection: Observation of One's Internal States

As with self-knowledge in any domain, information about the social and behavioral self can be derived from accurate awareness of interoceptive sensations, thoughts, and emotions. Recent work defining the self from a neuroscientific perspective suggests that at the base level of our self-concept, introceptive information derives from two processing streams: proprioceptive information about the position and movement of the body in space, and visceral information about physiologic state, particularly emotional, need, or drive states (Seeley & Sturm, 2006). Authors of other chapters in this volume will address the relationship between interoception and self-knowledge more comprehensively (see Craig, Chapter 4, this volume). However, it has been well-established that the translation of interoceptive information into awareness begins in the right anterior insula (Craig, 2003; Critchley, Wiens, Rotshtein, Ohman, & Dolan, 2004). This information is then fed forward to downstream structures such as the anterior cingulate and orbitofrontal cortex, which further contextualize these interoceptive signals and can initiate an appropriate behavioral response (Damasio, 1996). Higher-level processing of interior, psychological information such as thoughts and emotions, whether these belong to the self or another person, recruits structures primarily along the medial aspect of the frontal lobes (Gusnard, Akbudak, Shulman, & Raichle, 2001; Lieberman, 2007). Once it is processed at this higher level, interoceptive information can be translated into self-schemas, especially when these states are recognized as having continuity over time (e.g., "I frequently feel very angry.")

2. Exteroception: Observation of One's Own Behaviors

Information about one's social persona can also be derived from taking a third-person perspective on one's own behaviors. Information about the self that is observed via third-person observation appears to primarily recruit a lateral frontal-temporal-parietal network (Lieberman, 2007). For instance, viewing one's own face activates the lateral prefrontal and lateral parietal cortex (Platek et al., 2006) and the neural substrate of recognizing that an action is performed by oneself rather than another is the lateral parietal cortex, predominantly in the right inferior parietal area (Farrer et al., 2003; Ruby & Decety, 2001). These lateral regions process information derived from a focus on nonpsychological, physical characteristics of self and other, including labeling facial emotions (Lieberman et al., 2007), emotional reappraisal (Ochsner et al., 2004), and impersonal moral reasoning (Greene, Nystrom, Engell, Darley, & Cohen, 2004). Social identity theory (Tajfel, 1982) and social comparison theory (Festinger, 1954) both suggest that establishment of self-knowledge via exteroceptive observation has a powerful impact on self-schema when one compares oneself to group norms or rules (Marques, Abrams, Paez, & Martinez-Taboada, 1998), or to the performance of others in one's group (Gardner & Lisberger, 2002). Thus, a significant amount of self-knowledge comes from comparing and contrasting oneself with others in one's social environment (e.g., "I give more money to charities than my coworkers do; thus, I am generous." "I am Scottish, and Scottish people have quick tempers.")

3. Memory for Personal Semantic Information

One's self-concept is formed over time and projected over time (Wakslak, Nussbaum, Liberman, & Trope, 2008), and memory plays a critical role. The term "longitudinal self" has been used to refer to the collection of self-schema, personal narratives, and episodic memories that work together to form a self-concept that includes the dimension of time (Seeley & Sturm, 2006). While explicit memories for episodic events can contribute to its construction, the longitudinal self primarily forms via implicit, often procedural memories that develop over time to form stable personal semantic information about the self. In normal subjects, the process of making controlled, self-referential judgments about one's personality traits (i.e., determining whether a trait adjective matches one's semantic knowledge about oneself) activates medial prefrontal structures (Johnson et al., 2002; Ochsner et al., 2005). There is some evidence that more automatic aspects of self-knowledge involve more ventral regions of the medial frontal cortex (Lieberman, 2007; Lieberman, Jarcho, & Satpute, 2004; Pfeifer, Lieberman, & Dapretto, 2007).

Patients with profound amnesia due to hippocampal damage (e.g., patients with Alzheimer disease [AD]) can still demonstrate a remarkably consistent sense of themselves, not only because this experience of continuity developed prior to the onset of their anterograde amnesia, but also because the longitudinal self-concept relies on two processes unaffected by hippocampal damage. First, like any highly familiar nonpersonal semantic information, long-term semantic information about the self (e.g., "I am an introvert") is typically preserved until late in the AD process, though as early memories progressively break down, the strength and cohesiveness of patients' self-concept do weaken (Addis & Tippett, 2004). Second, autobiographical memories become increasingly consolidated and semanticized over time, and retrieval relies less on medial temporal and increasingly on left frontal networks (Eustache et al., 2004). Conversely, in a disease like semantic dementia, autobiographical memories appear to be equally affected across all but the most recent time epochs due to the loss of even semanticized personal information (Piolino et al., 2003), which may in turn weaken the strength of their sense of longitudinal self.

Even though patients with mild to moderate AD may retain substantial personal semantic memory, reliance on stable, long-term self-knowledge becomes a liability in situations where essential elements of one's personality or social self have recently changed, which is often the case in patients with neurodegenerative disease or brain injury. Even in cases where individuals are capable of accurate social self-monitoring and become aware that their current behavior is inconsistent with their longitudinal self-concept, hippocampally-mediated memory for this novel awareness is critical for the incorporation of this new knowledge into an updated self-schema. Without the ability to form new episodic memories, individuals will be unable to use information gathered from their own behavior monitoring to modify their longitudinal selves, which become frozen in time at the point they were last able to remember novel self-observations.

Self-Knowledge Derived from Others' Feedback

Whether it is derived from explicit or implicit feedback from others, reflected self-knowledge contributes to self-concept formation and maintenance. In fact, different individuals' opinions of us can be evoked as separate perspectives to be compared to our own self-schema (Ochsner et al., 2005).

1. Explicit Communication from Others

Though it is not common to receive direct, explicit feedback from others about how they perceive you, both praise and criticism can be very powerful in informing one's self-concept (Sachs-Ericsson, Verona, Joiner, & Preacher, 2006), primarily because they are more difficult to miss or ignore than any other source of self-related information (e.g., "He said I was being selfish by not offering to help him fold the laundry.") However, even normal individuals can discount or discredit explicit feedback from others if it is too discrepant from their self-schema, and this phenomenon is frequently observed in brain-injured individuals (Prigatano, 2005) and patients with neurodegenerative diseases (Mendez & Shapira, 2005). Patients who consistently reject explicit feedback about their behavior and personality are more likely to have had a multi-component breakdown of the self-monitoring systems.

2. Implicit Communication from Others

Implicit feedback about oneself from others is a much more quotidian social event, but it is more difficult to detect and correctly interpret than explicit feedback. It is derived primarily from any of three sources: *(1)* paralinguistic cues in the facial expression, voice prosody, or body posture/position of the other (e.g., "She laughed awkwardly and looked pointedly away from me—I think I just revealed too much information about myself and made her uncomfortable."), *(2)* the other's avoidant or distancing behavior (e.g., "He hasn't returned my calls since I made that joke about his friend."), and *(3)* the indirect content of conversational speech (e.g., "You must be terribly busy since you haven't had the chance to write those thank-you notes yet.") Widely divergent skills are necessary to derive self-related feedback from these subtle cues, including reading facial and prosodic emotions, detecting sarcasm, perspective taking, empathy, awareness of social norms, etc. Anatomic damage to any number of neuroanatomic circuits responsible for social and emotional signal detection can cause patients to either overlook or misinterpret these implicit cues. These likely include social and emotional processing regions in the non-dominant temporal lobe (Allison, Puce, & McCarthy, 2000; Olson, Plotzker, & Ezzyat, 2007) and regions throughout the frontal lobes implicated in interpretation of others' intentions.

Social Self-Awareness in Neurodegenerative Disease

The behavioral neurology of neurodegenerative disease has gained increased research attention during the past decade, and more psychometrically and neuroscientifically sophisticated methods have been brought to bear on the problem of measuring patients' altered social behavior and personality. While AD is the most prevalent of these diseases and has thus garnered the lion's share of attention in the past, interest in the atypical dementias has been steadily increasing. This is particularly relevant to the examination of anosognosia for personality change, because while early personality changes are minimal in typical presentations of AD, they can be drastic in other clinical syndromes like frontotemporal dementia.

This, in turn, provides an avenue for investigation of the relationship between altered social behavior and social self-awareness. "Loss of insight" is considered a common symptom in the atypical dementias, and this term typically refers not only to disease anosognosia or failure to recognize cognitive deficits, but also to the failure to self-monitor social behavior.

1. Altered Behavior in Neurodegenerative Disease

While not a focus of this chapter, disease-mediated alterations in social behavior are the backdrop against which patients' social self-assessments are performed. Without behavior changes, it is unclear whether a patient's report of static behavior over time reflects accurate self-knowledge and intact self-monitoring, or whether self-monitoring deficits are present but are invisible because there has never been an atypical behavior to notice and catalogue.

Neurodegenerative diseases fall into two categories with respect to changes in social behavior and personality. In the first category are diseases like AD, cerebrovascular disease (VascD), behavioral variant frontotemporal dementia (bvFTD), and semantic dementia (SemD), in which behavior changes have been well studied and in which there is a general clinical consensus about whether altered social behavior is a typical or atypical symptom of the disease. Ample evidence suggests that in typical forms of AD affecting predominantly posterior cortex, social behavior is comparatively preserved early in the disease (Chen, Borson, & Scanlan, 2000; Cummings, 1997; Hope et al., 1997), but that patients show a consistent pattern of increased neuroticism as well as decreases in extraversion, social assertiveness, openness to new experiences, and conscientiousness (Chatterjee, Strauss, Smyth, & Whitehouse, 1992; Rankin, Kramer, Mychack, & Miller, 2003; Siegler, Dawson, & Welsh, 1994; Siegler et al., 1991; Strauss, Pasupathi, & Chatterjee, 1993; Welleford, Harkins, & Taylor, 1994). In VascD, clinical presentations vary widely depending on the location, extent, and nature of the damage, but a subset of these patients appear to have significantly increased base rates of social deficits, such as disinhibited speech and behavior, poor judgment, irritability, and other personality changes (Aharon-Peretz, Daskovski, Mashiach, Kliot, & Tomer, 2003; Bathgate, Snowden, Varma, Blackshaw, & Neary, 2001; Rankin, 2008). The behavioral variant of FTD (bvFTD) is well-established to have early, dramatic changes to personality and behavior (Bathgate et al., 2001; Bozeat, Gregory, Ralph, & Hodges, 2000; Miller et al., 1991). bvFTD disproportionately affects the (right > left) insula, anterior cingulate, dorsomedial frontal lobes, and the ventral orbitofrontal cortex, as well as parts of the basal ganglia (Rosen et al., 2002). The clinical criteria for diagnosing bvFTD rely almost entirely on behavior symptoms, including early decline in interpersonal conduct, early decline in personal conduct, and early emotional blunting (Neary et al., 1998). The SemD subtype of frontotemporal lobar degeneration (FTLD) affects primarily the anterior temporal lobes and amygdalae, but it also affects the insula, anterior cingulate, subgenual cingulate/orbitofrontal cortex, and basal ganglia (Rosen et al., 2002). Though the Neary clinical criteria for diagnosing SemD focuses on language symptoms (Neary et al., 1998), SemD patients can show social withdrawal, loss of empathy, impaired judgment, bizarre behavior, denial of illness, and mental rigidity depending largely on their degree of right temporal pathology (Bathgate et al., 2001; Bozeat et al., 2000; Edwards-Lee et al., 1997; Miller, Chang, Mena, Boone, & Lesser, 1993; Perry et al., 2001).

The second category includes neurodegenerative diseases for which there is some information available concerning social behavior and personality, but clinical research on the topic is limited to case reports or small studies, and the nature and prevalence of social behavior changes is not well established. In this group are progressive supranuclear palsy (PSP), corticobasal degeneration (CBD), dementia with Lewy bodies (DLB), and progressive nonfluent aphasia (PNFA). Progressive supranuclear palsy is characterized by significant damage to brainstem and subcortical structures (Boxer et al., 2006). Clinically, in addition to atypical parkinsonism, PSP patients have significant cognitive deficits consistent with a frontal-subcortical disconnection syndrome (Litvan, 2002) and may also present with a frontal behavior syndrome that includes loss of insight (O'Keefe et al., 2007) and social disengagement (Litvan, Mega, Cummings, & Fairbanks, 1996). Corticobasal degeneration has many neuropathological similarities to both FTLD and PSP, and it presents with a variety of clinical syndromes affecting frontal and parietal cortex and white matter (Boxer et al., 2006). The aphasic subgroup is more likely to develop severely self-critical behaviors and depression as a result of the disease (Litvan, Cummings, & Mega, 1998), and a subset of CBD patients present with such substantial changes to personality, social behavior, and insight that they are clinically very similar to bvFTD patients (Kertesz, Martinez-Lage, Davidson, & Munoz, 2000; Mathuranath, Xuereb, Bak, & Hodges, 2000). Few formal studies of social behavior in DLB have been performed; however, clinical accounts suggest that some DLB patients experience increased anger and irritability, odd behavior, and other personality changes (McKeith et al., 2005). Similarly, PNFA patients' behavior is rarely studied, partly due to the difficulty of finding enough true PNFA patients (Gorno-Tempini et al., 2004), but also because anecdotal clinical evidence suggests that these patients have preserved social and emotional functioning (Mesulam, 2007).

2. Social Self-Knowledge in Neurodegenerative Disease

When patients with neurodegenerative disease show any alteration in their ability to recognize their level of functioning, it is typically labeled "loss of insight"; however, the affected domain of insight varies widely within and between diseases (Evers, Kilander, & Lindau, 2007), and the literature has unfortunately remained fairly imprecise on this topic.

Hundreds of studies have been performed to characterize loss of insight in AD (see Kaszniak and Edmonds, Chapter 11, this volume); however, these have nearly uniformly focused on awareness of disease and cognitive and functional deficits, rather than insight into alterations of personality and social behavior. A study by Onor, Trevisol, Negro, and Aguglia (2006) investigated behavioral self-monitoring in AD and mild cognitive impairment (MCI) patients by performing semistructured interviews with subjects and their caregiver-informants asking about behavioral symptoms such as hallucinations, unusual verbal and physical behavior, agitation, irritability, mood, emotion perception, and emotional expression. They found that both MCI and AD subjects underestimated their behavioral symptoms, and overestimated their ability to perceive their caregivers' emotions. Salmon and colleagues (2008) also found that AD subjects underestimated their degree of behavior disturbances, as did a more recent study by Banks and Weintraub (2008), though the specific manner in which they asked subjects to describe their behavior was unspecified, so it is not clear exactly what element of their behavior the patients were rating.

In a study performed by our lab (Rankin, Baldwin, Pace-Savitsky, Kramer, & Miller, 2005), AD patients were asked to describe their current personality using a questionnaire yielding information about eight personality traits such as extraversion, warmth, dominance, and arrogance. For six of the eight personality facets, AD patients' self-estimates (controlling for actual personality change) were no more discrepant from their informants' estimates than were those of healthy older control subjects. However, AD patients significantly underestimated the degree to which they behaved in a submissive, unassertive manner, and overestimated their level of extraversion, compared to informant reports. Importantly, the AD group's self-estimates in these discrepant domains were very similar to their caregivers' retrospective descriptions of how the patients' personality had appeared before the onset of neurodegenerative disease. This supports the hypothesis that in AD, inaccurate self-knowledge of personality may derive from a failure of online self-monitoring of recent personality change, resulting in a static self-concept that no longer matches reality as it is observed by others.

Loss of insight into behavioral and personality changes has been much more widely examined in bvFTD. It is an early hallmark of the disease and is even a part of the prevailing diagnostic criteria (Neary et al., 1998). There is some clinical overlap between the diagnoses of bvFTD and SemD (Liu et al., 2004) due to the fact that some patients from both categories have right temporal damage and the concomitant clinical symptoms. Thus, the literature on loss of insight in bvFTD sometimes explicitly examines SemD patients, and at other times it is relevant to this right temporal subset of SemD patients even when the group is not explicitly studied.

The data on the prevalence of loss of insight in bvFTD varies due to the different assessment methods and constructs measured. However, in an early study operationalizing insight in a manner consistent with the Neary consensus criteria, this was found to be one of the earliest and most highly prevalent symptoms of bvFTD, appearing in 59% of patients at presentation and 100% of patients at 2-year follow-up (Mendez & Perryman, 2002). In fact, this was the only core symptom (other than insidious onset and gradual progression) that was present in 100% of bvFTD patients after 2 years. In the same year, Diehl and Kurz (2002) examined neuropsychiatric symptoms in 30 bvFTD patients and found that loss of insight was the most prevalent symptom, occurring in 90% of their sample.

Loss of insight in bvFTD has been measured in a variety of different ways, but there is substantial evidence that the majority of bvFTD patients explicitly deny that their social behaviors are problematic and describe themselves in very positive terms, even when this is directly at odds with how others describe them (O'Keefe et al., 2007; Ruby et al., 2007). Eslinger and colleagues (2005) asked bvFTD, SemD, PNFA, and AD patients to rate themselves in the areas of cognition, behavior, emotion and empathy using three questionnaire rating scales. Patients with bvFTD substantially overrated their self-monitoring and empathic perspective-taking, along with cognitive abilities, while SemD patients overrated their self-monitoring, empathic concern, and empathic perspective-taking. Patients with AD overrated their memory but none of their social and personality behaviors, and PNFA patients were not significantly inaccurate on any self-assessments. All of the groups, however, underrated their level of apathy compared to ratings of control subjects. In our study specifically examining self-awareness of personality and personality change (Rankin et al., 2005), bvFTD patients showed a greater magnitude of inaccuracy in more domains of personality than AD patients. Also, they demonstrated significantly worse self-knowledge in the aspects of personality that had changed the most since the onset of their disease (i.e., coldness, introversion, and submissiveness).

In an alternative perspective on the issue of inaccurate self-knowledge in bvFTD, Miller et al. (2001) described a subset of bvFTD patients for whom a central symptom was a profound alteration of fundamental aspects of self (e.g., changing one's political, social, and religious affiliations and values). Patients were aware of these novel personalities and some could articulate their new beliefs and describe their behavioral routines, suggesting perhaps that online self-monitoring was not their primary deficit. All but one of these patients demonstrated disproportionate hypometabolism in the nondominant frontal lobe. The authors suggest that the disease may have caused the longitudinal self-concept to essentially disintegrate, allowing alternatives to gain ascendance. In support of this idea, there is evidence that unlike AD and SemD patients, who show a temporal gradient to their autobiographical memories, bvFTD patients show a uniform impairment of autobiographical memory across all epochs of their lives (Piolino et al., 2003). It is possible that at least some bvFTD patients not only lose the ability to derive information about themselves from online self-monitoring, but also lose track of who they were before the onset of their disease, in contrast to AD patients, who seem to return to their initially strong premorbid self-concept when self-monitoring of current behavior breaks down.

Qualitatively, some have suggested that what is often called loss of insight in bvFTD may actually be lack of distress over inappropriate behavior ("anosodia-phoria," or lack of concern), rather than a lack of awareness of these new symptoms. Mendez and Shapira (2005) provide the following observations of patient behavior to support this theory:

> One patient stated, "I am shallow now … this bothers other people but not me." Another patient would go into stores and restaurants and leave without paying for goods and services. She could describe these episodes and the potential consequences, but she was not distressed or concerned about her behavior. Several other patients conveyed the same lack of concern for doing the right thing despite knowing the difference.

However, this same study found that across their patient sample there was a mixed presentation of positron emission tomography (PET) hypometabolism across frontal and temporal lobes, as well as right and left hemispheres. Also, the study did not examine whether patients with this anosodiaphoria differed anatomically from subjects with true loss of self-knowledge. More recently, Evers and colleagues (2007) attempted to better operationalize loss of insight in a group of eight bvFTD patients, some of whom demonstrated predomi-nantly temporal atrophy and substantial naming deficits and may have over-lapped diagnostically with SemD. When the authors used unstructured, conversational interviews to examine patients' insight into their cognition, personality, functional status, and disease status, three of these patients had preserved insight. However, two of these three had temporal > frontal hypo-metabolism on a PET scan. While some anatomic studies have correlated loss of insight with frontal damage (Harwood et al., 2005; McMurtray et al., 2006; Mendez & Shapira, 2005), others have found it to correlate with either left or right temporal damage (Ruby et al., 2007; Thompson, Patterson, & Hodges, 2003). These qualitative differences in degree and quality of insight across bvFTD patients suggest that additional clarification is needed, most likely through combining a more fine-grained approach to measuring insight with more careful characterization of anatomic-behavioral correlates using both bvFTD and SemD patients.

Thus far, only one quantitative study of insight in CBD and PSP patients has been published, and it found that though their self-awareness of personality change was not as dramatically impaired as that of a comparison group of bvFTD patients, CBD and PSP patients did demonstrate poor insight into their behavioral characteristics (O'Keefe et al., 2007). One other study directly com-pared accuracy of self-knowledge in VascD patients against that of bvFTD patients and found that though the deficits in the VascD group were less severe, they did worsen over the course of the disease (Moretti et al., 2005). Unfortunately, no studies have yet been performed to address accuracy of social self-knowledge in DLB.

3. Social Self-Monitoring in Neurodegenerative Disease

If self-knowledge is derived from all of the different sources described in the first section of this chapter (e.g., interoception, exteroception, semantic self-knowledge, implicit and explicit social feedback), this suggests that different types of self-monitoring may be required to derive each particular type of self-knowledge. Thus, focal neurodegenerative conditions would be expected to have a differential impact on social self-monitoring depending on the affected anatomic circuits, resulting in the failure to update self-knowledge in divergent domains. However, careful examination of the process by which patients with neurodegenerative disease lose their ability to self-monitor their social persona is almost entirely missing from the current clinical literature, which thus far has been primarily limited to studying patients' loss of self-knowledge. In one relevant study, Banks and Weintraub (2008) asked AD, FTD, and PNFA patients to rate their "behavior" (though the authors never specify what questions were asked) before, and then after filling out the Frontal Behavioral Inventory (FBI) questionnaire describing themselves. Patients' self-ratings after being primed to think about themselves by completing the FBI did not differ significantly from their pre-FBI estimates, suggesting their self-knowledge of behavior did not change. More significantly, all three patient groups' post-evaluation self-ratings of behavior (i.e., their "self-monitoring") was more inaccurate for behavior than for eyesight or naming ability.

The near absence of examination of self-monitoring in neurodegenerative disease is particularly problematic, because loss of social self-monitoring can provide a fascinating window into the sources of behavioral self-regulation in a way that loss of cognitive self-monitoring cannot. When an AD patient demonstrates poor awareness of his or her memory deficits, it is logical to assume that the particular patterns of neural damage leading to the loss of insight are either separate from, or at least partly a result of, the memory loss. However, when an FTD patient demonstrates poor awareness of his or her behavior deficits, we cannot assume that the loss of insight and the social behavior changes are separate processes, or that the loss of insight is merely another symptom of the neural breakdown responsible for his or her inappropriate social behavior. In fact, theoretical models of social behavior suggest that self-monitoring may actually be required for normal social self-control (Eslinger et al., 2005; Miller et al., 2001). This implies that loss of insight may actually temporally precede and even play a causal role in patients' development of social dysdecorum.

Novel Studies of Social Self-Monitoring in Neurodegenerative Disease

Because of this substantial gap in the literature, we performed some experiments using different approaches to directly assess self-monitoring in neurodegenerative disease patients. Experiment 1 was a pilot study to determine whether the established method of assessing self-monitoring via post-test performance ratings could also effectively be applied to tests measuring social sensitivity. In Experiment 2, we obtained informant ratings of patients' social self-monitoring, and examined not only the differences across dementia groups but also investigated whether a causal relationship between disinhibited social behavior and loss of social insight could be inferred based on the timing of symptom onset.

Experiment 1

For this experiment, we piloted the use of the standard pre- and post-test self-rating paradigm, not with standard neuropsychological tests or behavior questionnaires, but with direct tests of social and emotional sensitivity. The goal was to elicit divergent patterns of self-ratings over time in different subject groups based on the accuracy and flexibility of their social self-concept when provided an opportunity for online monitoring of test performance.

Methods

Testing was performed on 39 subjects who included 11 bvFTDs, 3 SemDs (Neary et al., 1998), 9 AD patients (McKhann et al., 1984), 7 CBDs (diagnosed according to the criteria described in Boxer et al., 2006), 3 PSPs (Litvan et al., 2003), and 6 healthy older control subjects (NC) who had a normal neurologic exam and cognitive testing. Subjects were 20 men and 19 women, with an average age of 61.8 years (SD = 8.0), and an average education level of 15.5 years (SD = 3.0). No significant between-group differences were found for sex, age, or education.

At the beginning of the testing session, subjects were oriented to a graphic depicting a group of people organized across a normal curve and were taught how to point to the graphic to indicate where they believe they would rank on a skill in relation to "other people." The subjects' self-rankings were converted into percentile scores for analysis. They were asked to rank their ability on three occasions for each of the two tests: a pre-test rating (PRE) to estimate the accuracy of their predictive self-knowledge, a post-test rating (POST) to determine the degree to which they exhibited online self-monitoring of their performance, and a third rating at the very end of the test session (END) to determine if any new self-knowledge gained by observing their own performance on the tests was maintained after a delay interval. For each assessment, subjects were asked to rank their ability to *(1)* recognize what emotion someone was feeling by watching a video of that person, and *(2)* recognize when someone was speaking sarcastically.

The tests of social and emotional perception were from The Awareness of Social Inference Test (TASIT; McDonald, Flanagan, Rollins, & Kinch, 2003). For the Emotion Evaluation Test (EET) subtest, subjects watched brief (~20-second) videos of actors performing semantically neutral scripts portraying one of the seven basic emotions (happy, surprised, neutral, sad, anxious, frightened, revolted) and were asked to choose the correct emotion from a card on which the seven options are written. To reduce the effects of fatigue on our elderly, demented subjects, we administered only items 1–14, for a maximum score of 14. Subjects also performed the Social Inference-Minimal (SI-M) subtest, for which they watched ~30- to 45-second videos of actors expressing themselves in either a sincere or a sarcastic manner, again with semantically neutral, interchangeable scripts (e.g., "I'd be happy to do it. I've got plenty of time.") and were asked to answer four yes-no questions about the emotions and intent of the characters. The total score for this test was the sum of correct responses to questions about the two kinds of sarcastic items. Subjects' actual performance on these tests (ACTUAL) was standardized into percentile scores based on the performance of 22 healthy older controls who did not participate in this self-rating experiment.

Results

Subjects' results were analyzed using a mixed regression model (SAS: PROC MIXED), controlling for sex and age, to derive within-group and between-group comparisons across time. Values for PRE, ACTUAL, POST, and END percentile ranks across the six subject groups can be found in Table 14.1 and Figure 14.1.

Evidence from studies employing self-ratings of cognitive performance have shown that even normal subjects give widely variable, and often inaccurate, predictive ratings of how they will perform on a test, ostensibly because they do not have a clear idea of the task itself (Eslinger et al., 2005). Thus, we expected predictive ratings to differ from actual performance in all subject groups, including controls. For the emotion evaluation task, PRE ratings were significantly higher than ACTUAL scores in AD, CBD, bvFTD, NC, and SemD groups, but not in the PSP group. For the sarcasm detection task, PRE ratings were significantly higher than ACTUAL scores in the CBD, bvFTD, and SemD groups, but the predictions of the AD, NC, and PSP groups were not significantly higher than their actual scores. The PSP group's average prediction exactly matched their actual performance, both at the 49th percentile.

We hypothesized that after performing the emotion recognition and sarcasm recognition tasks, subjects with intact self-monitoring (e.g., NC subjects) would be able to give a more accurate estimate of their abilities in which their

Table 14.1 Differences across Subject Groups in Self-Ratings of Performance on Tests of Emotional and Social Sensitivity

Percentile (SD)	TASIT: Emotion Evaluation Test				TASIT: Sarcasm Task (SI-M)			
	Prediction	Postdiction	End of Session	Actual Score	Prediction	Postdiction	End of Session	Actual Score
NC (n = 6)	67.2 (17.6)	72.5 (12.9)	75.8 (13.9)	29.3 (39.1)	61.8 (11.2)	65.8 (17.4)	72.8 (13.0)	47.3 (30.0)
bvFTD (n = 11)	64.1 (23.1)	62.3 (19.0)	61.8 (20.4)	12.3 (17.7)	55.3 (18.2)	60.1 (21.2)	60.2 (19.1)	17.9 (23.4)
SemD (n = 3)	60.0 (17.3)	66.7 (28.9)	45.3 (37.2)	1.3 (0.6)	65.0 (21.2)	44.7 (38.3)	65.0 (21.2)	6.3 (9.2)
AD (n = 9)	57.8 (23.1)	59.8 (13.6)	63.6 (17.3)	15.3 (21.1)	53.1 (21.0)	60.1 (17.9)	59.3 (12.9)	34.4 (25.3)
CBD/PNFA (n = 7)	65.1 (16.7)	67.8 (18.0)	72.5 (19.4)	22.7 (29.7)	63.6 (24.4)	63.0 (26.3)	78.7 (11.8)	36.4 (23.0)
PSP (n = 3)	55.7 (12.4)	54.7 (7.4)	70.0 (18.0)	43.3 (32.3)	48.7 (4.0)	58.0 (10.8)	60.3 (12.7)	49.3 (14.7)

AD, Alzheimer's disease; bvFTD, behavioral variant of frontotemporal dementia; CBD/PNFA, corticobasal degeneration/progressive nonfluent aphasia; NC, normal control subjects; PSP, progressive supranuclear palsy; SemD, semantic dementia.

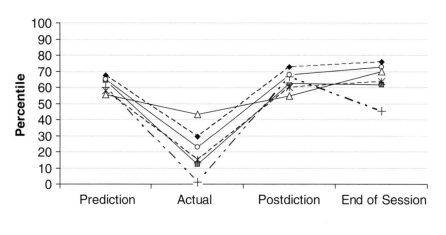

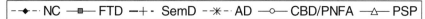

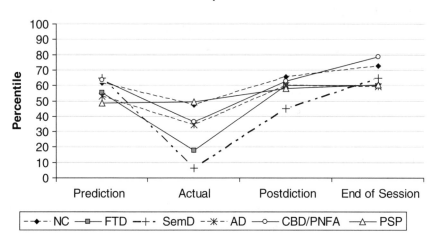

Figure 14.1 Graph of self-rating performance across diagnostic groups. AD, Alzheimer's disease; CBD/PNFA, corticobasal degeneration/progressive nonfluent aphasia; FTD, frontotemporal dementia; NC, normal control subjects; PSP, progressive supranuclear palsy; SemD, semantic dementia; TASIT, the awareness of social inference test (Mac Donald, 2003).

POST rating would be closer to their actual score (ACTUAL) than their PRE rating. Conversely, subjects with self-monitoring deficits (e.g., bvFTD patients) would not have adjusted their self-ratings to be closer to their actual performance, and instead would provide a POST rating very similar to their PRE rating. For the emotion evaluation task, however, no group showed any change from the PRE estimate to the POST estimate, and every group but the PSP subjects showed significantly higher POST estimates compared to their ACTUAL scores. On the sarcasm detection task, the same pattern was seen, with no significant differences between the PRE and POST estimates in any group, including controls.

We also hypothesized that for some subject groups with otherwise intact behavioral self-monitoring, some subjects would forget their actual performance by the end of the evaluation period (e.g., AD patients), in which case their END ratings would be more similar to their PRE ratings than their ACTUAL or POST ratings. Conversely, subjects capable of maintaining and incorporating the new information about their performance into their self-concept (e.g., NC subjects) would provide END ratings that were closer to their POST ratings than their PRE ratings, demonstrating that they had adjusted their self-knowledge to be more accurate based on their experience performing the tests. Contrary to our expectations, no group revised their self-estimate as of their POST assessment; thus, differences between POST and END ratings were not a meaningful way to see whether any revision of self-estimate was maintained over time. On the emotion evaluation task, no subject group showed significant differences between their POST and END ratings, with the exception of the SemD group, who rated themselves as significantly worse at END ratings than their POST ratings. No group showed a significant difference between POST and END ratings of their performance on the sarcasm detection task.

Experiment 1 Summary

We expected to see divergent patterns across groups of neurodegenerative disease patients as they rated their performances before and after a series of social and emotional awareness tasks. However, with the exception of a very small group of PSP patients ($n = 3$) on which few generalizations can be based, all subject groups including healthy older controls overestimated their ability to judge emotions and detect sarcasm, both before performing the corresponding tasks and immediately afterward. These data suggest that none of the groups demonstrated online self-monitoring of their ability to read social signals in response to these social sensitivity tasks, and all groups maintained an inaccurately inflated self-concept of their abilities despite implicit evidence to the contrary.

Experiment 2

Our attempt to obtain direct evidence of self-monitoring of social skills in a face-to-face testing paradigm was largely unsuccessful. However, we also attempted to obtain information on social self-monitoring in a somewhat more ecologically valid manner, by directly asking subjects and a first-degree relative informant about how well the subject recognized and used social feedback from others to alter their behavior.

Methods

For this study, a much larger group of subjects was enrolled (total $n = 155$: 35 bvFTD, 23 SemD, 42 AD, 14 CBD, 12 PSP, 9 primary progressive nonfluent aphasia [PNFA; Neary et al., 1998], and 20 NC subjects). Subjects included 78 males and 77 females (mean age 62.7 ± 7.8; mean education 16.2 ± 2.7). Among the nonnormal subjects, mean MMSE $= 22.9 \pm 6.1$, mean CDR $= 0.9 \pm 0.5$ (i.e., mild dementia).

Social self-monitoring behavior was assessed with the Revised Self-Monitoring Scale (RSMS; Lennox & Wolfe, 1984), a 13-item questionnaire that is a revision of the original Snyder Self-Monitoring Scale (Snyder, 1974). The first subscale, "Sensitivity to the expressive behavior of others," (RSMS-EX) is designed to assess awareness of subtle emotional and social cues specifically concerning one's own behavior (e.g., "I can usually tell I've said something inappropriate by reading it in the listener's eyes."). The second subscale, "Ability to modify self-presentation" (RSMS-SP), measures the ability to respond to social context and interpersonal signals and modify one's behavior to be more appropriate to the particular needs of the situation.

Spouses, relatives, or close friends were asked to fill out the RSMS questionnaire describing the subject's current characteristics. An informant report on the subject was considered to be a valid estimate of their daily social self-monitoring, because behaviors described by the RSMS all are observable, not only by the subject, but also by people who frequently interact with them. Though we expected some subjects groups to give divergent accounts of their self-monitoring on the RSMS compared to their informants, we still obtained RSMS self-reports from a subset of 123 subjects (NC $= 20$; bvFTD $= 30$; SemD $= 14$; PNFA $= 8$; AD $= 30$; CBD $= 10$; PSP $= 11$). This subset was biased toward inclusion of patients with fewer cognitive and language deficits who retained the capacity to fill out the questionnaires themselves, while informants were able to report on subjects with more severe cognitive deficits.

Informants also provided a report on the subjects' real-life social behaviors via the Neuropsychiatric Inventory (NPI) structured interview. The NPI Disinhibition subscale total score is a composite of the frequency and severity of socially inappropriate behaviors such as saying crude or hurtful things, touching or speaking to strangers inappropriately, inappropriately disclosing personal information, and acting or speaking impulsively.

Results

Subjects' results were analyzed using a general linear model (SAS: PROC GLM), and sex, age, and MMSE were used as covariates in all analyses.

bvFTD and SemD subjects were rated on both RSMS-EX and RSMS-SP scores as significantly lower than NC subjects, and no other groups were seen by their informants as having poorer social self-monitoring (Table 14.2).

Table 14.2 Differences across Subject Groups in Demographics and Scores on the Revised Self-Monitoring Scale (RSMS; Lennox, 1984), including Self-Ratings and Informant Ratings

M (SD)	NC (n = 20)	bvFTD (n = 35)	SemD (n = 23)	PNFA (n = 9)	AD (n = 42)	CBD (n = 14)	PSP (n = 12)
Age	61.2	61.8	63.5	66.0	61.3	65.1	66.3
	(10.2)	(7.0)	(5.8)	(8.9)	(8.2)	(6.9)	(5.4)
Sex (M/F)	(10/10)	(27/8)	(12/11)	(1/8)	(22/20)	(2/12)	(4/8)
Education	17.7	16.5	16.2	15.6	16.0	14.3	15.9
	(2.1)	(2.2)	(2.6)	(3.4)	(3.1)	(1.7)	(3.0)
CDR	0.05	1.1	0.9	0.5	0.8	0.6	1.0
	(0.16)	(0.5)	(0.5)	(0.4)	(0.3)	(0.5)	(0.5)
RSMS-EX (Sensitivity to Expressive Feedback)							
Informant	25.2	14.0	15.7	26.1	23.8	21.9	22.0
	(4.7)	(5.8)*	(7.0)*	(3.9)	(6.0)	(7.6)	(8.4)
Subject	26.4	24.8	21.4	26.8	23.5	27.7	24.3
	(4.5)	(6.6)	(5.2)	(2.6)	(5.9)	(4.5)	(7.8)*
RSMS-SP (Ability to Modify Self-Presentation)							
Informant	27.8	19.5	20.6	28.0	26.4	24.4	24.4
	(2.9)	(4.3)*	(4.7)*	(3.7)	(3.7)	(5.2)	(6.2)
Subject	27.3	28.3	26.2	26.4	26.6	27.5	22.2
	(2.5)	(6.1)	(3.9)	(5.5)	(4.7)	(6.3)	(7.0)

* Differs from NC group at $p < .05$ (Dunnett-Hsu post-hoc test controlling for sex and MMSE).
AD, Alzheimer's disease; bvFTD, behavioral variant of frontotemporal dementia; CBD, corticobasal degeneration; CDR, clinical dementia rating; NC, normal control subjects: PNFA, progressive nonfluent aphasia; PSP, progressive supranuclear palsy; SemD, semantic dementia.

However, when self-reports were examined, no group rated themselves as significantly worse than controls at sensitivity to other's expressive feedback (RSMS-EX), though SemD subjects showed a nonsignificant trend ($p = .072$). However, PSP subjects rated themselves significantly lower than controls on their ability to modify their own self-presentation as a result of social feedback (RSMS-SP). When self-informant difference scores were analyzed, the only group whose self-reports were significantly different from that of their informants was the bvFTD group.

Based on current models of metacognition (Eslinger et al., 2005), we hypothesized that deficits in behavioral self-monitoring would causally precede deficits in behavioral self-control. We examined the temporal relationship between social self-monitoring and self-control in social situations by analyzing informant reports of the RSMS in relation to NPI Disinhibition scores. These analyses were conducted in two parts. First, regressions were performed, controlling for sex, mini-mental state exam (MMSE), and diagnostic group, to determine if RSMS could significantly predict NPI Disinhibition scores. Both RSMS-EX and

RSMS-SP showed unique ability to predict Disinhibition ($p < .0001$). The standardized regression coefficients for both models were of similar magnitude (RSMS-EX beta $= -0.28$; RSMS-SP beta $= -0.34$), in models accounting for 47% and 44% of Disinhibition variance, respectively. When RSMS-EX and RSMS-SP are included in the same model, only RSMS-EX demonstrated a unique ability to predict Disinhibition, and RSMS-SP dropped out of the model. However, RSMS-EX and RSMS-SP were significantly correlated, controlling for sex and MMSE, at $r = 0.78$, suggesting that they have substantial collinearity in a regression analysis, and their relative independent relationships to Disinhibition could not be clearly delineated.

Next, to investigate the temporal relationship between loss of social self-monitoring and loss of social self-control, we performed crosstabs to examine the frequency with which patients showed independent versus comorbid impairments on the RSMS and NPI Disinhibition scales. Continuous scores on these scales were converted to binary "yes-no" values based on whether subjects showed clinically abnormal scores relative to controls. RSMS raw scores for patients ($n = 128$) were standardized using data from the older normal controls. Subjects obtaining RSMS subscale scores falling below $z = -1.30$ (i.e. less than 9th percentile, or borderline impaired) were considered to have deficits in self-monitoring. Subjects with NPI-Disinhibition scores equal to or greater than 5 were considered to have clinically significant disinhibition.

Thirty-seven percent of patients were not impaired in either self-monitoring or behavior. Patients who demonstrated deficits in sensitivity to social feedback (impaired RSMS-EX) were about as likely to be disinhibited (NPI-Disinhibition "yes": 25% of subjects) as to not be disinhibited (NPI-Disinhibition = "no": 34% of subjects). However, only 4% of subjects demonstrated no feedback sensitivity deficits (no impairment on RSMS-EX) but were considered disinhibited (NPI-Disinhibition = "yes"). This suggests that while it is common for patients to have problems monitoring social feedback without concurrent deficits in social self-control, it is very rare for socially disinhibited subjects not to have self-monitoring deficits. This same pattern was true in the RSMS-SP data, where patients were about evenly distributed across the combinations of RSMS-SP and Disinhibition symptoms, but only 5% of patients who were socially disinhibited were seen as having normal sensitivity to social feedback. When the analysis was limited to bvFTD patients, only 3% of socially disinhibited patients had normal RSMS-EX scores, and 5% had normal RSMS-SP scores.

Experiment 2 Summary

This experiment demonstrated that (1) bvFTD and SemD subjects are poorer at social self-monitoring than healthy older controls and other dementia control groups, (2) bvFTD patients have an explicitly inflated concept of their own ability to monitor social feedback from others, and (3) when social self-monitoring data are analyzed alongside of data on loss of social control, very few patients who behave in a socially inappropriate manner do not also have diminished social self-monitoring, while the converse is not true.

Discussion and Conclusions

Social Self-Monitoring: Normally Deficient?

It was particularly striking that in the very small sample represented in Experiment 1, our healthy normal control subjects overestimated their abilities and were impervious to performance-based feedback, demonstrating a pattern of poor self-monitoring similar to that of patients. Though one other study has employed a similar self-rating of behavior paradigm to assess self-monitoring, they did not ask control subjects to perform this element of the protocol (Banks & Weintraub, 2008). One of the difficulties employing self-ratings of performance with cognitive, rather than social, tasks is that many of the cognitive tasks show ceiling effects in healthy normal patients; thus, their predicted abilities and actual abilities match, and no updating of self-concept is required, or observed. However, when compared to a larger group of well-characterized, healthy older control subjects, two-thirds of control subjects in this study failed the emotion naming task, though all but one of them performed in the average range on the sarcasm detection task. The diverse and even impaired performance observed in the control group would suggest that ceiling effects were not an issue here, and that a subset of the control subjects should have had ample implicit evidence that they were having difficulty with the task, and thus should have revised their self-rating between PRE and POST assessment. It is possible that deficits in social sensitivity cosegregate with deficits in self-monitoring of social skills, so the fact that our small sample of normal controls performed decidedly abnormally on the emotion evaluation task may have been causally related to their abnormally flat self-ratings on the self-monitoring task. It remains to be seen whether a different pattern would occur in a larger group of normal control subjects. However, these results serve to highlight the fact that it is typical for self-appraisals to be positively biased (Robins & Beer, 2001; Taylor & Brown, 1988). It also shows that self-monitoring of performance on social and emotional sensitivity tasks is difficult, perhaps more difficult than self-monitoring of performance on cognitive tasks, since NC subjects are substantially more accurate monitoring their cognition (Eslinger et al., 2005).

The results of Experiment 1 also suggest that procedural alterations to the study method might be necessary to provide useful data with regard to self-monitoring of social and emotional functioning. Consistent with many studies employing the pre- and post-test rating methods for assessment of cognitive deficits (Banks & Weintraub, 2008; Eslinger et al., 2005; O'Keefe et al., 2007) we did not provide subjects with explicit feedback describing their performance on these emotion naming and sarcasm detection tasks. The implicit feedback subjects derived from their performance on the task may not have been adequate to cause them to alter their self-concept, perhaps because they did not realize that they were providing incorrect responses. In the future, a paradigm in which subjects are given explicit feedback about their performance (e.g., "You got four of those wrong.") before they are asked for their post-test ratings might yield the evidence of social self-monitoring and revisions of self-assessments that this experiment did not.

Self-Monitoring, Self-Control, and Anatomy: Complex Interrelationships

Both experiments provided rudimentary but intriguing evidence that the patterns of social self-monitoring may significantly diverge across dementias, particularly in the form of at least partly preserved self-monitoring in SemD and perhaps even PSP. While SemD patients have some anterior cingulate and orbitofrontal damage, the disease neuroanatomy typically leaves the rest of the frontal lobes intact, making them an excellent control group for bvFTD and AD subjects who typically have more widespread frontal involvement and show more self-monitoring deficits (Banks & Weintraub, 2008). Though AD, bvFTD, and SemD patients can all have deficits in social signal detection (Lavenu & Pasquier, 2005; Rosen et al., 2004), this does not seem adequate to explain the different patterns and degrees of altered self-monitoring across the groups. Additional processes are likely at work, such as altered awareness of interoceptive information and autobiographical self-awareness in bvFTD, or memory loss for exteroceptive behavioral observations in AD. Research is needed that will carefully characterize each of these elements of clinical phenomenology with respect to disease and anatomy.

While it is impossible to use this kind of cross-sectional, observational data to definitively establish a temporal sequence of onset between the two symptoms of decreased social self-monitoring and decreased social self-control, the data from Experiment 2 do suggest that loss of social self-control seldom, if ever, occurs outside of the context of loss of self-monitoring. This temporal relationship has already been suggested by cross-sectional symptom prevalence studies that demonstrate that impaired insight affects more bvFTD patients at initial visit than any other symptom, and that it is impaired in 100% of subjects a few years into the disease, whereas other symptoms do not affect all patients (Diehl & Kurz, 2002; Mendez & Perryman, 2002). A causal relationship makes intuitive, logical sense and has previously been suggested by various researchers (Eslinger et al., 2005; Miller et al., 2001). However, currently even specialists in bvFTD approach behavior change and loss of insight as if they are symptoms that are equally likely to occur first, and which are perhaps due to a common pathogenesis, rather than having any discernable temporal or causal relationship.

Certainly, more carefully designed analysis of the relationship between insight and social behavior is warranted, including longitudinal studies, and studies using more precise measures that discriminate among symptoms of altered self-knowledge, loss of online social self-monitoring, anosodiaphoria, and anosognosia for personality and social behavior. Evidence is multiplying that different diseases involving distinct neurological circuits cause very different patterns of metacognition and social behavior, and more attention must be focused on the diversity of processes underlying the derivation of social self-knowledge.

References

Addis, D. R., & Tippett, L. J. (2004). Memory of myself: Autobiographical memory and identity in Alzheimer's disease. *Memory, 12,* 56–74.

Aharon-Peretz, J., Daskovski, E., Mashiach, T., Kliot, D., & Tomer, R. (2003). Progression of dementia associated with lacunar infarctions. *Dementia and Geriatric Cognitive Disorders, 16*(2), 71–77.

Allison, T., Puce, A., & McCarthy, G. (2000). Social perception from visual cues: Role of the STS region. *Trends in Cognitive Sciences, 4*(7), 267–278.

Banks, S., & Weintraub, S. (2008). Self-awareness and self-monitoring of cognitive and behavioral deficits in behavioral variant frontotemporal dementia, primary progressive aphasia and probable Alzheimer's disease. *Brain and Cognition, 67* (1), 58–68.

Bathgate, D., Snowden, J. S., Varma, A., Blackshaw, A., & Neary, D. (2001). Behaviour in frontotemporal dementia, Alzheimer's disease and vascular dementia. *Acta Neurologica Scandinavica, 103*(6), 367–378.

Boxer, A. L., Geschwind, M. D., Belfor, N., Gorno-Tempini, M. L., Schauer, G. F., Miller, B., et al. (2006). Patterns of brain atrophy differentiate corticobasal degeneration from progressive supranuclear palsy. *Archives of Neurology, 63,* 81–86 .

Bozeat, S., Gregory, C. A., Ralph, M. A., & Hodges, J. R. (2000). Which neuropsychiatric and behavioural features distinguish frontal and temporal variants of frontotemporal dementia from Alzheimer's disease? *Journal of Neurology, Neurosurgery, and Psychiatry, 69*(2), 178–186.

Chatterjee, A., Strauss, M., Smyth, K. A., & Whitehouse, P. J. (1992). Personality changes in Alzheimer's disease. *Archives of Neurology, 49,* 486–491.

Chen, J. C., Borson, S., & Scanlan, J. M. (2000). Stage-specific prevalence of behavioral symptoms in Alzheimer's disease in a multi-ethnic community sample. *American Journal of Geriatric Psychiatry, 8*(2), 123–133.

Craig, A. D. (2003). Interoception: The sense of the physiological condition of the body. *Current Opinion in Neurobiology, 13*(4), 500–505.

Critchley, H. D., Wiens, S., Rotshtein, P., Ohman, A., & Dolan, R. J. (2004). Neural systems supporting interoceptive awareness. *Nature Neuroscience, 7*(2), 189–195.

Cummings, J. L. (1997). The Neuropsychiatric Inventory: Assessing psychopathology in dementia patients. *Neurology, 48*(5 Suppl 6), S10–16.

Damasio, A. R. (1996). The somatic marker hypothesis and the possible functions of the prefrontal cortex. *Philosophical Transactions of the Royal Society of London. Series B: Biological Sciences, 351*(1346), 1413–1420.

Diehl, J., & Kurz, A. (2002). Frontotemporal dementia: Patient characteristics, cognition, and behaviour. *International Journal of Geriatric Psychiatry, 17*(10), 914–918.

Edwards-Lee, T., Miller, B. L., Benson, D. F., Cummings, J. L., Russell, G. L., Boone, K., et al. (1997). The temporal variant of frontotemporal dementia. *Brain, 120*(Pt 6), 1027–1040.

Eslinger, P. J., Dennis, K., Moore, P., Antani, S., Hauck, R., & Grossman, M. (2005). Metacognitive deficits in frontotemporal dementia. *Journal of Neurology, Neurosurgery and Psychiatry, 76*(12), 1630–1635.

Eustache, F., Piolino, P., Giffard, B., Viader, F., De La Sayette, V., Baron, J. C., et al. (2004). 'In the course of time': A PET study of the cerebral substrates of autobiographical amnesia in Alzheimer's disease. *Brain, 127*(Pt 7), 1549–1560.

Evers, K., Kilander, L., & Lindau, M. (2007). Insight in frontotemporal dementia: Conceptual analysis and empirical evaluation of the consensus criterion "loss of insight" in frontotemporal dementia. *Brain and Cognition, 63*(1), 13–23.

Farrer, C., Franck, N., Georgieff, N., Frith, C. D., Decety, J., & Jeannerod, M. (2003). Modulating the experience of agency: A positron emission tomography study. *NeuroImage, 18*(2), 324–333.

Festinger, L. (1954). A theory of social comparison processes. *Human Relations, 7*, 117–140.

Gardner, J. L., & Lisberger, S. G. (2002). Serial linkage of target selection for orienting and tracking eye movements. *Nature Neuroscience, 5*(9), 892–899.

Gorno-Tempini, M. L., Dronkers, N. F., Rankin, K. P., Ogar, J. M., Phengrasamy, L., Rosen, H. J., et al. (2004). Cognition and anatomy in three variants of primary progressive aphasia. *Annals of Neurology, 55*, 335–346.

Greene, J. D., Nystrom, L. E., Engell, A. D., Darley, J. M., & Cohen, J. D. (2004). The neural bases of cognitive conflict and control in moral judgment. *Neuron, 44*(2), 389–400.

Gusnard, D. A., Akbudak, E., Shulman, G. L., & Raichle, M. E. (2001). Medial prefrontal cortex and self-referential mental activity: Relation to a default mode of brain function. *Proceedings of the National Academy of Sciences USA, 98*(7), 4259–4264.

Harwood, D. G., Sultzer, D. L., Feil, D., Monserratt, L., Freedman, E., & Mandelkern, M. A. (2005). Frontal lobe hypometabolism and impaired insight in Alzheimer disease. *American Journal of Geriatric Psychiatry, 13*(11), 934–941.

Hope, T., Keene, J., Gedling, K., Cooper, S., Fairburn, C., & Jacoby, R. (1997). Behavior changes in dementia 1: Point of entry data of a prospective study. *International Journal of Geriatric Psychiatry, 12*, 1062–1073.

Johnson, S. C., Baxter, L. C., Wilder, L. S., Pipe, J. G., Heiserman, J. E., & Prigatano, G. P. (2002). Neural correlates of self-reflection. *Brain, 125*(Pt 8), 1808–1814.

Kertesz, A., Martinez-Lage, P., Davidson, W., & Munoz, D. G. (2000). The corticobasal degeneration syndrome overlaps progressive aphasia and frontotemporal dementia. *Neurology, 55*(9), 1368–1375.

Lavenu, I., & Pasquier, F. (2005). Perception of emotion on faces in frontotemporal dementia and Alzheimer's disease: A longitudinal study. *Dementia and Geriatric Cognitive Disorders, 19*(1), 37–41.

Lennox, R., & Wolfe, R. (1984). Revision of the self-monitoring scale. *Journal of Personality and Social Psychology, 46,* 1349–1364.

Lieberman, M. D. (2007). Social cognitive neuroscience: A review of core processes. *Annual Review of Psychology, 58,* 259–289.

Lieberman, M. D., Eisenberger, N. I., Crockett, M. J., Tom, S. M., Pfeifer, J. H., & Way, B. M. (2007). Putting feelings into words: Affect labeling disrupts amygdala activity in response to affective stimuli. *Psychological Science, 18*(5), 421–428.

Lieberman, M. D., Jarcho, J. M., & Satpute, A. B. (2004). Evidence-based and intuition-based self-knowledge: An FMRI study. *Journal of Personality and Social Psychology, 87*(4), 421–435.

Litvan, I. (2002). Personality and behavioral changes with frontal-subcortical dysfunction. In D. G. Lichter & J. L. Cummings (Eds.), *Frontal-subcortical circuits in psychiatric and neurological disorders* (pp. 151–162). New York: The Guilford Press.

Litvan, I., Bhatia, K. P., Burn, D. J., Goetz, C. G., Lang, A. E., McKeith, I., et al. (2003). SIC task force appraisal of clinical diagnostic criteria for Parkinsonian disorders. *Movement Disorders, 18*(5), 467–486.

Litvan, I., Cummings, J. L., & Mega, M. (1998). Neuropsychiatric features of corticobasal degeneration. *Journal of Neurology, Neurosurgery, and Psychiatry, 65*(5), 717–721.

Litvan, I., Mega, M. S., Cummings, J. L., & Fairbanks, L. (1996). Neuropsychiatric aspects of progressive supranuclear palsy. *Neurology, 47*(5), 1184–1189.

Liu, W., Miller, B. L., Kramer, J. H., Rankin, K., Wyss-Coray, C., Gearhart, R., et al. (2004). Behavioral disorders in the frontal and temporal variants of frontotemporal dementia. *Neurology, 62*(5), 742–748.

Marques, J., Abrams, D., Paez, D., & Martinez-Taboada, C. (1998). The role of categorization and in-group norms in judgments of groups and their members. *Journal of Personality and Social Psychology, 75*(4), 976–988.

Mathuranath, P. S., Xuereb, J. H., Bak, T., & Hodges, J. R. (2000). Corticobasal ganglionic degeneration and/or frontotemporal dementia? A report of two overlap cases and review of literature. *Journal of Neurology, Neurosurgery, and Psychiatry, 68*(3), 304–312.

McDonald, S., Flanagan, S., Rollins, J., & Kinch, J. (2003). TASIT: A new clinical tool for assessing social perception after traumatic brain injury. *Journal of Head Trauma Rehabilitation, 18*(3), 219–238.

McKeith, I. G., Dickson, D. W., Lowe, D. M., Emre, M., O'Brien, J. T., Feldman, H., et al. (2005). Diagnosis and management of dementia with Lewy bodies: Third report of the DLB consortium. *Neurology, 65,* 1863–1872.

McKhann, G., Drachman, D., Folstein, M., Katzman, R., Price, D., & Stadlan, E. M. (1984). Clinical diagnosis of Alzheimer's disease: Report of the NINCDS-ADRDA Work Group under the auspices of Department of Health and Human Services Task Force on Alzheimer's Disease. *Neurology, 34*(7), 939–944.

McMurtray, A. M., Chen, A. K., Shapira, J. S., Chow, T. W., Mishkin, F., Miller, B. L., et al. (2006). Variations in regional SPECT hypoperfusion and clinical features in frontotemporal dementia. *Neurology, 66*(4), 517–522.

Mendez, M. F., & Perryman, K. M. (2002). Neuropsychiatric features of frontotemporal dementia: Evaluation of consensus criteria and review. *Journal of Neuropsychiatry and Clinical Neurosciences, 14*(4), 424–429.

Mendez, M. F., & Shapira, J. S. (2005). Loss of insight and functional neuroimaging in frontotemporal dementia. *Journal of Neuropsychiatry and Clinical Neurosciences Research, 17*(3), 413–416.

Mesulam, M. M. (2007). Primary progressive aphasia: A 25-year retrospective. *Alzheimer Disease and Associated Disorders, 21*(4), S8–S11.

Miller, B. L., Chang, L., Mena, I., Boone, K., & Lesser, I. M. (1993). Progressive right frontotemporal degeneration: Clinical, neuropsychological and SPECT characteristics. *Dementia, 4*(3–4), 204–213.

Miller, B. L., Cummings, J. L., Villanueva-Meyer, J., Boone, K., Mehringer, C. M., Lesser, I. M., et al. (1991). Frontal lobe degeneration: Clinical, neuropsychological, and SPECT characteristics. *Neurology, 41*(9), 1374–1382.

Miller, B. L., Seeley, W. W., Mychack, P., Rosen, H. J., Mena, I., & Boone, K. (2001). Neuroanatomy of the self: Evidence from patients with frontotemporal dementia. *Neurology, 57*(5), 817–821.

Miller, L. (2008). Stress and resilience in law enforcement training and practice. *International Journal of Emergency Mental Health, 10*(2), 109–124.

Moretti, R., Torre, P., Antonello, R. M., Cattaruzza, T., Cazzato, G., & Bava, A. (2005). Frontal lobe dementia and subcortical vascular dementia: A neuropsychological comparison. *Psychological Reports, 96*(1), 141–151.

Neary, D., Snowden, J. S., Gustafson, L., Passant, U., Stuss, D., Black, S., et al. (1998). Frontotemporal lobar degeneration: A consensus on clinical diagnostic criteria. *Neurology, 51*(6), 1546–1554.

Ochsner, K. N., Beer, J. S., Robertson, E. R., Cooper, J. C., Gabrieli, J. D., Kihsltrom, J. F., et al. (2005). The neural correlates of direct and reflected self-knowledge. *NeuroImage, 28*(4), 797–814.

Ochsner, K. N., Knierim, K., Ludlow, D. H., Hanelin, J., Ramachandran, T., Glover, G., et al. (2004). Reflecting upon feelings: An fMRI study of neural systems supporting the attribution of emotion to self and other. *Journal of Cognitive Neuroscience, 16* (10), 1746–1772.

O'Keefe, F. M., Murray, B., Coen, R. F., Dockree, P. M., Bellgrove, M. A., Garavan, H., et al. (2007). Loss of insight in frontotemporal dementia, corticobasal degeneration and progressive supranuclear palsy. *Brain, 130,* 753–764.

Olson, I. R., Plotzker, A., & Ezzyat, Y. (2007). The enigmatic temporal pole: A review of findings on social and emotional processing. *Brain, 130*(7), 1718–1731.

Onor, M. L., Trevisiol, M., Negro, C., & Aguglia, E. (2006). Different perception of cognitive impairment, behavioral disturbances, and functional disabilities between persons with mild cognitive impairment and mild Alzheimer's disease and their caregivers. *American Journal of Alzheimer's Disease and Other Dementias, 21*(5), 333–338.

Perry, R. J., Rosen, H. R., Kramer, J. H., Beer, J. S., Levenson, R. L., & Miller, B. L. (2001). Hemispheric dominance for emotions, empathy and social behaviour: evidence from right and left handers with frontotemporal dementia. *Neurocase, 7*(2), 145–160.

Pfeifer, J. H., Lieberman, M. D., & Dapretto, M. (2007). "I know you are but what am I?!": Neural bases of self- and social knowledge retrieval in children and adults. *Journal of Cognitive Neuroscience, 19*(8), 1323–1337.

Piolino, P., Desgranges, B., Belliard, S., Matuszewski, V., Lalevée, C., De la Sayette, V., et al. (2003). Autobiographical memory and autonoetic consciousness: Triple dissociation in neurodegenerative diseases. *Brain, 126*(Pt 10), 2203–2219.

Platek, S. M., Loughead, J. W., Gur, R. C., Busch, S., Ruparel, K., Phend, N., et al. (2006). Neural substrates for functionally discriminating self-face from personally familiar faces. *Human Brain Mapping, 27*(2), 91–98.

Prigatano, G. P. (2005). Impaired self-awareness after moderately severe to severe traumatic brain injury. *Acta Neurochirurgica Supplement, 93*, 39–42.

Rankin, K. P., Baldwin, E., Pace-Savitsky, C., Kramer, J. H., & Miller, B. L. (2005). Self-awareness and personality change in dementia. *Journal of Neurology, Neurosurgery, and Psychiatry, 75*(5), 632–639.

Rankin, K. P., Kramer, J. H., Mychack, P., & Miller, B. L. (2003). Double dissociation of social functioning in frontotemporal dementia. *Neurology, 60*(2), 266–271.

Rankin, K.P., Santos-Modesitt, W., Kramer, J.H., Pavlic, D., Beckman, V., & Miller, B.L. (2008). Spontaneous social behaviors discriminate behavioral dementias from psychiatric disorders and other dementias. *Journal of Clinical Psychiatry. 69*(1):60–73.

Robins, R. W., & Beer, J. S. (2001). Positive illusions about the self: Short-term benefits and long-term costs. *Journal of Personality and Social Psychology, 80*(2), 340–352.

Rosen, H. J., Gorno-Tempini, M. L., Goldman, W. P., Perry, R. J., Schuff, N., Weiner, M., et al. (2002). Patterns of brain atrophy in frontotemporal dementia and semantic dementia. *Neurology, 58*(2), 198–208.

Rosen, H. J., Pace-Savitsky, C., Perry, R. J., Kramer, J. H., Miller, B., & Levinson, R. W. (2004). Recognition of emotion in the frontal and temporal variants of frontotemporal dementia. *Dementia and Geriatric Cognitive Disorders, 17*(4), 277–281.

Ruby, P., & Decety, J. (2001). Effect of subjective perspective taking during simulation of action: A PET investigation of agency. *Nature Neuroscience, 4*(5), 546–550.

Ruby, P., Schmidt, C., Hogge, M., D'Argembeau, A., Collette, F., & Salmon, E. (2007). Social mind representation: Where does it fail in frontotemporal dementia? *Journal of Cognitive Neuroscience, 19*(4), 671–683.

Sachs-Ericsson, N., Verona, E., Joiner, T., & Preacher, K. J. (2006). Parental verbal abuse and the mediating role of self-criticism in adult internalizing disorders. *Journal of Affective Disorders, 93*(1–3), 71–78.

Salmon, E., Perani, D., Collette, F., Feyers, D., Kalbe, E., Holthoff, V., et al. (2008). A comparison of unawareness in frontotemporal dementia and Alzheimer's disease. *Journal of Neurology, Neurosurgery, and Psychiatry, 79*(2), 176–179.

Seeley, W. W., & Sturm, V. E. (2006). Self-representation and the frontal lobes. In B. L. Miller & J. L. Cummings (Eds.), *The human frontal lobes* (2nd edition, Vol. 1, pp. 317–334). New York: Guilford Press.

Siegler, I. C., Dawson, D. V., & Welsh, K. A. (1994). Caregiver ratings of personality change in Alzheimer's disease patients: A replication. *Psychology and Aging, 9*(3), 464–466.

Siegler, I. C., Welsh, K. A., Dawson, D. V., Fillenbaum, G. G., Earl, N. L., Kaplan, E. B., et al. (1991). Ratings of personality change in patients being evaluated for memory disorders. *Alzheimer's Disease and Associated Disorders, 5*, 240–250.

Snyder, M. (1974). Self-monitoring of expressive behavior. *Journal of Personality and Social Psychology, 30*, 526–537.

Strauss, M. E., Pasupathi, M., & Chatterjee, A. (1993). Concordance between observers in descriptions of personality change in Alzheimer's disease. *Psychology and Aging*, *8*(4), 475–480.

Tajfel, H. (1982). Social psychology of intergroup relations. In *Annual review of psychology* (Vol. 33, pp. 1–39). Annual Reviews Inc.

Taylor, S. E., & Brown, J. D. (1988). Illusion and well-being: A social psychological perspective on mental health. *Psychological Bulletin, 103*(2), 193–210.

Thompson, S. A., Patterson, K., & Hodges, J. R. (2003). Left/right asymmetry of atrophy in semantic dementia: Behavioral-cognitive implications. *Neurology, 61*(9), 1196–1203.

Uziel, L. (2007). Individual differences in the social facilitation effect: A review and meta-analysis. *Journal of Research in Personality, 41*(2007), 579–601.

Wakslak, C. J., Nussbaum, S., Liberman, N., & Trope, Y. (2008). Representations of the self in the near and distant future. *Journal of Personality and Social Psychology, 95*(4), 757–773.

Welleford, E. A., Harkins, S. W., & Taylor, J. R. (1994). Personality change in dementia of the Alzheimer's type: Relations to caregiver personality and burden. *Experimental Aging Research, 21*, 295–314.

15

Anosognosia and Error Processing in Various Clinical Disorders

Ian H. Robertson

Do I tend to talk too loudly? Would people consider me brash and insensitive? Am I fat? Am I clever? Am I forgetful? Would others consider me bad tempered? Am I nervous?

Much of modern psychology is based on asking individuals to self-evaluate in response to questions such as these, and the results obtained by such self-ratings are often replicable and predictive of real-life behavior tendencies (Manly, Robertson, Galloway, & Hawkins, 1999), as well as differential brain function (Fischer, Wik, & Fredrikson, 1997; Haas, Constable, & Canli, 2008). How, in the *mêlée* of everyday life, do we manage to observe ourselves sufficiently consistently as to come up with fairly reliable and at least partially valid quantitative and comparative ratings of our behaviors in a bewildering number of dimensions? One prerequisite for this must be adequate attention to key episodes and features of everyday behavior and the second some kind of memorial "running average" of these in the form of summary self-evaluations across a range of dimensions.

While there must be some degree of accuracy in self-evaluations in order to produce the replicable relationships that we observe, it is clear that the above attention-memory model cannot be the whole story. Under a number of circumstances, individuals can be inaccurate in their self-evaluations—for instance, underestimation of personal competence in depression (Voelz, Walker, Pettit, Joiner Jr., & Wagner, 2003), overestimation in mania (Leahy, 2005), overestimation of "fatness" in anorexia nervosa (Sachdev, Mondraty, Wen, & Gulliford, 2008), and underestimation of driving competence under the influence of alcohol (Barkley, Murphy, O'Connell, Anderson, & Connor, 2006).

Self-evaluation can be inaccurate, and following damage to the brain, this inaccuracy can extend to the extremes of anosognosia across virtually all the syndromes of disordered brain function outlined in the other chapters of this book. What is clear from these chapters is the many different ways in which awareness of a disability can break down, and the many different cognitive and brain processes that can contribute to the anosognosia. While recognizing the range and complexity of the ways in which self-awareness can break down, the purpose of this chapter is to review evidence for a central role of certain attentional and error-processing mechanisms that may be a common underpinning of many different types of disorders of self-evaluation.

Offline Self-Referential Thought versus Online Self-Evaluation

When people are asked to make judgments pertaining to their internal, emotional, or "self" states, medial prefrontal cortex activations (Johnson et al., 2002), and in particular dorsal medial prefrontal activations (Gusnard, Akbudak, Shulman, & Raichle, 2001) are commonly found. During attentionally demanding tasks requiring an external focus, these regions are typically inhibited and dorsolateral prefrontal areas show activations (Manly et al., 2003).

Such an "internal" focus—reflecting on the qualities of self and its attributes—may be conceptually separate from the processes involved in evaluating one's performance in various behavioral dimensions in the course of everyday life. The "offline" judgment as to whether I am, for example, a habitually careless person may depend on quite different cognitive processes from the "online" assessment, in the course of attentionally demanding activities, as to whether in this instance I have been careless. Is there any evidence to support such an assertion?

One major source of information about our moment-to-moment performance that contributes to self-evaluation is *error*. It is when we realize that we have closed the door with the key inside that we recognize our carelessness. The most careless among us may not realize the error until we arrive back home late at night and cannot get into our house. This is an everyday example of what could be referred to as a problem with vigilant attention.

My colleagues Hester and Garavan have shown that awareness of error is associated with dorsolateral prefrontal cortex functioning (Hester, Foxe, Molholm, Shpaner, & Garavan, 2005), supporting the view that online evaluation of personal performance draws on different dorsolateral cortical systems than offline self-referential thought. In this chapter, I will expand on this hypothesis, proposing that accurate self-evaluation depends on adequate levels of vigilant attention, and that intact error-processing mechanisms are a key contributor to this attention and, by implication, to self-evaluation.

Vigilant Attention

Vigilant attention is defined as "the capacity to maintain aware responding to routine stimuli and responses while avoiding automaticity and in the absence of external challenge, difficulty, novelty or emotional salience which would otherwise exogenously drive attention to the stimuli in question" (Robertson & Garavan, 2004).

Vigilant attention is closely linked to one of Posner and Petersen's (1990) three hypothetical supramodal attentional control systems: the *alerting* system. According to Posner and Petersen (1990), this is a noradrenergically driven system, which increases the signal-to-noise ratio of target stimuli and thus enhances target detection, albeit at a slightly increased level of false-positives. The locus coeruleus, with its stronger right than left hemisphere innervation (Oke, Keller, Mefford, & Adams, 1978), shows activity which is highly correlated with behavioral performance where monkeys have to detect relatively rare visual targets among foils, but optimal performance is achieved not at maximum levels of locus coeruleus activity, but rather at intermediate levels (Usher, Cohen, Servan-Schreiber, Rajkowski, & Aston-Jones, 1999).

The negative effects of noradrengeric depletion on performance in humans can be ameliorated by task difficulty (Arnsten & Contant, 1992), external noise (Smith & Nutt, 1996), and general "challenge" (see Robertson & Garavan, 2004). Vigilant attention therefore represents an attentional capacity that is distinct from the attentional resource conventionally measured in demanding attentional switching or control tasks involving fast responding and working memory load. Furthermore, it is *not* defined by time on task effects as is often assumed, as the attention to targets in routine situations fluctuates over periods of tens of seconds (Johnson et al., 2007; Whitehead, 1991); the time on task effects originally reported by Mackworth (1968), which occur over periods of tens of minutes, may reflect decreases in the arousal component of the vigilant attention system (Johnson et al., 2007; Paus et al., 1997).

Elaborating from Posner and Petersen's (1990) original concept of the alerting system, the vigilant attention system has two main interacting components: a bottom-up arousal system based in the locus coeruleus, and a top-down attention system based largely in the right dorsolateral prefrontal cortex, with the involvement also of areas of the right parietal cortex. As Paus and his colleagues (1997) have shown, these two systems are involved in vigilant attention, and interact, but are separable (Paus et al., 1997). Declining arousal due to circadian, drug, or brain impairment can be compensated for by the attention system, while bottom-up modulation of the arousal system by drugs, external noise, or challenge can enhance the performance of the right frontoparietal attention system (Robertson & Garavan, 2004).

Until recently, there was very little evidence from human participants of a linkage between vigilant attention and noradrenergic functioning. Recently our laboratory has shown in healthy people with different dosages of the DBH gene—believed to influence availability of noradrenalin in the cortex—that vigilant attention performance is significantly poorer in people with two copies of the gene (Greene, Bellgrove, Gill, & Robertson, 2009).

The right frontoparietal system is a strong candidate for distinguishing aware versus nonaware responses; this has been shown in change blindness studies, where right frontoparietal activation distinguishes stimuli where the change is detected from those where it is not (Beck, Rees, Frith, & Lavie, 2001), and in error processing studies as being a key part of a network that distinguishes errors which are consciously recognized versus those that are not (Hester et al., 2005). The hypothesis advanced in the present chapter—that the vigilant attention system and related error processing have a privileged role in mediating disorders of awareness—is consistent with the many papers that show a prevalence of right frontal pathologies linked to disorders of insight in Alzheimer's disease (Harwood et al., 2005), post-stroke hemiplegia (Pia, Neppi-Modona, Ricci, & Berti, 2004), and schizophrenia (Shad, Muddasani, & Keshavan, 2006).

"Unskilled and Unaware of It": Insight in the Normal Population

An intriguingly titled paper "Unskilled and unaware of it: How difficulties in recognizing one's own incompetence lead to inflated self-assessments" by Kruger and Dunning (1999) is just one of a considerable literature showing that normal, non-brain-impaired populations show consider levels of inaccuracy—usually overestimation—of their levels of attainment and competence across a broad range of domains. Furthermore, those judged objectively to be least competent in a particular domain (for instance, sense of humor) are the least accurate in self-evaluating their level of competence, showing high levels of overestimation. A few other examples of this phenomenon will suffice here: one review (Davis et al., 2006) of self-rated versus objectively assessed competence among physicians throughout the world reported: "A number of studies found the worst accuracy in self-assessment among physicians who were the least skilled and those who were the most confident." In general there was a very poor relationship between self-rated competence and actual competence. The facts that most drivers consider themselves to be "above average" in driving abilities (McKenna, Stanier, & Lewis, 1991) and that 94% of university/college teachers consider their work to be "above average" (Cross, 1977) drive home a point that is more fully made elsewhere (Dunning, Heath, & Suls, 2004).

Kruger and Dunning's (1999) findings of an *inverse* relationship between competence and accuracy of self-evaluation is echoed in several other studies and the explanation proposed is that incompetence robs people of the metacognitive resources to simultaneously perform the task and monitor their own performance at it. The question for the present chapter is whether we can better define the "metacognitive resource" that may underpin such inaccurate self-assessments.

To help address this question, we gave 79 healthy people between the ages of 18 and 53 a battery of neuropsychological tests as well as two self-rating scales: the Frontal Systems Behavior Scale (Grace & Malloy, 2001) and the Cognitive Failures Questionnaire (Broadbent, Cooper, FitzGerald, & Parkes, 1982). Their self-ratings were compared with the ratings of a close relative or friend, and discrepancy scores were calculated. We hypothesized—for the reasons outlined above, namely that online monitoring of performance requires intact vigilant attention to performance—that people who underestimated their level of error and disorganized behavior in everyday life would show impairment on tests of vigilant attention. This is indeed what we found: people who underestimated the level of disorganization in their lives had significantly higher errors on a test of vigilant attention compared to accurate estimators or overestimators (Hoerold et al., 2008).

Vigilant attention capacity, as predicted, is correlated with accuracy of self-evaluation. Vigilant attention is also known to be strongly associated with activation of the right dorsolateral prefrontal cortex (Manly et al., 2003; Paus et al., 1997): is this region also associated with accuracy of self-evaluation? In the next section, I will consider evidence from traumatic brain injury (TBI) and localized lesion studies to address this and related questions.

Insight and the Right Dorsolateral Prefrontal Cortex in Neuropsychiatric and Neurological Disorders

As Prigatano (see Chapter 12, this volume) has pointed out, TBI can result in a disabling deficit in self-evaluation, which can be a major obstacle to rehabilitation. A proportion of people with TBI underestimate their own deficits in comparison to the ratings of relatives (O'Keeffe, Dockree, & Robertson, 2004), and because of this, TBI self ratings of everyday attentional failures do not correlate with actual attentional performance on assessment; in contrast however, actual performance does correlate with the ratings of attentional failures made by relatives. (Robertson, Manly, Andrade, Baddeley, & Yiend, 1997).

As mentioned earlier, adequate vigilant attention—hypothesized in this chapter to be a necessary (but not necessarily sufficient) prerequisite for accurate online self-evaluation—is strongly linked to right dorsolateral prefrontal cortex activation. Is there any evidence that such activation is in turn associated with accurate self-assessment? An fMRI study of TBI individuals showed that indeed there is. Accuracy of self-evaluation was significantly correlated with functional activation of the right dorsolateral prefrontal cortex (Schmitz, Rowley, Kawahara, & Johnson, 2006). A recent study from our laboratory comparing people with right versus left prefrontal cortex lesions with posterior lesions found that people with right prefrontal cortex lesions showed significantly lower levels of online awareness of error during a sustained attention task in which they were required to verbally report errors.

As a final example, the level of insight in schizophrenia has been shown to be significantly correlated with right dorsolateral prefrontal cortex volume (see Shad et al., 2006, their figure 4). The right dorsolateral prefrontal cortex is strongly linked to impaired self-evaluation across a range of disorders, and this can also be observed in the neurodegenerative conditions the tau-opathies, namely frontotemporal dementia (FTD), corticobasal degeneration (CBD), and progressive supranuclear palsy (PSP). In a study carried out by my doctoral student Fiadhnait O'Keeffe, it emerged that among these conditions it was in the one most strongly affecting the prefrontal cortex—FTD—that the greatest level of unawareness existed, consistent with the view that unawareness does have a specific relationship to prefrontal cortex functioning. O'Keeffe found that—at around 20%—error awareness among FTD patients was less than half that of CBD and PSP individuals (O'Keeffe, Murray et al., 2007).

Awareness and Arousal

The ultimate states of impaired awareness are sleep, intoxication, coma, and death. Sleep, the most benign of these processes, is the end point of a continuum of alertness via various states of drowsiness. Measures of vigilant attention such as the Sustained Attention to Response Task (Robertson et al., 1997) have proved to be the most sensitive measures of degrees of cognitive impairment related to daytime drowsiness (Fronczek, Middelkoop, Dijk, & Lammers, 2006) and, supporting the vigilant attention-arousal-awareness link proposed in this chapter, sleep-related declines in arousal reduce awareness of errors and events (Makeig & Jung, 1996; Tsai, Young, Hsieh, & Lee, 2005).

Unilateral spatial neglect can be considered a canonical disorder of aware-ness. Heilman, Schwartz, and Watson (1978) proposed over 30 years ago that hypoarousal was a key element of neglect—and hence of impaired awareness. A number of studies have shown that arousal is a critical variable associated with level of awareness of the neglected side of space, for instance, showing decreases in awareness with declining levels of arousal (Manly, Dobler, Dodds, & George, 2005). O'Connell et al. (2007) have also shown that electroencephalography arousal measures (theta-beta ratios) correlate 0.48 with error awareness levels across healthy participants.

Such correlational studies are supported by research showing a causal link between arousal and awareness. We have shown that unpredictable auditory tones without informational value and which transiently increase arousal temporarily reduce—and in some cases abolish—the spatial deficit for about 1 second after their presentation (Robertson, Mattingley, Rorden, & Driver, 1998), this having been replicated in a developmental unilateral spatial neglect (Dobler, Manly, Verity, Woolrych, & Robertson, 2003). Training neglect patients to increase arousal by a self-alerting procedure also improves awareness for the neglected side (Robertson, Tegner, Tham, Lo, & Nimmo-Smith, 1995), and more recently, Manly and his colleagues have shown that the simple expedient of imposing a time limit during a cancellation task greatly improves awareness of the neglected side, likely as a result of the increased arousal induced by the challenge (George, Mercer, Walker, & Manly, 2008). In summary, the arousal component of the vigilant attention system seems to be causally implicated in levels of online awareness.

Role of Error in Mediating Awareness of Deficit

How do I know if I am talking too loud, have made a social faux pas, or have behaved absent-mindedly? The most common source of such information is from *error:* I see the look of discomfort on my interlocutor's face, or I remember as I close the door that my keys are on the table inside, for example. I may also detect incipient errors before full behavioral execution of them—freezing just as I am about to say something socially insensitive to the person or just catching myself before the door closes.

Some states of anosognosia may be exacerbated due to reduced sensory or proprioceptive input, or to disrupted corollary discharge, which shields the person from experiencing the errors that would contribute to their awareness of deficit. But apart from that, people must be sufficiently vigilant as to be able to recognize error as it occurs. Furthermore, the psychophysiological response to error may in turn enhance vigilant attention, possibly via enhanced arousal. Let me consider the evidence for some of these possibilities.

If people with impaired prefrontal cortex function arising from FTD or TBI are asked to verbally report when they make an error on simple vigilance tasks, they show a much higher rate of failure to notice errors than do age-matched controls (O'Keeffe, Dockree, Moloney, Carton, & Robertson, 2007; O'Keeffe, Murray et al., 2007) unless the task is unpredictable and challenging, in which case awareness rates in TBI patients is within the normal range (O'Keeffe, Dockree et al., 2007). Furthermore, in the TBI group, there was a significantly reduced electrodermal response to errors, even for errors of which they were fully aware (O'Keeffe et al., 2004). This is also true of another group with impaired prefrontal function—and in particular *right* prefrontal function (Castellanos et al., 1996)—attention-deficit/hyperactivity disorder (ADHD). O'Connell, Bellgrove, Dockree, and Robertson (2004) have shown that

ADHD children have reduced electrodermal responses to errors. Among the TBI group, there was also a 0.62 correlation between amplitude of Skin Conductance Response (SCR) to error and the overall level of error awareness.

Conclusions

Self-evaluation is the basis for insight, and accurate self-evaluation requires adequate online attention to ongoing performance in the routines of everyday life. The vigilant attention system is the system responsible for this routine monitoring, and it consists of a network that includes two interrelated but independent systems: a locus coeruleus, noradrenalin-based arousal system on the one hand, and a right dorsolateral prefrontal and parietal network on the other. These two subsystems mutually facilitate each other and can compensate for underperformance in the other. Errors are important cues to attention to performance underpinning self-evaluation, and a number of common clinical conditions impairing prefrontal cortex function show impaired error awareness but also impaired arousal response to aware errors. Vigilant attention and awareness share common neuroanatomical underpinnings, and they may be overlapping concepts. Some forms of anosognosia may arise because of reduced error awareness arising from sensory or corollary discharge factors, but impaired vigilant attention, arousal, and associated error responsivity are major factors in poor insight across many different clinical conditions, including TBI, ADHD, schizophrenia, and the tau-opathies, particularly FTD.

References

Arnsten, A. F. T., & Contant, T. A. (1992). Alpha-2 adrenergic agonists decrease distractibility in aged monkeys performing the delayed response task. *Psychopharmacology, 108,* 159–169.

Barkley, R. A., Murphy, K. R., O'Connell, T., Anderson, D., & Connor, D. F. (2006). Effects of two doses of alcohol on simulator driving performance in adults with attention-deficit/hyperactivity disorder. *Neuropsychology, 20*(1), 77–87.

Beck, D. M., Rees, G., Frith, C. D., & Lavie, N., (2001). Neural correlates of change detection and change blindness. *Nature Neuroscience, 4,* 645–650.

Broadbent, D. B., Cooper, P. F., FitzGerald, P., & Parkes, K. R. (1982). The Cognitive Failures Questionnaire (CFQ) and its correlates. *British Journal of Clinical Psychology, 21,* 1–16.

Castellanos, F. X., Giedd, J. N., Marsh, W. L., Hamburger, S. D., Vaituzis, A. C., Dickstein, D. P., et al. (1996). Quantitative brain magnetic-resonance-imaging in attention-deficit hyperactivity disorder. *Archives of General Psychiatry, 53*(7), 607–616.

Cross, P. (1977). Not can but *will* college teaching be improved. *New Directions for Higher Education, 17,* 1–15.

Davis, D. A., Mazmanian, P. E., Fordis, M., Van Harrison, R., Thorpe, K. E., & Perrier, L. (2006). Accuracy of physician self-assessment compared with observed measures of competence: A systematic review. *Journal of the American Medical Association, 296*(9), 1094–1102.

Dobler, V., Manly, T., Verity, C., Woolrych, J., & Robertson, I. H. (2003). Modulation of spatial attention in a child with developmental unilateral neglect. *Developmental Medicine & Child Neurology, 45*(4), 282–288.

Dunning, D., Heath, C., & Suls, J. M. (2004). Flawed self-assessment: Implications for health, education, and the workplace. *Psychological Science in the Public Interest, 5*(3), 69–106.

Fischer, H., Wik, G., & Fredrikson, M. (1997). Extraversion, neuroticism and brain function: A PET study of personality. *Personality and Individual Differences, 23*(2), 345–352.

Fronczek, R., Middelkoop, H., Dijk, J. V., & Lammers, G. (2006). Focusing on vigilance instead of sleepiness in the assessment of narcolepsy: High sensitivity of the Sustained Attention to Response Task (SART). *Sleep, 29,* 187–191.

George, M. S., Mercer, J. S., Walker, R., & Manly, T. (2008). A demonstration of endogenous modulation of unilateral spatial neglect: The impact of apparent time-pressure on spatial bias. *Journal of the International Neuropsychological Society, 14,* 33–41.

Grace, J., & Malloy, P. (2001). *Frontal Systems Behavior Scale professional manual.* Lutz: Florida: Psychological Assessment Resources.

Greene, C., Bellgrove, M. A., Gill, M., & Robertson, I. H. (2009). Noradrenergic genotype predicts lapses in sustained attention. *Neuropsychologia, 47,* 591–594.

Gusnard, D. A., Akbudak, E., Shulman, G. L., & Raichle, M. E. (2001). Medial pre-frontal cortex and self-referential mental activity: Relation to a default mode of brain function. *Proceedings of the National Academy of Sciences, USA, 98,* 4259–4264.

Haas, B. W., Constable, R. T., & Canli, T. (2008). Stop the sadness: Neuroticism is associated with sustained medial prefrontal cortex response to emotional facial expressions. *NeuroImage, 42*(1), 385–392.

Harwood, D. G., Sultzer, D. L., Feil, D., Monserratt, L., Freedman, E., & Mandelkern, M. A. (2005). Frontal lobe hypometabolism and impaired insight in Alzheimer disease. *American Journal of Geriatric Psychiatry, 13*(11), 934–941.

Heilman, K. M., Schwartz, H. D., & Watson, R. T. (1978). Hypoarousal in patients with the neglect syndrome and emotional indifference. *Neurology, 28*(3), 229–232.

Hester, R., Foxe, J. J., Molholm, S., Shpaner, M., & Garavan, H. (2005). Neural mechanisms involved in error processing: A comparison of errors made with and without awareness. *NeuroImage, 27*(3), 602–608.

Hoerold, D., Dockree, P., O'Keeffe, F., Bates, H., Pertl, M., & Robertson, I. (2008). Neuropsychology of self-awareness in young adults. *Experimental Brain Research, 186*(3), 509–515.

Johnson, K. A., Kelly, S. P., Bellgrove, M. A., Barry, E., Cox, M., Gill, M., et al. (2007). Response variability in attention deficit hyperactivity disorder: Evidence for neurop-sychological heterogeneity. *Neuropsychologia, 45,* 630–638.

Johnson, S. C., Baxter, L. C., Wilder, L. S., Pipe, J. G., Heiserman, J. E., & Prigatano, G. P. (2002). Neural correlates of self-reflection. *Brain, 125,* 1808–1814.

Kruger, J., & Dunning, D. (1999). Unskilled and unaware of it: How difficulties in recognizing one's own incompetence lead to inflated self-assessments. *Journal of Personality and Social Psychology, 77*, 1121–1134.

Leahy, R. L. (2005). Clinical implications in the treatment of mania: Reducing risk behavior in manic patients. *Cognitive and Behavioral Practice, 12*(1), 89–98.

Mackworth, J. F. (1968). Vigilance, arousal and habituation. *Psychological Review, 75*, 308–322.

Makeig, S., & Jung, T.-P. (1996). Tonic, phasic, and transient EEG correlates of auditory awareness in drowsiness. *Cognitive Brain Research, 4*(1), 15–25.

Manly, T., Dobler, V. B., Dodds, C. M., & George, M. A. (2005). Rightward shift in spatial awareness with declining alertness. *Neuropsychologia, 43*(12), 1721–1728.

Manly, T., Owen, A. M., Datta, A., Lewis, G., Scott, S., Rorden, C., et al. (2003). Enhancing the sensitivity of a sustained attention task to frontal damage. Convergent clinical and functional imaging evidence. *Neurocase, 9*, 340–349.

Manly, T., Robertson, I. H., Galloway, M., & Hawkins, K. (1999). The absent mind: Further investigations of sustained attention to response. *Neuropsychologia, 37*(6), 661–670.

McKenna, F. P., Stanier, R. A., & Lewis, C. (1991). Factors underlying illusory self-assessment of driving skill in males and females. *Accident Analysis and Prevention, 23*, 45–52.

O'Connell, R. G., Bellgrove, M. A., Dockree, P. M., & Robertson, I. H. (2004). Reduced electrodermal response to errors predicts poor sustained attention performance in attention deficit hyperactivity disorder. *Neuroreport, 15*, 2535–2538.

O'Connell, R. G., Dockree, P. M., Bellgrove, M. A., Kelly, P. S., Hester, R., Garavan, H., et al. (2007). The role of cingulate cortex in the detection of errors with and without awareness: A high-density electrical mapping study. *European Journal of Neuroscience, 25*(8), 2571–2579.

O'Keeffe, F. M., Dockree, P. M., Moloney, P., Carton, S., & Robertson, I. H. (2007). Characterising error-awareness of attentional lapses and inhibitory control failures in patients with traumatic brain injury. *Experimental Brain Research, 180*, 59–67.

O'Keeffe, F. M., Dockree, P. M., & Robertson, I. H. (2004). Poor insight in traumatic brain injury mediated by impaired error processing? Evidence from electrodermal activity. *Cognitive Brain Research, 22*, 101–112.

O'Keeffe, F. M., Murray, B., Coen, R. F., Dockree, P. M., Bellgrove, M. A., Garavan, H., et al. (2007). Loss of insight in frontotemporal dementia, corticobasal degeneration and progressive supranuclear palsy. *Brain, 130*(3), 753–764.

Oke, A., Keller, R., Mefford, I., & Adams, R. (1978). Lateralization of norepinephrine in human thalamus. *Science, 200*, 1411–1413.

Paus, T., Zatorre, R. J., Hofle, N., Caramanos, Z., Gotman, J., Petrides, M., et al. (1997). Time-related changes in neural systems underlying attention and arousal during the performance of an auditory vigilance task. *Journal of Cognitive Neuroscience, 9*, 392–408.

Pia, L., Neppi-Modona, M., Ricci, R., & Berti, A. (2004). The anatomy of anosognosia for hemiplegia: A meta-analysis. *Cortex, 40*, 367–377.

Posner, M. I., & Petersen, S. E. (1990). The attention system of the human brain. *Annual Review of Neuroscience, 13*, 25–42.

Robertson, I. H., & Garavan, H. (2004). Vigilant attention. In M. S. Gazzaniga (Ed.), *The Cognitive neurosciences* (3rd edition, pp. 563–578). Cambridge, MA: MIT Press.

Robertson, I. H., Manly, T., Andrade, J., Baddeley, B. T., & Yiend, J. (1997). Oops! Performance correlates of everyday attentional failures in traumatic brain injured and normal subjects: The Sustained Attention to Response Task (SART). *Neuropsychologia, 35*, 747–758.

Robertson, I. H., Mattingley, J. B., Rorden, C., & Driver, J. (1998). Phasic alerting of neglect patients overcomes their spatial deficit in visual awareness. *Nature, 395*(10), 169–172.

Robertson, I. H., Tegner, R., Tham, K., Lo, A., & Nimmo-Smith, I. (1995). Sustained attention training for unilateral neglect: Theoretical and rehabilitation implications. *Journal of Clinical and Experimental Neuropsychology, 17*, 416–430.

Sachdev, P., Mondraty, N., Wen, W., & Gulliford, K. (2008). Brains of anorexia nervosa patients process self-images differently from non-self-images: An fMRI study. *Neuropsychologia, 46*(8), 2161–2168.

Schmitz, T. W., Rowley, H. A., Kawahara, T. N., & Johnson, S. C. (2006). Neural correlates of self-evaluative accuracy after traumatic brain injury. *Neuropsychologia, 44*(5), 762–773.

Shad, M. U., Muddasani, S., & Keshavan, M. S. (2006). Prefrontal subregions and dimensions of insight in first-episode schizophrenia—A pilot study. *Psychiatry Research: Neuroimaging, 146*(1), 35–42.

Smith, A., & Nutt, D. (1996). Noradrenaline and attention lapses. *Nature, 380*, 291.

Tsai, L.-L., Young, H.-Y., Hsieh, S., & Lee, C.-S. (2005). Error monitoring after sleep deprivation. *Sleep, 28*, 707–713.

Usher, M., Cohen, J. D., Servan-Schreiber, D., Rajkowski, J., & Aston-Jones, G. (1999). The role of locus coeruleus in the regulation of cognitive performance. *Science, 283*, 549–553.

Voelz, Z. R., Walker, R. L., Pettit, J. W., Joiner Jr., T. E., & Wagner, K. D. (2003). Depressogenic attributional style: Evidence of trait-like nature in youth psychiatric inpatients. *Personality and Individual Differences, 34*(7), 1129–1140.

Whitehead, R. (1991). Right hemisphere processing superiority during sustained visual attention. *Journal of Cognitive Neuroscience, 3*, 329–335.

16

Emotional Awareness among Brain-Damaged Patients

Ricardo E. Jorge

More than a century ago, Babinski coined the term *anosognosia* to describe the puzzling presentation of patients who were unaware of their motor deficits associated with stroke. A similar phenomenon was also described among patients suffering from cortical blindness and other sensory deficits (Bisiach, Vallar, Perani, Papagno, & Berti, 1986). From its inception, it was clear that anosognosia could not be adequately explained purely on the basis of psychological terms and was related to the disruption of specific neural circuits in the brain (Heilman, Barrett, & Adair, 1998; Orfei et al., 2007; Ramachandran, 1996). More recently, this eminently neurological approach was applied to describe unawareness of deficits in other domains, such as memory and executive functions, as well as in complex processes regulating decision making and social interaction (Bechara, Damasio, Tranel, & Damasio, 1997, 2005; Boake, Freeland, Ringholz, Nance, & Edwards, 1995; Damasio, 1996; Levine, Calvanio, & Rinn, 1991; McGlynn & Schacter, 1989; Schacter, 1990). In addition, the spectrum of structural alterations of the brain was expanded to include traumatic injuries (Giacino & Cicerone, 1998; Hoofien, Gilboa, Vakil, & Barak, 2004; Prigatano & Schacter, 1991) and neurodegenerative disorders such as Alzheimer's disease (Souchay, 2007; Starkstein et al., 1996), Huntington's disease (Hoth et al., 2007), and frontotemporal dementia (Eslinger et al., 2005; Ruby et al., 2007; Salmon et al., 2008).

In the realm of psychiatry, loss of insight was a decisive criterion in the early conceptualization of mental illness, particularly with regard to major psychosis. During the last half of the nineteenth century, however, psychiatric investigators became aware that patients with psychiatric disorders varied with regard to the degree of awareness of their cognitive, volitional, and emotional deficits (Berrios, 1996). Later, at the time when the psychiatric field was revolutionized by the formulation of the psychoanalytic theory (Freud & Brill, 1938), awareness and insight were interpreted on the basis of psychodynamic concepts and defense mechanisms. However, both the neurological and psychiatric disciplines converge in the assumption that the clinical phenomena subsumed under the notions of unawareness, insight, and denial have significant prognostic and therapeutic implications and that their presence has a detrimental effect on patients' recovery.

Defining multidimensional concepts such as anosognosia, awareness of emotions, and insight is certainly a challenging task. For instance, although there is agreement with regard to the fact that these phenomena occur along a continuum and are better described within a dimensional perspective, it is unclear whether a categorical diagnosis would provide a more meaningful understanding of their functional repercussion, clinical course, and long-term prognosis (Markova & Berrios, 1995; Markova, Clare, Wang, Romero, & Kenny, 2005). In addition, investigators in this field have enriched the conceptual discussion of these phenomena by the identification of important differences between awareness and attribution processes (Russell, 2003), explicit versus implicit features (Lane, Ahern, Schwartz, & Kaszniak, 1997), as well as the opposition of intellectual and emotional awareness developed in the psychoanalytic tradition (Alford & Beck, 1994).

Markova and Berrios (1995) remind us that insight is an intentional concept and thus implies a specific object. In turn, the nature of this object will determine the clinical phenomenon and the method employed to assess it. This is particularly relevant in the case of emotions and affective symptoms, which are more difficult to be identified, described, and eventually measured. Consequently, operational definitions and quantitative assessments of unawareness are much more developed in the neurological and neuropsychological terrains than in the psychiatric arena. For instance, there are very few instruments assessing insight of affective illness, none of them with a clear-cut demonstration of their validity (Sturman & Sproule, 2003).

Studying mood disorders that occur in the aftermath of brain damage adds further complexity to this problem. Although multiple etiological factors contribute to the emergence of these types of mood disorders, it is accepted that the disruption of specific distributed neural networks encompassing the prefrontal cortex and the medial temporal lobe plays an important causal role and modifies their clinical presentation. For instance, mood disorders associated with cerebrovascular disease are characterized by the frequent occurrence of executive impairment and apathetic features. Insight and awareness of affective deficits are clinical phenomena that have been rarely studied among brain-injured patients and their neurobiological mechanism is largely unknown. However, we can hypothesize that abnormality in emotional regulation and metacognitive functions would have distinct clinical presentation among depressed patients with coexistent brain damage.

An extensive analysis of the psychological concepts related to emotional processing as well as a portrayal of the unrelenting progress of affective neuroscience research are clearly out of the scope of this chapter. However, I will briefly describe the constructs of emotional awareness and alexithymia, as well as the instruments that have been commonly used to assess them. Finally, I review recent studies on alexithymia associated with stroke and traumatic brain injury and report preliminary results of our work on this topic.

Emotional Awareness and Alexithymia

To some extent, the current conceptualization of emotional processing was fore-shadowed by the work of two major figures of psychological thought: William James and Ludwig Wittgenstein. James was among the first to emphasize the importance of somatic and autonomic sensory feedback, and of the resulting cortical representation of body states in the physiology of feelings and emotions. He also suggested that emotional experiences play a decisive role in modeling behavior (James, 1890). Although Wittgenstein was critical of many aspects of James' work (e.g., the method of introspection and the notion of an ostensive definition of psychological concepts), he acknowledged the importance of what became known as the James-Lange theory. However, Wittgenstein and Anscombe (1953) emphasized the importance of linguistic processing and of what he called *language games* in the delimitation of psychological concepts. Furthermore, according to his view, language is ultimately the expression of a particular form of life; it depends and develops on the basis of the interaction with the material and cultural aspects of our world (Wittgenstein & Anscombe, 1953). Language and other forms of symbolic representation become inextricably associated with the representation and expression of emotions, dissecting them as an anatomist and modeling them as a sculptor. In addition, Wittgenstein's emphasis on the inter-active (social) experiential aspects of language acquisition connotes the develop-mental nature of emotional awareness.

Functional neuroimaging studies on linguistic processing of emotional infor-mation have demonstrated that affect labeling modifies the limbic response to negative emotional images. In contrast to gender labeling of pictures, affect labeling increases activity in areas of the right prefrontal cortex, specifically the right ventrolateral prefrontal cortex and the medial prefrontal cortex. Furthermore, the fact that activity in these regions is inversely correlated with amygdala activity suggests that linguistic processing of emotions modulates more basic affective responses (Creswell, Way, Eisenberger, & Lieberman, 2007; Lieberman et al., 2007). More recent studies from the same investigators showed that repeated exposure to labeled aversive images produces greater autonomic reactivity attenuation than repeated exposure to nonlabeled aversive images. In addition, this greater attenuation is also observed 8 days after the initial exposure, even when the aversive stimuli were presented without their labels (Tabibnia, Lieberman, & Craske, 2008).

Interestingly, more than three decades ago, Sifneos et al. (1973) introduced the concept of alexithymia (literally *without words for mood*) to define an alteration in emotional processing characterized by the difficulty in identifying emotions and differentiating them from other physical states, difficulty in describing emotions, limited ability to represent or fantasize scenarios with significant emotional content, and a concrete cognitive style that disregards the complex emotional, motivational, and symbolic aspects of human behavior (Apfel & Sifneos, 1979; Sifneos, 1973, 1996; Taylor, Bagby, & Parker, 1993; Weinryb, Gustavsson, Asberg, & Rossel, 1992).

Alexithymic patients show altered processing of emotional information (e.g., the ability to identify facial expressions) (Parker, Taylor, & Bagby, 1993; Roedema & Simons, 1999) and deficient modulation of emotional responses that may result in impulsive behavior (Taylor & Bagby, 2004). In addition, alexithymia has been associated with changes in major personality dimensions, such as increased neuroticism and decreased openness to new experiences (Bagby, Taylor, & Parker, 1994). It has also been suggested that patients with alexithymia have a limited capacity to enjoy pleasurable and gratifying experiences (i.e., they tend to be anhedonic), as well as severe impairment in coping with stress (Bagby, Taylor, & Parker, 1994; Loas et al., 1998; Luminet, Bagby, Wagner, Taylor, & Parker, 1999). Furthermore, alexithymic patients are prone to express psychological distress in the form of somatic symptoms and, thus, are more vulnerable to develop psychosomatic disorders (Taylor, Bagby, & Parker, 1991). Finally, regarding the relationship of alexithymia with mental illness, previous studies have reported the presence of alexithymic features among patients with diverse psychopathological conditions such as depressive disorders (Marchesi, Bertoni, Cantoni, & Maggini, 2008; Saarijarvi, Salminen, & Toikka, 2006), post-traumatic stress disorder (Frewen, Pain, Dozois, & Lanius, 2006; Kupchik et al., 2007; Yehuda et al., 1997), eating disorders (Taylor, Parker, Bagby, & Bourke, 1996), and Cluster B personality disorders (Guttman & Laporte, 2002; Sayar, Ebrinc, & Ak, 2001).

There are several instruments designed to give a quantitative estimation of alexithymia. At the present time, the Toronto Alexithymia Scale (TAS) is the most widely used assessment device, with the most rigorous psychometric validation. A revised version consisting of 20 items (TAS-20) that cluster in three main factors has been consistently replicated in independent samples of healthy controls and various clinical populations (Bagby, Taylor, & Parker, 1994; Parker, Taylor, Bagby, & Thomas, 1991; Taylor, Bagby, & Parker, 2003). The first factor corresponds to the ability to identify emotions, the second factor is related to the ability to describe emotions, and the third factor assesses the concrete cognitive style observed among alexithymic patients. There is some controversy regarding the stability of the alexithymia construct and whether TAS-20 scores have significant correlations with conventional measures of the severity of depressive and anxious symptoms (de Timary, Luts, Hers, &

Luminet, 2008; Honkalampi, Hintikka, Saarinen, Lehtonen, & Viinamaki, 2000; Marchesi, Bertoni, Cantoni, & Maggini, 2008; Marchesi, Brusamonti, & Maggini, 2000; Subic-Wrana, Bruder, Thomas, Lane, & Kohle, 2005). Overall, the available evidence on this issue suggests that alexithymia, depression and anxiety are related but ultimately independent constructs with a different longitudinal course (Marchesi, Brusamonti, & Maggini, 2000). Finally, we must keep in mind that we can use a cut-off score on the TAS-20 scale in order to make a categorical diagnosis of alexithymia.

Lane, Quinlan, Schwartz, Walker, and Zeitlin (1990) have taken a different approach to assess awareness of emotions that resulted in the development of the Level of Emotional Awareness Scale (LEAS) (Lane et al., 1990). Rather than relying on self-reported information, as in the case of TAS-20, the LEAS attempts to objectively probe the extent and quality of emotional awareness. Basically, when completing this instrument, subjects are required to describe their feelings, as well as those of another person in response to different scenarios depicted in 20 vignettes of two to four sentences. The scoring system evaluates the structure of the experience focusing on the specificity, variety, and range of the emotional words used, as well as the degree of understanding of the different perspectives of the subjects involved in a particular situation. Of note, LEAS scores do not correlate with self-reported negative affect in the absence of anxiety or depressive disorders (Subic-Wrana et al., 2005). Greater emotional awareness is associated with greater impulse control consistent with a top-down regulation of more basic and implicit emotional responses. Consistent with this notion, patients with borderline personality disorder present lower LEAS scores (Levine, Marziali, & Hood, 1997). In addition, patients with PTSD (Frewen et al., 2008) and patients with psychosomatic disorders (Subic-Wrana et al., 2005) present lower LEAS scores than healthy controls.

Lane et al. (1990) used positron emission tomography (PET)—based emotional activation paradigms to identify brain regions that correlated with emotional awareness as measured by LEAS scores (Lane et al., 1998). They concluded that, in the case of visually induced emotion, LEAS scores showed a positive correlation with an activation cluster located in right midcingulate cortex, while for recall-induced emotion the region that showed the highest correlation with LEAS scores was the right anterior cingulate cortex (ACC). More important, both clusters overlapped in a discrete region of the dorsal ACC in the right hemisphere (Lane et al., 1998). A second study by the same group reported that these significant correlations were mainly observed in high arousal conditions and were greater for women (McRae, Reiman, Fort, Chen, & Lane, 2008).

As a result of research conducted with the help of the LEAS, and inspired by the work of Paul MacLean (1977, 1985), Lane (2008) proposed a hierarchical model of emotional awareness that was meant to provide a general framework for the study of psychosomatic illness (Lane, 2008). He emphasizes the developmental nature of this process and the progressive integration of specific schemata that configure emotional experience. According to Lane's (2008) model, emotional awareness develops through five levels of increasing complexity: awareness of physical sensations, action tendencies, single emotions, blend of emotions, and, finally, blends of blends of emotional experience. The first two levels rely on implicit (unconscious) processing of emotionally laden stimuli, while the remaining three levels correspond to a progressively complex explicit (conscious) elaboration of emotional experiences.

This model distinguishes between the neural components of implicit processing (e.g., the thalamus and the amygdala) (Doron & Ledoux, 1999; Doyere, Debiec, Monfils, Schafe, & LeDoux, 2007; Phelps, Delgado, Nearing, & LeDoux, 2004; Phelps & LeDoux, 2005; Rogan, Staubli, & LeDoux, 1997) and three components of the conscious experience of emotion: background feelings, focal attention to feelings, and reflective awareness. Background feelings give the basic emotional color to our experience, but they are not the focus of our attention (Damasio, 2003; Kawasaki et al., 2005). They are probably integrated in circuits that include, among other regions, structures that process interoceptive information such as the subgenual and pregenual ACC, the anterior insula, and the somatosensory associative areas in the parietal cortex of the right hemisphere (Adolphs, Damasio, Tranel, Cooper, & Damasio, 2000; Anderson & Phelps, 2002; Bechara, Damasio, Tranel, & Damasio, 2005; Damasio, 1996; Mesulam & Mufson, 1982). Attention to feelings and the activation of linguistic processing have been associated with the function of the dorsal ACC, a region known to mediate controlled rather than automatic behavioral responses, as well as error monitoring (Botvinick, Nystrom, Fissell, Carter, & Cohen, 1999; Brown & Braver, 2005; Bush et al., 2002; Carter et al., 1998; Critchley, 2005; Critchley, Wiens, Rotshtein, Ohman, & Dolan, 2004; Frankland, Bontempi, Talton, Kaczmarek, & Silva, 2004; Kalisch, Wiech, Critchley, & Dolan, 2006; Kerns et al., 2004; Sharot, Riccardi, Raio, & Phelps, 2007; Wang et al., 2005; Yamasaki, LaBar, & McCarthy, 2002). Finally, reflective awareness of emotions implies further cognitive operations on the emotional information that is proposed to be conducted in those prefrontal circuits that have evolved and specialized to represent mental states of the self and of others (i.e., theory of mind processes), particularly those involving the dorsomedial prefrontal cortex. The complex representation of these states corresponds to higher levels of emotional awareness and will modify the processing of ulterior emotional stimuli (D'Argembeau et al., 2007; Moran, Macrae, Heatherton, Wyland, & Kelley, 2006; Ochsner et al., 2004; Spreng, Mar, & Kim, 2008).

Alexithymia in Stroke

Disturbances of emotional perception and emotional expression associated with neurological illness have been studied for several decades. For instance, Tucker et al. (1977) reported that patients with right hemisphere damage (RHD) demonstrated defective emotional prosody (Tucker, Watson, & Heilman, 1977). This finding was replicated in a large number of empirical studies and aprosodia has been accepted as a relatively frequent neuropsychiatric complication of stroke (Borod et al., 2000; Heilman, Leon, & Rosenbek, 2004; Leon et al., 2005; Ross, Harney, deLacoste-Utamsing, & Purdy, 1981; Ross, Thompson, & Yenkosky, 1997). More recently, Bloom, Borod, Obler, and Gerstman (1992) observed that, when asked to describe emotional laden slides, patients with RHD elicited words of significantly less emotional content than patients with left hemisphere damage (LHD) or healthy controls (Bloom et al., 1992). Similarly, Borod et al. (1996) compared the discourse of patients with RHD, LHD, and normal volunteers and concluded that the emotional content of the discourse of subjects with RHD was significantly less than that observed among patients with LHD or controls (Borod et al., 1996). Other investigators, however, were not able to replicate these findings. For example, Blonder et al. (2005) reported opposite results when comparing the percentage of emotional words in the discourse of 14 aphasic patients (LHD) and 9 patients with aprosodia (RHD). These authors suggest that the deficits in emotional expression observed in patients with RHD are related to abnormalities in the encoding of nonverbal emotional expression rather than the inability to experience or conceptualize emotions (Blonder et al., 2005). The latter is consistent with previous clinical studies reporting that the frequency of major depression is not significantly different in stroke patients with anosognosia compared with stroke patients without anosognosia (Starkstein, Berthier, Fedoroff, Price, & Robinson, 1990).

An empirical evaluation of the alexithymia construct has rarely been done in the context of structural brain damage. However, early studies in cerebral commissurotomy patients proposed that alexithymia resulted from deficits in interhemispheric transfer of information by which emotional experiences integrated in the right hemisphere cannot access linguistic processing circuits located in the left (TenHouten, Hoppe, Bogen, & Walter, 1986). Recently, Spaletta et al. (2001) used the TAS-20 to assess alexithymic features in a group of 48 stroke patients, 21 with RHD and 27 with LHD (Spalletta et al., 2001). After controlling for the level of cognitive impairment and the severity of depression and anxiety symptoms, TAS-20 scores were significantly higher among patients with RHD, an effect driven by significantly higher scores in Factor 1 (identify emotions) and Factor 2 (describe emotions) of the TAS-20 scale. There was also a gender by side interaction by which men with RHD had significantly higher TAS-20 scores than men with LHD. Significant lateralized differences were not observed among women. Overall, these findings suggest that alexithymia may be a good indicator of unawareness of emotions among patients with stroke (Spalletta et al., 2001).

The same group of investigators examined whether alexithymia overlapped with unawareness of motor deficits (anosognosia) in an independent sample of 50 first-ever stroke patients with RHD (Spalletta et al., 2007). Alexithymia was diagnosed using a cut-off score in the TAS-20 (scores equal or greater than 61 determined a positive diagnosis) while anosognosia was assessed using the Bisiach Anosognosia Scale and neglect was evaluated through the neurological examination and appropriate neuropsychological tests such as the Line Bisection Test (Friedman, 1990). Of the 50 patients included in the study, 26% patients had anosognosia, 52% presented with neglect, and 52% were diagnosed as alexithymic. More important, there were cases where alexithymia occurred independently from anosognosia, suggesting that these conditions are mediated by different, although probably overlapping neural circuits. Consistent with this notion, patients with coexistent alexithymia and anosognosia had more extensive lesions and greater frontal dysfunction than patients with alexithymia without anosognosia (Spalletta et al., 2007). Finally, these investigators have examined the clinical course of 50 patients with post-stroke depression to determine whether TAS-20 scores that correspond to the three alexithymia factors change with antidepressant treatment (Spalletta, Ripa, Bria, Caltagirone, & Robinson, 2006). Out of these 50 patients, 18 had coexistent alexithymia while the remaining 32 patients were not alexithymic. As expected, a diagnosis of alexithymia was significantly associated with RHD. Patients with an alexithymia diagnosis showed a significant decline of Factor 1 and Factor 2 scores associated with antidepressant treatment. Such a decline was not observed in the group of patients without alexithymia. Interestingly, the change in the TAS-20 scores did not correlate with the change in Hamilton Depression Rating Scale (HDRS) scores and, thus, was not related to the magnitude of the antidepressant response (Spalletta et al., 2006). It is unclear whether changes in the activation of mood regulation areas associated with the effect of antidepressants (e.g., different areas of the cingulate cortex) contribute to the change in TAS-20 scores.

Although alexithymia has been consistently associated with RHD among patients with stroke, little has been done to further identify the lateralized circuits mediating emotional awareness. A recent report, however, described the case of a 61-year-old woman with an ischemic stroke in the territory of the right pericallosal artery who presented with reduced emotional responsiveness, impaired affect recognition, and prominent alexithymic features (TAS-20 score was 62) (Schafer et al., 2007). Magnetic resonance imaging (MRI) showed a lesion of the right ACC and the anterior corpus callosum that involved the dorsal ACC and extended into the ventral aspect of the medial superior frontal gyrus (Schafer et al., 2007). This is consistent with the model of emotional awareness previously described.

Alexithymia in Traumatic Brain Injury

Background

There are several reports on the association of traumatic brain injury (TBI) and alexithymia. Williams et al., evaluated 135 outpatients in a family practice setting for the presence of both TBI and alexithymia. They observed that those patients who had a positive history of TBI had significantly higher TAS-20 scores than patients without a history of TBI (Williams et al., 2001). Koponen et al. (2005) compared the frequency of alexithymia between 54 chronic TBI patients and a control group of similar demographic characteristics and comparable severity of depressive symptoms. Alexithymia was significantly more frequent among the TBI group (Odds Ratio = 2.64, Confidence Interval = 1.03—6.80) and was associated with greater psychopathology (Koponen et al., 2005). Another recent study by Henry, Phillips, Crawford, Theodorou, and Summers (2006) compared a group of 28 subjects with severe TBI with 31 healthy control subjects on the different factors of the TAS-20, self-reported measures of depression, anxiety, and quality of life, as well as fluency tasks of different complexity (Henry et al., 2006). As expected, TBI patients showed greater levels of alexithymia than controls. There was a strong association between the TAS-20 Factor 1 (identify emotions) and Factor 2 (describe emotions) and self-report measures of anxiety, depression, and quality of life. After controlling for the substantial effect of depression and anxiety symptoms, difficulty to identify emotions (Factor 1) was associated with reduced quality of life. This factor was the only variable related to deficit in executive functioning (Henry et al., 2006). Finally, Wood and Williams (2007) examined the prevalence and correlates of alexithymia in a larger group of TBI patients ($n = 121$) compared with 52 patients with orthopedic injuries. These investigators confirmed the higher frequency of alexithymia in the TBI group compared with the control group, as well as the presence of moderate correlations between TAS-20 scores and self-report measures of anxiety and depression. However, regression analysis revealed that depression and anxiety scores explained a small percentage of the variance in TAS-20 scores, suggesting that these constructs are overlapping, albeit distinct, constructs in the TBI population. There was not a significant association between alexithymia and severity of brain injury or executive dysfunction (Wood & Williams, 2007).

For the past few years we have studied the prevalence, duration, and clinical correlates of mood and anxiety disorders following TBI. Further details of this work can be found elsewhere (Jorge, 2005; Jorge et al., 2004; Jorge et al., 2005). In this chapter we will report our preliminary findings on alexithymia following TBI, as assessed with the use of the TAS-20.

Methods

Participants consisted of 91 consecutive patients with closed head injury admitted to the University of Iowa Hospitals and Clinics, Iowa City ($n = 60$) or the Iowa Methodist Medical Center, Des Moines ($n = 31$). Patients with penetrating head injuries or those with clinical or radiological findings suggesting spinal cord injury were excluded from the study. Sixty-eight (74.7%)

of the 91 patients with TBI were injured in a motor vehicle collision, 16 patients (17.6%) by a fall, 3 patients (3.3%) by assault, and 4 patients (4.4%) by other mechanisms (e.g., sport-related injuries). Severity of TBI was assessed using the 24-hour Glasgow Coma Scale (GCS) score (Teasdale & Jennett, 1976). The overall severity of the traumatic injury was assessed using the Abbreviated Injury Scale (MacKenzie, Shapiro, & Eastham, 1985). Using initial GCS scores and computed tomographic data, 40 patients (44.3%) were classified as mild TBI, 30 patients (32.5%) with moderate TBI, and 21 patients (23.2%) with severe TBI. The TAS-20 was included as part of the assessment battery several months after the study was initiated. Of the 91 TBI patients who were initially enrolled in this study, 74 (81.3%) completed the TAS-20 and constitute our study group.

Psychiatric assessment was conducted using the Structured Clinical Interview for *DSM-IV* diagnoses (Williams et al., 1992). Severity of depressive and anxiety symptoms were assessed using the Hamilton Depression Rating Scale (HDRS) (Hamilton, 1960) and the Hamilton Anxiety Scale (HARS) (Hamilton, 1959), respectively. Aggressive behavior was assessed using a modified version of the Overt Aggression Scale (OAS) (Silver & Yudofsky, 1991). To be categorized as aggressive, a patient had to have at least four episodes of significant aggressive behavior during the previous month and have an aggression score of 3 or more on the OAS. As aforementioned, the TAS-20 was used to evaluate alexithymic features. Scores equal or greater than 61 on this scale were considered indicative of alexithymia diagnosis.

The Mini-Mental State Examination (MMSE) (Folstein, Folstein, & McHugh, 1975) was used as a global measure of cognitive functioning. Impairment in activities of daily living was assessed using the Functional Independence Measure (Forer & Granger, 1987). Psychosocial adjustment was quantitatively assessed using the Social Functioning Examination and Social Ties Checklist (Starr, Robinson, & Price, 1983).

Neuropsychological assessment focused on memory and frontal-executive functioning, as assessed by the following six tests: Rey Auditory Verbal Learning Test (delayed recall trial) (Rey, 1964); Rey Complex Figure Test (delayed recall trial) (Rey, 1964); Trail Making Test (Time B) (Reitan, 1971); Multilingual Aphasia Examination (Controlled Oral Word Association Test total score) (Benton, Hamsher, & Sivan, 1994); Stroop Color-Word Interference Test (Golden, 1978); and Wisconsin Card-Sorting Test (the number of perseverative errors) (Heaton, Chelune, & Tailey, 1993).

In addition, a research MRI was obtained in a subgroup of these patients ($n = 31$) using a 1.5-Tesla scanner at the radiology department of the University of Iowa. The tools of a locally developed software package, BRAINS-2 (Department of Psychiatry, University of Iowa) were used to generate volumetric data (Andreasen et al., 1996). The validity and reproducibility of morphometric analysis using the aforementioned software has been reported in previous studies (Magnotta et al., 1999; Magnotta et al., 2002). In addition, the ACC was traced on segmented coronal images simultaneously inspecting the other image planes and surface reconstruction (McCormick et al., 2006). The ACC was further subdivided into four architectonically and functionally distinct sectors: dorsal, rostral, subcallosal, and subgenual (McCormick et al., 2006).

Results

Of the 74 patients included in this study, 17 (23%) met diagnostic criteria for alexithymia and were included in the alexithymia group (Alex), while the remaining 57 TBI patients were included in the nonalexithymia group (No-Alex). The background characteristics of both groups are summarized in Table 16.1. There were no differences between the Alex and the No-Alex groups in age, gender, socioeconomic status, and educational level or unemployment rates. In addition, there were not significant differences in the severity of brain injury, activities of daily living impairment, or social functioning.

Psychiatric findings are summarized in Table 16.2. When compared with the No-Alex group, ALEX patients had significantly higher frequency of alcohol misuse (Fisher Exact Test, $p = 0.0225$), drug misuse (Fisher Exact Test, $p = 0.027$), and aggressive behavior (Fisher Exact Test, $p = 0.0117$). We did not observe significant differences between the Alex and the No-Alex groups in the frequency of major depression or anxiety disorder with generalized features. In addition, we did not find significant differences between the groups in the severity of anxiety or depressive symptoms. We examined the correlation between TAS-20 total and factor scores with both HDRS and HARS total scores. There was a significant correlation between Factor 1 (ability to identify emotions) scores and both HDRS scores (Spearman Rho= 0.3180, $p = .0141$) and HARS scores (Spearman Rho = 0.3047, $p = .02$) and a trend for significance

Table 16.1 Background Characteristics

Variable	Alexithymia ($n = 17$)	No Alexithymia ($n = 57$)
Age [Mean (SD)]	35.3 (14.5)	37.9 (16.6)
Sex (% of females)	35.3	41.1
Years of education [Mean (SD)]	12.3 (3.2)	13.2 (2.5)
Socioeconomic status (% of Classes IV and V)	37.5	44
Employment (% of unemployed)	11.8	12.9
Glasgow Coma Scale (GCS) [Mean (SD)]	11.1 (3.5)	11.7 (2.8)
Abbreviated Injury Scale (AIS) [Mean (SD)]	18.1 (8.5)	16.5 (8.2)
Functional Independence Measure (FIM) [Mean (SD)]	62.1 (9.7)	63.5 (8.3)
Social Functioning Examination (SFE) [Mean (SD)]	170 (16.9)	166 (13.7)

Table 16.2 Psychiatric Assessment

Variable	Alexithymia (n = 17)	No Alexithymia (n = 57)
Mood disorder with major depression features (%)	40	22.5
Anxiety disorder with generalized anxiety features (%)	41.1	24.6
Alcohol abuse or dependence (%) * Fisher Exact Test, p = .0225	64.7	35.3
Drug abuse or dependence (%) * Fisher Exact Test, p = .027	41.2	15.8
Aggressive behavior (%) * Fisher Exact Test, p = .017	58.8	28.1
HAMD-17 scores [Mean (SD)]	11.9 (9.1)	8.1 (5.3)
HAMA scores [Mean (SD)]	11.8 (7.2)	10.1 (6.0)
Previous psychiatric history (%)	41.1	24.6

in the case of HDRS scores and Total TAS-20 scores (Spearman Rho = 0.2341, $p = .0743$). The rest of the correlations were not significant.

We also examined the relationship between alexithymia and neuropsychological performance in memory and executive functioning tests (see Table 16.3). Accounting for the fact that educational level as well as depression and anxiety

Table 16.3 Neuropsychological Variables

Variable	Alexithymia (n = 12)	No Alexithymia (n = 57)
Rey Auditory Verbal Learning Test (Delay recall) [Mean (SD)]	7.9 (3.4)	9.5 (3.1)
Rey Complex Figure Test (Delay recall) [Mean (SD)]	14.7 (4.3)	16.7 (5.6)
Control Oral Word Association Test (Total Score) [Mean (SD)]	36.9 (15.2)	40.0 (10.4)
Wisconsin Card Sorting Test (Number of perseverative errors) [Mean (SD)]	11.0 (5.8)	8.7 (5.6)
Trail Making Test (Time B) [Mean (SD)]	74.8 (27.9)	82.8 (48.0)
Stroop Test (Color/word interference) [Mean (SD)]	37.7 (10.6)	35.8 (10.9)
Mini Mental Status Examination (Total Score) [Mean (SD)]	27.8 (1.5)	27.4 (2.3)

might have influenced neuropsychological scores, we included these variables as covariates in the analysis of differences between the groups. Overall, we did not find significant differences between the Alex and No-Alex groups on any of the different neuropsychological measures assessing memory and executive functioning. Furthermore, neuropsychological scores were not significantly correlated with total or factor-specific TAS-20 scores.

We finally examined the relationship between alexithymia and neuroimaging findings. With regard to the initial radiological findings (those obtained immediately after TBI in clinical settings), there were no significant differences between the Alex and the No-Alex groups in the frequency of focal and diffuse patterns of injury, the frequency of focal identifiable lesions in the right or left hemisphere, or in the frequency of identifiable frontal, temporal, or parietal lesions.

The limited number of alexithymic patients with available volumetric MRIs ($n = 6$) precluded group analysis of research imaging data. Multiple regression analysis, however, was performed in the whole group of patients in whom we obtained a research MRI and had TAS-20 scores ($n = 31$). We built a multiple regression model using the total TAS-20 score as the dependent variable and the volume of the different regions of the ACC (McCormick et al., 2006), gender and GCS scores as independent variables. After adjusting for GCS, women presented lower alexithymia scores than men (F $(1, 27) = 5.8$, $p = .02$) and there was a statistical trend indicating that larger right dorsal cingulate cortex volume is associated with lower alexithymia scores (F$(1,27) = 3.8$, $p = 0.06$) (see Figure 16.1).

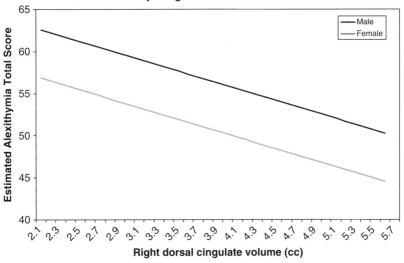

Figure 16.1 Relationship between alexithymia and dorsal anterior cingulate cortex volumes. GCS, Glasgow Coma Scale.

Comment

In summary, when compared with nonalexithymic TBI patients, TBI patients with alexithymia had significantly higher frequency of alcohol and drug misuse, as well as evidence of impulsive aggressive behavior. Difficulty in identifying emotions (TAS-20 Factor 1) was positively correlated with measures of the severity of depressive and anxiety symptoms and with aggression scores. In addition, there was some indication that alexithymia was related to reduced volumes of the right dorsal ACC. On the other hand, we did not observe an association between alexithymia and the severity of TBI, the presence of focal lesions of the right hemisphere, or the presence of focal lesions of the frontal lobes. Furthermore, there was no association between alexithymia and executive dysfunction as measured by usual neuropsychological tests.

An association between alexithymia, substance misuse, impulsivity, and aggression has been previously reported in previous studies of patients with addictive disorders (Evren & Evren, 2005; Evren et al., 2008; Loas, Otmani, Lecercle, & Jouvent, 2000; Speranza et al., 2004). We have also reported that there is significant overlap between mood disorders, alcohol misuse, and aggression among TBI patients during the first year following trauma (Jorge et al., 2004; Jorge et al., 2005).

These findings should be interpreted from the perspective of the known deregulation of emotional processing resulting from prefrontal dysfunction associated with TBI. Mood disorders may result from deactivation of more lateral and dorsal frontal cortex and increased activation in ventral limbic and paralimbic structures including the amygdala (Drevets, 1999; Mayberg et al., 1997; Mayberg et al., 1999). It is in this context of increased psychological distress and negative emotional arousal that coexistent alexithymic features would further contribute to impulsive behavior and aggression. Of course, alexithymia may be associated with multiple factors, including those related to previous emotional and personality development, personal history of addictive disorders, as well as structural and functional abnormalities of medial regions of the prefrontal cortex resulting from the TBI.

Final Remarks

Awareness of affective deficits among brain-injured patients has not been extensively studied. There is still controversy about the conceptualization of this clinical phenomenon and, more importantly, about the methods by which emotional awareness may be reliably assessed in this population. For instance, probably due to its more complex administration and scoring procedures, there are few studies that have used the LEAS with brain-injured subjects.

Emotional awareness is a hierarchical process that ultimately has a decisive impact on complex patterns of social interaction and personal fulfillment. It is not surprising that disruption of this process affects psychosocial adjustment and medical outcomes. For example, the impulsivity and lack of empathy frequently observed among TBI patients have a deleterious effect on their social functioning and quality of life. In addition, it is conceivable that the increased autonomic reactivity that can be observed in alexithymic patients may be associated with increased cardiovascular morbidity among stroke patients.

Future studies should contemplate the longitudinal assessment of alexithymic features in order to determine whether alexithymia and the level of emotional awareness are significant predictive factors of recovery and quality of life among patients with brain injury.

References

Adolphs, R., Damasio, H., Tranel, D., Cooper, G., & Damasio, A. R. (2000). A role for somatosensory cortices in the visual recognition of emotion as revealed by three-dimensional lesion mapping. *Journal of Neuroscience, 20*(7), 2683–2690.

Alford, B. A., & Beck, A. T. (1994). Cognitive therapy of delusional beliefs. *Behaviour Research & Therapy, 32*(3), 369–380.

Anderson, A. K., & Phelps, E. A. (2002). Is the human amygdala critical for the subjective experience of emotion? Evidence of intact dispositional affect in patients with amygdala lesions. *Journal of Cognitive Neuroscience, 14*(5), 709–720.

Andreasen, N. C., Rajarethinam, R., Cizadlo, T., Arndt, S., Swayze, V. W., II, Flashman, L. A., et al. (1996). Automatic atlas-based volume estimation of human brain regions from MR images. *Journal of Computer Assisted Tomography, 20*, 98–106.

Apfel, R. J., & Sifneos, P. E. (1979). Alexithymia: Concept and measurement. *Psychotherapy and Psychosomatics, 32*(1–4), 180–190.

Bagby, R. M., Parker, J. D., & Taylor, G. J. (1994). The twenty-item Toronto Alexithymia Scale—I. Item selection and cross-validation of the factor structure. *Journal of Psychosomatic Research, 38*(1), 23–32.

Bagby, R. M., Taylor, G. J., & Parker, J. D. (1994). The Twenty-item Toronto Alexithymia Scale—II. Convergent, discriminant, and concurrent validity. *Journal of Psychosomatic Research, 38*(1), 33–40.

Bechara, A., Damasio, H., Tranel, D., & Damasio, A. R. (1997). Deciding advantageously before knowing the advantageous strategy. *Science, 275*(5304), 1293–1295.

Bechara, A., Damasio, H., Tranel, D., & Damasio, A. R. (2005). The Iowa Gambling Task and the somatic marker hypothesis: Some questions and answers. *Trends in Cognitive Science, 9*(4), 159–162; discussion 162–154.

Benton, A. L., Hamsher, K., & Sivan, A. B. (1994). *Multilingual aphasia examination.* Iowa City, IA: AJA Associates.

Berrios, G. E. (1996). *The history of mental symptoms: Descriptive psychopathology since the nineteenth century.* Cambridge, England: Cambridge University Press.

Bisiach, E., Vallar, G., Perani, D., Papagno, C., & Berti, A. (1986). Unawareness of disease following lesions of the right hemisphere: Anosognosia for hemiplegia and anosognosia for hemianopia. *Neuropsychologia, 24*(4), 471–482.

Blonder, L. X., Heilman, K. M., Ketterson, T., Rosenbek, J., Raymer, A., Crosson, B., et al. (2005). Affective facial and lexical expression in aprosodic versus aphasic stroke patients. *Journal of the International Neuropsychological Society, 11*(6), 677–685.

Bloom, R. L., Borod, J. C., Obler, L. K., & Gerstman, L. J. (1992). Impact of emotional content on discourse production in patients with unilateral brain damage. *Brain and Language, 42*(2), 153–164.

Boake, C., Freeland, J. C., Ringholz, G. M., Nance, M. L., & Edwards, K. E. (1995). Awareness of memory loss after severe closed-head injury. *Brain Injury, 9*(3), 273–283.

Borod, J. C., Rorie, K. D., Haywood, C. S., Andelman, F., Obler, L. K., Welkowitz, J., et al. (1996). Hemispheric specialization for discourse reports of emotional experiences: Relationships to demographic, neurological, and perceptual variables. *Neuropsychologia, 34*(5), 351–359.

Borod, J. C., Rorie, K. D., Pick, L. H., Bloom, R. L., Andelman, F., Campbell, A. L., et al. (2000). Verbal pragmatics following unilateral stroke: Emotional content and valence. *Neuropsychology, 14*(1), 112–124.

Botvinick, M., Nystrom, L. E., Fissell, K., Carter, C. S., & Cohen, J. D. (1999). Conflict monitoring versus selection-for-action in anterior cingulate cortex. *Nature, 402* (6758), 179–181.

Brown, J. W., & Braver, T. S. (2005). Learned predictions of error likelihood in the anterior cingulate cortex. *Science, 307*(5712), 1118–1121.

Bush, G., Vogt, B. A., Holmes, J., Dale, A. M., Greve, D., Jenike, M. A., et al. (2002). Dorsal anterior cingulate cortex: A role in reward-based decision making. *Proceedings of the National Academy of Sciences USA, 99*(1), 523–528.

Carter, C. S., Braver, T. S., Barch, D. M., Botvinick, M. M., Noll, D., & Cohen, J. D. (1998). Anterior cingulate cortex, error detection, and the online monitoring of performance. *Science, 280*(5364), 747–749.

Creswell, J. D., Way, B. M., Eisenberger, N. I., & Lieberman, M. D. (2007). Neural correlates of dispositional mindfulness during affect labeling. *Psychosomatic Medicine, 69*(6), 560–565.

Critchley, H. D. (2005). Neural mechanisms of autonomic, affective, and cognitive integration. *Journal of Comparative Neurology, 493*(1), 154–166.

Critchley, H. D., Wiens, S., Rotshtein, P., Ohman, A., & Dolan, R. J. (2004). Neural systems supporting interoceptive awareness. *Nature Neuroscience, 7*(2), 189–195.

Damasio, A. (2003). Feelings of emotion and the self. *Annals of the New York Academy of Sciences, 1001*, 253–261.

Damasio, A. R. (1996). The somatic marker hypothesis and the possible functions of the prefrontal cortex. *Philosophical Transactions of the Royal Society of London B Biological Sciences, 351*(1346), 1413–1420.

D'Argembeau, A., Ruby, P., Collette, F., Degueldre, C., Balteau, E., Luxen, A., et al. (2007). Distinct regions of the medial prefrontal cortex are associated with self-referential processing and perspective taking. *Journal of Cognitive Neuroscience, 19* (6), 935–944.

de Timary, P., Luts, A., Hers, D., & Luminet, O. (2008). Absolute and relative stability of alexithymia in alcoholic inpatients undergoing alcohol withdrawal: Relationship to depression and anxiety. *Psychiatry Research, 157*(1–3), 105–113.

Doron, N. N., & Ledoux, J. E. (1999). Organization of projections to the lateral amygdala from auditory and visual areas of the thalamus in the rat. *Journal of Comparative Neurology, 412*(3), 383–409.

Doyere, V., Debiec, J., Monfils, M. H., Schafe, G. E., & LeDoux, J. E. (2007). Synapse-specific reconsolidation of distinct fear memories in the lateral amygdala. *Nature Neuroscience, 10*(4), 414–416.

Drevets, W. C. (1999). Prefrontal cortical-amygdalar metabolism in major depression. *Annals of the New York Academy of Sciences, 877,* 614–637.

Eslinger, P. J., Dennis, K., Moore, P., Antani, S., Hauck, R., & Grossman, M. (2005). Metacognitive deficits in frontotemporal dementia. *Journal of Neurology, Neurosurgery and Psychiatry, 76*(12), 1630–1635.

Evren, C., & Evren, B. (2005). Self-mutilation in substance-dependent patients and relationship with childhood abuse and neglect, alexithymia and temperament and character dimensions of personality. *Drug and Alcohol Dependence, 80*(1), 15–22.

Evren, C., Sar, V., Evren, B., Semiz, U., Dalbudak, E., & Cakmak, D. (2008). Dissociation and alexithymia among men with alcoholism. *Psychiatry and Clinical Neurosciences, 62*(1), 40–47.

Folstein, M. F., Folstein, S. E., & McHugh, P. R. (1975). Mini-Mental State: A practical method for grading the cognitive state of patients for the clinician. *Journal of Psychiatric Research, 12,* 189–198.

Forer, S., & Granger, C. V. (1987). *Functional independence measure.* Buffalo, NY: The Buffalo General Hospital State University of New York at Buffalo.

Frankland, P. W., Bontempi, B., Talton, L. E., Kaczmarek, L., & Silva, A. J. (2004). The involvement of the anterior cingulate cortex in remote contextual fear memory. *Science, 304*(5672), 881–883.

Freud, S., & Brill, A. A. (1938). *The basic writings of Sigmund Freud.* Translated and edited, with an introduction, by A. A. Brill. New York: Modern Library.

Frewen, P., Lane, R. D., Neufeld, R. W., Densmore, M., Stevens, T., & Lanius, R. (2008). Neural correlates of levels of emotional awareness during trauma script-imagery in posttraumatic stress disorder. *Psychosomatic Medicine, 70*(1), 27–31.

Frewen, P. A., Pain, C., Dozois, D. J., & Lanius, R. A. (2006). Alexithymia in PTSD: Psychometric and FMRI studies. *Annals of the New York Academy of Sciences, 1071,* 397–400.

Friedman, P. J. (1990). Spatial neglect in acute stroke: The line bisection test. *Scandinavian Journal of Rehabilitative Medicine, 22*(2), 101–106.

Giacino, J. T., & Cicerone, K. D. (1998). Varieties of deficit unawareness after brain injury. *Journal of Head Trauma Rehabilitation, 13*(5), 1–15.

Golden, C. J. (1978). *Stroop color and word test.* Chicago: Stoelting.

Guttman, H., & Laporte, L. (2002). Alexithymia, empathy, and psychological symptoms in a family context. *Comprehensive Psychiatry, 43*(6), 448–455.

Hamilton, M. (1959). The assessment of anxiety states by rating. *British Journal of Medical Psychology, 32*(1), 50–55.

Hamilton, M. A. (1960). A rating scale for depression. *Journal of Neurology, Neurosurgery, and Psychiatry, 23,* 56–62.

Heaton, R. K., Chelune, G. J., & Tailey, J. L. (1993). *The Wisconsin Card Sorting Test.* Odessa, FL: Psychological Assessment Resources.

Heilman, K. M., Barrett, A. M., & Adair, J. C. (1998). Possible mechanisms of anosognosia: A defect in self-awareness. *Philosophical Transactions of the Royal Society of London B Biological Sciences, 353*(1377), 1903–1909.

Heilman, K. M., Leon, S. A., & Rosenbek, J. C. (2004). Affective aprosodia from a medial frontal stroke. *Brain and Language, 89*(3), 411–416.

Henry, J. D., Phillips, L. H., Crawford, J. R., Theodorou, G., & Summers, F. (2006). Cognitive and psychosocial correlates of alexithymia following traumatic brain injury. *Neuropsychologia, 44*(1), 62–72.

Honkalampi, K., Hintikka, J., Saarinen, P., Lehtonen, J., & Viinamaki, H. (2000). Is alexithymia a permanent feature in depressed patients? Results from a 6-month follow-up study. *Psychotherapy and Psychosomatics, 69*(6), 303–308.

Hoofien, D., Gilboa, A., Vakil, E., & Barak, O. (2004). Unawareness of cognitive deficits and daily functioning among persons with traumatic brain injuries. *Journal of Clinical and Experimental Neuropsychology, 26*(2), 278–290.

Hoth, K. F., Paulsen, J. S., Moser, D. J., Tranel, D., Clark, L. A., & Bechara, A. (2007). Patients with Huntington's disease have impaired awareness of cognitive, emotional, and functional abilities. *Journal of Clinical and Experimental Neuropsychology, 29*(4), 365–376.

James, W. (1890). *The principles of psychology.* Vols 1 and 2. New York: Dover. Republished (1952). Chicago: Encyclopaedia Britannica.

Jorge, R. E. (2005). Neuropsychiatric consequences of traumatic brain injury: A review of recent findings. *Current Opinion in Psychiatry, 18*(3), 289–299.

Jorge, R. E., Robinson, R. G., Moser, D., Tateno, A., Crespo-Facorro, B., & Arndt, S. (2004). Major depression following traumatic brain injury. *Archives of General Psychiatry, 61*(1), 42–50.

Jorge, R. E., Starkstein, S. E., Arndt, S., Moser, D., Crespo-Facorro, B., & Robinson, R. G. (2005). Alcohol misuse and mood disorders following traumatic brain injury. *Archives of General Psychiatry, 62*(7), 742–749.

Kalisch, R., Wiech, K., Critchley, H. D., & Dolan, R. J. (2006). Levels of appraisal: A medial prefrontal role in high-level appraisal of emotional material. *NeuroImage, 30*(4), 1458–1466.

Kawasaki, H., Adolphs, R., Oya, H., Kovach, C., Damasio, H., Kaufman, O., et al. (2005). Analysis of single-unit responses to emotional scenes in human ventromedial prefrontal cortex. *Journal of Cognitive Neuroscience, 17*(10), 1509–1518.

Kerns, J. G., Cohen, J. D., MacDonald, A. W., III, Cho, R. Y., Stenger, V. A., & Carter, C. S. (2004). Anterior cingulate conflict monitoring and adjustments in control. *Science, 303*(5660), 1023–1026.

Koponen, S., Taiminen, T., Honkalampi, K., Joukamaa, M., Viinamaki, H., Kurki, T., et al. (2005). Alexithymia after traumatic brain injury: Its relation to magnetic resonance imaging findings and psychiatric disorders. *Psychosomatic Medicine, 67*(5), 807–812.

Kupchik, M., Strous, R. D., Erez, R., Gonen, N., Weizman, A., & Spivak, B. (2007). Demographic and clinical characteristics of motor vehicle accident victims in the community general health outpatient clinic: A comparison of PTSD and non-PTSD subjects. *Depression and Anxiety, 24*(4), 244–250.

Lane, R. D. (2008). Neural substrates of implicit and explicit emotional processes: A unifying framework for psychosomatic medicine. *Psychosomatic Medicine, 70*(2), 214–231.

Lane, R. D., Ahern, G. L., Schwartz, G. E., & Kaszniak, A. W. (1997). Is alexithymia the emotional equivalent of blindsight? *Biological Psychiatry, 42*(9), 834–844.

Lane, R. D., Quinlan, D. M., Schwartz, G. E., Walker, P. A., & Zeitlin, S. B. (1990). The Levels of Emotional Awareness Scale: A cognitive-developmental measure of emotion. *Journal of Personality Assessment, 55*(1–2), 124–134.

Lane, R. D., Reiman, E. M., Axelrod, B., Yun, L. S., Holmes, A., & Schwartz, G. E. (1998). Neural correlates of levels of emotional awareness. Evidence of an interaction between emotion and attention in the anterior cingulate cortex. *Journal of Cognitive Neuroscience, 10*(4), 525–535.

Leon, S. A., Rosenbek, J. C., Crucian, G. P., Hieber, B., Holiway, B., Rodriguez, A. D., et al. (2005). Active treatments for aprosodia secondary to right hemisphere stroke. *Journal of Rehabilitation Research and Development, 42*(1), 93–101.

Levine, D., Marziali, E., & Hood, J. (1997). Emotion processing in borderline personality disorders. *Journal of Nervous and Mental Disease, 185*(4), 240–246.

Levine, D. N., Calvanio, R., & Rinn, W. E. (1991). The pathogenesis of anosognosia for hemiplegia. *Neurology, 41*(11), 1770–1781.

Lieberman, M. D., Eisenberger, N. I., Crockett, M. J., Tom, S. M., Pfeifer, J. H., & Way, B. M. (2007). Putting feelings into words: Affect labeling disrupts amygdala activity in response to affective stimuli. *Psychological Sciences, 18*(5), 421–428.

Loas, G., Dhee-Perot, P., Chaperot, C., Fremaux, D., Gayant, C., & Boyer, P. (1998). Anhedonia, alexithymia and locus of control in unipolar major depressive disorders. *Psychopathology, 31*(4), 206–212.

Loas, G., Otmani, O., Lecercle, C., & Jouvent, R. (2000). Relationships between the emotional and cognitive components of alexithymia and dependency in alcoholics. *Psychiatry Research, 96*(1), 63–74.

Luminet, O., Bagby, R. M., Wagner, H., Taylor, G. J., & Parker, J. D. (1999). Relation between alexithymia and the five-factor model of personality: A facet-level analysis. *Journal of Personality Assessment, 73*(3), 345–358.

MacKenzie, E. J., Shapiro, S., & Eastham, J. N. (1985). The Abbreviated Injury Scale and Injury Severity Score. Levels of inter- and intrarater reliability. *Medical Care, 23*(6), 823–835.

MacLean, P. D. (1977). The triune brain in conflict. *Psychotherapy and Psychosomatics, 28*(1–4), 207–220.

MacLean, P. D. (1985). Brain evolution relating to family, play, and the separation call. *Archives of General Psychiatry, 42*(4), 405–417.

Magnotta, V., Heckel, D., Andreasen, N. C., Cizadlo, T., Westmoreland Corson, P., Ehrhardt, J., et al. (1999). Measurement of brain structures by artificial neural networks: Two-dimensional and three-dimensional applications. *Radiology, 211*, 781–790.

Magnotta, V. A., Harris, G., Andreasen, N. C., O'Leary, D. S., Yuh, W. T., & Heckel, D. (2002). Structural MR image processing using the BRAINS2 toolbox. *Computerized Medical Imaging and Graphics, 26*(4), 251–264.

Marchesi, C., Bertoni, S., Cantoni, A., & Maggini, C. (2008). Is alexithymia a personality trait increasing the risk of depression? A prospective study evaluating alexithymia before, during and after a depressive episode. *Psychological Medicine*, 1–6.

Marchesi, C., Brusamonti, E., & Maggini, C. (2000). Are alexithymia, depression, and anxiety distinct constructs in affective disorders? *Journal of Psychosomatic Research, 49*(1), 43–49.

Markova, I. S., & Berrios, G. E. (1995). Insight in clinical psychiatry revisited. *Comprehensive Psychiatry, 36*(5), 367–376.

Markova, I. S., Clare, L., Wang, M., Romero, B., & Kenny, G. (2005). Awareness in dementia: Conceptual issues. *Aging and Mental Health, 9*(5), 386–393.

Mayberg, H. S., Brannan, S. K., Mahurin, R. K., Jerabek, P. A., Brickman, J. S., Tekell, J. L., et al. (1997). Cingulate function in depression: A potential predictor of treatment response. *Neuroreport, 8*(4), 1057–1061.

Mayberg, H. S., Liotti, M., Brannan, S. K., McGinnis, S., Mahurin, R. K., Jerabek, P. A., et al. (1999). Reciprocal limbic-cortical function and negative mood: Converging PET findings in depression and normal sadness. *American Journal of Psychiatry, 156*(5), 675–682.

McCormick, L. M., Ziebell, S., Nopoulos, P., Cassell, M., Andreasen, N. C., & Brumm, M. (2006). Anterior cingulate cortex: An MRI-based parcellation method. *NeuroImage, 32*(3), 1167–1175.

McGlynn, S. M., & Schacter, D. L. (1989). Unawareness of deficits in neuropsychological syndromes. *Journal of Clinical and Experimental Neuropsychology, 11*(2), 143–205.

McRae, K., Reiman, E. M., Fort, C. L., Chen, K., & Lane, R. D. (2008). Association between trait emotional awareness and dorsal anterior cingulate activity during emotion is arousal-dependent. *NeuroImage, 41*(2), 648–655.

Mesulam, M. M., & Mufson, E. J. (1982). Insula of the old world monkey. III: Efferent cortical output and comments on function. *Journal of Comparative Neurology, 212*(1), 38–52.

Moran, J. M., Macrae, C. N., Heatherton, T. F., Wyland, C. L., & Kelley, W. M. (2006). Neuroanatomical evidence for distinct cognitive and affective components of self. *Journal of Cognitive Neuroscience, 18*(9), 1586–1594.

Ochsner, K. N., Knierim, K., Ludlow, D. H., Hanelin, J., Ramachandran, T., Glover, G., et al. (2004). Reflecting upon feelings: An fMRI study of neural systems supporting the attribution of emotion to self and other. *Journal of Cognitive Neuroscience, 16*(10), 1746–1772.

Orfei, M. D., Robinson, R. G., Prigatano, G. P., Starkstein, S., Rusch, N., Bria, P., et al. (2007). Anosognosia for hemiplegia after stroke is a multifaceted phenomenon: A systematic review of the literature. *Brain, 130*(Pt 12), 3075–3090.

Parker, J. D., Taylor, G. J., & Bagby, R. M. (1993). Alexithymia and the recognition of facial expressions of emotion. *Psychotherapy and Psychosomatics, 59*(3–4), 197–202.

Parker, J. D., Taylor, G. J., Bagby, R. M., & Thomas, S. (1991). Problems with measuring alexithymia. *Psychosomatics, 32*(2), 196–202.

Phelps, E. A., Delgado, M. R., Nearing, K. I., & LeDoux, J. E. (2004). Extinction learning in humans: Role of the amygdala and vmPFC. *Neuron, 43*(6), 897–905.

Phelps, E. A., & LeDoux, J. E. (2005). Contributions of the amygdala to emotion processing: from animal models to human behavior. *Neuron, 48*(2), 175–187.

Prigatano, G. P., & Schacter, D. L. (Eds.) (1991). *Awareness of deficit after brain injury: Clinical and theoretical issues.* New York: Oxford University Press.

Ramachandran, V. S. (1996). The evolutionary biology of self-deception, laughter, dreaming and depression: Some clues from anosognosia. *Medical Hypotheses, 47*(5), 347–362.

Reitan, R. M. (1971). Trail making test results for normal and brain-damaged children. *Perceptual Motor Skills, 33*(2), 575–581.

Rey, A. (1964). *L'examine clinique en psychologie.* Paris: Presses Universitaires de France.

Roedema, T. M., & Simons, R. F. (1999). Emotion-processing deficit in alexithymia. *Psychophysiology, 36*(3), 379–387.

Rogan, M. T., Staubli, U. V., & LeDoux, J. E. (1997). Fear conditioning induces associative long-term potentiation in the amygdala. *Nature, 390*(6660), 604–607.

Ross, E. D., Harney, J. H., deLacoste-Utamsing, C., & Purdy, P. D. (1981). How the brain integrates affective and propositional language into a unified behavioral function. Hypothesis based on clinicoanatomic evidence. *Archives of Neurology, 38*(12), 745–748.

Ross, E. D., Thompson, R. D., & Yenkosky, J. (1997). Lateralization of affective prosody in brain and the callosal integration of hemispheric language functions. *Brain and Language, 56*(1), 27–54.

Ruby, P., Schmidt, C., Hogge, M., D'Argembeau, A., Collette, F., & Salmon, E. (2007). Social mind representation: Where does it fail in frontotemporal dementia? *Journal of Cognitive Neuroscience, 19*(4), 671–683.

Russell, J. A. (2003). Core affect and the psychological construction of emotion. *Psychological Review, 110*(1), 145–172.

Saarijarvi, S., Salminen, J. K., & Toikka, T. (2006). Temporal stability of alexithymia over a five-year period in outpatients with major depression. *Psychotherapy and Psychosomatics, 75*(2), 107–112.

Salmon, E., Perani, D., Collette, F., Feyers, D., Kalbe, E., Holthoff, V., et al. (2008). A comparison of unawareness in frontotemporal dementia and Alzheimer's disease. *Journal of Neurology, Neurosurgery, and Psychiatry, 79*(2), 176–179.

Sayar, K., Ebrinc, S., & Ak, I. (2001). Alexithymia in patients with antisocial personality disorder in a military hospital setting. *Israel Journal of Psychiatry and Related Sciences, 38*(2), 81–87.

Schacter, D. L. (1990). Toward a cognitive neuropsychology of awareness: Implicit knowledge and anosognosia. *Journal of Clinical and Experimental Neuropsychology, 12*(1), 155–178.

Schafer, R., Popp, K., Jorgens, S., Lindenberg, R., Franz, M., & Seitz, R. J. (2007). Alexithymia-like disorder in right anterior cingulate infarction. *Neurocase, 13*(3), 201–208.

Sharot, T., Riccardi, A. M., Raio, C. M., & Phelps, E. A. (2007). Neural mechanisms mediating optimism bias. *Nature, 450*(7166), 102–105.

Sifneos, P. E. (1973). The prevalence of "alexithymic" characteristics in psychosomatic patients. *Psychotherapy and Psychosomatics, 22*(2), 255–262.

Sifneos, P. E. (1996). Alexithymia: Past and present. *American Journal of Psychiatry, 153* (7 Suppl.), 137–142.

Silver, J. M., & Yudofsky, S. C. (1991). The Overt Aggression Scale: Overview and guiding principles. *Journal of Neuropsychiatry and Clinical Neurosciences, 3*(2), S22–29.

Souchay, C. (2007). Metamemory in Alzheimer's disease. *Cortex, 43*(7), 987–1003.

Spalletta, G., Pasini, A., Costa, A., De Angelis, D., Ramundo, N., Paolucci, S., et al. (2001). Alexithymic features in stroke: Effects of laterality and gender. *Psychosomatic Medicine, 63*(6), 944–950.

Spalletta, G., Ripa, A., Bria, P., Caltagirone, C., & Robinson, R. G. (2006). Response of emotional unawareness after stroke to antidepressant treatment. *American Journal of Geriatric Psychiatry, 14*(3), 220–227.

Spalletta, G., Serra, L., Fadda, L., Ripa, A., Bria, P., & Caltagirone, C. (2007). Unawareness of motor impairment and emotions in right hemispheric stroke: A preliminary investigation. *International Journal of Geriatric Psychiatry, 22*(12), 1241–1246.

Speranza, M., Corcos, M., Stephan, P., Loas, G., Perez-Diaz, F., Lang, F., et al. (2004). Alexithymia, depressive experiences, and dependency in addictive disorders. *Substance Use and Misuse, 39*(4), 551–579.

Spreng, R. N., Mar, R. A., & Kim, A. S. (2008). The common neural basis of autobiographical memory, prospection, navigation, theory of mind and the default mode: A quantitative meta-analysis. *Journal of Cognitive Neuroscience, 21*(3), 489–510.

Starkstein, S. E., Berthier, M. L., Fedoroff, P., Price, T. R., & Robinson, R. G. (1990). Anosognosia and major depression in two patients with cerebrovascular lesions. *Neurology, 40*(9), 1380–1382.

Starkstein, S. E., Sabe, L., Vazquez, S., Teson, A., Petracca, G., Chemerinski, E., et al. (1996). Neuropsychological, psychiatric, and cerebral blood flow findings in vascular dementia and Alzheimer's disease. *Stroke, 27*(3), 408–414.

Starr, L. B., Robinson, R. G., & Price, T. R. (1983). Reliability, validity, and clinical utility of the social functioning exam in the assessment of stroke patients. *Experimental Aging Research, 9*(2), 101–106.

Sturman, E. D., & Sproule, B. A. (2003). Toward the development of a Mood Disorders Insight Scale: Modification of Birchwood's Psychosis Insight Scale. *Journal of Affective Disorders, 77*(1), 21–30.

Subic-Wrana, C., Bruder, S., Thomas, W., Lane, R. D., & Kohle, K. (2005). Emotional awareness deficits in inpatients of a psychosomatic ward: A comparison of two different measures of alexithymia. *Psychosomatic Medicine, 67*(3), 483–489.

Tabibnia, G., Lieberman, M. D., & Craske, M. G. (2008). The lasting effect of words on feelings: Words may facilitate exposure effects to threatening images. *Emotion, 8*(3), 307–317.

Taylor, G. J., & Bagby, R. M. (2004). New trends in alexithymia research. *Psychotherapy and Psychosomatics, 73*(2), 68–77.

Taylor, G. J., Bagby, R. M., & Parker, J. D. (1991). The alexithymia construct. A potential paradigm for psychosomatic medicine. *Psychosomatics, 32*(2), 153–164.

Taylor, G. J., Bagby, R. M., & Parker, J. D. (1993). Alexithymia—State and trait. *Psychotherapy and Psychosomatics, 60*(3–4), 211–214.

Taylor, G. J., Bagby, R. M., & Parker, J. D. (2003). The 20-Item Toronto Alexithymia Scale. IV. Reliability and factorial validity in different languages and cultures. *Journal of Psychosomatic Research, 55*(3), 277–283.

Taylor, G. J., Parker, J. D., Bagby, R. M., & Bourke, M. P. (1996). Relationships between alexithymia and psychological characteristics associated with eating disorders. *Journal of Psychosomatic Research, 41*(6), 561–568.

Teasdale, G., & Jennett, B. (1976). Assessment and prognosis of coma after head injury. *Acta Neurochirurgica (Wien), 34*(1–4), 45–55.

TenHouten, W. D., Hoppe, K. D., Bogen, J. E., & Walter, D. O. (1986). Alexithymia: An experimental study of cerebral commissurotomy patients and normal control subjects. *American Journal of Psychiatry, 143*(3), 312–316.

Tucker, D. M., Watson, R. T., & Heilman, K. M. (1977). Discrimination and evocation of affectively intoned speech in patients with right parietal disease. *Neurology, 27*(10), 947–950.

Wang, J., Rao, H., Wetmore, G. S., Furlan, P. M., Korczykowski, M., Dinges, D. F., et al. (2005). Perfusion functional MRI reveals cerebral blood flow pattern under psychological stress. *Proceedings of the National Academy of Sciences USA, 102*(49), 17804–17809.

Weinryb, R. M., Gustavsson, J. P., Asberg, M., & Rossel, R. J. (1992). The concept of alexithymia: An empirical study using psychodynamic ratings and self-reports. *Acta Psychiatrica Scandinavica, 85*(2), 153–162.

Williams, J. B., Gibbon, M., First, M. B., Spitzer, R. L., Davies, M., Borus, J., et al. (1992). The Structured Clinical Interview for DSM-III-R (SCID). II. Multisite test-retest reliability. *Archives of General Psychiatry, 49*(8), 630–636.

Williams, K. R., Galas, J., Light, D., Pepper, C., Ryan, C., Kleinmann, A. E., et al. (2001). Head injury and alexithymia: Implications for family practice care. *Brain Injury, 15*(4), 349–356.

Wittgenstein, L., & Anscombe, G. E. M. (1953). *Philosophical investigations: The German text, with a revised English translation* (3rd edition). Malden, MA,: Blackwell.

Wood, R. L., & Williams, C. (2007). Neuropsychological correlates of organic alexithymia. *Journal of the International Neuropsychological Society, 13*(3), 471–479.

Yamasaki, H., LaBar, K. S., & McCarthy, G. (2002). Dissociable prefrontal brain systems for attention and emotion. *Proceedings of the National Academy of Sciences USA, 99*(17), 11447–11451.

Yehuda, R., Steiner, A., Kahana, B., Binder-Brynes, K., Southwick, S. M., Zemelman, S., et al. (1997). Alexithymia in Holocaust survivors with and without PTSD. *Journal of Traumatic Stress, 10*(1), 93–100.

V

Anosognosia and Hysteria

17

Neuroanatomy of Impaired Body Awareness in Anosognosia and Hysteria: A Multicomponent Account

Roland Vocat and Patrik Vuilleumier

What is more disconcerting than someone who cannot move his arm and/or leg but is unaware of this deficit? Or someone who can move and walk normally but is nevertheless convinced of being paralyzed? How would it be possible to remain ignorant of one's own body state?

These questions have puzzled physicians and neurologists for more than a hundred years, and still remain a matter of debate. Both of these perplexing conditions have been commonly observed in medical practice for many centuries, and they are still frequent nowadays, respectively called *anosognosia* and *hysterical conversion* in our modern clinical terminology. Yet the underlying mental and physiological mechanisms of such impairments in bodily awareness are far from being understood.

The phenomenon of anosognosia occurs in patients with cerebral injuries such as stroke, most often involving the right hemisphere. In this condition, a severe neurological deficit, like hemianopia or hemiplegia, is not recognized by the patient, even after direct confrontation. The most common manifestation of anosognosia is anosognosia for hemiplegia (AHP), in spite of the fact that paralysis can be easily demonstrated to the patient and has profound consequences for his or her everyday life. However, anosognosia can affect other neurological domains, such as memory, blindness, aphasia, and so forth (see other chapters in this volume). Since the original description by Babinski (1914), it is well recognized that this neuropsychological syndrome cannot be simply explained by a general cognitive decline or dementia, but results from specific losses in sensorimotor awareness.

By contrast, hysterical conversion is in many ways a mirror condition, in which the patients experience a deficit of motor, sensory, or cognitive functions without any organic neurological damage, and without intentionally feigning it. Like anosognosia, patients with hysterical conversion frequently present with a weakness or paralysis of one or several limbs, but other common deficits may involve memory, vision, or language disturbances. This phenomenon was extensively studied by pioneer neurologists in the nineteenth century, including Babinski himself (Babinski & Dagnan-Bouveret, 1912) and his master Charcot (1892), but it then became essentially attributed to unconscious psychiatric factors following the work of Janet (1887, 1889, 1911) and Freud (Freud & Breuer, 1895).

In this chapter, we will review recent studies that investigated these two conditions using neuropsychological measures, as well as structural and functional brain imaging techniques. We will first describe data concerning anosognosia and then turn to hysterical conversion. Finally, we will consider whether similar mechanisms might be involved in both cases, and we will highlight the notion that distinct neural pathways are likely to contribute to different distortions of awareness for one's own bodily state.

Anosognosia for Hemiplegia

Anosognosia for hemiplegia (AHP) involves a failure to acknowledge a paralysis after brain damage (see Bottini et al., Chapter 2; Kranath & Baier, Chapter 3; and Heilman & Harciarek, Chapter 5, this volume), but the clinical manifestation of this phenomenon may take many different forms. Indeed, one of the most typical features of anosognosia is certainly its variability. It is likely that different types or different components of AHP might exist and show various expressions in different patients (see Marcel, Tegner, & Nimmo-Smith, 2004; for a review, see Vuilleumier, 2004).

First of all, anosognosia is often fluctuating in time. Patients may answer the same question about a particular function differently at different moments. Secondly, a lack of explicit report of the deficit is sometimes associated with discrepant remarks (e.g., "My arm is tired today") or behaviors (e.g., accepting to stay in bed) that suggest the existence of some acceptance or some implicit knowledge of the deficit. Thirdly, the default in awareness may concern different aspects of a deficit: its presence or its nature (e.g., "No, I am not paralyzed"), its cause (e.g., "I am in the hospital because I got a cold"), its consequences for a particular action (e.g., "my arm is weak but I am able to open this bottle"), or for the patient's everyday life (e.g. "I have to go back home because next Monday I have to go to work"), as well as the necessary adjustments (e.g. "At home, I will be able to dress and take a shower on my own"). These different domains are usually not affected at the same level. Finally, different deficits in the same patient can show different levels of awareness. Thus, anosognosia may be selective for a particular modality (e.g., a patient is anosognosic for his hemianopia but not his plegia or vice versa) and sometimes even more selective in a given modality (e.g., a patient is anosognosic for the plegia of his arm but not his leg).

These multiple manifestations of anosognosia make its characterization and measurement difficult. No standard comprehensive scale has been developed to take into account this whole complexity. Hence, anosognosia is often estimated along one particular dimension only, such as the severity of unawareness in relation to varying degrees of confrontation with the deficit (direct or indirect). For hemiplegia, the most commonly used scale is the four-level questionnaire developed by Bisiach, Perani, Vallar, and Berti (1986), which probes for an explicit verbal acknowledgment of the motor impairment. This scale grades the severity of AHP as a function of whether plegia is reported after a general question about health, after a specific question about the arm, after a motor confrontation or if it is not reported. Other questionnaires (Cutting, 1978; Feinberg, Roane, & Ali, 2000) also assess the existence of related phenomena such as somesthesic illusions or somatoparaphrenias, but in a purely descriptive and itemized manner rather than according to a systematic classification scheme (for review of assessment methods, see Orfei et al., 2007; Vuilleumier, 2000).

Frequency and Evolution

Anosognosia for hemiplegia is essentially an acute phenomenon that most often disappears within a few weeks after acute brain injury. A meta-analysis by Baier and Karnath (2005) noted that it was found in 10%–18% of stroke patients with hemiparesis. In a recent study conducted by our group (Vocat et al., in preparation), we found that among 58 right-hemispheric strokes with hemiplegia, one-third were associated with unawareness of the motor deficit when patients were examined 3 days after the stroke. One week post-stroke, one-fifth of the patients were still anosognosics, while this number decreased to 5% half a year later (see Figure 17.1). Hence, only in rare cases, anosognosia may persist beyond the acute phase and even become chronic.

In our study, we also asked patients to describe their awareness for the onset of their symptoms and their emotional reaction at this time. Answers to this question revealed that even some patients who were nosognosic 3 days after stroke during our examination could not report precisely nor lateralize their symptoms at onset, or showed an inappropriate emotional reaction. Thus, at this very early stage (a few hours after the stroke), two-thirds of the patients could presumably be classified as anosognosic. Moreover, this percentage is certainly underestimated, as patients had the opportunity to modify their initial memory according to the report of doctors or relatives. These observations suggest that anosognosia may not be an extraordinary state in such conditions, but a rather "normal" or at least typical phase following sudden neurological change (especially when involving certain areas in the right hemisphere). After acute insults such as a stroke, the brain probably needs sufficient time and new information to

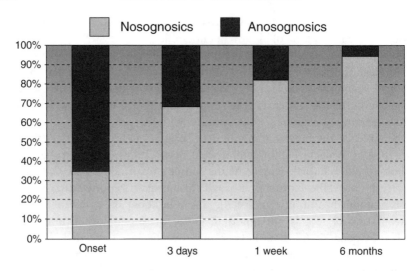

Figure 17.1 Evolution of awareness for motor deficits over time in our prospective study. The proportion of patients with/without AHP is shown for the day of stroke and then 3 days later, one week later, and 6 months later (n = 50, 50, 44 and 19 patients, respectively). Anosognosia at stroke onset is separated in two groups, reflecting either nosognosia or anosognosia, as estimated by the report from the patient (3 days post-stroke) concerning the installation of his neurological symptoms. For the three other periods, anosognosia was estimated according to the standard procedure of the Bisiach questionnaire (patients were considered as anosognosics with a Bisiach of 2 and 3 and nosognosics with a Bisiach of 0 and 1, as suggested by Baier & Karnath (2005)). The time-course indicates that anosognosia is essentially an acute phenomenon, concerning 2/3 of the patients at the stroke onset, but rapidly decreasing to 1/3 only three days later, and 1/5 one week later. After 6 months, severe anosognosia persists in a few rare cases.

adjust and reorganize itself. This period may therefore be particularly propitious for the emergence of anosognosia, while some unkown factors or specific deficits might lead to its persistence and cause related behavioral manifestations seen beyond the very acute stage.

   The consequences of anosognosia can be dramatic because it sometimes pre-vents the patients from looking for necessary treatments (or may delay emergency care such as thrombolysis). When these patients live alone at home, they can spend hours or days on the floor, without feeling the need to call for help or realizing the reason of their fall. Moreover, their anosognosia may even engender more danger and injury due to the patients trying to stand up and walk. Once hospitalized, another harmful consequence is the lack of participation in therapy (see Maeshima et al., 1997). As the patients believe that everything is fine, they sometimes see no utility to stay in the hospital and to participate in therapies (from drug treatment to physical therapy). Finally, a more general outcome of anosognosia is a lack of concern for new adjustments concerning their everyday life (work, family, house, etc.). Patients sometimes want to go on with their work and past activities, at the despair of their relatives. These unrealistic goals may even persist when patients appear more aware of the existence of physical deficits. Moreover, some patients may acknowledge their deficit but show no particular concern for it (anosodiaphoria). The social impact of these behaviors is also very important. All these consequences constitute well-known limitations for the treatment and recovery of stroke (Ownsworth & Clare, 2006; Ownsworth et al., 2007; Ownsworth & McKenna, 2004). Hence, a better understanding of the mechanisms of anosognosia and their clinical evolution are critical in order to act effectively upon them, so as to improve the management and rehabilitation of these patients.

Mechanisms and Comorbidity

Since the original description of AHP by Babinski (1914), more than 100 years of clinical research have highlighted both the regularities and oddities of this deficit, and several researchers have proposed a possible explanatory theory, yet there is still very little agreement on the exact neuropsychological mechanisms involved nor on their cerebral substrates. In fact, most of the existing theories have been counterattacked by clinical observations or inconsistencies arguing against them.

Many of the first attempts to understand anosognosia focused on the identification of a single cause for this phenomenon (see Table 17.1). Thus, among the most influential proposals, researchers have pointed to the possible role of a deficit in sensation or proprioception (Babinski, 1914), visuospatial neglect (Bisiach, Vallar, Perani, Papagno, & Berti, 1986), confabulations (Feinberg, 1997), memory impairments (Starkstein, Fedoroff, Price, Leiguarda, & Robinson, 1992), overestimation of self-performance and lack

Table 17.1 Summary of Classic Hypotheses on Anosognosia for Hemiplegia

Babinski (1914): sensory and/or proprioceptive feedback
Weinstein & Kahn (1955): denial and personality traits (e.g., perfectionism)
Bisiach et al. (1986): spatial or personal neglect/dyschiria
McGlynn & Schachter (1989): access to a specific conscious awareness system
Levine (1990): discovery theory (proprioception and cognitive impairment)
Heilman (1991): feedforward theory (motor initiation and preparation)
Starkstein et al. (1992): mental flexibility and memory abilities
Feinberg (1997): neglect and confabulation
Frith et al. (2000): deficit in comparing planned and executed action
Marcel et al. (2004): overestimation of self-performance and lack of mental flexibility
Vuilleumier (2004): ABC model (deficits in appreciation, beliefs, and checks)
Davies et al. (2005): two-factor theory (two deficits preventing the discovery)

of mental flexibility (Marcel et al., 2004), psychological defense mechanisms (Weinstein & Kahn, 1955), a default in the intentional planning of movement (Heilman, 1991), a failure to compare planned and executed action (Frith, Blakemore, & Wolpert, 2000; Vallar & Ronchi, 2006), or a disruption and/or disconnection of a specific module dedicated to motor awareness (McGlynn & Schacter, 1989).

However, none of these proposals has been found to be sufficient, by itself alone, to account for all the complex features of anosognosia. Hence, more recent models have proposed that AHP might result from a combination of different deficits, rather than from a single "core" deficit. For example, Levine proposed an interesting "discovery theory" (Levine, 1990), according to which anosognosia would appear when a deficit of proprioception or perception from a body part co-occurs with a global cognitive dysfunction that prevents a correct "inference" of the lack of function. A similar idea was proposed as an "ABC" model (Vuilleumier, 2004), where awareness relies on a set of neuropsychological functions mediating Appreciation, Belief, and Check processes. Thus, anosognosia might emerge due to various deficits affecting appreciation (due to different possible combinations of neurological and neuropsychological losses) together with deficits in other cognitive or affective functions necessary to change one's own beliefs and/or act upon signals of uncertainty. Importantly, in this perspective, anosognosia might represent a similar clinical endpoint caused by a constellation of distinct deficits, each of which having a different severity in different patients, but adding up to produce the same total effect. Likewise, more recently, Davies, Davies, and Coltheart (2005) proposed explicitly for the first time that anosognosia might emerge because of different "cocktails" of deficit. Thus, their two-factor theory asserts that a combination between a neuropsychological deficit (the first factor) along with a more general cognitive impairment (the second factor) can be sufficient to produce anosognosia. Nevertheless, the exact combination of factors necessary to produce AHP has not been directly demonstrated yet.

We recently conducted a large prospective study (Vocat et al., in preparation) in which we systematically looked at the neurological, neuropsychological, and psychological components associated with AHP, in a population of patients with a first acute right-hemisphere stroke. Among a series of 337 patients, 58 were recruited because of a significant unilateral motor weakness. Our assessment was made at three different time points: 3 days after stroke (hyperacute stage), 1 week later (post-acute stage), and 6 months later (chronic stage). Besides an assessment of AHP using the Bisiach scale (Bisiach, Vallar, Perani, Papagno, & Berti, 1986) and Feinberg questionnaire (Feinberg, Roane, & Ali, 2000), we tested for a wide range of neurological functions, including motor strength, sensation, proprioception, vision, and vigilance, as well as several neuropsychological domains such as perceptual and motor neglect, executive functions, memory, orientation, global cognitive functioning, and self-evaluation of both motor and cognitive tasks (Marcel et al., 2004), plus psychological variables such as mood, anxiety, irritability, and optimism. To take into account the different degrees of AHP and its fluctuations over time, we computed a single score of anosognosia based on the mean from two different evaluations on the Bisiach scale plus the Feinberg questionnaire (separated by intervening tests), for each of the assessments.

Our results (Vocat et al., in preparation) showed that, for the first two periods (at 3 days and 1 week), almost all neurological and neuropsychological tests were related to the severity of anosognosia. Hemianesthesia, impaired proprioception, reduced vigilance, hemianopia, visual and tactile extinction, spatiotemporal disorientation, visuospatial neglect, and poor anterograde memory were all found to show significant correlations with AHP. This pattern of data is consistent with the notion of a multifactorial disorder and the role of large brain lesions that are likely to disrupt several cognitive functions. There was no reliable correlation with the severity of motor weakness, or with "simple" frontal functions. A stepwise multiple regression analysis indicated that the degree of proprioceptive loss and extrapersonal spatial neglect were the strongest predictors of the severity of AHP. However, despite the frequent associations of some deficits, we could find several patients who showed a dissociation between the same deficits, including three who had AHP with severe neglect but no proprioceptive loss or vice versa, supporting the idea that AHP is not related to a unique set of deficits, but rather results from the sum of combined impairments whose relative severity may vary across patients (Vuilleumier, 2004).

Notably, our psychological testing (which attempts to assess depression, anxiety, anger, interest, optimism, etc.) failed to reveal any systematic association with AHP, for any of the testing periods. This result does not support the notion that premorbid personality factors or secondary affective reactions play a major role in the emergence of AHP.

Finally, we also examined the evolution over time of the different deficits, in relation to the evolution of AHP. We observed that anosognosia showed the same time course with a rapid decrease as the deficit of proprioception, visuospatial neglect, and temporospatial disorientation, between the hyperacute (3 days) and post-acute (1 week) stages. But at the final testing stage, 6 months after the stroke, only neuropsychological components were still linked with anosognosia, in particular visuospatial neglect, memory impairment, and temporospatial disorientation. Taken together, these results suggest that even if different combinations of neurological and neuropsychological deficits can be responsible for AHP, they may have a different impact on its persistence beyond the acute stage. While both neurological and neuropsychological impairments are involved in the emergence of AHP, the neuropsychological factors seem more determinant for chronic persistence.

Neuroanatomical Substrates

To understand the possible mechanisms underlying AHP, many researchers have tried to identify specific neuroanatomical correlates. Of course, such an approach necessarily implies that this syndrome is not purely due to some reactive psychological defense mechanisms, but represents a direct clinical manifestation of dysfunction in one or several brain regions.

In accord with this assumption, a first major anatomical characteristic of AHP is the hemispheric asymmetry that has been reported since the earliest descriptions of this phenomenon and has been subsequently observed by many investigators (see Heilman & Harciarek, Chapter 5, this volume). A greater frequency of both anosognosia and anosodiaphoria after right hemispheric stroke was already emphasized by Babinski himself (1914). More recently, experimental studies (Adair, Gilmore, Fennell, Gold, & Heilman, 1995; Breier et al., 1995; Gilmore, Heilman, Schmidt, Fennell, & Quisling, 1992; Lu et al., 1997; Lu et al., 2000) have used the Wada procedure in epileptic patients (i.e., injecting anesthetics such as amytal in one or the other hemisphere for presurgical testing of language laterality) and could thus confirm a relative dominance of the right hemisphere in the production of AHP during transient hemiplegia. In these studies, the limitations of testing due to language deficits after left hemispheric dysfunction could be overcome by preparing the patients before the injection of amytal so that they could expect the deficit and know how to communicate (via a nonverbal means) during the Wada test. This procedure allowed researchers to probe whether patients could acknowledge their paralysis, and also to obtain a verbal report following the complete remission of symptoms after the Wada test. The occurrence of AHP during the Wada test clearly demonstrates that a psychodynamic explanation of AHP is not sufficient, since patients know in advance about the temporary existence and provoked nature of their plegia but still deny it upon direct assessment.

Note however that even if this hemispheric asymmetry is well established, AHP can also be occasionally observed with left hemispheric lesions. Moreover, anosognosia of language disorders is frequently seen in patients with Wernicke's aphasia, which typically follows lesions in the left hemisphere (see Kertesz, Chapter 6; Cocchini & Della Sala, Chapter 7, this volume). These findings point to the fact that anosognosia, as a general phenomenon affecting different domains, does not relate to a single module located in a particular cerebral region that would be responsible for a generic knowledge about one's current health; but it can emerge after damage to distinct cognitive domains involving different lesion sites. Therefore, the hemispheric asymmetry usually described in anosognosia is undoubtedly dependent on the specific neurological function that is concerned (e.g., hemiplegia versus language deficits).

Another more general observation is that anosognosia usually occurs after large brain lesions (Feinberg, Haber, & Leeds, 1990; Hier, Mondlock, &

Caplan, 1983; Levine, Calvanio, & Rinn, 1991; Willanger, Danielsen, & Ankerhus, 1981). Nevertheless, some cases have been reported with a relatively focal lesion (Bisiach et al., 1986; House & Hodges, 1988). However, a variety of different brain areas have been held to be critically implicated, including the temporoparietal cortex, thalamus, basal ganglia, as well as their interconnecting pathways in the posterior deep white matter (for review, see Vuilleumier, 2000). A few case reports have also described the occurrence of AHP with intriguing noncortical lesions, involving, for example, the pons (Assenova, Benecib, & Logak, 2006; Bakchine, Crassard, & Seilhan, 1997; Evyapan & Kumral, 1999), together with some preexisting cognitive decline reported in some of these patients only (Bakchine et al., 1997). A disruption between frontal and parietal areas due to "diaschisis" has been suggested to explain these phenomena.

A more systematic investigation of lesions associated with AHP was recently conducted by using different types of statistical overlap analysis (see Bottini et al., Chapter 2, and Karnath & Baier, Chapter 3, this volume). Karnath et al. (Baier & Karnath, 2008; Karnath, Baier, & Nagele, 2005) suggested a key role for damage to the posterior insula, whereas Berti et al. (2005) found maximal overlap in premotor, motor, and sensory cortical areas. In addition, among two recent meta-analyses of previous anatomical studies, one pointed to the combination of parietal and frontal lesions and their possible impact on corticosubcortical circuits underlying awareness of motor acts (Pia, Neppi-Modona, Ricci, & Berti, 2004), whereas another (Orfei et al., 2007) underscored a predominant involvement of the prefrontal and parieto-temporal cortex, as well as of the insula and thalamus (see also Vuilleumier, 2000). However, these overlap studies present with a few methodological issues that may limit their interpretation. In particular, these techniques require a dichotomic classification separating the patients in two groups: anosognosics versus nosognosics. But from a clinical perspective, this cut-off does not reflect the multiple variations and fluctuations of anosognosia. Moreover, some patients may receive the same total score of anosognosia on Bisiach or Feinberg questionnaire, but have different combinations of causal deficits (as predicted by the ABC model, see above; Vuilleumier, 2004). Furthermore, patients with acute and more chronic forms of anosognosia are sometimes mixed in some studies.

To remedy some of these problems, in our own recent study of right-hemisphere stroke patients (Vocat et al., in preparation), we performed an overlap analysis of lesions that took into account the different degrees of anosognosia in different patients, as well as its evolution over time. We reconstructed the lesions for each of our patients on the basis of the cerebral scanner made 1 week after the stroke, in a blind manner. To analyze statistically the sites of maximal overlap, we applied a voxel-by-voxel lesion symptom mapping (VLSM) method as described elsewhere (Bates et al., 2003; Grandjean, Sander, Lucas, Scherer, & Vuilleumier, 2008), which allows taking into account the severity of anosognosia in different patients, by weighing the importance of each lesion by the mean score on Bisiach and Feinberg scales (calculated from the two successive assessments). Thus, this method highlights those voxels whose damage leads to the most severe cases of AHP.

In the hyperacute phase (3 days post stroke), the most common areas of damage in patients with a severe left AHP (relative to those without or with milder AHP) were found in the anterior insula, plus the anterior part of the claustrum and putamen, anterior internal capsule, head of caudate, and anterior paraventricular white matter within the right hemisphere (see Figure 17.2A). For patients with persisting AHP in the second phase 1 week later, several other regions of the right hemisphere were also selectively affected, now including the premotor cortex, temporo-parietal junction, frontal white matter in anterior internal capsule, as well as the hippocampus, and amygdala (see Figure 17.2B). Thus, while lesions in anterior insula and anterior subcortical structures were most distinctive for AHP in the hyperacute period (3 days after stroke), additional lesions in parietal, frontal, and/or temporal structures were needed to

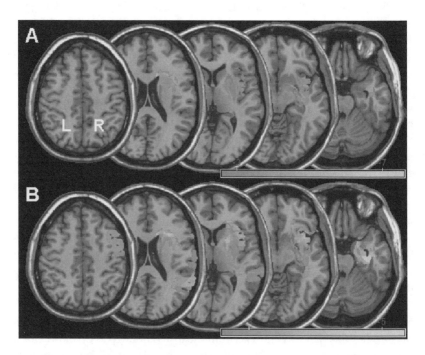

Figure 17.2 Results of statistical anatomical lesion analysis in our prospective study of AHP. Voxelwise mapping of brain areas correlating with anosognosia scores in the hyperacute phase (*A:* 3 days after stroke) and in the post-acute phase (*B:* 1 week after stroke). The voxels highlighted are those that show a significant difference (*p* < .01) in the severity of anosognosia between patients with/without a lesion in these voxels. (See Color Plate 17.2)

produce a more sustained AHP (1 week later). Taken together, these anatomical data do not only converge with the notion that AHP is likely to result from multiple component deficits but also point to several possible mechanisms underlying these deficits such as those entailing impairments in appreciation, belief, and check processes.

On the one hand, our findings in hyperacute stage (3 days after stroke) converge with the report of frequent insula damage by Karnath & Baier (Chapter 3, this volume). The insula might be involved in feelings of body ownership and agency (Karnath, Baier, & Nagele, 2005), but its anterior sector is also implicated in error monitoring (Magno, Foxe, Molholm, Robertson, & Garavan, 2006; Taylor, Stern, & Gehring, 2007), in representing internal body states (Critchley, Wiens, Rotshtein, Ohman, & Dolan, 2004), and in processing uncertainty, in concert with prefrontal cortices and basal ganglia (Harris, Sheth, & Cohen, 2008). The latter structure also plays a key role in performance monitoring and behavioral adjustments (Ullsperger & von Cramon, 2006) and was also more frequently damaged in our patients with AHP, together with white-matter connections in subcortical frontal regions. Damage to these circuits may therefore disrupt the neural systems normally responsible for the monitoring of motor actions and errors (and for implementing a subsequent "switch" in behavior).

On the other hand, our findings in the post-acute stage (1 week after stroke) converge with those of Berti et al. (2005), suggesting a crucial role for lesions in premotor cortex. Premotor areas do not only mediate motor initiation and preparation but are also thought to be responsible for generating a corollary discharge that can be used to monitor and adjust movements, according to sensory and proprioceptive feedback (see the feedforward model of action control proposed by Blakemore, Wolpert, & Frith, 2002). Accordingly, a recent study of Fotopoulou et al. (2008), in which a rubber hand was used to simulate movement of the left paralyzed arm, showed that anosognosic patients can accurately discriminate between the presence/absence of movement of the rubber hand, as long as they are not instructed to imagine themselves doing this movement. When a motor intention is generated (by having to imagine to move), a movement of the rubber hand is incorrectly reported even if it was motionless. This intriguing study shows the importance of motor intention and preparation in the anosognosic phenomenon, which can dominate actual sensory information. However, such findings are not readily compatible with other observations, suggesting that a lack of motor intention might play a causal role in abolishing motor awareness in anosognosia (Gold, Adair, Jacobs, & Heilman, 1994; see also Heilman & Harciarek, Chapter 5, this volume).

We also found that other brain regions were important in the maintenance of anosognosia during the post-acute phase (1 week after stroke), including the temporo-parietal junction (TPJ) and the amygdalo-hippocampal complex. Numerous studies have shown that the right TPJ is critically linked to spatial attention (see Halligan, Fink, Marshall, & Vallar, 2003, for a recent review), and damage to this region typically produces left hemispatial neglect (Mort et al., 2003). In keeping with this, neglect has often been suspected to play an important role in AHP (Bisiach et al., 1986; Cutting, 1978; Hier, Mondlock, & Caplan, 1983; Starkstein, Fedoroff, Price, Leiguarda, & Robinson, 1992; Vuilleumier, 2000), and our own study also revealed that extrapersonal neglect was one of the major neuropsychological disorders correlating with both the severity and time-course of AHP (Vocat et al., in preparation).

Finally, a less expected finding was the correlation of AHP with damage to the amygdalo-hippocampal complex in medial temporal lobe. These regions are known to play a key role in memory and emotion. The hippocampus subserves the encoding of events in episodic memory (Squire, 1992), and lesions in this area prevent any integration of new information into current knowledge. The amygdala is a structure critically implicated in emotional processing and learning (see Phelps & LeDoux, 2005, for a review), with a particular importance for fear (Ohman & Mineka, 2001) and, more generally, for the detection and appraisal of self-relevant stimuli (Sander, Grafman, & Zalla, 2003). Thus, lesions to this structure may cause a loss of fear responses (Adolphs et al., 2005) as well as an incapacity to take into account various forms of feedback that are relevant for subsequent behavioral adjustments (Ousdal et al., 2008). In the case of anosognosia, it is tempting to speculate that damage of these two structures could lead to more superficial processing of the abnormal or threatening feedback generated by a paralyzed limb and motor failures, as well as to greater forgetfulness of these events. Consistent with this hypothesis, our results (Vocat et al., in preparation) also indicated a mild but significant correlation between memory difficulties and anosognosia in the post-acute (1 week) and chronic (6 months) phases.

To sum up, our results help reconcile the apparent discrepancies between previous studies on the neural bases of anosognosia (Berti et al., 2005; Bisiach et al., 1986; Karnath et al., 2005). We show that no single brain area seems to be sufficient by itself to produce AHP. Indeed, no single brain area appears to be damaged in 100% of anosognosic patients. Rather, a complex network of interacting cerebral regions seems likely to be implicated in the occurrence and persistence of this syndrome. The critical lesions might also act by disconnecting white-matter pathways between subcortical and posterior brain regions to more anterior areas in the frontal lobe. This widespread network appears to encompass not only proprioception and spatial attention but also motor planning, action monitoring, memory, and affective relevance detection. Each of these functions might potentially be affected in AHP, but perhaps to different degrees in different patients.

A Multicomponent and Multifocal Disorder

Both the neuropsychological and anatomical analyses reviewed above clearly converge to indicate that AHP is likely to represent a multicomponent syndrome, associated with multifocal brain damage as typically seen in large stroke lesions. Different combinations of deficits might add up to produce similar behavioral outcome or interact together to produce different forms of AHP.

Thus, consistent with our ABC hypothesis (Vuilleumier, 2004), a severe impairment in one or many of the "appreciation" components (such as proprioception and spatial attention) might be sufficient to cause AHP in the presence of mild impairments in the "check" components (such as action monitoring or affective appraisal). But conversely, in another case, AHP might primarily arise due to a severe disruption of check components despite minor losses in proprioception and a lack of neglect. This ABC combinatorial rule would be consistent with occasional observations of striking dissociations between AHP and some deficits that are otherwise known to be strongly correlated with AHP (e.g., spatial neglect).

However, the exact cognitive processes underlying each of the ABC components and their neuroanatomical correlates still remain to be better characterized. Further studies are needed to test a range of abilities associated not only with sensory and motor functions but also related to reasoning, belief formation, error monitoring, affective processing, and so forth. Below we speculate on a few specific dimensions of self-awareness and self-monitoring that might potentially offer valuable avenues for future investigations of AHP.

Evidence for a Multiple Parallel System Account

Which combination of neurological and/or neuropsychological deficit is crucial to produce anosognosia is still unknown. As noted above, it is possible that several different factors are involved, and that a particular "cocktail" of deficits is necessary to explain the emergence and/or the persistence of anosognosia after brain damage, consistent with our results showing the co-existence of multiple cognitive and anatomical correlates. In addition, different forms or different degrees of anosognosia might exist and reflect different components in the syndrome. Here we briefly review a number of cognitive and affective processes that have been identified in other neuropsychological disorders as well as during normal performance in healthy subjects and that might potentially play some role in the behavioral manifestations of anosognosia.

Implicit and Explicit Processing

Clinical observations suggest that there are essentially four types of possible reactions when confronted with a neurological deficit such as plegia after cerebral injury. The first case is a full awareness of the deficit. Patients can describe their deficit and the handicap that will affect their life. A second case is a superficial description of the symptom (usually with some minimization of its impact), but the patients fail to take their condition into account when projecting themselves in the future or when making decisions. This corresponds to the notion of anosodiaphoria (i.e., a lack of affective concern for the deficit with a preserved sensory and cognitive appreciation), and it accords with the frequent disorders seen in patients with traumatic brain injury (TBI), typically attributed to frontal lobe syndrome (Levine, Dawson, Boutet, Schwartz, & Stuss, 2000; Levine et al., 1998; Prigatano & Altman, 1990). Third, patients may present with a classic and full form of anosognosia. They do not spontaneously report their deficit, deny it even after motor confrontations, behave as if they could go on with their past life without changes, and show no clear understanding of the reasons why they are currently investigated in the hospital or attribute their illness to a more abstract and causal level without direct reference to the deficit (i.e., they may acknowledge a diagnosis of stroke or heart attack but have no paralysis). Such patients may even hallucinate accurate movement with their affected limb and report that actions made on request have been correctly executed despite the lack of any visible movements, resembling a form of motor confabulation (Feinberg, 1997). However, a fourth case concerns anosognosic patients who seem to have some unconscious knowledge of their paralysis (corresponding to the notion of "dunkle Erkenntnis" described by Anton (1898)). These patients are compliant and stay calmly in the hospital, have compensatory movements to adjust to their paralysis, and participate in therapy without opposition, but they show no clear knowledge of what is wrong with them. After confrontations with their motor weakness, these patients may confess that they did not reach the demanded state but justify their failure by false but "plausible" reasons like "my arm is tired," "today it doesn't work as I want," "it takes more time than usual," "my arm is not paralyzed, but a little sleepy now," "my arm is not sufficiently warmed up," or "I don't want to do this now" (and so forth). These justifications might reflect some trace of "implicit" detection of the deficit, at least to the point where the outcome of a specific goal is not adequately realized. Nevertheless, these patients appear unable to integrate this mismatch and new information related to their condition so as to infer the existence of their (seemingly unnoticed) deficit.

Based on these observations, it would be tempting to distinguish between at least two levels or two types of "awareness of the deficit": namely, an implicit and an explicit aspect. Most current accounts of AHP and assessment procedures assume that these two levels lie on a continuum of severity, and therefore conflate them into a single score. However, we believe that they might reflect different aspects of sensori-motor monitoring, and that it might be useful to separate these different behavioral manifestations by using distinct measures. In keeping with this, a recent study (Nardone, Ward, Fotopoulou, & Turnbull, 2007) showed that patients with AHP showed slower reaction times to visual targets preceded by a word related to their motor deficit (arm, hand) verus another neutral body part (eye, back). Because this slowing was the most severe in the two patients with the most severe anosognosia, these authors concluded that AHP might reflect an active suppression mechanism. However, other mechanisms underlying a disso-ciation between implicit and explicit knowledge of the paralysis might potentially produce a similar pattern. Also consistent with this hypothesis, it has been reported that patients with AHP might report some knowledge of their deficit after manipulation reducing spatial neglect such as vestibular stimulation (Bisiach, Rusconi, & Vallar, 1991; Ramachandran, 1995; Rode et al., 1992; Vallar, Guariglia, & Rusconi, 1997), or are hypothesized to do so when reporting their dreams after sleeping (Ramachandran, 1996).

Moreover, a number of observations suggesting a dissociation between unconscious and conscious processing have been described in other domains in neuropsychology (De Gelder, De Haan, & Heywood, 2002). In particular, in visual perception, many phenomena can reveal the existence of information processing in the absence of conscious verbal report. This may happen, for example, for stimuli in the left hemifield in patients with spatial neglect (Marshall & Halligan, 1988; Vuilleumier, Schwartz, Clarke, Husain, & Driver, 2002); or even more impressive, in patients with blindsight after visual field loss (Stoerig & Cowey, 1997). These examples show that, in conditions where perception is very incomplete and poor (due to deficit of attention or primary sensory processing), some processes in the brain may still "detect" sensory features that are not available to conscious report. Nevertheless, this residual subliminal processing can have indirect effects on the patient's behavior, by influencing his or her responses or choices even without him being aware of it, as shown in neglect patients who prefer a stimulus over another based on unseen cues (Marshall & Halligan, 1988). Even in normal subjects, unconscious priming by an undetected, briefly presented stimulus can facilitate its reproces-sing during a later supraliminal presentation (Dehaene et al., 2001) or produce subsequent biases in accessing its semantic field (Ortells, Daza, & Fox, 2003).

Based on these observations, it is therefore possible to imagine that, in condi-tion of altered sensori-motor feedbacks, the brain might still detect some mis-match between a planned action and its real outcome despite a lack of conscious awareness. This might exist in some patients but not all of them, resulting in different subtypes of AHP, as suggested by the clinical observations described above. However, the exact neural substrates for these effects still remain to be explored.

Action Monitoring and Error-Related Processing

Neuroscience research in healthy subjects has identified a specific neurophysio-logical marker for the detection of any mismatch between expected and actual motor outcome. This has been studied in various paradigms investigating the EEG responses evoked by error detection, and it led to the discovery of a specific waveform after error commission, known as the error-related negativity (ERN; see Falkenstein, Hoormann, Christ, & Hohnsbein, 2000, for a review). This

EEG component shows up 50 to 100 ms after a motor error and has neural sources located primarily in the anterior cingulate cortex (ACC; Dehaene, Posner, & Tucker, 1994; van Veen & Carter, 2002). Importantly, the very short latency of the ERN after an error suggests that it cannot simply result from processing the sensory consequences of an erroneous response. Rather, it is likely to be generated by some internal comparator mechanisms operating on a representation of the motor command or response selection itself, and thus might arise prior to conscious awareness of the error.

Accordingly, elegant experiments using antisaccade tasks in normal subjects (Endrass, Reuter, & Kathmann, 2007; Nieuwenhuis, Ridderinkhof, Blom, Band, & Kok, 2001) have shown that a clear ERN can be elicited when errors are made but not verbally reported. Thus, incorrect saccades with small movements in the wrong directions did not reach consciousness but nevertheless were detected by internal monitoring processes. Similar results have been found with other paradigms such as the Stroop task (Hester, Foxe, Molholm, Shpaner, & Garavan, 2005; O'Connell et al., 2007). On the contrary, a study by Larson, Kaufman, Schmalfuss, and Perlstein (2007) reported that TBI patients were aware of errors in a Stroop task (as much as control participants) but showed a decrease in the amplitude of the ERN. However, these patients showed no difference in another error-related component, the Pe, a positive waveform that arises later (300 to 500 ms post-onset, possibly reflecting some kind of P300 component), and that is thought to reflect conscious processing of errors. Other studies also confirmed that the generation of ERN does not depend on awareness of errors. For example, Stemmer, Segalowitz, Witzke, and Schonle (2004) showed that patients with damage to the anterior cingulate cortex had a diminished ERN, but with a preserved awareness of errors. These findings suggest that regions other than ACC are important for conscious monitoring.

Brain regions involved in error processing have been further established by the work of Ullsperger, von Cramon, and Muller (2002). These authors investigated three groups of patients with different lesion sites (in orbitofrontal, lateral frontal, or temporal cortex) during a speeded task and found that the lateral frontal cortex was the only region where damage abolished the ERN component. Remarkably, in almost all of these patients, the lesions also extended to the anterior insula, a region highlighted in our lesion analysis of patients with AHP (see above; Vocat et al., in preparation) and frequently activated in error monitoring tasks (Klein et al., 2007; Magno, Foxe, Molholm, Robertson, & Garavan, 2006; Taylor, Stern, & Gehring, 2007). In addition, other studies have been conducted in Parkinson's disease patients (Stemmer, Segalowitz, Dywan, Panisset, & Melmed, 2007; but see Holroyd, Praamstra, Plat, & Coles, 2002), who are impaired at detecting their motor errors (see also Prigatano & Maier, Chapter 9, this volume) and show a reduced amplitude in the ERN.

Taken together, these results clearly suggest that error detection relies on several neural pathways, related to at least two distinct levels of awareness: an implicit and

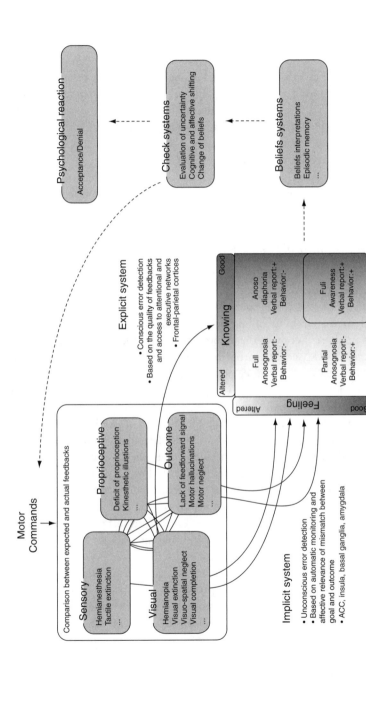

Figure 17.3 A multicomponent model of anosognosia for hemiplegia. ACC, anterior cingulate cortex.

automatic stage, with an early latency, reflected by the ERN component, which is presumably generated in the ACC but may depend on information processed in lateral prefrontal areas and possibly the anterior insula; as well as a more explicit stage, with a later latency and distinct neural generators (Vocat, Pourtois, & Vuilleumier, 2008). It remains to be determined how these neurophysiological markers of action monitoring (ERN and Pe) might relate to the behavioral manifestations of anosognosia, and whether they might correlate with differences in the level of awareness in these patients, reflecting implicit detection versus explicit verbal report of their deficits, respectively. Normally, these two monitoring systems are likely to be interconnected and integrated, but they might be differentially affected due to the cerebral lesion and the loss of internal feedbacks representations. In the following section, we briefly outline how these two parallel monitoring systems, implicit and explicit, might make distinct contributions to AHP and other related disorders (see Figure 17.3).

Motor Error Monitoring and Unawareness of Deficit

Every movement begins with the generation of a motor goal and ends with a produced effect. Models of motor control (e.g., Blakemore, Wolpert, & Frith, 2002) assume that the brain computes the movement parameters needed to reach the desired state by planning and executing motor commands and then comparing an efferent copy of these commands with the actual outcome based on ongoing feedback (sensory, proprioceptive, visual), in order to allow online motor adjustments (see Bottini et al., Chapter 2, this volume). In hemiplegic patients, the motor command itself might be disrupted by the lesion, which might then suppress internal signals to other brain structures implicated in the monitoring of movement (see feedforwad theory of AHP in Heilman & Harciarek, Chapter 5, this volume). In addition, feedback information might also be reduced by sensory disturbances, including hemianesthesia and tactile extinction, as well as by proprioceptive loss, spatial neglect, visual deficits such as hemianopia and visual extinction, or even visual completion and kinesthetic illusions. Thus, information about the actual outcome of an action might be affected by more than a single deficit, and even more so by a combination of different deficits. Importantly, it is possible that such losses might affect the implicit, explicit, or both monitoring systems.

Explicit awareness of motor impairment presumably arises through an integration of several channels (i.e., visual, proprioceptive, tactile, or motor signals) that carry feedback information about movements and become represented in a mental "global workspace" possibly mediated by a reverberant state of neurophysiological synchronization between fronto-parietal areas and other modality-specific regions (Dehaene, Changeux, Naccache, Sackur, & Sergent, 2006; Dehaene & Naccache, 2001; Dehaene, Sergent, & Changeux, 2003; Rodriguez et al., 1999; Tallon-Baudry & Bertrand, 1999). Access of information to these large-scale networks might result in a conscious "knowing" about the deficit, selective orienting of attention, verbal report, as well as appropriate goal-directed behavior. Lesions in fronto-parietal networks or their afferent input connections might (partly or totally) deprive the explicit action monitoring system from reliable feedback or feedforward signals necessary to consciously evaluate motor performance (Davies et al., 2005; Vuilleumier, 2004), consistent with the pattern of lesion we found to be associated with sustained AHP in the post-acute stage after stoke (1 week later; see earlier discussion). However, as previously noted, impaired access of sensorimotor information to conscious awareness may not necessarily prevent a parallel implicit monitoring system to detect anomalies in the current motor or sensory state.

On the other hand, implicit monitoring or motor error processing might be mediated by distinct neural pathways, including not only the ACC (which is thought to produce the ERN component in EEG studies) but also other regions implicated in motor action monitoring such as the anterior insula (see Craig, Chapter 4, this volume) and basal ganglia. These brain regions might contribute to more automatic and "unconscious" processing of error signals, based on the comparison between expected and actual feedback for the planned movement (through motor, proprioceptive, tactile, and/or visual inputs). Activation of implicit error processing systems could result in a more diffuse "feeling" about the deficit, perhaps including emotional and arousal dimensions. A lesion, disconnection, or degradation affecting sensorimotor feedback to these pathways might therefore suppress any kind of implicit warning signal when an incorrect motor action occurs. Our lesion analysis (Vocat et al., in preparation) showed no lesion in ACC correlating with anosognosia, but the anterior insula and basal ganglia were found to be consistently damaged, together with the anterior white matter possibly connecting motor areas to ACC (see Figure 17.2B), for both the hyperacute (3 days) and post-acute (1 week) stages.

In addition, our results also revealed that post-acute AHP correlated with damage to the amygdala and hippocampus, that is, brain structures critically implicated in the detection of affectively relevant stimuli and memory formation. Deficits in either of these components could further contribute to an inability to learn about the motor deficits, and hence to adjust behavior or awareness accordingly, despite preserved detection of sensorimotor errors during confrontation.

Different degrees of disturbances along both the explicit and implicit monitoring systems might correspond to the four different clinical types of awareness disorders that are observed in patients (as summarized in Figure 17.3). When both systems are functionally intact, the patients have a "full awareness" of their motor performance (normal or impaired). When both systems are dysfunctional, the patients may present with total unawareness or "full anosognosia." Not only can they not report their deficit even after confrontation, but they behave as if nothing is wrong and take risky behavior, such as trying to get up and walk despite hemiplegia. Typically, they are unable to accept the reasons for being admitted to the hospital. By contrast, when explicit monitoring is impaired but implicit monitoring is intact, the deficit might not be reported, yet patients present with indirect behavioral manifestations reflecting some unconscious knowledge or "feeling" of it. Although they deny the deficits, they may sometimes act appropriately, give awkward interpretations in response to confrontations to their weakness, or misattribute their failures to other illnesses. These patients will stay in their bed and accept medical exams or therapy. On the contrary, when explicit monitoring is preserved and implicit systems are damaged, a deficit can be verbally admitted (e.g. during confrontation), but because there is no other "feeling of wrongness," the importance of the deficit is minimized or overlooked in more spontaneous conditions. Such patients may fail to adapt to their new conditions despite apparent nosognosia. This kind of disorder is common in TBI patients (see Langevin & Le Gall, 1999, for a review) but also occurs in stroke patients, and it bears some resemblance with anosodiaphoria (Babinski, 1914). For example, one of our patient was a physician and could very precisely describe the onset of his neurological weakness (a total hemiplegia) and knew that it was caused by a stroke; however, he did not feel the need to call for help or go to hospital for treatment, and he made implausible plans to play golf with his son on weekends.

Of course, this schematic typology of four different categories of awareness is not always as strict and clear in clinical practice, possibly because both monitoring systems can be affected at different degrees in different patients. Nevertheless, we believe that this may help to better characterize the behavioral manifestations of AHP, and it should encourage further empirical investigations of the neuropsychological correlates of anosognosia (see Cocchini & Della Sala, Chapter 7; Orfei et al., Chapter 19, this volume).

Interpretations, Beliefs, and Belief Changes

Both the implicit "feeling" and explicit "knowing" about motor performance should normally be integrated in a single coherent appreciation, based on the convergence of the different feedback and feedfoward signals, which can be consciously manifested and verbally expressed by the patient. We hypothesize that this function might take place in the left hemisphere and reflect the "interpreter" processes that have been observed in split brain patients (Gazzaniga, 2000). Rational or delusional elaborations under the control of the left hemisphere interpreter could induce the formation of false beliefs that may combine with old or "default" beliefs about one's health, or with stereotypical biases in self-evaluation. For instance, it is a normal tendency of healthy individuals to overestimate their well-being and underestimate their risk for diseases (Weinstein, 1984, 1987, 1989). A role for this integrative interpreter might underlie the frequent rationalization or even confabulations expressed by some patients when they explain away their failures (Assal, 1983; Ramachandran, 1995).

However, the existence of biased interpretations or false beliefs may not be sufficient to account for all aspects of anosognosia, since repeated confrontations with the deficit (or at least its consequences) should eventually elicit some signals of uncertainty that could then prompt for an appropriate verification and revision of current beliefs based on new experience. These uncertainty signals might result from cognitive or affective processes activated by monitoring systems, or from higher-level executive systems that are recruited when information provided by the monitoring systems is incongruent or insufficient (Norman & Shallice, 1986). Indeed, a striking feature of anosognosic patients is that such a tendency to check and modify current beliefs seems often to be missing. Despite recurrent confrontations and encounters with caregivers or doctors, they may stick to their interpretation rather than call it into question, despite the obvious self-relevance and emotional significance of a potential deficit. In some sense, these patients behave exactly opposite to those patients with somatoform disorders (e.g. hypochondria) who have exaggerated fears about a possible illness; rather, they appear remarkably easy and unworried about incongruent or missing information concerning their current bodily state. This suggests that cognitive or affective processes necessary for updating old beliefs might also be altered by the lesion.

In a recent study (Vocat et al., in preparation), we specifically tested for the ability of patients to change beliefs by asking them to guess a word according to a series of five successive clues, which provided a progressive informative content about the target word. After each clue (even for the first very general one), patients had to propose a word and give their level of confidence from 0 (not sure at all) to 8 (completely sure). We found that anosognosic patients were much more confident for responses to the initial clues than nosognosic patients. Moreover, they tended to perseverate with a first wrong answer even when faced with the incongruency of subsequent clues, typically providing some "plausible" but largely irrelevant connections between their chosen word and the given clues. Nevertheless, after the fifth and last clue, which provided the most specific information about the target word, anosognosic and nosognosic patients were equally successful at finally resolving the riddles, indicating that anosognosics did not have general reasoning deficits but rather that they tended to remain stuck to their false beliefs and failed to modify them, unless clearly incongruent information was given. These findings therefore clearly demonstrate for the first time that anosognosia correlates with a specific disturbance to modify current beliefs, even when these do not rely on sensorimotor feedback and do not concern their motor performance or health.

Based on our neuropsychological and anatomical lesion overlap (Vocat et al., in preparation), we speculate that deficits in changing beliefs in anosognosia might be associated with lesions in the hippocampus and amygdala, possibly together with connections to medial prefrontal areas involved in self-monitoring (Norman & Shallice, 1986). Damage to these structures might disrupt the encoding of important new information in memory and reduce the normal affective drive to adjust behavior in the face of self-relevant, potentially threatening situations. Damage to the insula and ventromedial prefrontal regions might also play a role in belief formation and belief changes by suppressing affective signals necessary to trigger belief changes (Naqvi & Bechara, 2009). Interestingly, in a recent imaging study that examined decisions based on various beliefs in healthy subjects, activation of the ventromedial prefrontal cortex was associated with accepted beliefs, whereas activation in insula correlated with disbelief and activation in ACC correlated with uncertainty (Harris, Sheth, & Cohen, 2008). In any case, the exact neural substrates of belief systems and impairment thereof will need further investigations.

Psychological Reaction

While there is no doubt that anosognosia is the direct result of a multifactorial organic brain dysfunction, it is important to keep in mind that this does not entirely exclude a role for purely psychological dimensions that can influence how individuals will cope with a sudden severe deficit. Defense mechanisms are well known to operate in healthy people, and there is no reason to think that they should always cease to work in stroke patients. The sudden loss of motor and sensory capacities for one's hemibody and its consequences obviously constitute a major traumatic event, likely to require some psychological coping and defense mechanisms. A phase of acceptance of the deficit and its implications is needed (see O'Callaghan, Powell, & Oyebode, 2006).

In addition, another intriguing possibility is that some lesions might affect the recruitment or the efficacy of these defense mechanisms, in either a positive or negative way (Schilder, 1935; Turnbull & Solms, 2007). For example, it is possible that some frontal lesions might abolish an inhibition that normally refrains the use of "denial," or conversely the lesions might suppress a motivational incentive to refute the acceptance of a deficit. How these psychological factors interact with neuropsychological impairments and modulate the clinical manifestations of AHP is still largely ignored, but they should not be minimized, even though it is certainly obvious that they cannot explain all anosognosic manifestations.

Outlook for Future Research on Anosognosia for Hemiplegia

To conclude this section on AHP, we would like to underscore that future models of anosognosia should incorporate a role for several distinct components that do not only relate to sensorimotor processing and cognitive appreciation of hemiplegia but should also take into account the role of parallel monitoring systems that encode error signals at different levels of awareness, as well as emotional systems that respond to these error signals and serve to adjust behavior or beliefs based on self-relevant information. Existing data converge to suggest that AHP is likely to result from a combination of several deficits affecting different domains (including proprioception, neglect, memory, belief formation, or verification), with corresponding multifocal neural correlates (including fronto-parietal cortex, premotor areas, insula, and anterior subcortical white-matter), but the exact combination responsible for the different aspects and the different types of AHP still remain to be clarified by large, systematic neuropsychological studies testing specific hypotheses.

Conversion and Hysterical Paralysis

Hysteria is a condition characterized by the report of subjective neurological symptoms (e.g., motor paralysis) without any damage to the nervous system, and thus it presents with a number of features that seemingly mirror the manifestations of anosognosia. Whereas AHP involves a lack of awareness, misbeliefs, or denial concerning a "real" deficit due to organic brain damage, and does not result from a more general cognitive impairment or confusion, on the contrary, hysterical paralysis implies a conscious experience, illusion, or conviction of a deficit that is not caused by any organic illness, yet not explained by voluntarily simulation or psychotic delusions (Vuilleumier, 2005, 2009). Hysteria is classified among psychiatric disorders, but many modern views on this condition are derived from the early work of neurologists who also studied anosognosia and pioneered neuropsychological accounts of awareness in the nineteenth century—particularly Charcot (1892) and Janet (1894). Babinski and Dagnan-Bouveret (1912) theorized about the role of emotional triggers in producing motor hysteria prior to Babinski's seminal case report on anosognosia of hemiplegia (Babinski, 1914), and he actually described the classic eponymous plantar reflex as a new clinical sign to distinguish between organic and hysterical paralysis (see Okun & Koehler, 2004). The contemporaneous work by Freud and Breuer (1895) similarly insisted on a transformation of unconscious emotional disturbances into physical complaints, eventually leading to the current diagnostic category of "conversion" (American Psychiatric Association, 1994) that has nowadays replaced the terminology of hysteria in psychiatry textbooks.

However, the exact cognitive and emotional processes underlying such conversion of psychological motives into physical symptoms, as well as their neurophysiological substrates, remain poorly known (Kozlowska, 2005; Vuilleumier, 2005, 2009). Unlike other psychiatric conditions, hysterical conversion has been only rarely studied using neurophysiological or neurocognitive approaches. In this section, we will review those theoretical accounts that have attempted to attribute conversion disorders to a dysfunction of specific neural circuits and, most particularly, summarize a few recent studies that applied brain imaging techniques to identify the functional neural correlates of hysterical paralysis.

Hysterical Conversion in Neurology

Hysterical conversion is still encountered by neurologists and represents 1%–4% of patients admitted to neurological wards (Krem, 2004). Different studies conducted in different periods and different hospitals have revealed a relatively stable rate across decades since the early half of the past century, despite changes in some of the predominant clinical manifestations (Frei, 1984; Mace, 1992; Perkin, 1989; Trimble, 1981). Like anosognosia, conversion most often involves motor or sensory functions, such as hemiplegia, paraplegia, or anesthesia, but also visual loss, amnesia, or even language disturbances and pseudo-dementia (e.g., Ganser syndrome). Moreover, several studies have suggested that motor conversion involves left limbs much more frequently than right limbs (Galin, Diamond, & Braff, 1977; Stern, 1983), just like AHP, suggesting that conversion symptoms might reflect an interaction in hemispheric asymmetries for motor control, emotional processing, and consciousness (Flor-Henry, 1978; Miller, 1984). However, other recent studies did not replicate this asymmetry (Stone et al., 2002; Stone, Warlow, Carson, & Sharpe, 2003) and motor symptoms may be observed on either side (Vuilleumier, 2005; Vuilleumier et al., 2001). Further, as emphasized by Freud, neurological symptoms in conversion hysteria may not respect the topographical organization of the nervous systems but more subjective or symbolic representations, and thus produce distinct atypical clinical manifestations such as glove anesthesia or tubular vision.

Although several neurological signs might be used to distinguish between organic and nonorganic deficits, including Babinski sign (Okun & Koehler, 2004) or Hoover sign (Koehler & Okun, 2004), there is no straightforward criteria or reliable "objective" sign to establish the diagnosis of conversion symptoms (Krem, 2004). In particular, the notion that conversion patients often present with a good acceptance of their symptoms (so called "belle indifference") has been shown to be relatively nonspecific (Vuilleumier, 2009). In fact, many of these patients may present with some emotional distress rather than emotional indifference; furthermore, a lack of concern is also frequent in anosognosic patients who do have a severe deficit. In addition, although hysterical symptoms are generally thought to result from a response to stressful situations or emotional eliciting factors (Binzer, Andersen, & Kullgren, 1997; Roelofs, Spinhoven, Sandijck, Moene, & Hoogduin, 2005), assessing their importance and relation to the symptoms may be highly dependent on subjective judgments by the clinician, and their causal role (or even existence) is therefore sometimes difficult to ascertain. Conversely, many patients with organic neurological diseases may also report stressful conditions preceding a "real" neurological illness, as shown for instance for stroke (House, Dennis, Mogridge, Hawton, & Warlow, 1990) or multiple sclerosis (Mohr, Hart, Julian, Cox, & Pelletier, 2004). Thus, the diagnosis of conversion is typically made after an exclusion of various potential organic diseases, requiring negative findings from a large range of clinical exams, including magnetic resonance imaging (MRI), electroencephalogram (EEG), electromyogram (EMG), transcranial magnetic stimulation (TMS), cerebrospinal fluid (CSF) tap, blood tests, and so forth. A better understanding of the cognitive and neurobiological mechanisms of conversion might therefore be useful to improve the assessment of these patients, because the accrual of many negative tests may not only cause discomfort but also worsen psychological distress and fears in these patients; and diagnosis by exclusion may prove difficult in some situations with mixed pathologies (Krem, 2004; Vuilleumier, 2009).

This is all the more problematic since a mixture of conversion hysteria with a "true" organic neurological disease may sometimes occur. For example, the presence of "typical" psychogenic conversion symptoms has been reported in patients with acute stroke (Gould, Miller, Goldberg, & Benson, 1986), multiple sclerosis (Nicolson & Feinstein, 1994), or after closed head injuries (Eames, 1992). These symptoms included exaggerated or non-neurological complaints, changing deficit, patchy or inconsistent distribution, as well as lack of concern. Interestingly, a large study in 167 patients found that such symptoms were most often seen in patients who had diffuse brain lesions (e.g., closed head injury, anoxia, encephalitis) or subcortical focal strokes, and correlated with the presence of extrapyramidal motor disorders (Eames, 1992), suggesting that a disconnection of cortico-subcortical pathways might contribute to produce dissociative experiences in the conscious motor control of these patients. A coexistence of hysterical conversion and organic neurological disease is also frequently seen in patients with epilepsy who may occasionally present with pseudo-seizures (Devinsky, 1998), possibly reflecting an influence of their past neurological illness on their response to emotional distress (Brown, 2004; Miller, 1987). Such mixture of organic and psychogenic symptoms obviously complicates the clinical diagnosis of conversion made on exclusion criteria only.

Importantly, although early studies reported that some patients with hysteria symptoms may develop a real neurological disease after several years (Mace & Trimble, 1996), a number of careful follow-up studies have clearly shown that such evolution is very uncommon (Crimlisk et al., 1998; Stone, Sharpe, Rothwell, & Warlow, 2003). Very few patients (<2%–5%) eventually develop a medical disorder which, in hindsight, could have explained the original presentation. In contrast, psychiatric comorbidity is relatively high, including frequent associations with other somatoform disorders, dissociative disorders, or depression (Binzer, Eisemann, & Kullgren, 1998). An appropriate diagnosis and rapid behavioral management seem particularly important to avoid a persistence of symptoms and poor psychiatric prognosis.

Neurophysiological Accounts of Hysterical Conversion

Whereas the Freudian theory of hysterical conversion did not make reference to any specific cerebral mechanisms underlying the production of physical symptoms, earlier accounts by Charcot and Janet as well as several other theorists after them proposed a number of neural pathways by which certain psychological states might affect sensorimotor function in these patients (see Table 17.2). However, these accounts were most often speculations based on clinical observations and existing knowledge of the nervous system at different times during the past century, rather than based on more empirical studies.

For instance, Charcot proposed that the functioning of the nervous system could be altered without any visible pathology under the influence of powerful ideas or suggestions, in a manner similar to the effect of hypnosis (Charcot, 1892). His student Janet (1894) considered that such effects could reflect a dissociation between conscious and unconscious processes that are normally integrated to control perception or behavior, and that such dissociation was caused by the impact of strong emotions on integrative processes coordinating

Table 17.2 Summary of Classic Hypotheses on Motor Conversion

Sydenham (1697): bodily effects of strong emotion
Charcot (1892): motor function altered by imagination, suggestions (neurosis)
Janet (1894): fixed idea but unconscious, dissociation from conscious volition
Freud & Breuer (1895); Freud (1909): affective motives, symbolic conversion
Babinski & Dagnan-Bouveret (1912): suggestion, triggered by emotion, interpretation and predisposition
Pavlov (1933): cortical inhibition (frontal) after overexcitation (subcortical)
Kretschmer (1948): primitive adaptive/reflexive behavior
Whitlock (1967): exaggerated patterns of adaptation to stress (psychological or organic)
Ludwig (1972): thalamic gating of afferent stimulation (vs. hypochondria)
Sackheim et al. (1979): selective block of sensory processing from awareness (motivation based)
Stern (1983): distortion of (left) sensory/motor inputs due to right hemisphere affective processes
Flor-Henry et al. (1981): left hemisphere dysfunction with transcallosal right hemisphere disinhibition
Spiegel (1991): attentional focusing (cingulate) and dissociation
Marshall et al. (1997): inhibition of motor action (orbitofrontal and cingulate cortex)
Oakley (1999): ongoing sensory/motor representation excluded from self-awareness (by central attentional system)
Damasio (2003): false representation in internal body maps (via "as-if" system)

these two levels of control. Later, other accounts (Kretschmer, 1948; Whitlock, 1967) proposed that conversion might represent a pathological exaggeration of some primitive forms of reflexive behavior elicited by psychological or physical stressors, similar to the motor arrest, feigned death, or flurry behaviors exhibited by many animal species in threatening situations. Along these lines, Pavlov (1941) speculated that an overexcitation of "subcortical centers" caused by strong emotions might lead to a compensatory response of cortical inhibitory processes (tentatively located in frontal lobe), whose regulatory action could then overflow to other systems and somehow "switch off" sensorimotor functions. Similarly, several subsequent theorists suggested that the pseudo-neurological deficits in hysterical conversion (such as paralysis, anesthesia, or blindness) might result from a selective "blockade" or "gating" of sensorimotor inputs, produced by motivational factors at the level of the thalamus (Ludwig, 1972; Sackeim, Nordlie, & Gur, 1979) or through the action of attentional mechanisms mediated by anterior cingulate or parietal cortex (Marshall, Halligan, Fink, Wade, & Frackowiack, 1997; Sierra & Berrios, 1999; Spiegel, 1991). Instead, other more recent accounts have suggested a disconnection between self-awareness processes mediated by central executive systems in prefrontal cortex and the ongoing sensory or motor representation in more posterior brain regions (Oakley, 1999), or a distortion of these sensory or motor representations due to emotional states or past traumatic experiences (Brown, 2004; Damasio, 2003).

However, until recently, very few studies have used direct neurophysiological measures such as EEG, magnetoencephalography (MEG), or functional brain imaging to provide direct support for these neurobiological accounts of conversion (for review, see Black, Seritan, Taber, & Hurley, 2004; Vuilleumier, 2005, 2009). A first study was published by Tiihonen, Kuikka, Viinamaki, Lehtonen, and Partanen (1995), who used single photon emission computed tomography (SPECT) in a single female patient with left arm anesthesia and reported an abnormal hemispheric asymmetry in brain activity with decreases in right parietal areas and increases in right frontal areas during left sensory stimulation. But no specific causal mechanism was suggested to explain these changes. A second influential study was conducted by Marshall and colleagues (1997) in another single patient. The latter suffered from chronic leg weakness for a few years and was asked to attempt to move one or the other leg on command during positron emission tomography (PET) imaging. Unlike the normal activation of left motor areas during executed movements with the right leg, the attempts of movement with the left/paralyzed leg were not only associated with a lack of activation in right motor cortex but also accompanied by an increased activation of orbitofrontal and anterior cingulate areas instead. This finding was taken to suggest that voluntary actions were prevented due to an active inhibition of motor pathways by orbitofrontal and cingulate areas in ventromedial prefrontal cortex.

Subsequently, several other studies using fMRI have also reported decreased activations in motor (Burgmer et al., 2006; Kanaan, Craig, Wessely, & David, 2007; Stone et al., 2007), sensory regions (Ghaffar, Staines, & Feinstein, 2006; Mailis-Gagnon et al., 2003), or visual regions (Werring, Weston, Bullmore, Plant, & Ron, 2004) in small groups ($n = 1$ to 8) of hysterical conversion patients with paralysis, anesthesia, or blindness, respectively, often together with concomitant increases in medial, ventral, or dorsolateral prefrontal areas. In a recent intriguing study of a woman with hysterical hemiplegia, Kanaan et al. (2007) observed that activity in the motor cortex was selectively reduced when the patient was exposed to auditory excerpts describing the traumatic events that supposedly triggered her symptoms (relative to neutral autobiographical events), and this reduction was associated with concomitant increases in medial temporal lobe, including amygdala and hippocampus. The authors suggested that the retrieval of traumatic memories via amygdalo-hippocampic structures could trigger some emotional processes in limbic regions that could in turn inhibit activity in motor cortex and hence produce hysterical paralysis. However, the exact neural pathways mediating such inhibition were not clearly specified.

Two other recent studies examined covert motor activation in patients with motor conversion while they watched video clips of hand movements (Burgmer et al., 2006) or while they performed a mental rotation task on pictures of hands (de Lange, Roelofs, & Toni, 2007). Whereas the former found reduced motor activation during movement observation, the latter found no anomalies in motor areas but increased activation in ventral cingulate cortex. The latter region was deactivated during task performance in normal subjects, but it could not be linked to inhibitory processes, as proposed by Marshall and colleagues (1997), because motor cortex was normally activated by the mental rotation task in the conversion patients and their performance indicated normal motor imagery. Hence, de Lange and colleagues (2007) attributed the activation of ventral cingulate cortex to increased self-monitoring processes, in agreement with a previous event-related potential (ERP) study in which components associated with action monitoring were enhanced during a motor-selection task in conversion patients (Roelofs, de Bruijn, & Van Galen, 2006). By contrast, a PET study comparing four patients with motor conversion and simulators found no difference in motor cortex during a simple motor task, but it found reduced activation in left dorsolateral prefrontal cortex for conversion and in right dorsolateral prefrontal cortex for simulation (Spence, Crimlisk, Cope, Ron, & Grasby, 2000). Left prefrontal changes were attributed to disturbances in mechanisms underlying conscious will and the generation of motor intentions (Spence, 1999).

Intact activation of motor and sensory cortices was also found in our own SPECT study, which included a group of seven patients with unilateral hysterical motor losses (Vuilleumier et al., 2001). These patients were administered a passive vibratory stimulation at two different times, first while they presented with their hysterical symptoms, and then several months later after they recovered. However, by comparing the symptomatic and recovery period, we found a selective hypoactivation of the thalamus and basal ganglia (caudate and putamen) in the hemisphere contralateral to the limbs affected by hysterical symptoms (see Figure 17.4).

These findings suggest that motor outputs might be suppressed by an inhibition of subcortical motor pathways, at the level of the cortico-striato-thalamic loops, rather than at the level of the primary motor cortex. Similar subcortical decreases have been found in patients with motor neglect after focal hemispheric stroke (Fiorelli, Blin, Bakchine, Laplane, & Baron, 1991). In addition, a functional network analysis in our conversion patients (Vuilleumier et al., 2001) indicated that subcortical decreases in contralateral hemisphere were selectively coupled with concomitant changes in ventral prefrontal areas (BA 11/ BA 45), suggesting that the latter brain regions might be responsible for a modulation of the basal ganglia-thalamic loops that could influence voluntary movement (Haber, 2003). However, ventral and medial prefrontal areas have been linked

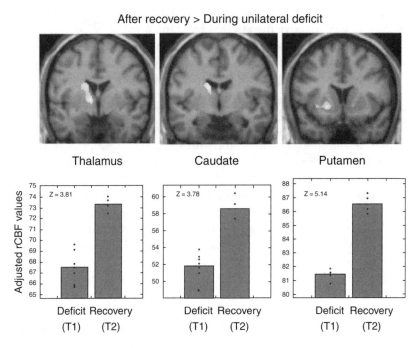

Figure 17.4 Brain regions showing decreased activity in the hemisphere contralateral to unilateral sensori-motor loss due to conversion hysteria ($n = 7$ patients). Comparing activation after recovery and during symptoms revealed significant changes in caudate nucleus, putamen, and thalamus, corresponding to major relays within the basal ganglia-thalamo-cortical loops that control movement initiation. (Adapted from Vuilleumier et al., 2001, with permission from Oxford University Press, *Brain, 124*, 1077–1090.) (See Color Plate 17.4)

to various functions, including not only behavioral inhibition (Lhermitte, Pillon, & Serdaru, 1986) but also emotional control (Bush, Luu, & Posner, 2000), self-referential memory (D'Argembeau et al., 2005), and belief judgments (Harris, Sheth, & Cohen, 2008). The exact role of cingulate and ventromedial prefrontal activity in hysterical conversion therefore remains to be further clarified.

In a recent single case study, we specifically tested for a contribution of active motor inhibition processes during hysterical paralysis (Cojan, Waber, Caruzzo, & Vuilleumier, 2009), by designing a new go-nogo task that allowed us to compare different motor processes for both the normal and affected limb, including motor preparation, execution, and inhibition. The patient was a young woman with a left hand weakness following a minor illness occurring in a period with several stressful life events. She underwent fMRI during a simple motor task, in which each trial began with the presentation of a picture of a hand (left or right), instructing the patient to prepare a movement on the corresponding side, which was then followed by either a go signal (requiring execution of the prepared movement) or a nogo signal (requiring inhibition of the prepared movement). This design allowed us to determine any similarities between a failure to move the affected hand (on a left go trial) and a normal voluntary inhibition of movement (on left or right nogo trials). A large body of literature in neuroimaging and neuropsychology has linked motor inhibition to the right inferior frontal gyrus (rIFG), for both motor and nonmotor cognitive tasks (Aron, 2007; Xue, Aron, & Poldrack, 2008), such that rIFG was predicted to be specifically activated by motor inhibition at least during nogo trials. In our patient, preparation induced a normal and symmetric pattern of activation of the contralateral motor cortex (Figure 17.5B), just like healthy controls (Figure 17.5A). This finding confirms intact motor imagery and intact motor intentions despite hysteria. During execution, the patient showed normal motor activation for the intact hand, but no activation in motor cortex for the affected limb (and no actual movement). Critically, she did not activate the rIFG on the left-go trials, even though she did not make any movement, whereas the rIFG was normally activated by inhibition on nogo trials in her case (with the right hand) as well as in healthy controls (for both their right and left hands). Importantly, this result reveals that the left hand paralysis did not recruit voluntary inhibitory processes mediated by rIFG. However, unlike healthy controls, the patient also selectively activated anterior and posterior midline brain regions, including the ventromedial prefrontal cortex (vmPFC) during execution attempts with the affected hand (left go trials), and both the ventromedial PFC and precuneus during preparation of left hand movements. In addition, connectivity analysis again revealed that the vmPFC was specifically coupled with the right motor cortex (contralateral to the paralyzed hand) but not with the left motor cortex (contralateral to the intact hand). Finally, we investigated a group of healthy volunteers who were asked to feign a left hand paralysis during the same task (Cojan, Waber,

Caruzzo, & Vuilleumier, 2009). However, the simulation of paralysis on left-go trials was found to produce exactly the same pattern of brain activity as the voluntary withholding a response on nogo trials (see Figure 17.5C), clearly demonstrating that hysterical paralysis was distinct from simulation.

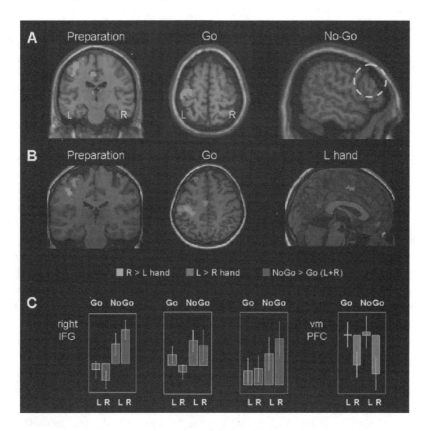

Figure 17.5 Brain regions activated during a go-nogo motor task performed with either hand. In a group of 12 healthy subjects *(A)* and a patient with left hysterical paralysis *(B)*, preparing a movement activated the contralateral motor cortex symmetrically for both the right and left hand. Motor cortex was also activated by execution (go trials) with either hand in healthy subjects, and with the intact right hand in the patient; however, a failure to move the hand on left go trails in the patient produced no increase in motor cortex but selective activation in precuneus and prefrontal areas. Importantly, the right inferior frontal gyrus (IFG) was activated by motor inhibition on nogo trials in healthy subjects but not during failures of movement on left go trials in the patient. The precuneus and ventromedial prefrontal cortex (PFC) were selectively activated by left-hand trials compared to right-hand trials. *(C)* Activation is plotted for the right IFG (shown in *A*) in normal controls, subjects simulating a left-hand paralysis, and the patient with left motor conversion (three panels from left to right, respectively); and for the ventromedial PFC (shown in *B*) in the patient. (Adapted from Cojan et al., 2009, with permission from Elsevier, *NeuroImage*, 47(3), 1026–1037.) (See Color Plate 17.5)

We also compared this pattern of activation in conversion with another situation where left arm paralysis was induced by hypnosis in a group of healthy volunteers who then had to perform the same go-nogo task in different states (Cojan et al., 2009). Changes in brain activity were clearly different between conversion and hypnosis for vmPFC (increased for all left hand actions in conversion) and for rIFG (increased for all conditions in hypnosis), while there was a similar increase of precuneus activity for all left hand actions during both hypnosis and conversion. These data suggest that hypnosis may also involve mental imagery and self-related memory processes that are sub-served by the precuneus (Cavanna & Trimble, 2006; Lou et al., 2004), but they imply a distinct modulation of executive monitoring systems in right IFG. Interestingly, activity in the precuneus has also been related to unconscious intentional biases in choices and actions (den Ouden, Frith, Frith, & Blakemore, 2005; Soon, Brass, Heinze, & Haynes, 2008). Another study also reported an activation of anterior cingulate cortex during hypnotic suggestion of paralysis (Halligan, Athwal, Oakley, & Frackowiak, 2000), but this was interpreted as the source of inhibition on motor actions.

Taken together, these imaging studies therefore converge to demonstrate that conversion symptoms may lead to functional changes in brain areas concerned with the affected sensorimotor domain, and they clearly differ from mere simu-lation. Conversion paralysis may involve a suppression of motor processes in basal ganglia-thalamic loops through the influence of medial parietal or ventro-medial prefrontal areas, which could in turn impact on primary motor cortex depending on the exact task requirements. Because motor cortex can still be activated by intentions and imagery, a suppression of activity in downstream basal ganglia loops might correspond to the subjective feeling of patients that their volition is preserved, but their execution is "blocked." In addition, conver-sion paralysis does not seem to result from an active inhibition by the right inferior prefrontal cortex as seen in classic nogo tasks, but rather it involves an increased activity and increased coupling with precuneus and ventromedial PFC. As the latter regions are thought to be particularly involved in self-related representations, imagery, belief checks, and emotion regulation, these results suggest that the primary motor cortex and afferent pathways might be abnor-mally influenced by internal processes related to self-processing rather than by the normal premotor mechanisms in dorsolateral and dorsomedial prefrontal regions.

Conclusions

Anosognosia and conversion hysteria have raised a number of fascinating ques-tions on the mind–brain relationship for more than a century, and both still are puzzling clinical conditions in neurology. Various hypotheses have been put forward to account for the striking dissociation between self-awareness and body states observed in these two disorders, but often on the basis of theoretical speculations rather than empirical investigations. With the advent of new neuroimaging techniques for advanced anatomical lesion analyses and functional brain mapping, we are now just beginning to unravel the interaction of multiple cognitive and affective processes that are likely to jointly contribute to produce such distortion in awareness.

In this review, we have argued that distinct patterns of AHP might result from losses in sensorimotor feedback combined with lesions affecting neural pathways responsible for different types of monitoring of motor errors, possibly operating at either explicit or implicit levels, together with additional lesions in cognitive and affective systems responsible for appropriate behavioral adjustment and learning (hence contributing to deficits in complex mental processes underlying belief formation, verification, or self-concern). This constellation corresponds to the presence of multifocal neural correlates (e.g., in parietal cortex, premotor areas, insula, etc.) typically caused by large lesions or dysfunction after stroke. We have also suggested that this obdurate unawareness for motor deficits in AHP might be mirrored by the seemingly imaginary experience of motor impairment in conversion hysteria. We showed that the latter might involve functional changes in cortico-subcortical motor pathways, combined with an activation of limbic regions and midline frontoparietal areas (including ventral prefrontal regions, ACC, precuneus, and perhaps amygdalo-hippocampal structures), which have previously been associated with self-related representations in imagery, memory and belief state presentation, and memory, and could impose inhibitory or modulatory influences on the motor pathways due to some emotional states in patients with conversion hysteria. However, it remains to be determined whether the mirror symptoms in anosognosia and conversion hysteria might correspond at least partly to mirror changes in some brain regions, and which neural networks and cognitive mechanisms might be concerned by both conditions, if any.

Based on our framework proposed to account in AHP, it would be tempting to extend the putative mechanisms responsible for losses of awareness to mirror disturbances resulting in productive symptoms rather than losses (see Figure 17.6). Thus, implicit monitoring processes conveying unconscious signals of motor errors might not only fail to activate in the presence of a deficit (as in AHP) but also produce abnormal signals in the absence of a corresponding deficit, leading to kinesthetic illusions (Feinberg et al., 2000; Lackner & DiZio, 1992; Naito et al., 2007) and limb reduplication syndromes (Halligan, Marshall, & Wade, 1993; Vuilleumier, Reverdin, & Landis, 1997) when explicit monitoring remains intact; or leading to frank somatoparaphrenia when explicit awareness of the deficit is lacking (Critchley, 1964; Halligan, Marshall, & Wade, 1995; Vallar & Ronchi, 2009). Conversely, a false perception of motor deficit might be delivered to conscious awareness by explicit

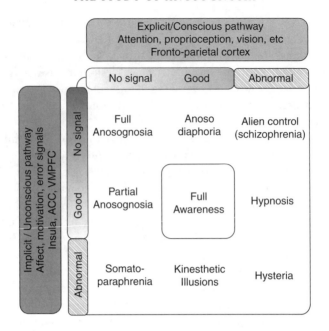

Figure 17.6 A schematic classification of impaired body awareness in different conditions. A putative role is shown for explicit/conscious and implicit/unconscious monitoring processes in relation to each condition, as an attempt to extend our account of motor monitoring deficits in anosognosia for hemiplegia to hysteria and other disorders. Both conscious and unconscious systems can possibly show different degrees of activity resulting in either abolished, normal, or abnormal signals about body states. ACC, anterior cingulate cortex; VMPFC, ventromedial prefrontal cortex.

monitoring processes during conversion hysteria or hypnosis, perhaps with a concomitant abnormal error signal in implicit pathways in hysteria (Sackeim, Nordlie, & Gur, 1979; Vuilleumier, 2005) but not hypnosis (corresponding to the typical dissociative state observed in the latter case); whereas abnormal motor signals in awareness with a loss of implicit motor error signal might possibly correspond to the delusion of alien motor control in schizophrenia and other psychosis (Spence, 2002). However, such a classification remains speculative and will need further systematic investigations to be verified and refined.

In summary, neuropsychology and neuropsychiatry encompass a vast number of disorders that imply a distortion in self-awareness and self-monitoring, ranging from insufficient or absent appraisal of current bodily states to exaggerated or even illusory experiences. We believe that a better understanding of mechanisms underlying such disorders is necessary not only to gain insight into some of the most fascinating facets of human consciousness but also to improve the clinical assessment, management, and rehabilitation strategies for these patients.

Acknowledgments

This work was supported by grants from the Swiss National Foundation (32003B-108367 and 32003B-114014) and Geneva Academic Society to PV, as well as a fellowship from the Foundation Boninchi to RV. We thank Fabienne Staub, Julien Bogousslavksy, and Theodor Landis for their support during our work.

References

Adair, J. C., Gilmore, R. L., Fennell, E. B., Gold, M., & Heilman, K. M. (1995). Anosognosia during intracarotid barbiturate anesthesia: Unawareness or amnesia for weakness. *Neurology, 45*(2), 241–243.

Adolphs, R., Gosselin, F., Buchanan, T. W., Tranel, D., Schyns, P., & Damasio, A. R. (2005). A mechanism for impaired fear recognition after amygdala damage. *Nature, 433*(7021), 68–72.

American Psychiatric Association. (1994). *Diagnostic and statistical manual of mental disorders* (4th ed.). Washington, DC: Author.

Anton, G. (1898). Ueber Herderkrankungen des Gehirns, welche vom Patienten selbst nicht wahrgenommen werden. *Wiener Klinische Wochenschrift, 11*, 227–229.

Aron, A. R. (2007). The neural basis of inhibition in cognitive control. *Neuroscientist, 13* (3), 214–228.

Assal, G. (1983). [No, I am not paralyzed, it's my husband's hand]. *Schweizer Archiv für Neurologie Neurochirurgie und Psychiatrie, 133*(1), 151–157.

Assenova, M., Benecib, Z., & Logak, M. (2006). [Anosognosia for hemiplegia with pontine infarction]. *Revue Neurologique (Paris), 162*(6–7), 747–749.

Babinski, J. (1914). Contribution à l'étude des troubles mentaux dans l'hémiplégie organique (anosognosie). *Revue Neurologique, 27*, 845–848.

Babinski, J., & Dagnan-Bouveret, J. (1912). Emotion et hystérie. *Journal de Psychologie, 9*(2), 97–146.

Baier, B., & Karnath, H. O. (2005). Incidence and diagnosis of anosognosia for hemiparesis revisited. *Journal of Neurology, Neurosurgery and Psychiatry, 76*(3), 358–361.

Baier, B., & Karnath, H. O. (2008). Tight link between our sense of limb ownership and self-awareness of actions. *Stroke, 39*(2), 486–488.

Bakchine, S., Crassard, I., & Seilhan, D. (1997). Anosognosia for hemiplegia after a brainstem haematoma: A pathological case. *Journal of Neurology, Neurosurgery and Psychiatry, 63*(5), 686–687.

Bates, E., Wilson, S. M., Saygin, A. P., Dick, F., Sereno, M. I., Knight, R. T., et al. (2003). Voxel-based lesion-symptom mapping. *Nature Neuroscience, 6*(5), 448–450.

Berti, A., Bottini, G., Gandola, M., Pia, L., Smania, N., Stracciari, A., et al. (2005). Shared cortical anatomy for motor awareness and motor control. *Science, 309*(5733), 488–491.

Binzer, M., Andersen, P. M., & Kullgren, G. (1997). Clinical characteristics of patients with motor disability due to conversion disorder: A prospective control group study. *Journal of Neurology, Neurosurgery and Psychiatry, 63*, 83–88.

Binzer, M., Eisemann, M., & Kullgren, G. (1998). Illness behavior in the acute phase of motor disability in neurological disease and in conversion disorder: A comparative study. *Journal of Psychosomatic Research, 44*(6), 657–666.

Bisiach, E., Perani, D., Vallar, G., & Berti, A. (1986). Unilateral neglect: Personal and extra-personal. *Neuropsychologia, 24*(6), 759–767.

Bisiach, E., Rusconi, M. L., & Vallar, G. (1991). Remission of somatoparaphrenic delusion through vestibular stimulation. *Neuropsychologia, 29*(10), 1029–1031.

Bisiach, E., Vallar, G., Perani, D., Papagno, C., & Berti, A. (1986). Unawareness of disease following lesions of the right hemisphere: Anosognosia for hemiplegia and anosognosia for hemianopia. *Neuropsychologia, 24*(4), 471–482.

Black, D. N., Seritan, A. L., Taber, K. H., & Hurley, R. A. (2004). Conversion hysteria: Lessons from functional imaging. *Journal of Neuropsychiatry and Clinical Neurosciences, 16*(3), 245–251.

Blakemore, S. J., Wolpert, D. M., & Frith, C. D. (2002). Abnormalities in the awareness of action. *Trends in Cognitive Science, 6*(6), 237–242.

Breier, J. I., Adair, J. C., Gold, M., Fennell, E. B., Gilmore, R. L., & Heilman, K. M. (1995). Dissociation of anosognosia for hemiplegia and aphasia during left-hemisphere anesthesia. *Neurology, 45*(1), 65–67.

Brown, R. J. (2004). Psychological mechanisms of medically unexplained symptoms: An integrative conceptual model. *Psychological Bulletin, 130*(5), 793–812.

Burgmer, M., Konrad, C., Jansen, A., Kugel, H., Sommer, J., Heindel, W., et al. (2006). Abnormal brain activation during movement observation in patients with conversion paralysis. *NeuroImage, 29*(4), 1336–1343.

Bush, G., Luu, P., & Posner, M. (2000). Cognitive and emotional influences in anterior cingulate cortex. *Trends in Cognitive Science, 4*(6), 215–222.

Cavanna, A. E., & Trimble, M. R. (2006). The precuneus: A review of its functional anatomy and behavioural correlates. *Brain, 129*(Pt 3), 564–583.

Charcot, J. M. (1892). *Leçons du Mardi à la Salpêtrière* (1887–1888): Bureau du Progrès Médical.

Cojan, Y., Waber, L., Carruzzo, A., & Vuilleumier, P. (2009). Motor inhibition in hysterical conversion paralysis. *NeuroImage, 47*(3), 1026–1037.

Crimlisk, H. L., Bhatia, K., Cope, H., David, A., Marsden, C. D., & Ron, M. A. (1998). Slater revisited: 6 year follow up study of patients with medically unexplained motor symptoms. *British Medical Journal, 316*, 582–586.

Critchley, H. D., Wiens, S., Rotshtein, P., Ohman, A., & Dolan, R. J. (2004). Neural systems supporting interoceptive awareness. *Nature Neuroscience, 7*(2), 189–195.

Critchley, M. (1964). Psychiatric symptoms and parietal disease: Differential diagnosis. *Proceedings of the Royal Society of Medicine, 57*, 422–428.

Cutting, J. (1978). Study of anosognosia. *Journal of Neurology, Neurosurgery, and Psychiatry, 41*(6), 548–555.

Damasio, A. R. (2003). *Looking for Spinoza: Joy, sorrow and the feeling brain.* New York: Harcourt.

D'Argembeau, A., Collette, F., Van der Linden, M., Laureys, S., Del Fiore, G., Degueldre, C., et al. (2005). Self-referential reflective activity and its relationship with rest: A PET study. *NeuroImage, 25*(2), 616–624.

Davies, M., Davies, A. A., & Coltheart, M. (2005). Anosognosia and the two-factor theory of delusions. *Mind and Language, 20*(2), 209–236.

De Gelder, B., De Haan, E. H., & Heywood, C. A. (2002). *Out of mind: Varieties of unconscious processes.* Oxford, England: Oxford University Press.

Dehaene, S., Changeux, J. P., Naccache, L., Sackur, J., & Sergent, C. (2006). Conscious, preconscious, and subliminal processing: A testable taxonomy. *Trends in Cognitive Science, 10*(5), 204–211.

Dehaene, S., & Naccache, L. (2001). Towards a cognitive neuroscience of consciousness: Basic evidence and a workspace framework. *Cognition, 79*(1–2), 1–37.

Dehaene, S., Naccache, L., Cohen, L., Bihan, D. L., Mangin, J. F., Poline, J. B., et al. (2001). Cerebral mechanisms of word masking and unconscious repetition priming. *Nature Neuroscience, 4*(7), 752–758.

Dehaene, S., Posner, M. I., & Tucker, D. M. (1994). Localization of a neural system for error detection and compensation. *Psychological Science, 5*(5), 303–305.

Dehaene, S., Sergent, C., & Changeux, J. P. (2003). A neuronal network model linking subjective reports and objective physiological data during conscious perception. *Proceedings of the National Academy of Sciences U S A, 100*(14), 8520–8525.

de Lange, F. P., Roelofs, K., & Toni, I. (2007). Increased self-monitoring during imagined movements in conversion paralysis. *Neuropsychologia, 45*(9), 2051–2058.

den Ouden, H. E., Frith, U., Frith, C., & Blakemore, S. J. (2005). Thinking about intentions. *NeuroImage, 28*(4), 787–796.

Devinsky, O. (1998). Nonepileptic psychogenic seizures: Quagmires of pathophysiology, diagnosis, and treatment. *Epilepsia, 39*(5), 458–462.

Eames, P. (1992). Hysteria following brain injury. *Journal of Neurology, Neurosurgery, and Psychiatry, 55*(11), 1046–1053.

Endrass, T., Reuter, B., & Kathmann, N. (2007). ERP correlates of conscious error recognition: Aware and unaware errors in an antisaccade task. *European Journal of Neuroscience, 26*(6), 1714–1720.

Evyapan, D., & Kumral, E. (1999). Pontine anosognosia for hemiplegia. *Neurology, 53* (3), 647–649.

Falkenstein, M., Hoormann, J., Christ, S., & Hohnsbein, J. (2000). ERP components on reaction errors and their functional significance: A tutorial. *Biological Psychology, 51*(2–3), 87–107.

Feinberg, T. E. (1997). Anosognosia and confabulations. In T. E. Feinberg & M. J. Farah (Eds.), *Behavioral neurology and neuropsychology* (pp. 369–390). New York: McGraw-Hill.

Feinberg, T. E., Haber, L. D., & Leeds, N. E. (1990). Verbal asomatognosia. *Neurology, 40*(9), 1391–1394.

Feinberg, T. E., Roane, D. M., & Ali, J. (2000). Illusory limb movements in anosognosia for hemiplegia. *Journal of Neurology, Neurosurgery, and Psychiatry, 68*(4), 511–513.

Fiorelli, M., Blin, J., Bakchine, S., Laplane, D., & Baron, J. C. (1991). PET studies of cortical diaschisis in patients with motor hemi-neglect. *Journal of the Neurological Sciences, 104*(2), 135–142.

Flor-Henry, P. (1978). Gender, hemispheric specialization and psychopathology. *Social Science and Medicine, 12*(3B), 155–162.

Flor-Henry, P., Fromm-Auch, D., Tapper, M., & Schopflocher, D. (1981). A neuropsychological study of the stable syndrome of hysteria. *Biological Psychiatry*, 16, 601–616.

Fotopoulou, A., Tsakiris, M., Haggard, P., Vagopoulou, A., Rudd, A., & Kopelman, M. (2008). The role of motor intention in motor awareness: An experimental study on anosognosia for hemiplegia. *Brain*, 131(12), 3432–3442.

Frei, J. (1984). Hysteria: Problems of definition and evolution of the symptomatology. *Schweizer Archiv für Neurologie Neurochirurgie und Psychiatrie*, 134(1), 93–129.

Freud, S., & Breuer, J. (1895). *Studies on hysteria* (1955 ed.). New York: Basic Books/ Hogarth Press.

Frith, C. D., Blakemore, S. J., & Wolpert, D. M. (2000). Abnormalities in the awareness and control of action. *Philosophical Transactions of the Royal Society of London B: Biological Sciences*, 355(1404), 1771–1788.

Galin, D., Diamond, R., & Braff, D. (1977). Lateralization of conversion symptoms: More frequent on the left. *American Journal of Psychiatry*, 134(578–580).

Gazzaniga, M. S. (2000). Cerebral specialization and interhemispheric communication: Does the corpus callosum enable the human condition? *Brain*, 123(Pt 7), 1293–1326.

Ghaffar, O., Staines, W. R., & Feinstein, A. (2006). Unexplained neurologic symptoms: An fMRI study of sensory conversion disorder. *Neurology*, 67(11), 2036–2038.

Gilmore, R. L., Heilman, K. M., Schmidt, R. P., Fennell, E. M., & Quisling, R. (1992). Anosognosia during Wada testing. *Neurology*, 42(4), 925–927.

Gold, M., Adair, J. C., Jacobs, D. H., & Heilman, K. M. (1994). Anosognosia for hemiplegia: An electrophysiologic investigation of the feed-forward hypothesis. *Neurology*, 44(10), 1804–1808.

Gould, R., Miller, B. L., Goldberg, M. A., & Benson, D. F. (1986). The validity of hysterical signs and symptoms. *Journal of Nervous and Mental Disorders*, 174, 593–597.

Grandjean, D., Sander, D., Lucas, N., Scherer, K. R., & Vuilleumier, P. (2008). Effects of emotional prosody on auditory extinction for voices in patients with spatial neglect. *Neuropsychologia*, 46(2), 487–496.

Haber, S. N. (2003). The primate basal ganglia: Parallel and integrative networks. *Journal of Chemical Neuroanatomy*, 26(4), 317–330.

Halligan, P. W., Athwal, B. S., Oakley, D. A., & Frackowiak, R. S. (2000). Imaging hypnotic paralysis: Implications for conversion hysteria. *Lancet*, 355(9208), 986–987.

Halligan, P. W., Fink, G. R., Marshall, J. C., & Vallar, G. (2003). Spatial cognition: Evidence from visual neglect. *Trends in Cognitive Science*, 7(3), 125–133.

Halligan, P. W., Marshall, J. C., & Wade, D. T. (1993). Three arms: A case study of supernumarery phantom limb after right hemisphere stroke. *Journal of Neurology, Neurosurgery, and Psychiatry*, 56, 159–166.

Halligan, P. W., Marshall, J. C., & Wade, D. T. (1995). Unilateral somatoparaphrenia after right hemisphere stroke: A case description. *Cortex*, 31(1), 173–182.

Harris, S., Sheth, S. A., & Cohen, M. S. (2008). Functional neuroimaging of belief, disbelief, and uncertainty. *Annals of Neurology*, 63(2), 141–147.

Heilman, K. M. (1991). Anosognosia: Possible neuropsychological mechanisms. In G. Prigatano & D. L. Schacter (Eds.), *Awareness of deficit after brain injury: Clinical and theoretical issues.* (pp. 53–62). New York: Oxford Universitary Press.

Hester, R., Foxe, J. J., Molholm, S., Shpaner, M., & Garavan, H. (2005). Neural mechanisms involved in error processing: A comparison of errors made with and without awareness. *NeuroImage, 27*(3), 602–608.

Hier, D. B., Mondlock, J., & Caplan, L. R. (1983). Behavioral abnormalities after right hemisphere stroke. *Neurology, 33*(3), 337–344.

Holroyd, C. B., Praamstra, P., Plat, E., & Coles, M. G. (2002). Spared error-related potentials in mild to moderate Parkinson's disease. *Neuropsychologia, 40*(12), 2116–2124.

House, A., Dennis, M., Mogridge, L., Hawton, K., & Warlow, C. (1990). Life events and difficulties preceding stroke. *Journal of Neurology, Neurosurgery and Psychiatry, 53* (12), 1024–1028.

House, A., & Hodges, J. (1988). Persistent denial of handicap after infarction of the right basal ganglia: A case study. *Journal of Neurology, Neurosurgery, and Psychiatry, 51* (1), 112–115.

Janet, P. (1887). L'anesthésie systématisée et la dissociation des phénomènes psychologiques. *Revue Philosophique, 1*, 449.

Janet, P. (1889). *L'automatisme psychologique* (1973 ed.). Paris: Société Pierre Janet et CNRS.

Janet, P. (1894). *L'état mental des hystériques.* Paris: Rueff.

Janet, P. (1911). *L'état mental des hystériques.* Paris: Félix Alcan.

Kanaan, R. A., Craig, T. K., Wessely, S. C., & David, A. S. (2007). Imaging repressed memories in motor conversion disorder. *Psychosomatic Medicine, 69*(2), 202–205.

Karnath, H. O., Baier, B., & Nagele, T. (2005). Awareness of the functioning of one's own limbs mediated by the insular cortex? *Journal of Neuroscience, 25*(31), 7134–7138.

Klein, T. A., Endrass, T., Kathmann, N., Neumann, J., von Cramon, D. Y., & Ullsperger, M. (2007). Neural correlates of error awareness. *NeuroImage, 34*(4), 1774–1781.

Koehler, P. J., & Okun, M. S. (2004). Important observations prior to the description of the Hoover sign. *Neurology, 63*(9), 1693–1697.

Kozlowska, K. (2005). Healing the disembodied mind: Contemporary models of conversion disorder. *Harvard Review of Psychiatry, 13*(1), 1–13.

Krem, M. M. (2004). Motor conversion disorders reviewed from a neuropsychiatric perspective. *Journal of Clinical Psychiatry, 65*(6), 783–790.

Kretschmer, E. (1948). *Hysteria: Reflex and instinct.* London: Peter Owen.

Lackner, J. R., & DiZio, P. (1992). Gravitoinertial force level affects the appreciation of limb position during muscle vibration. *Brain Research, 592*(1–2), 175–180.

Langevin, P., & Le Gall, D. (1999). L'anosognosie secondaire à une atteinte frontale. In M. Van der Linden, X. Seron, D. Le Gall, & P. Andrès (Eds.), *Neuropsychologie des lobes frontaux* (pp. 289–307). Marseille, France: Solal.

Larson, M. J., Kaufman, D. A., Schmalfuss, I. M., & Perlstein, W. M. (2007). Performance monitoring, error processing, and evaluative control following severe TBI. *Journal of the International Neuropsychological Society, 13*(6), 961–971.

Levine, B., Dawson, D., Boutet, I., Schwartz, M. L., & Stuss, D. T. (2000). Assessment of strategic self-regulation in traumatic brain injury: Its relationship to injury severity and psychosocial outcome. *Neuropsychology, 14*(4), 491–500.

Levine, B., Stuss, D. T., Milberg, W. P., Alexander, M. P., Schwartz, M., & Macdonald, R. (1998). The effects of focal and diffuse brain damage on strategy application: Evidence from focal lesions, traumatic brain injury and normal aging. *Journal of the International Neuropsychological Society, 4*(3), 247–264.

Levine, D. N. (1990). Unawareness of visual and sensorimotor defects: A hypothesis. *Brain and Cognition, 13*(2), 233–281.

Levine, D. N., Calvanio, R., & Rinn, W. E. (1991). The pathogenesis of anosognosia for hemiplegia. *Neurology, 41*(11), 1770–1781.

Lhermitte, F., Pillon, B., & Serdaru, M. (1986). Human autonomy and the frontal lobes. Part I: Imitation and utilization behavior: A neuropsychological study of 75 patients. *Annals of Neurology, 19*(4), 326–334.

Lou, H. C., Luber, B., Crupain, M., Keenan, J. P., Nowak, M., Kjaer, T. W., et al. (2004). Parietal cortex and representation of the mental self. *Proceedings of the National Academy of Sciences USA, 101*(17), 6827–6832.

Lu, L. H., Barrett, A. M., Cibula, J. E., Gilmore, R. L., Fennell, E. B., & Heilman, K. M. (2000). Dissociation of anosognosia and phantom movement during the Wada test. *Journal of Neurology, Neurosurgery, and Psychiatry, 69*(6), 820–823.

Lu, L. H., Barrett, A. M., Schwartz, R. L., Cibula, J. E., Gilmore, R. L., Uthman, B. M., et al. (1997). Anosognosia and confabulation during the Wada test. *Neurology, 49* (5), 1316–1322.

Ludwig, A. M. (1972). Hysteria: A neurobiological theory. *Archives of General Psychiatry, 27,* 771–777.

Mace, C. J. (1992). Hysterical conversion. I: A history; II: A critique. *British Journal of Psychiatry, 161*(369), 369–377; 378–389.

Mace, C. J., & Trimble, M. R. (1996). Ten-year prognosis of conversion disorder. *British Journal of Psychiatry, 169*(3), 282–288.

Maeshima, S., Dohi, N., Funahashi, K., Nakai, K., Itakura, T., & Komai, N. (1997). Rehabilitation of patients with anosognosia for hemiplegia due to intracerebral haemorrhage. *Brain Injury, 11*(9), 691–697.

Magno, E., Foxe, J. J., Molholm, S., Robertson, I. H., & Garavan, H. (2006). The anterior cingulate and error avoidance. *Journal of Neuroscience, 26*(18), 4769–4773.

Mailis-Gagnon, A., Giannoylis, I., Downar, J., Kwan, C. L., Mikulis, D. J., Crawley, A. P., et al. (2003). Altered central somatosensory processing in chronic pain patients with "hysterical" anesthesia. *Neurology, 60*(9), 1501–1507.

Marcel, A. J., Tegner, R., & Nimmo-Smith, I. (2004). Anosognosia for plegia: Specificity, extension, partiality and disunity of bodily unawareness. *Cortex, 40* (1), 19–40.

Marshall, J. C., & Halligan, P. W. (1988). Blindsight and insight in visuo-spatial neglect. *Nature, 336*(6201), 766–767.

Marshall, J. C., Halligan, P. W., Fink, G. R., Wade, D. T., & Frackowiack, R. S. J. (1997). The functional anatomy of a hysterical paralysis. *Cognition, 64,* B1–B8.

McGlynn, S. M., & Schacter, D. L. (1989). Unawareness of deficits in neuropsychological syndromes. *Journal of Clinical and Experimental Neuropsychology, 11*(2), 143–205.

Miller, E. (1987). Hysteria: Its nature and explanation. *British Journal of Clinical Psychology, 26*(Pt 3), 163–173.

Miller, L. (1984). Neuropsychological concepts of somatoform disorders. *International Journal of Psychiatry in Medicine, 14*(1), 31–46.

Mohr, D. C., Hart, S. L., Julian, L., Cox, D., & Pelletier, D. (2004). Association between stressful life events and exacerbation in multiple sclerosis: A meta-analysis. *British Medical Journal, 328*(7442), 731.

Mort, D. J., Malhotra, P., Mannan, S. K., Rorden, C., Pambakian, A., Kennard, C., et al. (2003). The anatomy of visual neglect. *Brain, 126*(Pt 9), 1986–1997.

Naito, E., Nakashima, T., Kito, T., Aramaki, Y., Okada, T., & Sadato, N. (2007). Human limb-specific and non-limb-specific brain representations during kinesthetic illusory movements of the upper and lower extremities. *European Journal of Neuroscience, 25*(11), 3476–3487.

Naqvi, N. H., & Bechara, A. (2009). The hidden island of addiction: The insula. *Trends in Neuroscience, 32*(1), 56–67.

Nardone, I. B., Ward, R., Fotopoulou, A., & Turnbull, O. H. (2007). Attention and emotion in anosognosia: Evidence of implicit awareness and repression? *Neurocase, 13*(5), 438–445.

Nicolson, R., & Feinstein, A. (1994). Conversion, dissociation, and multiple sclerosis. *Journal of Nervous and Mental Disease, 182*(11), 668–669.

Nieuwenhuis, S., Ridderinkhof, K. R., Blom, J., Band, G. P., & Kok, A. (2001). Error-related brain potentials are differentially related to awareness of response errors: Evidence from an antisaccade task. *Psychophysiology, 38*(5), 752–760.

Norman, D. A., & Shallice, T. (1986). Attention to action: Willed and automatic control of behaviour. In R. J. Davidson, G. E. Schwartz, & D. Shapiro (Eds.), *Consciousness and self-regulation: Advances in research and theory* (pp. 1–18). New York: Plenum Press.

Oakley, D. A. (1999). Hypnosis and conversion hysteria: A unifying model. *Cognitive Neuropsychiatry, 4*, 3.

O'Callaghan, C., Powell, T., & Oyebode, J. (2006). An exploration of the experience of gaining awareness of deficit in people who have suffered a traumatic brain injury. *Neuropsychological Rehabilitation, 16*(5), 579–593.

O'Connell, R. G., Dockree, P. M., Bellgrove, M. A., Kelly, S. P., Hester, R., Garavan, H., et al. (2007). The role of cingulate cortex in the detection of errors with and without awareness: A high-density electrical mapping study. *European Journal of Neuroscience, 25*(8), 2571–2579.

Ohman, A., & Mineka, S. (2001). Fears, phobias, and preparedness: Toward an evolved module of fear and fear learning. *Psychological Review, 108*(3), 483–522.

Okun, M. S., & Koehler, P. J. (2004). Babinski's clinical differentiation of organic paralysis from hysterical paralysis: Effect on US neurology. *Archives of Neurology, 61*(5), 778–783.

Orfei, M. D., Robinson, R. G., Prigatano, G. P., Starkstein, S., Rusch, N., Bria, P., et al. (2007). Anosognosia for hemiplegia after stroke is a multifaceted phenomenon: A systematic review of the literature. *Brain, 130*(Pt 12), 3075–3090.

Ortells, J. J., Daza, M. T., & Fox, E. (2003). Semantic activation in the absence of perceptual awareness. *Perception & Psychophysics, 65*(8), 1307–1317.

Ousdal, O. T., Jensen, J., Server, A., Hariri, A. R., Nakstad, P. H., & Andreassen, O. A. (2008). The human amygdala is involved in general behavioral relevance detection:

Evidence from an event-related functional magnetic resonance imaging go-nogo task. *Neuroscience, 156*(3), 450–455.

Ownsworth, T., & Clare, L. (2006). The association between awareness deficits and rehabilitation outcome following acquired brain injury. *Clinical Psychology Review, 26*(6), 783–795.

Ownsworth, T., Fleming, J., Strong, J., Radel, M., Chan, W., & Clare, L. (2007). Awareness typologies, long-term emotional adjustment and psychosocial outcomes following acquired brain injury. *Neuropsychological Rehabilitation, 17*(2), 129–150.

Ownsworth, T., & McKenna, K. (2004). Investigation of factors related to employment outcome following traumatic brain injury: A critical review and conceptual model. *Disability and Rehabilitation, 26*(13), 765–783.

Pavlov, I. P. (1941). *Lectures on conditioned reflexes. Vol. 2: Conditioned reflexes and psychiatry* (H. W. Gantt, trans.). New York: International Publishers.

Pavlov, J. (1933). Essai d'une interprétation physiologique de l'hystérie. Encéphale, 285–293.

Perkin, G. D. (1989). An analysis of 7836 succesive new outpatient referrals. *Journal of Neurology, Neurosurgery, and Psychiatry, 52,* 447–448.

Phelps, E. A., & LeDoux, J. E. (2005). Contributions of the amygdala to emotion processing: From animal models to human behavior. *Neuron, 48*(2), 175–187.

Pia, L., Neppi-Modona, M., Ricci, R., & Berti, A. (2004). The anatomy of anosognosia for hemiplegia: A meta-analysis. *Cortex, 40*(2), 367–377.

Prigatano, G. P., & Altman, I. M. (1990). Impaired awareness of behavioral limitations after traumatic brain injury. *Archives of Physical Medicine and Rehabilitation, 71* (13), 1058–1064.

Ramachandran, V. S. (1995). Anosognosia in parietal lobe syndrome. *Consciousness and Cognition, 4*(1), 22–51.

Ramachandran, V. S. (1996). The evolutionary biology of self-deception, laughter, dreaming and depression: Some clues from anosognosia. *Medical Hypotheses, 47*(5), 347–362.

Rode, G., Charles, N., Perenin, M. T., Vighetto, A., Trillet, M., & Aimard, G. (1992). Partial remission of hemiplegia and somatoparaphrenia through vestibular stimulation in a case of unilateral neglect. *Cortex, 28*(2), 203–208.

Rodriguez, E., George, N., Lachaux, J. P., Martinerie, J., Renault, B., & Varela, F. J. (1999). Perception's shadow: Long-distance synchronization of human brain activity. *Nature, 397*(6718), 430–433.

Roelofs, K., de Bruijn, E. R., & Van Galen, G. P. (2006). Hyperactive action monitoring during motor-initiation in conversion paralysis: An event-related potential study. *Biological Psychology, 71*(3), 316–325.

Roelofs, K., Spinhoven, P., Sandijck, P., Moene, F. C., & Hoogduin, K. A. (2005). The impact of early trauma and recent life-events on symptom severity in patients with conversion disorder. *Journal of Nervous and Mental Disease, 193*(8), 508–514.

Sackeim, H. A., Nordlie, J. W., & Gur, R. C. (1979). A model of hysterical and hypnotic blindness: Cognition, motivation, and awareness. *Journal of Abnormal Psychology, 88*(5), 474–489.

Sander, D., Grafman, J., & Zalla, T. (2003). The human amygdala: An evolved system for relevance detection. *Reviews of Neuroscience, 14*(4), 303–316.

Schilder, P. (1935). Psycho-analysis of space. *International Journal of Psycho-analysis, 16*, 274–295.

Sierra, M., & Berrios, G. E. (1999). Towards a neuropsychiatry of conversive hysteria. In P. W. Halligan & A. S. David (Eds.), *Conversion hysteria: Towards a cognitive neuropsychological account (Special Issue of the Journal Cognitive Neuropsychiatry)* (pp. 267–287). Hove, England: Psychology Press Publication.

Soon, C. S., Brass, M., Heinze, H. J., & Haynes, J. D. (2008). Unconscious determinants of free decisions in the human brain. *Nature Neuroscience, 11*(5), 543–545.

Spence, S. A. (1999). Hysterical paralyses as disorders of action. In P. W. Halligan & A. S. David (Eds.), *Conversion hysteria: Towards a cognitive neuropsychological account (Special Issue of the Journal Cognitive Neuropsychiatry)* (pp. 203–226). Hove, England: Psychology Press Publication.

Spence, S. A. (2002). Alien motor phenomena: A window on to agency. *Cognitive Neuropsychiatry, 7*(3), 211–220.

Spence, S. A., Crimlisk, H. L., Cope, H., Ron, M. A., & Grasby, P. M. (2000). Discrete neurophysiological correlates in prefrontal cortex during hysterical and feigned disorder of movement. *Lancet, 355*, 1243–1244.

Spiegel, D. (1991). Neurophysiological correlates of hypnosis and dissociation. *Journal of Neuropsychiatry Clinical Neurosciences, 3*, 440–445.

Squire, L. R. (1992). Memory and the hippocampus: A synthesis from findings with rats, monkeys, and humans. *Psychological Review, 99*(2), 195–231.

Starkstein, S. E., Fedoroff, J. P., Price, T. R., Leiguarda, R., & Robinson, R. G. (1992). Anosognosia in patients with cerebrovascular lesions. A study of causative factors. *Stroke, 23*(10), 1446–1453.

Stemmer, B., Segalowitz, S. J., Dywan, J., Panisset, M., & Melmed, C. (2007). The error negativity in nonmedicated and medicated patients with Parkinson's disease. *Clinical Neurophysiology, 118*(6), 1223–1229.

Stemmer, B., Segalowitz, S. J., Witzke, W., & Schonle, P. W. (2004). Error detection in patients with lesions to the medial prefrontal cortex: An ERP study. *Neuropsychologia, 42*(1), 118–130.

Stern, D. B. (1983). Psychogenic somatic symptoms on the left side: Review and interpretation. In M. S. Myslobodsky (Ed.), *Hemisyndromes: Psychobiology, neurology, psychiatry* (pp. 415–445). New York: Academic Press.

Stoerig, P., & Cowey, A. (1997). Blindsight in man and monkey. *Brain, 120 (Pt 3)*, 535–559.

Stone, J., Sharpe, M., Carson, A., Lewis, S. C., Thomas, B., Goldbeck, R., et al. (2002). Are functional motor and sensory symptoms really more frequent on the left? A systematic review. *Journal of Neurology, Neurosurgery, and Psychiatry, 73*(5), 578–581.

Stone, J., Sharpe, M., Rothwell, P. M., & Warlow, C. P. (2003). The 12 year prognosis of unilateral functional weakness and sensory disturbance. *Journal of Neurology, Neurosurgery, and Psychiatry, 74*(5), 591–596.

Stone, J., Warlow, C., Carson, A., & Sharpe, M. (2003). A systematic review of the laterality of hysterical hemiplegia. *Journal of Neurology, Neurosurgery, and Psychiatry, 74*(8), 1163–1164.

Stone, J., Zeman, A., Simonotto, E., Meyer, M., Azuma, R., Flett, S., et al. (2007). fMRI in patients with motor conversion symptoms and controls with simulated weakness. *Psychosomatic Medicine, 69*(9), 961–969.

Sydenham, T. (1697). Discourse concerning hysterical and hypochondriacal distempers. In Dr. Sydenham's Complete Method of Curing almost All Diseases, and Description of their Symptoms. To Which Are Now Added Five Discourses of the Same Author Concerning Pleurisy, Gout, Hysterical Passion, Dropsy and Rheumatism (3rd ed.). 149, London: Newman and Parker.

Tallon-Baudry, C., & Bertrand, O. (1999). Oscillatory gamma activity in humans and its role in object representation. *Trends in Cognitive Science, 3*(4), 151–162.

Taylor, S. F., Stern, E. R., & Gehring, W. J. (2007). Neural systems for error monitoring: Recent findings and theoretical perspectives. *Neuroscientist, 13*(2), 160–172.

Tiihonen, J., Kuikka, J., Viinamaki, H., Lehtonen, J., & Partanen, J. (1995). Altered cerebral blood flow during hysterical paresthesia. *Biological Psychiatry, 37*(2), 134–135.

Trimble, M. R. (1981). *Neuropsychiatry*. Chichester, England: J. Wiley & Sons.

Turnbull, O. H., & Solms, M. (2007). Awareness, desire, and false beliefs: Freud in the light of modern neuropsychology. *Cortex, 43*(8), 1083–1090.

Ullsperger, M., & von Cramon, D. Y. (2006). The role of intact frontostriatal circuits in error processing. *Journal of Cognitive Neurosciences, 18*(4), 651–664.

Ullsperger, M., von Cramon, D. Y., & Muller, N. G. (2002). Interactions of focal cortical lesions with error processing: Evidence from event-related brain potentials. *Neuropsychology, 16*(4), 548–561.

Vallar, G., Guariglia, C., & Rusconi, M. L. (1997). Modulation of the neglect syndrome by sensory stimulation. In P. Thier & H. O. Karnath (Eds.), *Parietal lobe contributions to orientation in 3D space* (pp. 555–578). Heidelberg, Germany: Springer-Verlag.

Vallar, G., & Ronchi, R. (2006). Anosognosia for motor and sensory deficits after unilateral brain damage: A review. *Restorative Neurology and Neuroscience, 24*(4–6), 247–257.

Vallar, G., & Ronchi, R. (2009). Somatoparaphrenia: A body delusion. A review of the neuropsychological literature. *Experimental Brain Research, 192*(3), 533–551.

van Veen, V., & Carter, C. S. (2002). The anterior cingulate as a conflict monitor: fMRI and ERP studies. *Physiology and Behavior, 77*(4–5), 477–482.

Vocat, R., Pourtois, G., & Vuilleumier, P. (2008). Unavoidable errors: A spatio-temporal analysis of time-course and neural sources of evoked potentials associated with error processing in a speeded task. *Neuropsychologia, 46*(10), 2545–2555.

Vuilleumier, P. (2000). Anosognosia. In J. Bogousslavsky, & J. L. Cummings (Eds.), *Behavior and mood disorders in focal brain lesions* (pp. 465–519). Cambridge, England: Cambridge University Press.

Vuilleumier, P. (2004). Anosognosia: The neurology of beliefs and uncertainties. *Cortex, 40*(1), 9–17.

Vuilleumier, P. (2005). Hysterical conversion and brain function. *Progressive Brain Research, 150*, 309–329.

Vuilleumier, P. (2009). The neurophysiology of self-awareness disorders in conversion hysteria. In S. Laureys and G. Tononi (Eds.), *The neurology of consciousness* (pp. 282–302). London: Elsevier Ltd.

Vuilleumier, P., Chicherio, C., Assal, F., Schwartz, S., Slosman, D., & Landis, T. (2001). Functional neuroanatomical correlates of hysterical sensorimotor loss. *Brain, 124*(Pt 6), 1077–1090.

Vuilleumier, P., Reverdin, A., & Landis, T. (1997). Four legs: Illusory reduplication of the lower limbs after bilateral parietal lobe damage. *Archives of Neurology, 54*, 1543–1547.

Vuilleumier, P., Schwartz, S., Clarke, K., Husain, M., & Driver, J. (2002). Testing memory for unseen visual stimuli in patients with extinction and spatial neglect. *Journal of Cognitive Neuroscience, 14*(6), 875–886.

Weinstein, E. A., & Kahn, R. L. (1955). *Denial of illness: Symbolic and physiological aspects.* Springfield, IL: Charles C. Thomas.

Weinstein, N. D. (1984). Why it won't happen to me: Perceptions of risk factors and susceptibility. *Health Psychology, 3*(5), 431–457.

Weinstein, N. D. (1987). Unrealistic optimism about susceptibility to health problems: conclusions from a community-wide sample. *Journal of Behavioral Medicine, 10*(5), 481–500.

Weinstein, N. D. (1989). Optimistic biases about personal risks. *Science, 246*(4935), 1232–1233.

Werring, D. J., Weston, L., Bullmore, E. T., Plant, G. T., & Ron, M. A. (2004). Functional magnetic resonance imaging of the cerebral response to visual stimulation in medically unexplained visual loss. *Psychological Medicine, 34*(4), 583–589.

Whitlock, F. A. (1967). The aetiology of hysteria. *Acta Psychiatrica Scandinavica, 43*, 144–162.

Willanger, R., Danielsen, U. T., & Ankerhus, J. (1981). Denial and neglect of hemiparesis in right-sided apoplectic lesions. *Acta Neurologica Scandinavica, 64*(5), 310–326.

Xue, G., Aron, A. R., & Poldrack, R. A. (2008). Common neural substrates for inhibition of spoken and manual responses. *Cerebral Cortex, 18*(8), 1923–1932.

VI

Measurement Issues and Technology

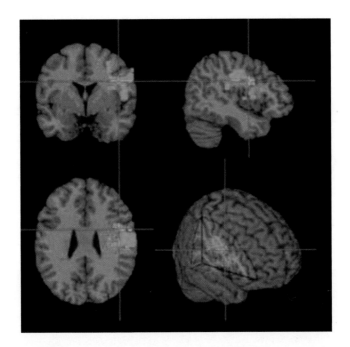

Plate 2.1 Brain areas with lesions associated with anosognosia (From Berti et al., 2005, reprinted with permission from the Association for the Advancement of Science, *Science, 309*(5733), 488–491.) (See Figure 2.1)

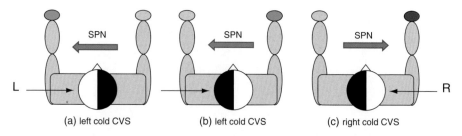

(a) left cold CVS   (b) left cold CVS   (c) right cold CVS

Plate 2.3 Effects of cold caloric vestibular stimulation (CVS) on tactile hemianesthesia in right brain–damaged and left brain–damaged patients as a consequence of the stimulation side (contralesional versus ipsilesional ear stimulation). The damaged hemisphere is colored in black. L, left; R, right; SPN, slow-phase nystagmus; green: positive effect (recovery) of tactile perception; red: no effect on tactile perception. (See Figure 2.3)

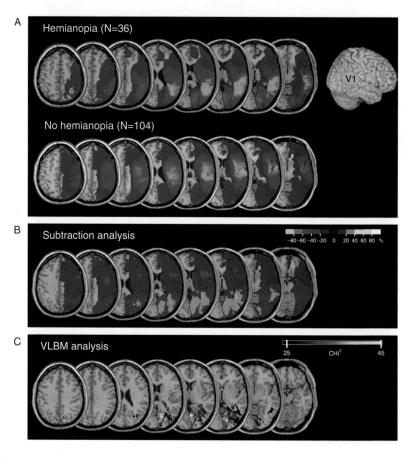

Plate 3.1 (See Box 3.1 for narrative associated with this plate)

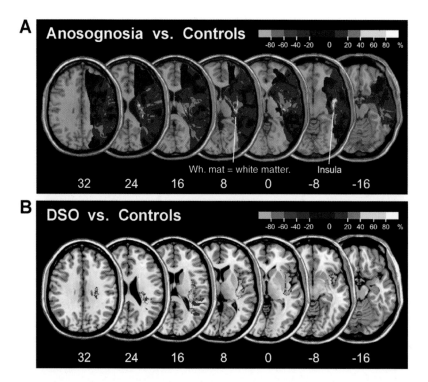

Plate 3.2 *(A)* Overlay plot of the subtracted superimposed lesions of a group of right brain damaged patients with anosognosia for hemiparesis/-plegia (AHP) minus a group of patients without AHP (control group). Wh. mat. = white matter. (Adapted from Karnath et al., 2005, with permission from The Society for Neuroscience, *The Journal of Neuroscience, 25*(31), 7134–7138.) *(B)* Overlay plot of the subtracted superimposed lesions of a patient group showing a disturbed sense of limb ownership (DSO) and AHP minus a control group without the disorder. (From Baier & Karnath, 2008, with permission from the American Heart Association, *Stroke, 39*, 486–488.) In each panel, the percentage of overlapping lesions of the anosognosia patients after subtraction of controls is illustrated by five colors coding increasing frequencies from dark red (difference = 1% to 20%) to white-yellow (difference = 81% to 100%). Each color represents 20% increments. The colors from dark blue (difference = –1% to –20%) to light blue (difference = –81% to –100%) indicate regions damaged more frequently in control patients. MNI z-coordinates of each transverse slice are given. In concordance, the two independent patient samples and analyses *(A and B)* revealed that the right insula is commonly damaged in patients with AHP and DSO but is significantly less affected in patients without these disorders. (See Figure 3.2)

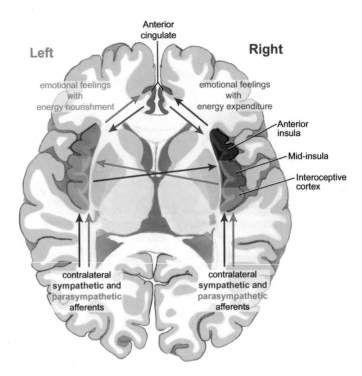

Plate 4.1 A schematic view of the integration of sympathetic (from lamina I) and parasympathetic (from NTS) afferent activity from the contralateral side of the body in the posterior (interoceptive) and middle portions of the insula, each of which becomes lateralized in the right (sympathetic) and left (parasympathetic) anterior insula of the human brain. The "core network" formed by the anterior insular cortex (AIC) and the anterior cingulate cortex (ACC) on both sides is also indicated. Drawing produced by the Neuroscience Publication office of Barrow Neurological Institute ©. (See Figure 4.1)

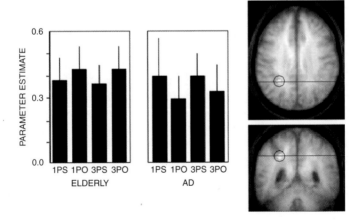

Plate 10.6 Activation clusters in the intra-parietal sulcus in the AD group as compared to elderly controls. 1PS = first person perspective on self, 1PO = first person perspective on other, 3PS = third person perspective on self, 3PO = third person perspective on other. (From Ruby et al., 2008, reprinted with permission from Elsevier, *Neurobiology of Aging*, 30: 1637–51.) (See Figure 10.6)

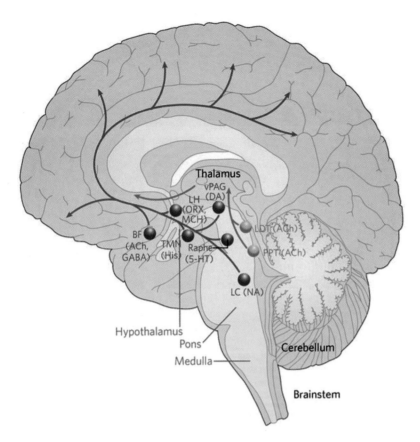

Plate 12.2 A summary diagram of the ascending arousal system. The cholinergic system, shown in yellow, provides the main input to the relay and reticular nuclei of the thalamus from the upper brainstem. This inhibits the reticular nucleus and activates the thalamic relay nuclei, putting them into transmission mode for relaying sensory information to the cerebral cortex. The cortex is activated simultaneously by a series of direct inputs, shown in red. These include monoaminergic inputs from the upper brainstem and posterior hypothalamus, such as noradrenaline (NA) from the locus coeruleus (LC), serotonin (5-HT) from the dorsal and median raphe nuclei, dopamine (DA) from the ventral periaqueduetal gray matter (vPAG), and histamine (His) from the tuberomammillary nucleus (TMN); petidergic inputs from the hypothalamus such as orexin (ORX) and melanin-concentrating hormone (MCH) both from the lateral hypothalamus (LH); and both cholinergic (ACH) and gamma-aminobulyric acid (GABA)-ergic inputs from the basal forebrain (BF). Activation of the brainstem yellow pathway in the absence of the red pathways occurs during rapid eye movement (REM) sleep, resulting in the cortex entering a dreaming state. LDT, laterodorsal tegmental nuclei; PPT, pedunculopontine. (From Saper, CB, Scammell, TE, Lu J. Hypothalamic regulation of sleep and circadian rhythms. *Nature* 437: 1257–1263, 2005. Reprinted with permission from Macmillan Publishers LTD) (See Figure 12.2)

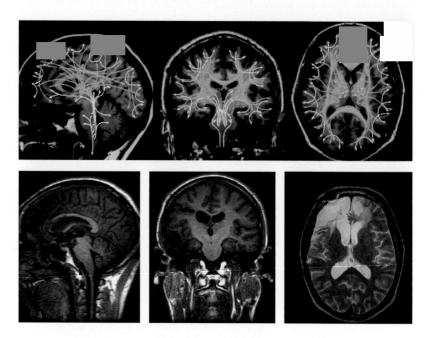

Plate 12.3 Top part of the figure is an over-simplified and theoretical representation of how three vectors of consciousness may be distributed in an overlapping fashion in the adult brain. Bottom part of the figure represents encephalomalacia associated with severe TBI. It is presented for comparison purposes to see how different vectors of consciousness may be differentially affected depending on the brain regions that are affected following severe TBI. (See Figure 12.3)

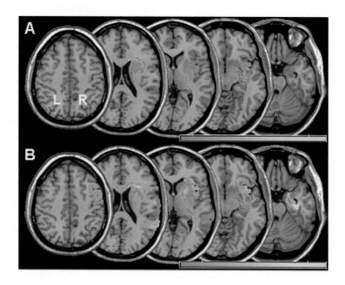

Plate 17.2 Results of statistical anatomical lesion analysis in our prospective study of AHP. Voxelwise mapping of brain areas correlating with anosognosia scores in the hyperacute phase (*A:* 3 days after stroke) and in the post-acute phase (*B:* 1 week after stroke). The voxels highlighted are those that show a significant difference ($p < .01$) in the severity of anosognosia between patients with/without a lesion in these voxels. (See Figure 17.2)

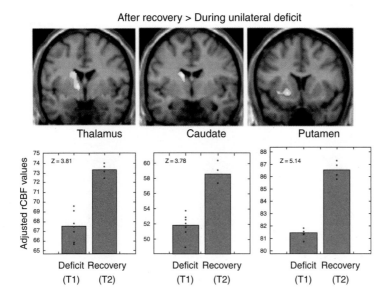

Plate 17.4 Brain regions showing decreased activity in the hemisphere contralateral to unilateral sensori-motor loss due to conversion hysteria ($n = 7$ patients). Comparing activation after recovery and during symptoms revealed significant changes in caudate nucleus, putamen, and thalamus, corresponding to major relays within the basal ganglia-thalamo-cortical loops that control movement initiation. (Adapted from Vuilleumier et al., 2001, with permission from Oxford University Press, *Brain, 124*, 1077–1090.) (See Figure 17.4)

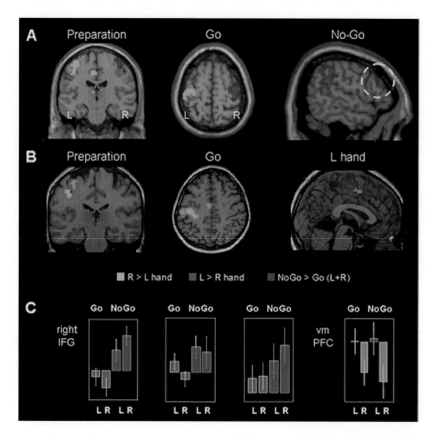

Plate 17.5 Brain regions activated during a go-nogo motor task performed with either hand. In a group of 12 healthy subjects *(A)* and a patient with left hysterical paralysis *(B)*, preparing a movement activated the contralateral motor cortex symmetrically for both the right and left hand. Motor cortex was also activated by execution (go trials) with either hand in healthy subjects, and with the intact right hand in the patient; however, a failure to move the hand on left go trails in the patient produced no increases in motor cortex but selective activation in precuneus and prefrontal areas. Importantly, the right inferior frontal gyrus (IFG) was activated by motor inhibition on nogo trials in healthy subjects but not during failures of movement on left go trials in the patient. The precuneus and ventromedial prefrontal cortex (PFC) were selectively activated by left-hand trials compared to right-hand trials. *(C)* Activation is plotted for the right IFG (shown in *A*) in normal controls, subjects simulating a left-hand paralysis, and the patient with left motor conversion (three panels from left to right, respectively); and for the ventromedial PFC (shown in *B*) in the patient. (Adapted from Cojan et al., 2009, with permission from Elsevier, *NeuroImage*, 47(3), 1026–1037.) (See Figure 17.5)

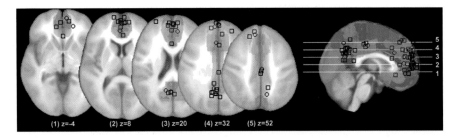

Plate 18.1 Loci of activations resulting from multiple neuroimaging task domains that require introspective appraisal of stimuli with self-relevant features. Squares indicate appraisal of one's own personality traits, personal morals, opinions, attitudes, visuospatial perspective, personal preferences (Craik et al., 1999; Cunningham, Raye, & Johnson, 2004; Greene, Nystrom, Engell, Darley, & Cohen, 2004; Greene, Sommerville, Nystrom, Darley, & Cohen, 2001; Jacobsen, Schubotz, Hofel, & Cramon, 2006; Johnson et al., 2002; Johnson et al., 2005; Kelley et al., 2002; Moll et al., 2002; Schmitz & Johnson, 2006; Schmitz et al., 2004; Seger, Stone, & Keenan, 2004; Vogeley et al., 2004; Zysset, Huber, Ferstl, & von Cramon, 2002; Zysset, Huber, Samson, Ferstl, & von Cramon, 2003). Circles indicate appraisal of reaction to affective stimulus content (Gusnard et al., 2001; Moll et al., 2002; Ochsner et al., 2004). (Adapted with permission from Schmitz & Johnson, 2007, with permission from Elsevier, *Neuroscience and Biobehavioral Reviews*, *31*(4), 585–596.) (See Figure 18.1)

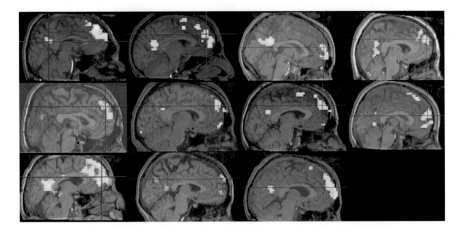

Plate 18.2 Midsagittal view of each participant showing prefrontal activation during self-reflective thought. The activations are superimposed on top of each participant's anatomical scan. Note the consistent activation of the prefrontal cortex across subjects. For the purposes of this display, the statistical threshold was set to an uncorrected *p*-value of .0005. These results are prior to any spatial standardization. (Adapted from Johnson et al., 2002, with permission from Oxford University Press, *Brain*, *125*(Pt 8), 1808–1814.) (See Figure 18.2)

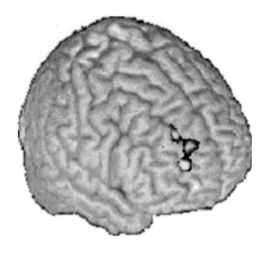

Plate 18.3 Random-effects group analysis indicating greater blood oxygen level–dependent (BOLD) signal during self-evaluation versus other evaluation. The main effect of activation occurred in the right dorsolateral prefrontal cortex (maxima $t = 7.44$, corrected false discover rate $= 0.013$; x, y, $z = 26$, 52, 16; cluster $= 202$). (Adapted from Schmitz et al., 2004, with permission from Elsevier, *NeuroImage*, 22(2), 941–947.) (See Figure 18.3)

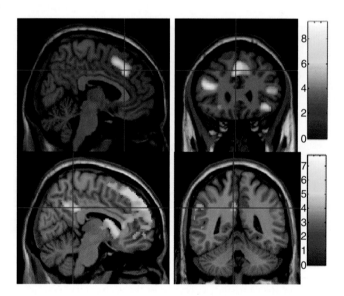

Plate 18.4 Statistical Parametric Map in 16 subjects during subjective decisions. *(Top)* Ambiguous/subjective vs. nonsubjective color similarity decision making. *(Bottom)* Preferential subjective versus ambiguous/subjective decisions. (Adapted from Johnson et al., 2005, with permission from MIT Press, *Journal of Cognitive Neuroscience*, 17(12), 1897–1906.) (See Figure 18.4)

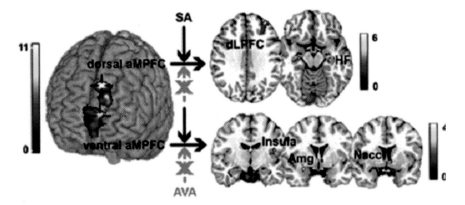

Plate 18.5 A group analysis ($n = 15$) of activation on the Self Appraisal task. Functional connectivity analysis allows one to use a seed region (i.e., the MPFC) and determine regions elsewhere in the brain where signal changes are highly correlated with the seed on the SA task condition but not the other. The ventral MPFC demonstrated coupling with nucleus accumbens, left amygdala, and insula, whereas the dorsal MPFC was selectively coupled with the right dorsolateral prefrontal cortex (dLPFC) and anterior hippocampus bilaterally. Amg, amygdala; aMPFC, anterior medial prefrontal cortex; HF, hippocampus; Nacc, nucleus acumbens. (Adapted from Schmitz & Johnson, 2006, with permission from Elsevier, *NeuroImage*, *30*, 1050–1058.) (See Figure 18.5)

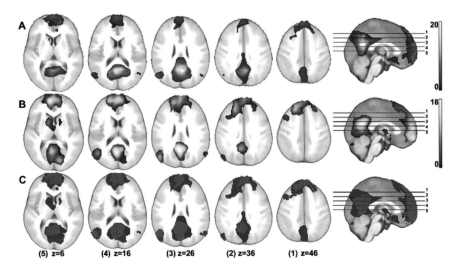

Plate 18.6 Neuroanatomic overlap of functional magnetic resonance imaging activity during a self-appraisal and functional connectivity during "resting" scans (*A and B*: $p_{FWE} > .001$): *(A)* functional connectivity map using posterior cingulate cortex seed region, *(B)* main effect of self-appraisal task, *(C)* map from *(A)* overlaid on map from *(B)*. Blue: regions showing only self-appraisal main effect; red: regions showing only functional connectivity with posterior cingulate cortex; purple: areas of overlap. (From Johnson & Ries, unpublished data.) (See Figure 18.6)

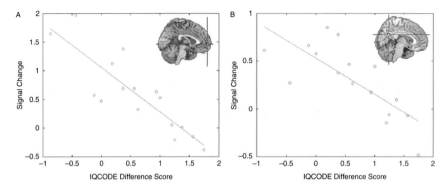

Plate 18.7 Relationship between cortical midline structures BOLD signal change during self-appraisal and a measure of anosognosia (i.e., IQCODE difference score) in MCI patients. *(A)* Plot of the negative correlation (r = −0.83, *p*FDR <0.05) between BOLD signal change during self-appraisal and IQCODE difference score in ventral MPFC cluster. *(B)* Plot of the negative correlation (r = −0.76, *p*FDR <0.05) between BOLD signal change during self-appraisal and IQCODE difference score in PCC of MCI participants. BOLD, blood oxygen level dependent; FDR, false discovery rate; MCI, mild cognitive impairment; MPFC, medial prefrontal cortex; PCC, posterior cingulated cortex. (Adapted from Ries et al., 2007, with permission from Cambridge University Press, *Journal of the International Neuropsychological Society*, 13(3), 450–461.) (See Figure 18.7)

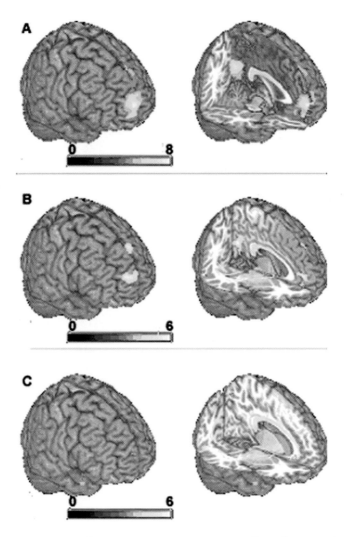

Plate 18.8 *(A)* Traumatic brain injury (TBI) group: main effect of activity during self-appraisal (FDR corrected *p* value < .01). *(B)* Control group: Activity during self-appraisal (FDR corrected *p* value < .01). *(C)* Two sample *t*-tests comparing TBI versus control group BOLD activity during self-appraisal. The TBI group showed greater signal change in the anterior cingulate cortex, precuneus, and right anterior temporal pole (uncorrected *p* value < .001). BOLD, bood oxygen level dependent; FDR, false discovery rate. (Adapted from Schmitz et al., 2006, with permission from Elsevier, *Neuropsychologia*, *44*(5), 762–773.) (See Figure 18.8)

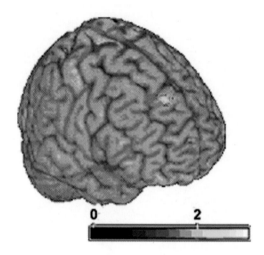

Plate 18.9 Region of significant correlation between BOLD response to self-appraisal and PCRS accuracy (uncorrected *p* value = .005) is in the right dorsal frontal lobe. BOLD, blood oxygen level dependent; PCRS, Patient Competency Rating Scale. (Adapted from Schmitz et al., 2006, with permission from Elsevier, *Neuropsychologia*, *44*(5), 762–773.) (See Figure 18.9)

18

Functional Imaging of Self-Appraisal

Sterling C. Johnson and Michele L. Ries

Ideas or schemas that one possesses about his or her own capabilities, aptitudes, and traits constitute an aspect of personal semantic knowledge that is integral for selecting adaptive and appropriate goal-directed behavior (Showers & Zeigler-Hill, 2003). The study of such first-person schemas and their development has been a long-standing area of psychological inquiry (James, 1890; Kagan, 1982; Leary & Price Tangney, 2003; Nelson & Fivush, 2004). Other chapters of this book are primarily concerned about self-schemas that were once, but are no longer accurate due to brain injury or disease. In contrast, the primary focus of this chapter is the use of functional imaging methods to examine the normative capacity for reflective thought and appraisal of self-schemas. This capacity is metacognitive in the sense that William James described it—the "I" experiences and evaluates the "me" (James, 1890).

In a prior review (Schmitz & Johnson, 2007) we described evidence from a wide range of affective, cognitive, and social neuroimaging research converging on a system of brain regions important broadly for appraising the self, self-relevant features of the environment, the contents of mind, and social interaction (see also Amodio & Frith, 2006). In that previously presented framework, we described the literature regarding overlapping and interacting brain networks in these kinds of self-appraisal. The anterior cingulate, ventromedial prefrontal cortex, insula, basal forebrain, and other subcortical regions were presented as a network responsible for bottom-up detection of salient, self-relevant intero- and exteroceptive stimuli. We had also proposed that dorsal aspects of anterior cingulate, medial prefrontal cortex (MPFC) extending along a ventral-dorsal axis, and the posterior cingulate instantiate top-down metacognitive evaluation of one's own behaviors, the behavior of others, and the interpretation of dynamic feedback during social interaction (see Figure 18.1, which is adapted from Schmitz & Johnson, 2007). In the present chapter we describe in more detail this latter metacognitive proposal and summarize experiments from our functional imaging laboratory and the wider literature that identify brain regions involved in self-appraisal.

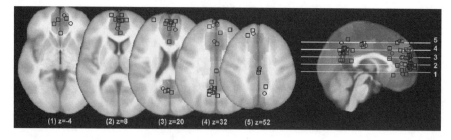

Figure 18.1 Loci of activations resulting from multiple neuroimaging task domains that require introspective appraisal of stimuli with self-relevant features. Squares indicate appraisal of one's own personality traits, personal morals, opinions, attitudes, visuospatial perspective, personal preferences (Craik et al., 1999; Cunningham, Raye, & Johnson, 2004; Greene, Nystrom, Engell, Darley, & Cohen, 2004; Greene, Sommerville, Nystrom, Darley, & Cohen, 2001; Jacobsen, Schubotz, Hofel, & Cramon, 2006; Johnson et al., 2002; Johnson et al., 2005; Kelley et al., 2002; Moll et al., 2002; Schmitz & Johnson, 2006; Schmitz et al., 2004; Seger, Stone, & Keenan, 2004; Vogeley et al., 2004; Zysset, Huber, Ferstl, & von Cramon, 2002; Zysset, Huber, Samson, Ferstl, & von Cramon, 2003). Circles indicate appraisal of reaction to affective stimulus content (Gusnard et al., 2001; Moll et al., 2002; Ochsner et al., 2004). (Adapted with permission from Schmitz & Johnson, 2007, with permission from Elsevier, *Neuroscience and Biobehavioral Reviews*, *31*(4), 585–596.) (See Color Plate 18.1)

In the following sections, we first discuss the way in which results of functional neuroimaging studies provide information complementary to that derived from lesion studies. Together these experimental approaches can yield a more comprehensive understanding of the brain substrate of self-evaluative processes. Second, we present results of functional magnetic resonance imaging (fMRI) studies from our research on self-appraisal. For details of the participants, task parameters, and statistical analysis in all studies presented, the reader is referred to the original papers, which are cited. Third, we present task-dependent and functional connectivity findings that provide insight into putative brain networks supporting self-appraisal. Fourth, we show how we have extended our findings from normative fMRI studies to the investigation of functional brain changes that accompany anosognosia in traumatic brain injury (TBI) and amnestic mild cognitive impairment patients. Since the work presented in this chapter is heavily dependent on functional MRI (fMRI) methodology, the chapter closes with a discussion of task design and interpretive considerations in fMRI research—both in the study of normative self-appraisal and in patients with anosognosia.

Functional Neuroimaging and Lesion Studies

Studies of patients with neurologic damage and functional neuroimaging studies of both cognitively healthy and neurologically impaired people provide complementary information for understanding the brain substrates of accurate self-appraisal and anosognosia. Most of what we know about brain–behavior relationships has been rooted in lesion work—with functional neuroimaging serving an attendant role in adding to this body of knowledge. However, functional neuroimaging (including blood oxygen level–dependent [BOLD] fMRI) offers the unique ability to assess brain correlates of behavior in the *intact* brain. Furthermore, examples exist in which functional neuroimaging has arguably been the foremost method responsible for furthering knowledge of localized brain functions. One example of this is the contribution of fMRI to our current knowledge regarding the posterior cingulate cortex's (PCC) involvement in self-appraisal—as well as this region's related role in episodic recognition memory. Before the advent of functional neuroimaging, it was difficult to assess PCC function in humans, largely due to the rarity of selective pathological lesions in this brain region (Valenstein et al., 1987; Vogt & Laureys, 2005; Vogt, Vogt, & Laureys, 2006). Functional neuroimaging in cognitively healthy adults over the past decade has rapidly propelled our understanding of the PCC's role in self-appraisal—showing reliable evidence that this region, together with the MPFC, is active during fMRI tasks in which people appraise their own traits, opinions, attitudes, and preferences (see Figure 18.1).

Imaging tools such as fMRI promise not only to inform us about the functional specialization of brain regions, but they are also uniquely suited to provide information about how regions across the brain may operate in synchrony (i.e., condition-dependent connectivity and functional connectivity) in service of behavioral functions such as self-appraisal. This approach to understanding behavioral phenomena such as self-appraisal and anosognosia in terms of networks of brain activity is critical since brain regions do not operate in isolation—the activity (and/or degeneration) of one brain region affects the function of other interconnected brain regions. In subsequent sections of this chapter, we will describe how functional connectivity is measured, and the implications it may have for understanding self-appraisal and anosognosia.

Functional Magnetic Resonance Imaging Studies of Self-Appraisal in the Intact Brain

Brain Activity during Self-Evaluation

When a patient is asked to describe his or her symptoms, he or she is essentially being asked to make a self-evaluative decision that is metacognitive. Similarly, self-report surveys of mood or physical symptoms require an evaluation or appraisal of some aspect of oneself on specific symptom dimensions. An initial study from our lab investigated fMRI activity associated with self-reflection (Johnson et al., 2002) in 11 right-handed cognitively healthy adults (mean age: 35 years). The experimental condition of the fMRI task required participants to rate themselves on simple statements regarding traits, attributes, and abilities

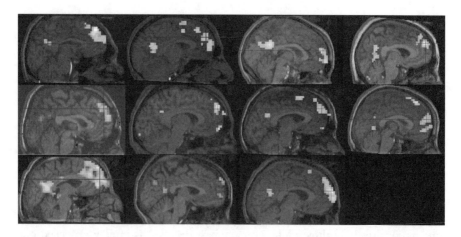

Figure 18.2 Midsagittal view of each participant showing prefrontal activation during self-reflective thought. The activations are superimposed on top of each participant's anatomical scan. Note the consistent activation of the prefrontal cortex across subjects. For the purposes of this display, the statistical threshold was set to an uncorrected *p*-value of .0005. These results are prior to any spatial standardization. (Adapted from Johnson et al., 2002, with permission from Oxford University Press, *Brain, 125*(Pt 8), 1808–1814.) (See Color Plate 18.2)

that required a yes/no decision and were in the style of questions found on the Minnesota Multiphasic Personality Inventory. The control condition involved retrieval of general factual knowledge. Functional magnetic resonance imaging was performed at Barrow Neurological Institute on a 1.5 Tesla scanner.

The results revealed a pattern of brain activation that was strikingly robust in single participants and highly consistent across participants (i.e., the kind of consistency one might see with a language or sensory motor paradigm was also observed in this self-appraisal paradigm). Figure 18.2 depicts a midsagittal slice from each of the 11 subjects. Strong BOLD signal was consistently observed in the anterior medial frontal lobe and posterior cingulate. Despite the robust fMRI signal, the behavioral phenomenon associated with this signal required further definition: it was unclear at this point whether fMRI activity associated with this task was primarily associated with self-reflection or represented more general metacognitive processes. Further, it was unclear whether the subjective/ambiguous nature of the self-appraisal condition was driving the result. We therefore constructed other fMRI tasks to address these issues.

Self-Evaluation versus Other Evaluation: Similarities and Distinctions in Regional Brain Activity

In a second study (Schmitz, Kawahara-Baccus, & Johnson, 2004), our goal was to determine similarities and distinctions in brain response during evaluation of oneself versus evaluation of a significant other (e.g., a close friend or relative). The paradigm employed in this study required the 19 young adult, cognitively healthy participants to make yes/no responses to trait adjectives to questions in three conditions: *(1)* self-evaluative (does the word describe me?), *(2)* other-evaluative (does the word describe my close friend?), *(3)* semantic (is the word positive?).

First, we found a highly similar pattern of results involving the MPFC and PCC when compared to the Johnson et al. (2002) study (see also Craik et al., 1999). This finding held regardless of whether the subject was appraising characteristics of oneself or a significant other. Ostensibly this suggests a more general metacognitive role for these structures that was not necessarily specific to the self. However, simulation theory would suggest that making inferences about a close other person still invokes self-referential processes (for an excellent description of this idea, see Mitchell, Banaji, & Macrae, 2005). Using a similar paradigm to the one we used, D'Argembeau et al. (2008) asked healthy subjects to appraise the self and significant other for a current time period and for a time period in the past. Similar to our result and supportive of Mitchell's hypothesis, they found cortical midline activations for all four conditions, though a greater degree of activation was found during the current self-appraisal condition.

The second major finding from Schmitz et al. (2004) was that when the "self" versus "other" conditions were directly compared, greater activity was observed in the right prefrontal cortex (see Figure 18.3, see also Kaplan, Aziz-Zadeh, Uddin, & Iacoboni, 2008) consistent with anosognosia lesion studies reviewed elsewhere

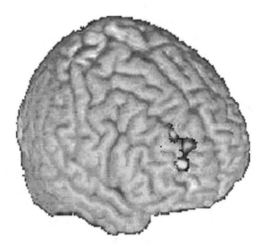

Figure 18.3 Random-effects group analysis indicating greater blood oxygen level–dependent (BOLD) signal during self-evaluation versus other evaluation. The main effect of activation occurred in the right dorsolateral prefrontal cortex (maxima $t = 7.44$, corrected false discover rate $= 0.013$; x, y, $z = 26$, 52, 16; cluster $= 202$). (Adapted from Schmitz et al., 2004, with permission from Elsevier, *NeuroImage*, 22(2), 941–947.) (See Color Plate 18.3)

in this book. This is supportive of the idea that the right more than the left frontal cortex contributes to self-representation.

Are Medial Prefrontal Cortex and Posterior Cingulate Cortex Activations Explained by Subjective Decisions That Are Not Necessarily Related to Self-Evaluation?

In Johnson et al. (2005) we examined the question of whether subjective decision making alone can account for the results in the anterior MPFC and PCC reported above. An important psychological factor that had been common to many prior experiments activating the MPFC is subjective evaluation—that is, making a decision when there may not be an externally verifiable correct answer. This subjectivity factor, regardless of self-relevance or emotional connotation, needed to be ruled out as the explanatory source of midline activation in our prior studies. To address this, we performed a study in 16 healthy young adults. The task required participants to decide which of two colored squares best matched a target square under different conditions. In condition 1, the decision was external and based on the color similarity between the target and the choice alternatives. This was an objective decision and was rather easy. In condition 2, the decision, though still external regarding color similarity, was difficult and subjective. In fact, the two choice alternatives were equally distant in color hue and intensity from the target color square. The equivalence among the choice alternatives meant that the answer was ambiguous, and the decision would be entirely subjective. A third condition was presented in which the participant was asked to rate which of the two choice colors was preferred with the target color. This was also a subjective choice, but now the reference was *internal* (a personal self-preference), rather than *external* (color similarity). The participants were cognitively healthy young adults (mean age: 23 years) who were able to understand the instructions and completed the task without difficulty.

The results indicated the following: the similarity decision (external: ambiguous versus easy) resulted in activations in the midcingulate and lateral parietal lobes (intraparietal sulcus), and inferior frontal and lateral orbital frontal lobes (the midcingulate activation is highlighted in the top panel of Figure 18.4). The MPFC and posterior cingulate cortices were *not* active in that contrast. The preference decision versus the ambiguous similarity decision (both conditions required subjective decisions, but differed with regard to the referent) revealed differential activation in the left MPFC and posterior cingulate and bilateral head of caudate nucleus (the posterior cingulate activation is highlighted in the bottom panel of Figure 18.4). These results—derived from an fMRI task that controlled for subjective decision making in the comparison condition—indicate that anterior MPFC and PCC responsivity was driven by an evaluation that requires processing about oneself and not simply subjective decision making.

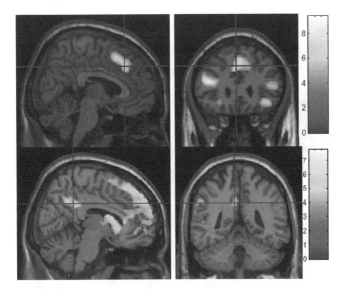

Figure 18.4 Statistical Parametric Map in 16 subjects during subjective decisions. *(Top)* Ambiguous/subjective vs. nonsubjective color similarity decision making. *(Bottom)* Preferential subjective versus ambiguous/subjective decisions. (Adapted from Johnson et al., 2005, with permission from MIT Press, *Journal of Cognitive Neuroscience*, 17(12), 1897–1906.) (See Color Plate 18.4)

Functional Magnetic Resonance Imaging Condition-Dependent and Functional Connectivity: Two Methods Informing Normative Brain Activity Important for Self-Appraisal

Condition-Dependent Connectivity during Self-Appraisal

Results from our lab and others show that the MPFC is consistently active during personally salient decision making (e.g., Figure 18.1, see also Northoff et al., 2006)—MFPC activity elicited in fMRI tasks targeting this psychological construct using diverse stimuli (from pain to reward to physical attractiveness) (Northoff et al., 2006; Schmitz & Johnson, 2007). However, networks of brain regions that exhibit condition-dependent relationships during self-reflective tasks (i.e., condition-dependent connectivity) are less defined. In one fMRI self-appraisal study (Schmitz & Johnson, 2006), we examined condition- and region- dependent correlations with more-distant brain regions. Using a self-appraisal decision-making task with two conditions (self-evaluative versus semantic decision), we presented trait adjectives and asked participants to decide whether the word described them (self-evaluative condition), or whether the word had a semantic positive connotation

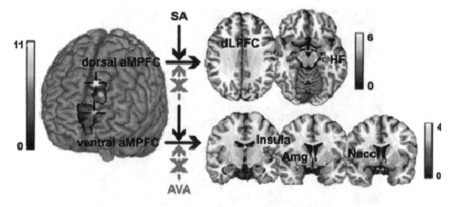

Figure 18.5 A group analysis ($n = 15$) of activation on the Self Appraisal task. Functional connectivity analysis allows one to use a seed region (i.e., the MPFC) and determine regions elsewhere in the brain where signal changes are highly correlated with the seed on the SA task condition but not the other. The ventral MPFC demonstrated coupling with nucleus accumbens, left amygdala, and insula, whereas the dorsal MPFC was selectively coupled with the right dorsolateral prefrontal cortex (dLPFC) and anterior hippocampus bilaterally. Amg, amygdala; aMPFC, anterior medial prefrontal cortex; HF, hippocampus; Nacc, nucleus acumbens. (Adapted from Schmitz & Johnson, 2006, with permission from Elsevier, *NeuroImage, 30,* 1050–1058.) (See Color Plate 18.5)

(semantic condition). The results revealed task-dependent relationships between the *ventral* anterior MPFC and the amygdala, insula, and nucleus accumbens; we also showed dorsal anterior MPFC condition-dependent connectivity with dorso-lateral prefrontal cortex (PFC) and bilateral hippocampi (see Figure 18.5). In the context of our self-appraisal task, the term "condition-dependent connectivity" means that these regions showed correlated activity during the self-appraisal condition, but not the comparison (semantic decision) condition. This type of effect reflects an interaction in the way that brain regions correlate with each other as a function of task. The MPFC networks identified in this study may subserve distinct contributory processes inherent to self-appraisal decisions, specifically a dorsally mediated cognitive and a ventrally mediated affective/self-relevance network. This proposition regarding regional functional specialization within the MPFC is consistent not only with the results of other neuroimaging studies but also with a large literature on the behavioral effects of lesions localized to ventral versus dorsal medial frontal lobe (Schmitz & Johnson, 2007).

Functional Connectivity: Overlap in Brain Regions Showing Activity during Self-Appraisal and "Default Mode" Connectivity

In healthy adults, several networks of functionally related brain regions show spontaneous and coherent low-frequency fluctuations in BOLD signal (i.e.,

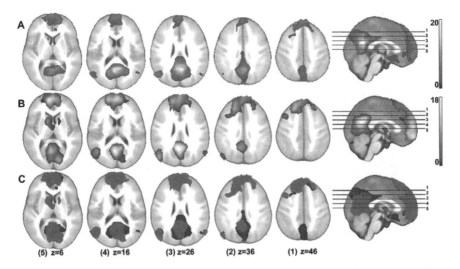

Figure 18.6 Neuroanatomic overlap of functional magnetic resonance imaging activity during a self-appraisal and functional connectivity during "resting" scans *(A and B:* pFWE > .001): *(A)* functional connectivity map using posterior cingulate cortex seed region, *(B)* main effect of self-appraisal task, *(C)* map from *(A)* overlaid on map from *(B)*. Blue: regions showing only self-appraisal main effect; red: regions showing only functional connectivity with posterior cingulate cortex; purple: areas of overlap. (From Johnson & Ries, unpublished data.) (See Color Plate 18.6)

functional connectivity). One such functional network, often termed the "default mode network" (DMN), comprises dorsomedial and ventromedial prefrontal cortex, anterior and posterior cingulate cortices, retrosplenial cortex, precuneus, lateral parietal cortices, and mesial temporal lobes (Greicius, Krasnow, Reiss, & Menon, 2003; Raichle et al., 2001; Raichle & Snyder, 2007). Based on the overlap of cortical midline regions showing fMRI activity during self-referential processing and regions showing DMN connectivity (see Figure 18.6), several behavioral neuroscientists have posited that functional connectivity within DMN regions reflects evaluative processing regarding oneself and monitoring one's relation to the outside world (Gusnard, Akbudak, Shulman, & Raichle, 2001; Gusnard & Raichle, 2001; Raichle et al., 2001). Results of a recent, well-behaviorally-controlled investigation of fMRI "rest" conditions suggest that both MPFC and PCC activity during low-cognitive-demand conditions relates to intentionally balancing attention between the external environment and the appraisal and regulation of one's behavior in the MRI scanner environment itself (Gilbert, Simons, Frith, & Burgess, 2006). Those results suggest that people "resting" in the scanner are engaged in self-referential processes (such as the self-regulation required to keep still in a confining loud space—the bore of the MRI) during so called "low-level" states.

To add to published data assessing the claim that DMN functional connectivity relates to self-evaluative processing, we collected "resting" fMRI data (i.e., scan data acquired while participants lay still in the scanner with eyes closed) in 22 cognitively healthy adults. This yielded data for DMN functional connectivity analysis. We also collected data from a block-design fMRI self-appraisal task in 91 cognitively healthy adults. A primary goal of our study was to more directly examine the neuroanatomic overlap between the statistical parametric map of DMN functional connectivity and the statistical map of fMRI response to the self-appraisal task.

We used a seed-region-based approach for our functional connectivity analysis of "resting" data. In this type of analysis, BOLD signal is extracted from a region of interest. Using this extracted data, a Pearson's product-moment correlation coefficient is calculated between the regional mean of seed region time courses and the time course for each voxel in the whole brain. We defined two seed regions in cortical midline regions shown to be active during self-appraisal: the posterior cingulate cortex and MPFC.

The self-appraisal fMRI task consisted of two conditions and was identical to the one described above (Schmitz & Johnson, 2006). In the self-appraisal (SA) condition, participants viewed trait adjectives and made yes/no button press responses to the question: "Does the word describe me?" In the semantic decision (SEM) comparison condition, participants viewed trait adjectives and made button press responses to the question: "Is the word positive?" The statistical contrast of interest in our random effects analysis (a one-group t test) examined the group effect of self-appraisal (SA > SEM).

Our main results—depicted in Figure 18.6—indicate that there is striking neuroanatomic overlap between regions active during self-appraisal and regions of DMN functional connectivity. Figure 18.6A shows DMN functional connectivity using the PCC seed; Figure 18.6B shows fMRI activity associated with self-appraisal, and Figure 18.6C shows regions of overlap between these maps (overlap in purple).

The data presented here in the context of the existing literature suggest that PCC-MPFC functional connectivity—a central aspect of the DMN—may reflect intrinsic brain activity important for intact self-referential processing. This hypothesis has yet to be fully tested. One way to test this hypothesis is to study the degree to which DMN connectivity is diminished in individuals with anosognosia. We are currently studying this hypothesis.

Extending Results of Normative Self-Appraisal Studies to Anosognosia in Patients

Mild Cognitive Impairment

As noted by Starkstein and Power (Chapter 10, this volume), anosognosia for impairment of cognitive and functional abilities is present in many patients with Alzheimer's disease. Recent research suggests that anosognosia for cognitive impairment in mild cognitive impairment (MCI) patients may be an important prognostic index, with one report indicating that MCI patients lacking awareness of cognitive and functional deficits show increased incidence of progressing to Alzheimer's disease over a 2-year period than those who show awareness (Tabert et al., 2002).

In a recent fMRI study, we (Ries et al., 2007) investigated MCI participants' brain activity associated with self-referential processing. As noted earlier in this chapter, the MPFC and PCC—cortical midline structures—are strongly implicated in this metacognitive function. In Ries et al. (2007), it was hypothesized that MCI participants' activation of cortical midline structures during self-appraisal would covary with their level of insight into their cognitive difficulties.

The study examined the correlation between awareness of deficit in amnestic MCI patients and BOLD response during a self-appraisal fMRI task. In this fMRI study, we used a blocked-design fMRI task that reliably evokes cortical midline activity in healthy controls (i.e., the same task used in our analysis of condition-dependent connectivity). Our behavioral evaluation of participants' level of awareness was based on a discrepancy score between two parallel forms of the Informant Questionnaire on Cognitive Decline in the Elderly (IQCODE). This questionnaire contains items querying changes (ranging from "much improved" to "much worse") over the past 10 years in one's memory ability (e.g., "Remembering things that have happened recently") and daily problem-solving ability and adaptive functioning (e.g., "making decisions on everyday matters"). One form was given to a relative or friend who had known the participant for 10 years or more (Jorm, 1994; Jorm, Christensen, Korten, Jacomb, & Henderson, 2000). We devised a second form with identical questions that was administered to the MCI participant.

Our MCI participants showed a wide range of insight into their cognitive difficulties, spanning from intact insight and concern about their memory to clear anosognosia. Results of our analysis of fMRI data revealed a highly significant relationship between cortical midline BOLD response during a self-appraisal task and self-awareness of deficit in MCI. Cortical midline regions included both MPFC (see Figure 18.7A) and PCC (see Figure 18.7B). A whole-brain voxel-based morphometry analysis of these participants showed no significant relationship between awareness and brain volume; MCI participants also did not show attenuated brain volume compared to an age-matched control group. The fMRI result suggests that impaired awareness shown by a subset of MCI patients is accompanied by a decrease in activity in structures that support accurate self-appraisal in healthy adults.

Traumatic Brain Injury

As reviewed by Prigatano (Chapter 12, this volume), anosognosia for impaired cognitive and social abilities is common in patients with moderate to severe TBI,

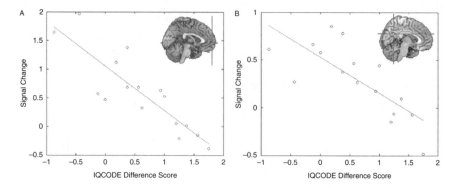

Figure 18.7 Relationship between cortical midline structures BOLD signal change during self-appraisal and a measure of anosognosia (i.e., IQCODE difference score) in MCI patients. *(A)* Plot of the negative correlation ($r = -0.83$, $p\text{FDR} < 0.05$) between BOLD signal change during self-appraisal and IQCODE difference score in ventral MPFC cluster. *(B)* Plot of the negative correlation ($r = -0.76$, $p\text{FDR} < 0.05$) between BOLD signal change during self-appraisal and IQCODE difference score in PCC of MCI participants. BOLD, blood oxygen level dependent; FDR, false discovery rate; MCI, mild cognitive impairment; MPFC, medial prefrontal cortex; PCC, posterior cingulated cortex. (Adapted from Ries et al., 2007, with permission from Cambridge University Press, *Journal of the International Neuropsychological Society*, *13*(3), 450–461.) (See Color Plate 18.7)

with approximately 45% of TBI patients exhibiting disparities between their self-appraised versus actual level of functioning (Flashman & McAllister, 2002). The accuracy of insight into one's post-injury self will impact one's ability to function effectively in the world. A brain-injured patient for whom self-awareness is compromised may hold ideas about the self that are no longer accurate or congruent with what others observe (Prigatano, 1999; Stuss, 1991). This is perhaps because they have not yet, or are not able to accommodate new post-injury experiences into the previously crystallized schemata. For example, a brain-injured patient may feel he or she can competently return to the same level of employment when a family member, who has observed the patient's current abilities, indicates otherwise. Prigatano (1996) has observed that when asked, brain-injured patients often underestimate their own emotional dysregulation, cognitive difficulties, and interpersonal deficits relative to a family member's rating of their abilities. Inaccurate self-knowledge can significantly impede efforts to rehabilitate brain-injured patients, since they may not appreciate the need for such treatment (Sherer et al., 1998a, 1998b).

Damage or selective degeneration of the anterior prefrontal regions has been associated with impaired self-awareness for the appropriateness of social interactions, judgment, and planning difficulties (Flashman et al., 2001; Miller et al., 2001; Prigatano & Schacter, 1991; Stuss, 1991), as well as impaired awareness of the mental states of others (i.e., "theory of mind";

Stone, Baron-Cohen, & Knight, 1998; Stuss, Gallup, & Alexander, 2001). Impaired self-awareness appears to occur more frequently following damage to the prefrontal cortex (Damasio, Tranel, & Damasio, 1990) and may be more sensitive to damage on the right (Happe, Brownell, & Winner, 1999; Levine et al., 1998; Stone et al., 1998).

In an fMRI study of anosognosia in TBI (Schmitz, Rowley, Kawahara, & Johnson, 2006), we used the same self-appraisal fMRI task described above that has been validated in cognitively healthy adults. In this study, the first analysis compared differences in the main effect of self-appraisal between TBI patients and controls. A second analysis of data from the TBI group used regression to examine the relationship between accuracy of self-appraisal and brain activity during the fMRI self-appraisal task. To assess accuracy we used Prigatano's Patient Competency Rating Scale (PCRS) and examined the discrepancy between patient and relative ratings. This analysis of the TBI data was guided by the hypothesis that fMRI activity in the MPFC (preferentially right hemisphere) would covary with accuracy of self-appraisal.

Results of this fMRI study indicated that both TBI (Figure 18.8a) and control groups (Figure 18.8b) showed significant cortical midline BOLD response during this self-appraisal task. Cortical midline regions showing activity included both dorsal and ventral medial prefrontal as well as the retrosplenial cortex. Direct comparison of the groups indicated that TBI patients show greater response in the right temporal pole, anterior cingulate, and retrosplenial cortex (Figure 18.8c).

Consistent with a primary hypothesis of this study, the regression analysis of the TBI patients' data showed that accuracy of self-appraisal as measured by the PCRS covaries positively with BOLD response to the self-appraisal task in right anterior superior frontal gyrus (Figure 18.9). This is consistent with findings from previous lesion studies implicating this frontal lobe region in accurate self-appraisal and insight (Adair et al., 1995; Belyi, 1987; Joseph, 1999; Miller et al., 2001).

Functional Neuroimaging Methodological Considerations

Since the data reviewed in this chapter are from fMRI experiments, this section discusses challenges that occur when studying self-referential processes and anosognosia in the fMRI environment. To provide a broad background, we briefly review the BOLD signal, the index of brain activity used in the vast majority of fMRI experiments. We present fMRI experimental design issues, with an emphasis on the study of self-appraisal. Last, we review challenges to interpreting the BOLD signal in patient populations with particular regard to hemodynamic and structural brain changes—considerations that are critical to the interpretation of fMRI studies of anosognosia.

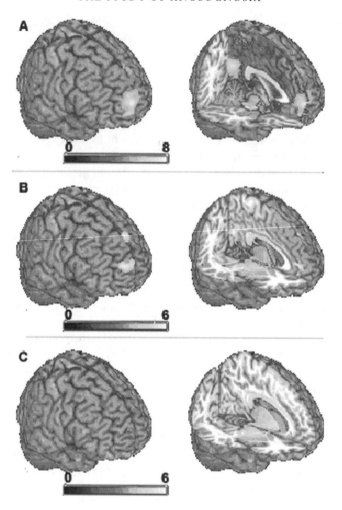

Figure 18.8 *(A)* Traumatic brain injury (TBI) group: main effect of activity during self-appraisal (FDR corrected *p* value < .01). *(B)* Control group: Activity during self-appraisal (FDR corrected *p* value < .01). *(C)* Two sample *t*-tests comparing TBI versus control group BOLD activity during self-appraisal. The TBI group showed greater signal change in the anterior cingulate cortex, precuneus, and right anterior temporal pole (uncorrected *p* value < .001). BOLD, bood oxygen level dependent; FDR, false discovery rate. (Adapted from Schmitz et al., 2006, with permission from Elsevier, *Neuropsychologia*, *44*(5), 762–773.) (See Color Plate 18.8)

The Blood Oxygen Level–Dependent Signal

Functional MRI offers a method of examining brain regions while those regions are functionally engaged in a specific task compared to a reference task. In most

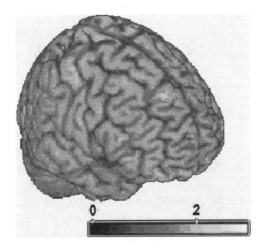

Figure 18.9 Region of significant correlation between BOLD response to self-appraisal and PCRS accuracy (uncorrected p value = .005) is in the right dorsal frontal lobe. BOLD, blood oxygen level dependent; PCRS, Patient Competency Rating Scale. (Adapted from Schmitz et al., 2006, with permission from Elsevier, *Neuropsychologia*, *44*(5), 762–773.) (See Color Plate 18.9)

fMRI studies, brain activity is indexed by the BOLD response, an increase in the ratio of oxygenated to deoxygenated hemoglobin that is correlated with neural activity. This phenomenon is due to the fact that: *(a)* local oxygen delivery is well beyond the metabolic need, and *(b)* that deoxyhemoglobin is paramagnetic. Although the neural response to stimulation is rapid (<100 ms), the BOLD response is much slower. Following an increase in neural activity, the typical BOLD signal gradually increases to its peak magnitude over approximately 6 seconds and decreases back to baseline over the next 6–8 seconds.

Important Factors in Functional Magnetic Resonance Imaging Experimental Design

A number of factors influence the results of fMRI experiments. Here we discuss two factors that have a significant impact on the way in which fMRI results are interpreted with regard to self-referential paradigms: *(1)* choice of the fMRI task conditions and *(2)* choice of overall experimental design.

Choice of Functional Magnetic Resonance Imaging Task Conditions

The goal of fMRI experiments is to assess brain activity associated with a particular behavioral construct of interest—such as self-appraisal. In order to do this, the difference in BOLD response between two behavioral conditions is measured. The experimental condition targets the behavioral construct of interest. In a study of anosognosia, the experimental condition might require a research participant to appraise characteristics or abilities that he or she currently possesses. Ideally, the comparison (or baseline) condition is constructed to be similar to the experimental condition in all features other than the behavioral construct of interest. If the two conditions were to differ in only one behavioral feature, then the difference in BOLD signal between the two conditions could be attributed to that feature (however, see Price, Moore, & Friston, 1997 for discussion of limits to the logic of cognitive subtraction). Our following discussion gives an example of such a task and highlights the importance of the choice of the comparison condition.

One self-appraisal task discussed in several sections of this chapter consists of an experimental (self) condition and a comparison (semantic decision) condition. In the self condition, trait adjectives are presented, and participants press a button to make yes/no decisions about whether each word describes him/her. In the semantic decision condition, participants are presented with the same trait adjectives seen during the self condition; however, in this comparison condition participants indicate whether each word was positive by pressing a button. Of note, the experimental and comparison conditions of this task are identical in terms of the adjectives presented (i.e., keeping language and visual processing aspects of the two tasks the same), the timing of stimulus presentation, and the button press response required by participants. Also the novelty of word stimuli was counterbalanced across condition. By keeping behavioral requirements of noninterest relatively constant across the experimental and comparison conditions (i.e., visual processing, language processing, attention, novelty, response timing, and motoric response), a comparison of these conditions allows the investigator to focus on the construct of self-appraisal and associated brain activity.

The lack of behavioral focus and definition is a major difficulty with studies that use low-level controls conditions such as "resting" or a fixation cross. Descriptors of cognitive operations that have been uncritically ascribed to the condition in which participants view a fixation cross include "default," "rest," "passive task," and "baseline." However, recent evidence (some alluded to above) strongly suggests that this terminology is not appropriately applied to one's *cognitive* state while lying still in an MRI scanner viewing a fixation cross, as it implies a state of baseline activity which has often been interpreted in fMRI research as "zero-activity" from which an experimental task can produce an activation or deactivation. The assumption of zero cognitive activity is not valid given results from our research and others that strongly suggest that the cognitive state of an individual lying in the scanner during such a low-level condition is active and self-regulatory. Because "rest" is associated with significant self-regulatory cognitive activity, it is a particularly poor choice of cognitive comparison condition in studies aiming to study self-appraisal or other self-referential functions. By using a "resting" comparison condition, one is likely to inadvertently mask activity in brain regions critical to the cognitive or metacognitive construct of interest.

Before leaving this topic, we do want to emphasize that there can be good reason to use "resting" or fixation-cross comparison condition in the service of examining a particular physiologic brain state (for discussion of this, the reader is referred to Raichle & Snyder, 2007); it is interpretation of brain–*behavior* relationships that we strongly caution against when a "resting" condition is employed and assumed to be an inert cognitive state.

Choice of Overall Experimental Design

The results of fMRI experiments are typically reported in terms of the magnitude of the BOLD signal (how much of a difference is there in BOLD signal between the experimental and comparison conditions) in a particular brain region. In some cases, authors report on the extent of BOLD activation (how large of a brain area shows fMRI activity exceeding a given statistical threshold). It is important to note that these fMRI results depend on not only researcher's ability to adequately measure the behavioral construct of interest but also the efficiency of the fMRI experimental design (i.e., how sensitively an fMRI experiment tests a specific hypothesis). Many factors influence design efficiency, but one of the most important factors is choice of a blocked, event-related, or mixed design. As discussed below, choice of the optimal design depends on the goals of the fMRI experiment.

In blocked-design experiments, trials from each task condition (i.e., experimental or comparison condition) are grouped together in the time series to form blocks (e.g., alternating a group of 10 trials of a "self" condition and 10 trials of a comparison condition). Blocked designs are the most efficient or sensitive designs—and for the testing of many hypotheses about self-appraisal and anosognosia, there can be good reason to use this experimental design. First, the blocked design's high efficiency or power to detect BOLD signal means that the experiment can be shorter—and therefore better tolerated by patients. Second, because one is examining aggregate BOLD response over several trials, fewer assumptions are needed regarding the precise magnitude and timing of the BOLD response than in event-related studies.

In an event-related experiment, trials from each task condition are presented in a random order rather than being grouped together. Event-related designs generally require the task to be longer, and they assume a more precise model of the BOLD response. Furthermore, event-related designs introduce much greater design complexity (e.g., requiring careful coordination of stimulus presentation timing with MRI scanning parameters such as jittering) and/or signal processing steps (e.g., slice-time correction). However, there are times when an event-related design is necessary. For example, if a researcher is interested in examining fMRI response when participants make a specific type of response (e.g., an error in self-appraisal), an event-related design is necessary to do this analysis.

Challenges to Interpreting the Blood Oxygen Level–Dependent Signal in Patients with Brain Injury or Neurodegeneration

The valid interpretation of fMRI comparisons between a patient group and controls rests on some important assumptions. The first assumption is not unique to the fMRI environment: in order to ensure construct validity of the behavior one is measuring, patients must be able to understand and adequately perform the task. Thus, collection of reaction time and accuracy data (when applicable) is critical to the interpretation of the study. Valid interpretation of fMRI results also relies on the assumption that patients and control participants have similar brain volume in the region of experimental focus. If volume is dissimilar, then brain volume must be accounted for in the statistical analysis. A last critical assumption underlying the interpretation of patient fMRI data is that neurovascular coupling (i.e., the relationship between neural activity and the sluggish hemodynamic response) is the same between controls and patients—across age groups and across individuals with varying vascular health. The hemodynamic response can be assessed empirically to see if this assumption is being met.

Summary

In this chapter we have reviewed studies of self-referential processes in healthy subjects and demonstrated application of this approach to TBI and MCI patient groups. The studies and topics reviewed here were selective and focused on the prior and ongoing work from our research lab. The general findings from these and other studies suggest that a supramodal network involving the MPFC and PCC are highly engaged during interospective and self-referential processes. We have also pointed out that this system may not be specific to explicit retrieval of personal semantic knowledge (metacognition) but may also be engaged during self regulation and monitoring of behavior, such as when an individual is making an effort to hold still during an MRI scan. Indeed, "rest" during an MRI scan has a higher degree of self-monitoring behavior when compared to rest in unobserved, private, casual, and familiar situations. When the researcher thinks of the baseline state as "holding still" rather than "rest," the self-referential implications become obvious.

This issue of epiphenomenal self-referential processes that occur in the context of being a research study participant or a patient receiving a functional imaging exam would benefit from further study, both in normal subjects and anosognosics. In this regard we have hypothesized that the brain imaging exam imposes a psychological context that is explicitly self-referential, thus engaging the same CNS structures that are involved during self-appraisal (Schmitz & Johnson, 2007).

Acknowledgments

This work was supported by the U.S. Department of Veterans Affairs Merit Review research grants to SCJ, the National Institutes of Health R01 MH65723, R01 AG021155, and with the facilities and resources of the Wm. S. Middleton Memorial Veterans Hospital, Madison, WI.

References

Adair, J. C., Na, D. L., Schwartz, R. L., Fennell, E. M., Gilmore, R. L., & Heilman, K. M. (1995). Anosognosia for hemiplegia: Test of the personal neglect hypothesis. *Neurology, 45*(12), 2195–2199.

Amodio, D. M., & Frith, C. D. (2006). Meeting of minds: The medial frontal cortex and social cognition. *Nature Reviews Neuroscience, 7*(4), 268–277.

Belyi, B. I. (1987). Mental impairment in unilateral frontal tumours: Role of the laterality of the lesion. *International Journal of Neuroscience, 32*(3–4), 799–810.

Craik, F. I. M., Moroz, T. M., Moscovitch, M., Stuss, D. T., Winocur, G., Tulving, E., & Kapur, S. (1999). In search of the self: A positron emission tomography study. *Psychological Science, 10*(1), 26–34.

Cunningham, W. A., Raye, C. L., & Johnson, M. K. (2004). Implicit and explicit evaluation: FMRI correlates of valence, emotional intensity, and control in the processing of attitudes. *Journal of Cognitive Neuroscience, 16*(10), 1717–1729.

Damasio, A. R., Tranel, D., & Damasio, H. (1990). Individuals with sociopathic behavior caused by frontal damage fail to respond autonomically to social stimuli. *Behavioural Brain Research, 41*(2), 81–94.

D'Argembeau, A., Feyers, D., Majerus, S., Collette, F., Van der Linden, M., Maquet, P., & Salmon, E. (2008). Self-reflection across time: Cortical midline structures differentiate between present and past selves. *Social, Cognitive, and Affective Neuroscience, 3*(3), 244–252.

Flashman, L. A., & McAllister, T. W. (2002). Lack of awareness and its impact in traumatic brain injury. *NeuroRehabilitation, 17*(4), 285–296.

Flashman, L. A., McAllister, T. W., Johnson, S. C., Rick, J. H., Green, R. L., & Saykin, A. J. (2001). Specific frontal lobe subregions correlated with unawareness of illness in schizophrenia: A preliminary study. *Journal of Neuropsychiatry and Clinical Neuroscience, 13*(2), 255–257.

Gilbert, S. J., Simons, J. S., Frith, C. D., & Burgess, P. W. (2006). Performance-related activity in medial rostral prefrontal cortex (area 10) during low-demand tasks. *Journal of Experimental Psychology: Human Perception and Performance, 32*(1), 45–58.

Greene, J. D., Nystrom, L. E., Engell, A. D., Darley, J. M., & Cohen, J. D. (2004). The neural bases of cognitive conflict and control in moral judgment. *Neuron, 44*(2), 389–400.

Greene, J. D., Sommerville, R. B., Nystrom, L. E., Darley, J. M., & Cohen, J. D. (2001). An fMRI investigation of emotional engagement in moral judgment. *Science, 293* (5537), 2105–2108.

Greicius, M. D., Krasnow, B., Reiss, A. L., & Menon, V. (2003). Functional connectivity in the resting brain: A network analysis of the default mode hypothesis. *Proceedings of the National Academy of Sciences USA, 100*(1), 253–258.

Gusnard, D. A., Akbudak, E., Shulman, G. L., & Raichle, M. E. (2001). Medial prefrontal cortex and self-referential mental activity: Relation to a default mode of brain function. *Proceedings of the National Academy of Sciences USA, 20*, 20.

Gusnard, D. A., & Raichle, M. E. (2001). Searching for a baseline: Functional imaging and the resting human brain. *Nature Reviews Neuroscience, 2*(10), 685–694.

Happe, F., Brownell, H., & Winner, E. (1999). Acquired "theory of mind" impairments following stroke. *Cognition, 70*(3), 211–240.

Jacobsen, T., Schubotz, R. I., Hofel, L., & Cramon, D. Y. (2006). Brain correlates of aesthetic judgment of beauty. *NeuroImage, 29*(1), 276–285.

James, W. (1890). *Principles of psychology.* New York: Holt.

Johnson, S. C., Baxter, L. C., Wilder, L. S., Pipe, J. G., Heiserman, J. E., & Prigatano, G. P. (2002). Neural correlates of self-reflection. *Brain, 125*(Pt 8), 1808–1814.

Johnson, S. C., Schmitz, T. W., Kawahara-Baccus, T. N., Rowley, H. A., Alexander, A. L., Lee, J., & Davidson, R. J. (2005). The cerebral response during subjective choice with and without self-reference. *Journal of Cognitive Neuroscience, 17*(12), 1897–1906.

Jorm, A. F. (1994). A short form of the Informant Questionnaire on Cognitive Decline in the Elderly (IQCODE): Development and cross-validation. *Psychological Medicine, 24*(1), 145–153.

Jorm, A. F., Christensen, H., Korten, A. E., Jacomb, P. A., & Henderson, A. S. (2000). Informant ratings of cognitive decline in old age: Validation against change on cognitive tests over 7 to 8 years. *Psychological Medicine, 30*(4), 981–985.

Joseph, R. (1999). Frontal lobe psychopathology: Mania, depression, confabulation, catatonia, perseveration, obsessive compulsions, and schizophrenia. *Psychiatry, 62* (2), 138–172.

Kagan, J. (1982). The emergence of self. *Journal of Child Psychology and Psychiatry, 23*, 363–381.

Kaplan, J. T., Aziz-Zadeh, L., Uddin, L. Q., & Iacoboni, M. (2008). The self across the senses: An fMRI study of self-face and self-voice recognition. *Social, Cognitive and Affective Neuroscience, 3*(3), 218–223.

Kelley, W. M., Macrae, C. N., Wyland, C. L., Caglar, S., Inati, S., & Heatherton, T. F. (2002). Finding the self? An event-related fMRI study. *Journal of Cognitive Neuroscience, 14*(5), 785–794.

Leary, M., & Price Tangney, J. (2003). The self as an organizing construct in the behavioral and social sciences. In M. Leary & J. Price Tangney (Eds.), *Handbook of self and identity* (pp. 3–14). New York: Guilford Press.

Levine, B., Black, S. E., Cabeza, R., Sinden, M., McIntosh, A. R., Toth, J. P., Tulving, E., & Stuss, D. T. (1998). Episodic memory and the self in a case of isolated retrograde amnesia. *Brain, 121*(Pt 10), 1951–1973.

Miller, B. L., Seeley, W. W., Mychack, P., Rosen, H. J., Mena, I., & Boone, K. (2001). Neuroanatomy of the self: Evidence from patients with frontotemporal dementia. *Neurology, 57*(5), 817–821.

Mitchell, J. P., Banaji, M. R., & Macrae, C. N. (2005). The link between social cognition and self-referential thought in the medial prefrontal cortex. *Journal of Cognitive Neuroscience, 17*(8), 1306–1315.

Moll, J., de Oliveira-Souza, R., Eslinger, P. J., Bramati, I. E., Mourao-Miranda, J., Andreiuolo, P. A., & Pessoa, L. (2002). The neural correlates of moral sensitivity: A functional magnetic resonance imaging investigation of basic and moral emotions. *Journal of Neuroscience, 22*(7), 2730–2736.

Nelson, K., & Fivush, R. (2004). The emergence of autobiographical memory: A social cultural developmental theory. *Psychological Review, 111*(2), 486–511.

Northoff, G., Heinzel, A., de Greck, M., Bermpohl, F., Dobrowolny, H., & Panksepp, J. (2006). Self-referential processing in our brain—A meta-analysis of imaging studies on the self. *NeuroImage, 31*, 440–457.

Ochsner, K. N., Knierim, K., Ludlow, D. H., Hanelin, J., Ramachandran, T., Glover, G., & Mackey, S. C. (2004). Reflecting upon feelings: An fMRI study of neural systems supporting the attribution of emotion to self and other. *Journal of Cognitive Neuroscience, 16*(10), 1746–1772.

Price, C. J., Moore, C. J., & Friston, K. J. (1997). Subtractions, conjunctions, and interactions in experimental design of activation studies. *Human Brain Mapping, 5* (4), 264–272.

Prigatano, G. (1996). Behavioral limitations TBI patients tend to underestimate: A replication and extension to patients with lateralized dysfunction. *The Clinical Neuropsychologist, 10*, 191–201.

Prigatano, G. (1999). Disorders of self-awareness after brain injury. In *Principles of neuropsychological rehabilitation.* New York: Oxford University Press.

Prigatano, G., & Schacter, D. (Eds.). (1991). *Awareness of deficit after brain injury: Clinical and theoretical implications.* New York: Oxford University Press.

Raichle, M. E., MacLeod, A. M., Snyder, A. Z., Powers, W. J., Gusnard, D. A., & Shulman, G. L. (2001). A default mode of brain function. *Proceedings of the National Academy of Sciences USA, 98*(2), 676–682.

Raichle, M. E., & Snyder, A. Z. (2007). A default mode of brain function: A brief history of an evolving idea. *NeuroImage, 37*(4), 1083–1090; discussion 1097–1089.

Ries, M. L., Jabbar, B. M., Schmitz, T. W., Trivedi, M. A., Gleason, C. E., Carlsson, C. M., Rowley, H. A., Asthana, S., & Johnson, S. C. (2007). Anosognosia in mild cognitive impairment: Relationship to activation of cortical midline structures involved in self-appraisal. *Journal of the International Neuropsychological Society, 13*(3), 450–461.

Schmitz, T. W., & Johnson, S. C. (2006). Self-appraisal decisions evoke dissociated dorsal-ventral aMPFC networks. *NeuroImage, 30*, 1050–1058.

Schmitz, T. W., & Johnson, S. C. (2007). Relevance to self: A brief review and framework of neural systems underlying appraisal. *Neuroscience and Biobehavioral Reviews, 31*(4), 585–596.

Schmitz, T. W., Kawahara-Baccus, T. N., & Johnson, S. C. (2004). Metacognitive evaluation, self-relevance, and the right prefrontal cortex. *NeuroImage, 22*(2), 941–947.

Schmitz, T. W., Rowley, H. A., Kawahara, T. N., & Johnson, S. C. (2006). Neural correlates of self-evaluative accuracy after traumatic brain injury. *Neuropsychologia, 44*(5), 762–773.

Seger, C. A., Stone, M., & Keenan, J. P. (2004). Cortical activations during judgments about the self and another person. *Neuropsychologia, 42*(9), 1168–1177.

Sherer, M., Bergloff, P., Levin, E., High, W. M., Jr., Oden, K. E., & Nick, T. G. (1998a). Impaired awareness and employment outcome after traumatic brain injury. *Journal of Head Trauma Rehabilitation, 13*(5), 52–61.

Sherer, M., Boake, C., Levin, E., Silver, B. V., Ringholz, G., & High, W. M., Jr. (1998b). Characteristics of impaired awareness after traumatic brain injury. *Journal of the International Neuropsychological Society, 4*(4), 380–387.

Showers, C., & Zeigler-Hill, V. (2003). Organization of self-knowledge: Features, functions, and flexibility. In M. Leary & J. Price Tangney (Eds.), *Handbook of self and identity*. New York: Guilford Press.

Stone, V. E., Baron-Cohen, S., & Knight, R. T. (1998). Frontal lobe contributions to theory of mind. *Journal of Cognitive Neuroscience, 10*(5), 640–656.

Stuss, D. (1991). Disturbance of self-awareness after frontal system damage. In G. Prigatano & D. Schacter (Eds.), *Awareness of deficit following brain injury: Clinical and theoretical issues* (pp. 63–83). New York: Oxford University Press.

Stuss, D. T., Gallup, G. G., & Alexander, M. P. (2001). The frontal lobes are necessary for "theory of mind." *Brain, 124*(Pt 2), 279–286.

Tabert, M. H., Albert, S. M., Borukhova-Milov, L., Camacho, Y., Pelton, G., Liu, X., Stern, Y., & Devanand, D. P. (2002). Functional deficits in patients with mild cognitive impairment: Prediction of AD. *Neurology, 58*(5), 758–764.

Valenstein, E., Bowers, D., Verfaellie, M., Heilman, K. M., Day, A., & Watson, R. T. (1987). Retrosplenial amnesia. *Brain, 110*(Pt 6), 1631–1646.

Vogeley, K., May, M., Ritzl, A., Falkai, P., Zilles, K., & Fink, G. R. (2004). Neural correlates of first-person perspective as one constituent of human self-consciousness. *Journal of Cognitive Neuroscience, 16*(5), 817–827.

Vogt, B. A., & Laureys, S. (2005). Posterior cingulate, precuneal and retrosplenial cortices: Cytology and components of the neural network correlates of consciousness. *Progressive Brain Research, 150*, 205–217.

Vogt, B. A., Vogt, L., & Laureys, S. (2006). Cytology and functionally correlated circuits of human posterior cingulate areas. *NeuroImage, 29*(2), 452–466.

Zysset, S., Huber, O., Ferstl, E., & von Cramon, D. Y. (2002). The anterior frontomedian cortex and evaluative judgment: An fMRI study. *NeuroImage, 15*(4), 983–991.

Zysset, S., Huber, O., Samson, A., Ferstl, E. C., & von Cramon, D. Y. (2003). Functional specialization within the anterior medial prefrontal cortex: A functional magnetic resonance imaging study with human subjects. *Neuroscience Letters, 335*(3), 183–186.

19

The Behavioral Measurement of Anosognosia as a Multifaceted Phenomenon

M. Donata Orfei, Carlo Caltagirone, and Gianfranco Spalletta

Since the first formal discussion on anosognosia by Babinski (1914), the term *anosognosia* has referred to the unawareness of sensorimotor deficits following a brain injury (Davies, Davies & Coltheart, 2005). Thus, typical clinical descriptions of anosognosia report cases of patients with paralysis, hemiparesis, hemianesthesia, hemianopia, or aphasia who deny their deficit, overestimate their abilities, claim that they are moving their handicapped limb and do not differ from other people, or partially admit difficulties but ascribe them to other causes (i.e., arthritis, tiredness, etc.), persisting in their beliefs despite contradictory objective evidence and external remarks by caregivers and physicians. Notably, anosognosics often do appear aware of all the other facets of their lives or admit other actual symptoms. In addition, some subjects show various forms of bodily delusions called somatoparaphrenias, for instance, the delusional belief that a body part is not owned by themselves and/or is owned by a certain other person (Marcel, Tegner & Nimmo-Smith, 2004). Anosognosia is typically modality specific, since a patient can be unaware of his or her hemiparesis but recognize his or her memory difficulties. However, anosognosia is not an all-or-nothing phenomenon but, on the contrary, can show various levels of complexity and severity.

A very salient issue concerns the hypothesis of a dissociation between conscious awareness and implicit knowledge of deficit. Ramachandran (1995) wondered whether it was conceivable that anosognosic subjects "...even though (they) deny their paralysis verbally, are aware at some deeper level that they are in fact paralyzed? And if such tacit knowledge does indeed exist, for what types of output is it available?" (p. 28). On the basis of a series of experiments with patients with anosognosia aimed to let a somewhat drowned awareness of the motor deficit emerge, Ramachandran (1995) came to the conclusion that patients either had no tacit knowledge of their paralysis or could not access it. He also underlined that neither the absence of frustration or distress while trying a bilateral action, nor the lack of learning in spite of repeated attempts, would support the hypothesis that anosognosia runs deep. On the contrary, clinical practice has highlighted a frequent discrepancy between implicit and explicit knowledge (Bisiach & Geminiani, 1991; Schacter, 1990), since some patients with anosognosia show contradictory behaviors, for instance, complaining they are paralyzed and yet attempting bilateral actions, while others deny paralysis but accept to stay in bed or in a wheelchair. In addition to this, some experimental trials support the hypothesis of implicit knowledge in anosognosia. For instance, vestibular stimulation was shown to induce a transient remission of anosognosia for hemiplegia and/or other unawareness phenomena, such as neglect (Cappa, Sterzi, Vallar & Bisiach, 1987; Vallar, Sterzi, Bottini, Cappa & Rusconi, 1990). While a recent study (Marcel et al., 2004) contrasted first- versus third-person knowledge of deficit, finding that a significant proportion of the subjects were more likely to give correct evaluations when asked in third person. These findings suggest that patients may have a covert knowledge of the impairment that is not consciously accessible. Schacter (1990) showed that in various neuropsychological conditions, such as amnesic syndrome, prosopagnosia, alexia, neglect, and blindsight, an underlying knowledge can be hypothesized. He and McGlynn (McGlynn & Schacter, 1989; Schacter, 1990) proposed that conscious experiences of perceiving, knowing, and remembering require the activation of the conscious awareness system (CAS), which can be activated by episodic memories or nonepisodic knowledge, such as lexical, conceptual, or spatial elements. In the former case, the result consists of a conscious memory for a recent event, while in the latter case the result is represented by the conscious awareness of knowing specific information. The CAS can interact with modular-level processors. While the activation at a modular level would determine an effect in behavior, the awareness of the action itself necessarily requires the interaction between CAS and modular processors. The disconnection between the output of a module and the CAS would therefore determine an implicit knowledge without a corresponding explicit awareness, as observed in anosognosia. Thus, anosognosia is a very complex and even apparently paradoxical phenomenon. In fact, since the first descriptions, the concept of lack of awareness of deficit has evolved from a one-dimensional phenomenon to a multidimensional and composite issue. The multifaceted nature of anosognosia is supported by the majority of recent neuropsychological pathogenic models of unawareness of deficit based on a modular structure including a wider range of related factors. For instance, Crosson et al., (Crosson, Barco, Velozo, Bolesta, Cooper et al., 1989) synthesized in his pyramidal model the possible levels of impairment of awareness, with different behavioral and rehabilitative implications: *(a)* intellectual

awareness (i.e., evident when the patient admits to having a particular difficulty), *(b)* emergent awareness (i.e., the deficit becomes evident to the patient
only in the course of action), and *(c)* anticipatory awareness (i.e., the patient is
able to consider the functional implications of the deficit and therefore his or her
limits). Thus, a patient can admit verbally to having a deficit but may fail to
recognize the deficit as it occurs, or ascribe it to an erroneous cause (emergent
awareness deficit at level b). Again, the patient can admit verbally to having a
deficit, realize the difficulty as it occurs, but fail to foresee realistically the
functional implications of the deficit (anticipatory awareness deficit at level c).
Also Schacter's (1990) model, to which we have already referred, implies a
modular system to explain anosognosia. A first-order theoretical account entails
postulating damage to, or disconnection of, a system or process that generates
awareness across multiple domains. A second-order account does not postulate
disruption of a cross-domain awareness mechanism, but instead appeals to
difficulties in gaining access to particular kinds of domain-specific information
that are associated with expressions of awareness in individual domains.
Analogously, the ABC model proposed by Vuilleumier (2004) describes a modular concept of anosognosia, underpinned by the cognitive dimensions involved
in anosognosia, that is, *(a)* appreciation, the ability to detect the presence of a
deficit, *(b)* belief, which refers to the beliefs about the self, and *(c)* check operation, which consists in the ability to monitor the performance. A deficit involving
one of these dimensions would result in different forms of anosognosia.
Synofzik, Vosgerau & Newen (2008) have proposed a multilevel conceptual
framework of self-awareness phenomena focusing on sense of ownership (i.e.,
the registration that my own arm is moving, rather than an arm belonging to
somebody else) and sense of agency (i.e., the registration that I am the initiator of
my actions, rather than someone else). Specifically, these two dimensions would
be based on complex mechanisms underlain by several functional levels, namely
a nonanalyzable level (including only an implicit self-representation), a conceptual level, at which properties can be systematically ascribed to different objects
(including the explicitly represented self), and a meta-representational level,
where mental representations can themselves be represented (and attributed to
the self or to others). In this perspective, anosognosia is described primarily as a
defect in sense of agency, but also as a defect in judgement of agency, that is, the
ability to interpret and correct beliefs about sense of agency. Finally, Synofzik
and colleagues (2008) traced back other delusional phenomena, such as asomatognosia and somatoparaphrenia, to defects in sense of ownership. A recent
paper by Spinazzola, Pia, Folegatti, Marchetti and Berti (2008) links different
unawareness phenomena to different modular brain circuitries. In particular,
anosognosia for motor impairment seems to be related to a defect in the activity
of areas connected with motor programming and motor monitoring, whereas
anosognosia for hemianesthesia seems to be related to an impairment in brain
areas involved in sensory-spatial processing. The authors assert that multilevel

dissociations between various unawareness phenomena (e.g., denial effect on proprioceptive anesthesia, anosognosia for hemianesthesia dissociation from unilateral extrapersonal and personal neglect) are the effect of a corresponding modular brain organization.

All these models have various advantages, namely the inclusion of metacognitive abilities, such as self-monitoring, anticipation of result, and the location of deficits at various levels. Thus, they provide helpful indications for specific rehabilitative intervention. As a consequence, an adequate assessment procedure is required in order to completely investigate this phenomenon. While a lack of comprehensive diagnostic procedures may potentially prevent the development of specific and efficient rehabilitation programs, the gathering of epidemiological data (Orfei, Robinson, Prigatano, Starkstein, Rüsch et al., 2007) and the acquisition of deeper knowledge concerning awareness processes and impairments are crucial. Thus, it is necessary to draw attention to a number of factors in anosognosia assessment in order to encourage the development of new and more efficient diagnostic procedures that can catch the several dimensions and components highlighted by our modern conceptualizations of awareness deficits.

The Most-Used Questionnaires for Anosognosia

In the last 30 years, a number of high-quality measures have been proposed for the assessment of anosognosia in stroke and traumatic brain injury (TBI). Especially with regard to stroke, these scales focus on some specific aspects and show a fair homogeneity in purposes and items. The best-known scales dealing with this approach are as follows:

1. Cutting's Questionnaire (Cutting, 1978), a clinician-rated scale that includes some questions about a general awareness of the deficit and reserves some additional items for possible concurrent phenomena, such as anosodiaphoria, that is, lack of interest in the deficit, and misoplegia, that is, hatred toward the paretic limb. The scale allows clinicians to state whether the patient is aware of his or her motor impairment, relying on a yes/no scale, but gives no information about which components of awareness are defective and to what extent.

2. Bisiach Scale (Bisiach, Vallar, Perani, Papagno & Berti, 1986), a clinician-rated scale that evaluates awareness of motor, sensorial, and visual-field deficits (specifically neglect) separately through verbal questions and simple neurological trials. Although definite questions are not provided by the authors, the trend consists in a progressively increasing specificity of the questions asked to the patient, corresponding to a decreasing level of awareness of deficit. Thus, score 0 is assigned to a patient who reports his or her deficit spontaneously or after a general question about health conditions. If the patient does not answer properly, the physician asks him or her general questions about his or her limbs or sight. If the patient answers correctly, he or she gets a score of 1; otherwise he or she is asked a specific question about the defective limb or sight. If he or she is

still unable to admit the deficit, the physician tries to make the deficit evident through some simple neurological trials. If not even this demonstration suffices to make the patient aware, he or she gets a score of 3 (severe unawareness). As we can see, the Bisiach Scale provides a more detailed scoring, discriminating four degrees of unawareness of deficit (i.e., absent, mild, moderate and severe). Although a score of 1 already indicates reduced awareness, Baier and Karnath (2005) suggested that the diagnosis of anosognosia is more properly defined by a score of at least 2. In fact, the authors hypothesize that subjects who score 1, though affected by a mild sensorimotor deficit, might subjectively judge other concurrent neurological symptoms as more prominent. So they would pay little attention to the sensorimotor deficit and would mention it only after a specific question. In this case, awareness of deficit per se would not actually be impaired, but in the assessment procedure might result as moderately impaired. In addition, Baier and Karnath (2005) found that patients scoring 0 and 1 showed very similar features with regard to variables such as age, severity of hemiparesis, neglect, etc. Conversely, patients scoring 1 showed significantly different features with respect to those scoring 2 or 3. In turn, patients scoring 2 and 3 showed several similarities. In other words, mild anosognosia graded as 1 would be an overinterpretation of the concept, which would not justify the actual diagnosis of anosognosia.

3. Anosognosia Questionnaire (Starkstein, Fedoroff, Price, Leiguarda, & Robinson, 1992) is conceptually and structurally similar to the Bisiach Scale. It provides six initial questions asked by the clinician to the patient, which explore the patient's awareness at a superficial level. If he or she does not admit the deficit, the patient is further compelled to face it by being asked five additional specific questions and requested to perform some actions with the handicapped limb. A global score is assigned at the end of the trial on a four-point scale based on the same criterion as the Bisiach Scale.

4. Anosognosia for Hemiplegia Questionnaire (Feinberg, Roane & Ali, 2000) consists of 10 items exclusively concerning left arm disability. However, it can be adapted for other motor deficits. Questions are asked by the clinician and each item is evaluated on a three-point scale (0 = full awareness, 0.5 = partial awareness, 1 = full unawareness), both before and during the demonstration of the deficit to obtain a total sum score ranging from 0 to 10 at the end of the questionnaire. The patient is repeatedly and openly confronted with the deficit and with his or her false beliefs by alternating questions and simple clinical trials.

All of these scales have been widely validated and are frequently used for assessing deficit of awareness in stroke. They have been developed strictly on the basis of the monodimensional and most salient phenomenological aspects of unawareness of deficit, that is, on sensorimotor impairment. Furthermore, they provide similar items and have analogous structure. However, a questionnaire recently developed for stroke patients, the Structured Awareness Interview (SAI; Marcel et al., 2004), differentiates and provides innovative characteristics, developed in order to investigate motor and sensorial deficits, functional abilities, and some delusional phenomena, such as somatoparaphrenia. It provides a numeric score for each item, which reflects the patient's self-evaluation of his or her own deficit (1 = severe, 2 = moderate/severe, 3 = no deficit), and a nominal classification, which reflects the adequacy of each answer (aware, unaware, inapplicable). In addition, the patient is asked to evaluate his or her ability in performing some unimanual, bimanual, and bipedal activities, in particular when he or she verbally overestimates his or her abilities. The authors suggest phrasing these last questions in a dual form, that is, making the patient reflect on him/herself (first-person questions: "In your present condition, how well can you . . . ?") and then to reflect on another person (third-person questions: "If I were in your present condition, how well could I . . . ?"). In fact, as previously hinted, a possible difference in the adequateness of the patient's answers must be recorded, since it could allow an implicit awareness (Marcel et al., 2004; Ramachandran, 1996; Vallar & Ronchi, 2006) of the deficit to emerge. Thus, this interview is quite articulated and discriminative for different aspects of anosognosia and allows clinicians to go beyond mere denial of deficit.

In other medical conditions, such as TBI, dementia, or psychosis, the investigation of unawareness of illness usually includes a wider range of issues, such as causal attribution, evaluation of functional implications in activities of daily living, measures of cognitive and behavioral deficits, need of treatment, and expectations of recovery. Furthermore, questionnaires are variously structured, allowing clinicians to administer the more appropriate and informative measure for the specific clinical picture. Definitively, it is fruitful to look at the assessment procedures adopted in neuropsychiatric conditions other than stroke, such as TBI, psychosis, and dementias, in order to explore the associated behavioral and cognitive dimensions in anosognosic patients. Thus, on the one side, unawareness of illness, regardless of the specific neuropsychiatric disorder, shows similar behavioral patterns (Lele & Joglekar, 1998), namely: *(a)* disavowal of the symptoms; *(b)* causal misattribution; *(c)* disavowal of the presence of a pathological process; *(d)* positive correlation between awareness of illness and depressive mood and between unawareness of illness and lack of concern; *(e)* modality specificity; *(f)* various levels of severity of unawareness and poor compliance with the rehabilitative or therapeutic course; and *(g)* a negative relationship with prognosis and recovery (Cairns, Maddock, Buchanan, David, Hayward et al., 2005; Jehkonen, Laihosalo & Kettunen, 2006a; Rüsch & Corrigan, 2002).

In spite of this, some additional elements prevent us from considering awareness disorders in the different neuropsychiatric conditions as expression of an individual cause. Indeed, Markovà and Berrios (1992; 2006) stressed that awareness is always awareness of something, insomuch that it is defined and shaped by the object that it refers to. Thus, it is necessary to go beyond the mere phenomenological dimension. Therefore, the manifestations of unawareness of illness in different disorders should be strictly traced back to the specific impaired domain (sensorimotor, cognitive, affective). In addition to this, awareness impairments may show very different courses. For instance, while anosognosia in stroke and TBI mostly recovers within a few days to 3 months, either spontaneously, or faster after rehabilitation treatment, in psychosis unawareness is chronic, often even if adequately treated, and in dementia it is even irreversible.

We do not have enough data about etiopathogenic mechanisms. Although some similar etiopathogenetic features of unawareness can be found through various neuropsychiatric disorders (such as a frequent involvement of right hemisphere, and in particular of frontal cortical areas as well as parieto-temporal areas), a number of additional heterogeneous findings within each disorder, as well as between various disorders, present a high heterogeneity (Orfei, Robinson, Bria, Caltagirone & Spalletta, 2008). However, keeping in mind all these considerations, some stimulating and fruitful conclusions from the assessment procedures for unawareness of illness in psychosis, dementia, and TBI can be drawn in order to improve and make the evaluation of anosognosia in stroke more exhaustive and consistent with the new multidimensional concept of this disorder.

With regard to TBI, which in some respects is phenomenologically closer to stroke, some interesting scales are as follows:

1. Self-Awareness of Deficit Interview (SADI; Fleming, Strong & Ashton, 1996), a clinician-rated scale that investigates three major areas, that is, self-awareness of deficit, self-awareness of functional implications of deficits, and ability to set realistic goals. For each domain, general questions are asked, followed by some specific prompts. Each area is evaluated on a four-point scale (0 = good awareness; 3 = poor awareness). While apparently generic, this semi-structured interview allows clinicians to assess the patient's understanding of the nature and the severity of the brain injury and of his or her present condition, and to explore the awareness of deficit and the cognitive ability to evaluate its functional consequences. In particular, it requires the patient to project his or her thoughts into the future, thus compelling him or her also to make an effort to think abstractly. This ability clearly requires a realistic awareness and a correct understanding of the injury.

2. Patient Competency Rating Scale (PCRS; Prigatano, Fordyce, Zeiner, Roueche, Pepping et al., 1986), a self-report questionnaire developed for the brain-injured population, which has also been used satisfactorily with stroke patients (Barskova & Wilz, 2006; Fischer, Gauggel & Trexler, 2004a). The patient is asked to evaluate him/herself on a list of 30 items referring to four domains of ability, namely activities of daily living, emotion, interpersonal relationships, and cognition. The same items are administered to the caregiver to judge the patient's competency. Each item is evaluated on a 5-point Likert scale (1 = the patient cannot perform the activity; 5 = the patient can perform the activity with ease). Thus, it seems to be highly discriminative. The last step consists of subtracting the caregiver's score from patient's score, so that the more negative the difference, the lower the patient's awareness. It has demonstrated

satisfactory factorial validity, test-retest reliability, internal consistency, and adequateness for longitudinal studies (Barskova & Wilz, 2006).
3. Awareness Questionnaire (Sherer, Bergloff, Boake, High, & Levin, 1998), which provides three self-report equivalent forms: one for the patient, one for the caregiver, and one for the clinician. It may be very informative because it consists of 17 items that require the comparison of patient's level of ability in emotional, physical, and cognitive areas before and after injury. The scoring provides a 5-point Likert scale, spanning from 1, meaning much worse, to 5, meaning much better. The analysis is conducted on the final total scores and item by item, where necessary. Also, in this case a relevant negative difference between patient's self-report and the other two evaluations is indicative of a defect in self-awareness.

These questionnaires are more comprehensive, consider a number of domains, and rely not only on a clinician's judgment but also on a caregiver's evaluation, which can provide additional information on the patient's experience previous to the brain injury. However, some considerations are required, that is: (a) some scales do not provide uniform cut-off scores, except for PCRS and AQ (Sherer, Hart & Nick, 2003) and for the SAI (Marcel et al., 2004; Nimmo-Smith, Marcel & Tegner, 2005); (b) it is not infrequent that stroke patients are not correctly informed about their condition by their relatives. Levine and colleagues (Levine, Warrenburg, Kerns, Schwartz, Delaney et al., 1987) clearly point out the risk to take lack of information for denial of illness (or anosognosia). We cannot underestimate this aspect, since a patient's ability to evaluate prognosis and functional implications can be disguised by missing or altered information given to the patient, especially when the deficit is mild to moderate; and (c) a reliable caregiver could not be available to get information about a patient's daily life. Moreover, this wider spectrum of items included in the scales to assess anosognosia in TBI mirrors the more complex clinical picture frequently following this medical condition. In fact, moderate to severe TBI is frequently accompanied by loss of consciousness and bilateral and asymmetrical lesions throughout the brain (Prigatano, Altman & O'Brien, 1990) and therefore with much less definite borders. As a consequence, TBI patients can show a wide range of impairments, such as motor, cognitive, affective, and behavioral deficits. In particular, social behavior can be altered (Bach & David, 2006; Borgaro, Prigatano, Kwasnica, Alcott & Cutter, 2004; Mathias & Coats, 1999; Prigatano, 2005). Most authors agree that unawareness in TBI concerns primarily cognitive, behavioral, and psychosocial deficits, and secondarily physical impairments (Fischer et al., 2004a; Gasquoine, 1992; Hart, Sherer, Whyte, Polansky & TA, 2004; Pagulayan, Temkin, Machamer & Dikmen, 2007; Prigatano et al., 1990). So TBI patients often lack awareness of cognitive deficits, are not able to monitor their own behavior, and have poor awareness about their impaired interpersonal skills and their impact on others (Bogod, Mateer & MacDonald, 2003). Although less evident and frequent, these features can nonetheless be present in stroke, and as such they require specific attention when assessing anosognosia in stroke as well.

A Multidimensional Assessment for a Multifaceted Phenomenon

Physicians generally realize a lack of awareness of a deficit in the course of clinical examination. For instance, in stroke or TBI patients anosognosia for motor impairment becomes evident when they are asked to use their paralyzed or weak limb, or to compare their paretic movements with analogous movements of the healthy limb (Lu, Barrett, Cibula, Gilmore, Fennell et al., 2000; Marcel et al., 2004; Nimmo-Smith et al., 2005). However, these procedures simply allow clinicians to detect the presence of anosognosia for the motor deficit; they give no information about specific phenomenological characteristics, extent of anosognosia, and "non-anosognosia-associated dimensions." On the contrary, referring to the modern neuropsychological models developed to explain anosognosia and drawing on cues from other medical conditions, in particular TBI, an exhaustive evaluation of unawareness of deficit in stroke has to investigate a number of highly informative dimensions. First, the anosognosic characteristic modality-specificity represents one of the most specific features of anosognosia in brain injury. In fact, as previously pointed out, unawareness can affect some functional domains but not others (Bach & David, 2006). Thus, the pool of questions assessing awareness has to span a number of functional areas. In addition to classical sensorimotor domain, it should include non-anosognosia-associated dimensions such as cognition, neuropsychiatric conditions, and behavior. In fact, stroke patients can also suffer from cognitive impairment (Patel, Coshall, Rudd & Wolfe, 2003; Spalletta, Guida, De Angelis & Caltagirone, 2002), mood disorders (Robinson, 2003; Spalletta & Caltagirone, 2008; Spalletta et al., 2002; Spalletta, Ripa & Caltagirone, 2005), and other behavioral disorders (Hama, Yamashita, Shigenobu, Watanabe, Hiramoto et al., 2007; Kim, Choi, Kwon & Seo, 2002; Spalletta, Pasini, Costa, De Angelis, Ramundo et al., 2001; Spalletta, Ripa, Bria, Caltagirone & Robinson, 2006; Starkstein, Fedoroff, Price, Leiguarda & Robinson, 1992). Concurrent unawareness phenomena, such as neglect, confabulations, bodily delusions, misoplegia, or anosodiaphoria, deserve a specific series of questions, for instance, concerning anomalous sensations or unrealistic beliefs about one's own limbs. Some classical anosognosia scales include items about these issues, but they generally are not sufficiently thorough or discriminating. In particular, the specific diagnosis of neglect requires attention (e.g., visual, tactile, personal, spatial, extinction; Gainotti & Tiacci, 1971; Gainotti, Messerli, Tissat, 1972; Brozzoli, Dematte, Pavani, Frassinetti & Farne, 2006; Spalletta, Serra, Fadda, Ripa, Bria et al., 2007), in order to clarify whether some of them are related to specific dimensions of anosognosia and to better define the still-debated matter of the co-occurrence of these two phenomena.

With regard to the awareness of the accident, causal attribution is a fundamental dimension to explore. Indeed, the patient can be aware of the deficit but ignore the real causes, or displace attention to nonrelevant causes or again attribute relevant symptoms to benign causes. Also, he or she might admit the causal pathological event but be unable to evaluate its actual severity. In the assessment of this point, clinicians have to take the patient's education, background, and cognitive level into account and make sure that the patient has received correct information. Analogously, expectations of recovery can inform us about the patient's altered perception of the pathological event and of the actual consequences. Frequently, anosognosic patients assert they are sane and expect to be discharged (Fischer et al., 2004a), or, if they partially admit a deficit, expect to recover fully and very soon, minimizing unrealistically threat to life or the severity of the disability. Ratings are to be based upon the degree to which unfavorable prognosis is distorted or changed to a more favorable one. Again, the evaluation must consider what medical information the patient has been given.

Another remarkable indicator of a realistic evaluation by the patient of his or her own condition is the admittance of need for treatment. Patients with anosognosia can show partial or full confidence in taking care of themselves, express disinterest in prolonged medical care/rehabilitation, or even refuse to attend the rehabilitative programs and clinicians' prescriptions. Similarly, awareness of functional implications represents a dimension to investigate, and specific questions in this area can reveal possible inconsistencies between a patient's expressed confidence in his or her abilities and the realistic limitations and uncertainties imposed by the pathological event. Thus, the patient might admit the seriousness of the deficit, yet assert that he or she is able to perform some limited actions, or even that he or she is capable of doing everything he or she could do before injury. For instance, a hemiplegic subject, though admitting to being hemiplegic, might assert that he or she is able to drive a car.

An exhaustive investigation of the phenomenon of anosognosia definitely has to take into consideration implicit knowledge, that is, the inconsistency between patients' verbal answers and behaviors (Fleming et al., 1996; Marcel et al., 2004; Schacter, 1990). In fact, as previously stressed, the inclusion of both verbal and nonverbal items is essential to bring a possible dissociation between explicit and implicit knowledge to light. For instance, with regard to motor deficits, the request to perform some actions, such as simply lifting the plegic arm/leg and comparing it with the normal one, or choosing between unimanual and bimanual/bipedal tasks, can be very informative. In fact, an anosognosic patient is expected to choose a bimanual task, while an underlying implicit knowledge of the deficit would compel him/her to privilege unimanual tasks (Ramachandran, 1995). Also, the already described alternate use of first/third-person questions about the deficit can be used. In fact, some anosognosic patients tend to answer more correctly when asked to evaluate the deficit as referred to another person than when referred to him/herself. A third method is the evaluation of a patient's discrepancy between predicted and actual performance in a task (Fischer, Trexler & Gauggel, 2004b; Hart, Giovannetti, Montgomery & Schwartz, 1998). This method may reveal a gap between intellectual and emergent awareness.

Finally, the possible overlap and interaction of the psychological defensive mechanism of denial with anosognosia should be considered also in stroke patients, although it has been studied mostly in TBI patients, where it is more frequent. Weinstein and Kahn (1955) were the first to raise the issue of what role motivation and psychological defense might play in unawareness of physical deficits. In other words, they wondered whether defective awareness of physical impairment might protect patients from depression or other forms of reaction (House & Hodges, 1988). Indeed, anosognosia and denial produce the same effect, that is, the disavowal or the minimization of the deficit, but on closer examination some salient behavioral differences emerge (Kortte, Wegener & Chwalisz, 2003; Prigatano & Klonoff, 1998). Prigatano (Prigatano & Klonoff, 1998; Prigatano, 2005), studying primarily TBI patients, noted that brain-injured subjects with anosognosia for cognitive deficits appear to lack information about themselves, show perplexity when receiving information about their deficits, and even indifference when asked to manage it. On the contrary, patients with denial demonstrate a resistance and sometimes an angry reaction when given feedback about their disability. Furthermore, anosognosia for motor impairment may be less chronic but more stable in its manifestations than denial. Indeed, patients in denial tend to ignore for a longer period of time the threatening information about their motor deficit. However, denial and anosognosia for motor deficit are not mutually exclusive and may interact and overlap over time. Thus, especially in the case of a mild to moderate deficit (Havet-Thomassin, Gardey, Aubin & Legall, 2004), possible motivational elements should always be weighed.

Remarks on the Structure of Questionnaires for Anosognosia

The high variability in the phenomenology of anosognosia in stroke patients requires reflection on some methodological choices, concerning namely the following:

1. *The objective standard to compare the patient's perceptions of the deficit.* Classical stroke anosognosia scales rely on clinical ratings, that is, the clinician judges whether patient's answers are consistent with his or her actual medical condition. In contrast, awareness questionnaires for TBI and dementia mostly rely upon the comparison between the patient's answers and informant/staff's

reports. Thus, subtracting the patient's evaluations from the caregiver's evaluation, a total score is obtained, which is supposed to reflect the degree of
awareness of the patient (Marcel et al., 2004; Ramachandran, 1996).
However, the reliability of this approach is debated which is also the case in
TBI patients. On the one hand, self/significant other comparisons can be quite
informative, since significant others have intimate knowledge of the patient
(Fleming et al., 1996); on the other hand, in the very acute stage following brain
injury this methodology may be not fully reliable, since relatives and significant
others can still have little information, not to mention the possible effects of
stress, anxiety (Prigatano, Borgaro, Baker & Wethe, 2005), and denial on their
judgment (Bogod et al., 2003; Fleming et al., 1996; Godfrey, Harnett, Knight,
Marsh, Kesel et al., 2003).

Some authors have developed measures to be used in TBI that consider these
aspects, such as the PCRS-R (Prigatano et al., 2005). In comparison to the
original PCRS, three additional items have been included, which ask the caregiver to list the current and main difficulties of the patient, to estimate on a
10-point Likert scale his or her own level of stress in taking care of the patient
(0 = no stress, 10 = severe stress), and to estimate the patient's level of awareness
again on a 10-point Likert scale (0 = no awareness, 10 = full awareness). The
authors of the scale hypothesize that a correlation between the judgment of
patient's awareness and the level of caregiver's distress can reflect a possible
effect of the latter on the former, although a causal effect can only be hypothesized. Even more complex, the Head Injury Behaviour Scale (HIBS; (Godfrey
et al., 2003) is a 20-item questionnaire where both the patient and the caregiver
indicate the presence of a list of behavioral difficulties that can follow a brain
injury, such as anger, impulsivity, poor decision making, and diminished
interest in things. In addition, the HIBS asks the caregiver to estimate on a
4-point Likert scale how stressful the patient's problematic behaviors are to
him/her (1 = no stress, 4 = severe stress). Thus, the HIBS provides an estimation
of the patient's awareness, which can be inferred by subtracting the patient's
score from the caregiver's score, and also provides an estimation of the caregiver's level of stress.

While a recent trial to test the differential efficacy of various methodologies in
anosognosia assessment in dementia has been carried out (Hannesdottir &
Morris, 2007), to our knowledge an analogous study to determine which
approach is more efficient in brain injury patients, and particularly in stroke,
has not yet been performed.

2. *Likert scales seem to be the most reliable for measuring depth of awareness,
   since, as pointed out, anosognosia can be characterized by various degrees.* Four
   degrees, as in the Bisiach Scale, seem to be reliable for an adequate evaluation of
   awareness of deficit, while a higher number of degrees runs the risk of being
   redundant and dispersive.

3. *Specific procedures for aphasic subjects.* Patients with global or severe comprehension aphasia cannot be tested on their awareness of language disorders, but
   even behavioral observation can provide some information about awareness of
   sensorimotor deficits. On the contrary, productive aphasia can be handled with

some specific administration devices. At a very simple level, the clinician can read aloud the answer alternatives and arrange with the aphasic patient specific gestures to indicate his or her own choice, or ask the patient to fill in the questionnaires on his or her own. Cocchini and Della Sala (in Chapter 7, this volume) illustrate in detail procedures and strategies appropriate for the assessment of anosognosia in aphasic patients. Notably, a number of studies on anosognosia mention generic inadequate linguistic abilities or severe language impairment as criteria of exclusion, while few do not mention the issue at all, leaving the reader at a loss (Orfei, Caltagirone & Spalletta, 2009).

Suggestions for Research That May Have a Strong Impact for Clinical Practice

A fair variability in the composition of the populations considered in different studies has emerged in a recent review (Orfei et al., 2009). In turn, this can account for the high variability in findings, specifically in epidemiological studies, and makes data hard to compare. Thus, clear and well-defined criteria for inclusion of patients in studies on anosognosia must be described. In particular, some features gain importance, first of all brain injury etiology. In fact, in a recent review (Orfei et al., 2009), in which we selected 43 studies on anosognosia following brain injury, spanning from 1986 to 2007, 47% of studies recruited only stroke patients, 37% only TBI subjects, and 16% combined various medical conditions, such as stroke, TBI, neoplastic pathologies, etc. The analysis of a heterogeneous sample can blur data, since in spite of phenomenological similarities, unawareness deficits can imply very different processes in different patient populations (Orfei et al., 2008). On the contrary, the direct comparison of anosognosia between homogeneous populations may spotlight differential and/or shared aspects of the awareness disorder in various medical conditions. Another possibly confounding factor is time elapsed from the acute event. Anosognosia can evolve rapidly, within a few days or months (Prigatano & Schacter, 1991; Starkstein et al., 1992) and more rarely can last for several years post-injury (Bogod et al., 2003; Leathem, Murphy & Flett, 1998; Murrey, Hale & Williams, 2005; Prigatano & Schacter, 1991; Starkstein et al., 1992). Notably, acute and chronic patients require differential assessment trials, depending on specific medical conditions (Orfei et al., 2009). In addition to this, the inclusion of acute and chronic patients in the same sample can be misleading. Heterogeneous timing of testing in different studies may contribute to the high variability in incidence rates (Orfei et al., 2007). Thus, it is necessary to stress target temporal terms, and results obtained with acute patients should be analyzed separately from those of chronic subjects. Specifically, given the high and rapid fluctuations of anosognosia in stroke, it is important to discriminate very acute patients, at least ranging from 1 to 7 days from injury, from acute patients, for instance, ranging from 8 to 29 days after stroke; finally, from 1 month on patients might be considered chronic and express different phenom- enological characteristics.

Laterality of lesion is another remarkable factor of interest. In fact, most studies include both right- and left-stroke patients, while a minority concern right patients only and no study recruits exclusively left-injured subjects (Orfei et al., 2009). Indeed, left-injured patients can be more difficult to assess because of possible aphasic deficits, so they tend not to be studied (Fleming et al., 1996; Jehkonen, Laihosalo & Kettunen, 2006b; Pedersen, Jørgensen, Nakayama, Raaschou & Olsen, 1996; Pia, Neppi-Modona, Ricci & Berti, 2004). However, the a priori exclusion may cause some confusion due to the under- estimation of rates of anosognosia in the total brain injury population.

Finally, longitudinal studies can be very informative in following the course of anosognosia that usually evolves as time goes by. Thus, the frequency of assessment should be rather high, especially in the acute phase. For instance, where possible, patients should be assessed within days after the brain injury, then at regular intervals. Furthermore, we stress the need to administer differ- ential procedures in the two stages of illness. In spite of this, Jehkonen and colleagues (2006a) reported that in 70% of studies no follow-up was carried out, which are data supported by our review (Orfei et al., 2009). A number of reasons can account for this trend. Possibly, the lack of follow-up procedures may express the prevalent interest for diagnosis and incidence, rather than for evolution of anosognosia. In addition, some pragmatic factors prevent a fre- quent assessment approach, especially in the very acute stage. Firstly, clinical practice and ward routine hardly deal with frequent questionnaire administra- tions, especially in the very acute stage. Also, fatigability, patient's pain, and reduced concentration can be salient problems. Secondly, early after brain injury the patient may not yet have had the chance to put his or her sensorimotor abilities to the test, and a reliable self-evaluation of cognitive abilities is unlikely, as they can be less salient to the patient than a physical deficit. Analogously, questions about functional implications of the deficit can be misleading and therefore should be limited. At this stage, questions about prognosis can be avoided for the objective lack of information. Thus, in the first days after brain injury, in order not to exhaust the subject and to obtain a reliable evaluation of the actual awareness of the patient, assessment should focus strictly on a few essential issues concerning mainly or exclusively evident impairments.

A Multilevel Approach to Anosognosia

Anosognosia cannot be considered as an isolated disorder; rather, it must be explored in a comprehensive view of the patient. In fact, as Prigatano (see Chapter 12, this volume) emphasizes, the specific phenomenology of anosognosia can depend on some pre-injury personality traits as well as be affected by some post-injury factors. Thus, we need to associate to the peculiar anosognosia assessment procedure the evaluation of different dimensions, firstly the level of cognitive impairment. In reality, the relationship between anosognosia and global cognitive level, as measured for instance by the Mini-Mental State Examination (Folstein, Folstein & McHugh, 1975) or Wechsler Intelligence subscales (Wechsler, 1981) is still controversial, since some authors assert that cognitive impairment can determine or contribute heavily to awareness deficits, while others disconfirm the causal role of cognitive deterioration in anosognosia, admitting at the most a worsening effect (Bogod et al., 2003; Davies et al., 2005; Levine, Calvanio & Rinn, 1991; Marcel et al., 2004; Starkstein et al., 1992). Also, mnestic functions play a controversial role in anosognosia. In fact, unawareness of deficit has been interpreted in some studies as the result of a mnestic failure, specifically of the inability to integrate new episodic experiences into long-term memory or one's self image (Marcel et al., 2004; Noé, Ferri, Caballero, Villodre, Sanchez et al., 2005). However, these data are not definite and require further in-depth examinations. Analogously, in some studies, performance at phonemic and semantic tasks in verbal fluency were positively related to anosognosia (Spalletta et al., 2007), although it is still to be explained how and to what extent language functions can affect awareness of deficit, or alternatively, if they are related by a third mechanism. In addition to this, it is important that executive functions, namely attention control, inhibition function, set shifting, and cognitive flexibility, as measured by tests such as the Wisconsin Card Sorting Test and the Stroop Test, have to be investigated in anosognosic patients. In fact, these neuropsychological functions showed significant positive correlations with anosognosia in TBI (Bogod et al., 2003; Noé et al., 2005). Furthermore, deficits of awareness of illness in schizophrenia and dementia were frequently found to be associated with poor performances in frontal tasks (Kashiwa, Kitabayashi, Narumoto, Nakamura, Ueda et al., 2005; Michon, Deweer, Pillon, Agid & Dubois, 1994; Shad, Muddasani, Prasad, Sweeney & Keshavan, 2004; Subotnik, Nuechterlain, Irzhevsky, Kitchen, Woo et al., 2005). Thus, it would be interesting to deepen these relationships and their functional role in anosognosia. As noted earlier, neuropsychiatric symptoms also represent a frequent consequence of stroke, so it is necessary to ascertain the relationship between them and anosognosia. For instance, depression and/or anxiety (Fleming, Strong & Ashton, 1998; Spalletta et al., 2006; Starkstein et al., 1992), apathy (Brodaty, Sachdev, Withall, Altendorf, Valenzuela et al., 2005; Hama et al., 2007), anger and hostility (Ghika-Schmid & Bogousslavsky, 1997; Kim et al., 2002), and unawareness of emotions (Spalletta et al., 2001; Spalletta et al., 2007) in anosognosic patients require further investigation, given their controversial relationship with awareness of illness and patient's outcome (Fleming et al., 1998; Kortte et al., 2003; Noé et al., 2005; Prigatano & Klonoff, 1998; Santos, Caeiro, Ferro, Albuquerque & Luisa Figueira, 2006; Weinstein & Kahn, 1955).

Last but not least, neuroimaging studies should be part and parcel of the diagnostic trial. In fact, a combination of data from conventional or, more interestingly, nonconventional structural magnetic resonance imaging (MRI) measures, such as diffusion tensor imaging (DTI) or tractography with behavioral data could provide relevant information about brain circuits involved in specific dimensions of self-awareness and their deficits, analogously to the investigations carried out in other pathological conditions (Flashman, McAllister, Johnson, Rick, Green et al., 2001; Ruby, Schmidt, Hogge, D'Argembeau, Collette et al., 2007; Shad, Muddasani & Keshavan, 2006). Currently, these methods are still not completely automated and require the supervision of technical experts. However, the information they provide, despite the time they require, might help clinicians to optimize individual rehabilitation programs in the near future. Also, advanced methods for studying structural indices in the cortex, such as thickness, in association with methods for studying functional and/or metabolic activity, such as positron emission tomography (PET), permit us to follow the process of cerebral plasticity following the recovery from awareness deficits (Schaechter, Moore, Connell, Rosen & Dijkhuizen, 2006). This might explain, if opportunely validated, why patients may fully recover within a few hours or instead become chronic.

Conclusions

There is a general consensus on the multidimensionality and complexity of the phenomenon of anosognosia in stroke and TBI, confirmed by the development of multicomponent neuropsychological models. The clarification of this issue is of great interest, and its importance is raised by the fact that unawareness of deficit has a high incidence rate and is associated with negative effect on prognosis and recovery of anosognosia. Moreover, self-awareness is one of the highest level functions of the human mind, and as such, it cannot be investigated without considering the subject in his or her wholeness. Thus, analogously to what happens in other multifaceted fields, such as neuropsychology or psychopathology, a comprehensive assessment procedure for anosognosia is necessary. Present diagnostic questionnaires, in spite of their reliability, still tend to reflect a monodimensional concept of anosognosia, intended mostly as unawareness of a deficit per se. Recent studies have contributed to a deeper knowledge of anosognosia, casting light on the involvement of a number of complex dimensions and superior cognitive abilities. Such a wide perspective on anosognosia requires an evolution in assessment, in order to gain a more definite diagnosis, to develop specific rehabilitation programs, and to understand awareness and related superior neuropsychological processes more deeply. Thus, we have outlined the main dimensions that should be included in a flexible and comprehensive assessment procedure for anosognosia (see Table 19.1).

Table 19.1 Dimensions to Investigate in Anosognosia and Related Measures

Dimension	Investigation Devices	Existing Scales Investigating the Dimension
Anosognosia		
Awareness of motor and/or sensorial deficits	Structured questions aimed at comparing patient's awareness with objective evidence	Bisiach scale, SAI, SADI, PCRS, Anosognosia Questionnaire (Starkstein et al., 1992), Anosognosia for Hemiplegia Questionnaire (Feinberg et al., 2000)
Awareness of cognitive deficits	Requests to esteem the ability in cognitive performances in daily activities	PCRS, AQ, SADI, Impaired Self-Awareness Scale (Prigatano & Klonoff, 1998)
Awareness of emotional and/or interpersonal deficits	Structured questions to compare with psychopathological and behavioral scales and with caregiver's reports	PCRS, AQ, HIBS, SADI
Implicit knowledge	Clinical trials and requests to perform actions, in order to compare verbal and procedural knowledge	SAI, Anosognosia Questionnaire
Evaluation of functional implications	Structured questions addressed to the patient to compare with objective evidence	SADI, PCRS, AQ, HIBS
Causal attribution	Structured questions about causes of deficits (verify information given to the patient)	SADI, SAI, LDIS
Evaluation of prognosis	Structured questions about timing and degree of recovery (verify information given to the patient)	SADI, LDIS
Compliance to rehabilitation	Structured questions addressed to the patient and to compare with staff's and caregiver's reports	LDIS
Degree of unawareness	Four-degree Likert scales	SADI, PCRS, AQ, SAI, Anosognosia Questionnaire, Anosognosia for Hemiplegia Questionnaire
Associated Phenomena		
Neglect	Specific tests to assess specific forms of neglect	Line crossing, letter cancellation, figure and shape copying, and line bisection tests, trials to assess nonvisual neglect forms (Lindell, Jalas, Tenovuo, Brunila, Voeten et al., 2007)
Somatoparaphrenias, misoplegia, anosodiaphoria, confabulation	Structured questions aimed at letting emerge possible bodily delusional phenomena, inconsistent feelings, or erroneous verbal admissions about the deficit	SAI, Anosognosia Questionnaire, Anosognosia for Hemiplegia Questionnaire

(*continued*)

Table 19.1 (Continued)

Dimension	Investigation Devices	Existing Scales Investigating the Dimension
Differential signs of anosognosia and/or psychological denial	Structured questions to let emerge possible peculiar behavioral aspects of psychological denial	Clinician's Rating Scale for Evaluating Impaired Self-Awareness and Denial of Disability (Prigatano & Klonoff, 1998), LDIS
Cognition		
Cognitive level	Tests to assess global cognitive impairment	MMSE, WAIS-R, Raven's Colored Progressive Matrices Test,
Mnestic functions	Tests to assess short- and long-term memory, and working memory	Digit Span, Corsi Block Test, Rey Auditory Verbal Learning Test, "n-back" tasks (Oliveri, Turriziani, Carlesimo, Koch, Tomaiuolo et al., 2001; Spalletta, Tomaiuolo, Di Paola, Trequattrini, Bria et al., 2008)
Language functions	Tests to assess associated language disorders	Phonological and semantic verbal fluency tests
Executive functions and attention	Tests to assess attention impairments	WCST, Stroop Test
Behavior		
Alexithymia	Scale to assess unawareness of emotions	TAS-20
Mood, anxiety and apathy symptoms, anger, and aggressiveness	Semi-structured scales to assess severity of depression, anxiety states, and apathy	HAM-D, HAM-A, Apathy Evaluation Scale (Marin, Biedrzycki & Firinciogullari, 1991), STAXI

AQ, Awareness Questionnaire (Sherer, Bergloff, Boake, High & Levin, 1998); HAM-A, Hamilton Anxiety Scale (Hamilton, 1959); HAM-D, Hamilton Depression Scale (Hamilton, 1960); HIBS, Head Injury Behaviour Scale (Godfrey et al., 2003); LDIS, Levine Denial of Illness Scale (Levine et al., 1987); MMSE, Mini-Mental State Examination; PCRS, Patient Competency Rating Scale (Prigatano et al., 1986); SADI, Self-Awareness of Deficit Interview (Fleming et al., 1996); SAI, Structured Awareness Interview (Marcel et al., 2004); STAI, State Trait Anxiety Inventory (Spielberger, Gorsuch & Lurshene, 1970); STAXI, State Trait Anger Expression Inventory (Spielberger, 1988); TAS-20, Toronto Alexithymia Scale (Bagby, Taylor & Parker, 1994); WAIS-R, Wechsler Adult Intelligence Scale Revised; WCST, Wisconsin Card Sorting Test.

Another remarkable issue is the specificity of various clinical situations that require partially different assessment modalities. For instance, for acute-phase subjects and in general for patients showing vigilance deficits, severe cognitive impairment, noncompliance, severe language disturbances, or behavioral disorders, a basic set of measures is more appropriate. On the other hand, patients showing persistent anosognosia have to be monitored regularly and as frequently as possible to detect progression of anosognosia, which in brain-injured subjects can be very sudden. For instance, an assessment administered at an acute stage, such as within 3 to 6 days of brain injury, has to be followed by regular consecutive assessments. Finally, research data are often inconsistent and hardly comparable because of a lack of uniformity in selection criteria and methodological choices. In the future these issues have to be clarified with appropriate methodologies.

In conclusion, we need to progress step by step toward a more definite, reliable, and valid diagnostic methodology, which should be structured considering the multifaceted expression of "specific anosognosia characteristics," the complexity of its interactions with "non-anosognosia-associated dimensions," such as behavior and cognition, and with other sociodemographic and clinical aspects.

References

Babinski, J. (1914). Contribution à l'étude de troubles mentaux dans l'hémiplegie organique cérébrale. *Revue Neurologique, 27,* 845–7.

Bach, L. J. & David, A. S. (2006). Self-awareness after acquired and traumatic brain injury. *Neuropsychological Rehabilitation, 16,* 397–414.

Bagby, R. M., Taylor, G. J. & Parker, J. D. (1994). The Twenty-item Toronto Alexithymia Scale–II. Convergent, discriminant, and concurrent validity. *Journal of Psychosomatic Research, 38,* 33–40.

Baier, B. & Karnath, H. O. (2005). Incidence and diagnosis of anosognosia for hemiparesis revisited. *Journal of Neurology, Neurosurgery and Psychiatry, 76,* 358–61.

Barskova, T. & Wilz, G. (2006). Psychosocial functioning after stroke: psychometric properties of the Patient Competency Rating Scale. *Brain Injury, 20,* 1431–7.

Bisiach, E. & Geminiani, G. (1991). Anosognosia related to hemiplegia and hemianopia. In G. P. Prigatano & D. L. Schacter, *Awareness of deficit after brain injury: Clinical and theoretical issues* (pp 17–39). New York: Oxford University Press.

Bisiach, E., Vallar, G., Perani, D., Papagno, C. & Berti, A. (1986). Unawareness of disease following lesions of the right hemisphere: anosognosia for hemiplegia and anosognosia for hemianopia. *Neuropsychologia, 24,* 471–82.

Bogod, N. M., Mateer, C. A. & MacDonald, S. W. S. (2003). Self-awareness after traumatic brain injury: A comparison of measures and their relationship to executive functions. *Journal of the International Neuropsychological Society, 9,* 450–58.

Borgaro, S. R., Prigatano, G. P., Kwasnica, C., Alcott, S. & Cutter, N. (2004). Disturbances in affective communication following brain injury. *Brain Injury, 18,* 33–9.

Brodaty, H., Sachdev, P. S., Withall, A., Altendorf, A., Valenzuela, M. J. & Lorentz, L. (2005). Frequency and clinical, neuropsychological and neuroimaging correlates of apathy following stroke – the Sydney Stroke Study. *Psychological Medicine, 35,* 1707–16.

Brozzoli, C., Dematte, M. L., Pavani, F., Frassinetti, F. & Farne, A. (2006). Neglect and extinction: within and between sensory modalities. *Restorative Neurology and Neuroscience, 24,* 217–32.

Cairns, R., Maddock, C., Buchanan, A., David, A. S., Hayward, P. & Richardson, G. (2005). Prevalence and predictors of mental incapacity in psychiatric in-patients. *British Journal of Psychiatry, 187,* 379–385.

Cappa, S., Sterzi, R., Vallar, G. & Bisiach, E. (1987). Remission of hemineglect and anosognosia during vestibular stimulation. *Neuropsychologia, 25*, 775–82.

Crosson, C., Barco, P. P., Velozo, C., Bolesta, M. M., Cooper, P. V., Werts, D., et al. (1989). Awareness and compensation in postacute head injury rehabilitation. *Journal of Head Trauma Rehabilitation, 4*, 46–54.

Cutting, J. (1978). Study of anosognosia. *Journal of Neurology, Neurosurgery and Psychiatry, 41*, 548–55.

Davies, M., Davies, A. A. & Coltheart, M. (2005). Anosognosia and the two-factor theory of delusions. *Mind and Language, 20*, 209–236.

Feinberg, T. E., Roane, D. M. & Ali, J. (2000). Illusory limb movements in anosognosia for hemiplegia. *Journal of Neurology, Neurosurgery and Psychiatry, 68*, 511–3.

Fischer, S., Gauggel, S. & Trexler, L. E. (2004a). Awareness of activity limitations, goal setting and rehabilitation outcome in patients with brain injuries. *Brain Injury, 18*, 547–62.

Fischer, S., Trexler, L. E. & Gauggel, S. (2004b). Awareness of activity limitations and prediction of performance in patients with brain injuries and orthopedic disorders. *Journal of International Neuropsychology Society, 10*, 190–9.

Flashman, L. A., McAllister, T. W., Johnson, S. C., Rick, J. H., Green, R. L. & Saykin, A. J. (2001). Specific frontal lobe subregions correlated with unawareness of illness in schizophrenia: a preliminary study. *Journal of Neuropsychiatry and Clinical Neuroscience, 13*, 255–7.

Fleming, J. M., Strong, J. & Ashton, R. (1996). Self-awareness of deficits in adults with traumatic brain injury: how best to measure? *Brain Injury, 10*, 1–15.

Fleming, J. M., Strong, J. & Ashton, R. (1998). Cluster analysis of self-awareness levels in adults with traumatic brain injury and relationship to outcome. *Journal of Head Trauma Rehabilitation, 13*, 39–51.

Folstein, M. F., Folstein, S. E. & McHugh, P. R. (1975). "Mini-mental state". A practical method for grading the cognitive state of patients for the clinician. *Journal of Psychiatric Research, 12*, 189–98.

Gainotti, G. & Tiacci, C. (1971). The relationships between disorders of visual perception and unilateral spatial neglect. *Neuropsychologia, 9*, 451–8.

Gainotti, G., Messerli, P. & Tissot, R. (1972). Qualitative analysis of unilateral spatial neglect in relation to laterality of cerebral lesions. *Journal of Neurology, Neurosurgery and Psychiatry, 35*, 545–50.

Gasquoine, P. G. (1992). Affective state and awareness of sensory and cognitive effects after closed head injury. *Neuropsychology, 6*, 187–96.

Ghika-Schmid, F. & Bogousslavsky, J. (1997). Affective disorders following stroke. *European Neurology, 38*, 75–81.

Godfrey, H. P. D., Harnett, M. A., Knight, R. G., Marsh, N. V., Kesel, D. A., Partridge, F. M., et al. (2003). Assessing distress in caregivers of people with a traumatic brain injury (TBI): a psychometric study of the Head Injury Behaviour Scale. *Brain Injury, 17*, 427–35.

Hama, S., Yamashita, H., Shigenobu, M., Watanabe, A., Hiramoto, K., Kurisu, K., et al. (2007). Depression or apathy and functional recovery after stroke. *International Journal of Geriatric Psychiatry, 22*, 1046–51.

Hamilton, M. (1959). The assessment of anxiety states by rating. *The British Journal of Medical Psychology, 32*, 50–55.

Hamilton, M. (1960). A rating scale for depression. *Journal of Neurology, Neurosurgery and Psychiatry, 12*, 56–62.

Hannesdottir, K. & Morris, R. G. (2007). Primary and secondary anosognosia for memory impairment in patients with Alzheimer's disease. *Cortex, 43*, 1020–30.

Hart, T., Giovannetti, T., Montgomery, M. W. & Schwartz, M. F. (1998). Awareness of errors in naturalistic action after traumatic brain injury. *Journal of Head Trauma Rehabilation, 13*, 16–28.

Hart, T., Sherer, M., Whyte, J., Polansky, M. & Novack, T. (2004). Awareness of Behavioral, Cognitive, and Physical Deficits in Acute Traumatic Brain Injury. *Archives of Physical Medicine and Rehabiliattaion, 85*, 1450–56.

Havet-Thomassin, V., Gardey, A. M., Aubin, G. & Legall, D. (2004). Several factors to distinguish anosognosia from denial after a brain injury. *Encephale, 30*(2), 171–81.

House, A. & Hodges, J. (1988). Persistent denial of handicap after infarction of the right basal ganglia: a case study. *Journal of Neurology, Neurosurgery and Psychiatry, 51*, 112–5.

Jehkonen, M., Laihosalo, M. & Kettunen, J. (2006a). Anosognosia after stroke: assessment, occurrence, subtypes and impact on functional outcome reviewed. *Acta Neuroligica Scandinavica, 114*, 293–306.

Jehkonen, M., Laihosalo, M. & Kettunen, J. E. (2006b). Impact of neglect on functional outcome after stroke: a review of methodological issues and recent research findings. *Restorative Neurology and Neuroscience, 24*, 209–15.

Kashiwa, Y., Kitabayashi, Y., Narumoto, J., Nakamura, K., Ueda, H. & Fukui, K. (2005). Anosognosia in Alzheimer's disease: association with patient characteristics, psychiatric symptoms and cognitive deficits. *Psychiatry and Clinical Neuroscience, 59*, 697–704.

Kim, J. S., Choi, S., Kwon, S. U. & Seo, Y. S. (2002). Inability to control anger or aggression after stroke. *Neurology, 58*, 1106–8.

Kortte, K. B., Wegener, S. T. & Chwalisz, K. (2003). Anosognosia and denial: their relationship to coping and depression in acquired brain injury. *Rehabilitation Psychology, 48*, 131–6.

Leathem, J. M., Murphy, L. J. & Flett, R. A. (1998). Self- and informant-ratings on the Patient Competency Rating Scale in patients with traumatic brain injury. *Journal of Clinical and Experimental Neuropsychology, 20*, 694–705.

Lele, M. V. & Joglekar, A. S. (1998). Poor insight in schizophrenia: neurocognitive basis. *Journal of Postgraduate Medicine, 44*, 50–5.

Levine, D. N., Calvanio, R. & Rinn, W. E. (1991). The pathogenesis of anosognosia for hemiplegia. *Neurology, 41*, 1770–81.

Levine, J., Warrenburg, S., Kerns, R., Schwartz, G., Delaney, R., Fontana, A., et al. (1987). The role of denial in recovery from coronary heart disease. *Psychosomatic Medicine, 49*, 109–17.

Lindell, A. B., Jalas, M. J., Tenovuo, O., Brunila, T., Voeten, M. J. & Hamalainen, H. (2007). Clinical assessment of hemispatial neglect: evaluation of different measures and dimensions. *The Clinical Neuropsychologist, 21*, 479–97.

Lu, L. H., Barrett, A. M., Cibula, J. E., Gilmore, R. L., Fennell, E. B. & Heilman, K. M. (2000). Dissociation of anosognosia and phantom movement during the Wada test. *Journal of Neurology, Neurosurgery and Psychiatry, 69*, 820–3.

Marcel, A. J., Tegner, R. & Nimmo-Smith, I. (2004). Anosognosia for plegia: specificity, extension, partiality and disunity of bodily unawareness. *Cortex, 40*, 19–40.

Marin, R. S., Biedrzycki, R. C. & Firinciogullari, S. (1991). Reliability and validity of the Apathy Evaluation Scale. *Psychiatry Research, 38*, 143–62.

Marková, I. S. & Berrios, G. E. (1992). The meaning of insight in clinical psychiatry. *British Journal of Psychiatry, 160*, 850–60.

Marková, I. S. & Berrios, G. E. (2006). Approaches to the assessment of awareness: conceptual issues. *Neuropsychological Rehabilitation, 16*, 439–55.

Mathias, J. L. & Coats, J. L. (1999). Emotional and cognitive sequelae to mild traumatic brain injury. *Journal of Clinical and Experimental Neuropsychology, 21*, 200–15.

McGlynn, S. M. & Schacter, D. L. (1989). Unawareness of deficits in neuropsychological syndromes. *The Journal of Clinical and Experimental Neuropsychology, 11*, 143–205.

Michon, A., Deweer, B., Pillon, B., Agid, Y. & Dubois, B. (1994). Relation of anosognosia to frontal lobe dysfunction in Alzheimer's disease. *Journal of Neurology, Neurosurgery and Psychiatry, 57*, 805–9.

Murrey, G. J., Hale, F. M. & Williams, J. D. (2005). Assessment of anosognosia in persons with frontal lobe damage: Clinical utility of the Mayo-Portland adaptability inventory (MPAI). *Brain Injury, 19*, 599–603.

Nimmo-Smith, I., Marcel, A. J. & Tegner, R. (2005). A diagnostic test of unawareness of bilateral motor task abilities in anosognosia for hemiplegia. *Journal of Neurology, Neurosurgery and Psychiatry, 76*, 1167–9.

Noé, E., Ferri, J., Caballero, M. C., Villodre, R., Sanchez, A. & Chirivella, J. (2005). Self-awareness after acquired brain injury. Predictors and rehabilitation. *Journal of Neurology, 252*, 168–75.

Oliveri, M., Turriziani, P., Carlesimo, G. A., Koch, G., Tomaiuolo, F., Panella, M., et al. (2001). Parieto-frontal interactions in visual-object and visual-spatial working memory: evidence from transcranial magnetic stimulation. *Cerebral Cortex, 11*, 606–18.

Orfei, M. D., Caltagirone, C. & Spalletta, G. (2009). The Evaluation of Anosognosia in Stroke Patients. *Cerebrovascular Diseases, 27*, 280–289.

Orfei, M. D., Robinson, R. G., Bria, P., Caltagirone, C. & Spalletta, G. (2008). Unawareness of illness in neuropsychiatric disorders: phenomenological certainty versus etiopathogenic vagueness. *Neuroscientist, 14*, 203–22.

Orfei, M. D., Robinson, R. G., Prigatano, G. P., Starkstein, S., Rüsch, N., Bria, P., et al. (2007). Anosognosia for hemiplegia after stroke is a multifaceted phenomenon: a systematic review of the literature. *Brain, 130*, 3075–90.

Pagulayan, K. F., Temkin, N. R., Machamer, J. E. & Dikmen, S. S. (2007). The measurement and magnitude of awareness difficulties after traumatic brain injury: A longitudinal study. *Journal of the International Neuropsychological Society, 13*, 561–70.

Patel, M., Coshall, C., Rudd, A. G. & Wolfe, C. D. (2003). Natural history of cognitive impairment after stroke and factors associated with its recovery. *Clinical Rehabilitation, 17*, 158–66.

Pedersen, P. M., Jørgensen, H. S., Nakayama, H., Raaschou, H. O. & Olsen, T. S. (1996). Frequency, determinants and consequences of anosognosia in acute stroke. *Journal of Neurology and Rehabilitation, 40*, 367–77.

Pia, L., Neppi-Modona, M., Ricci, R. & Berti, A. (2004). The anatomy of anosognosia for hemiplegia: a meta-analysis. *Cortex, 40*, 367–77.

Prigatano, G. P. (2005). Disturbances of self-awareness and rehabilitation of patients with traumatic brain injury: a 20-year perspective. *Journal of Head Trauma Rehabilation, 20*, 19–29.

Prigatano, G. P., Altman, I. M. & O'Brien, K. P. (1990). Behavioral limitations that traumatic-brain injured tend to underestimate. *The Clinical Neuropsychologist, 4*, 163–76.

Prigatano, G. P., Borgaro, S., Baker, J. & Wethe, J. (2005). Awareness and distress after traumatic brain injury: a relative's perspective. *Journal of Head Trauma Rehabilation, 20*, 359–67.

Prigatano, G. P., Fordyce, D. J., Zeiner, H. K., Roueche, J. R., Pepping, M. & Wood, B. C. (1986). *Neuropsychological rehabilitation after brain injury.* Baltimore, MD: John's Hopkins University Press.

Prigatano, G. P. & Klonoff, P. S. (1998). A Clinician's Rating Scale for evaluating impaired self-awareness and denial of disability after brain injury. *The Clinical Neuropsychologist, 12*, 56–67.

Prigatano, G. P. & Schacter, D. L. (Eds.) (1991). *Awareness of deficit after brain injury: Clinical and Theoretical issues.* New York: Oxford University Press.

Ramachandran, V. S. (1995). Anosognosia in parietal lobe syndrome. *Consciousness and Cognition, 4*, 22–51.

Ramachandran, V. S. (1996). The evolutionary biology of self-deception, laughter, dreaming and depression: some clues from anosognosia. *Medical Hypotheses, 47*, 347–62.

Robinson, R. G. (2003). Poststroke depression: prevalence, diagnosis, treatment, and disease progression. *Biological Psychiatry, 54*, 376–87.

Ruby, P., Schmidt, C., Hogge, M., D'Argembeau, A., Collette, F. & Salmon, E. (2007). Social mind representation: where does it fail in frontotemporal dementia? *Journal of Cognitive Neuroscience, 19*, 671–83.

Rüsch, N. & Corrigan, P. W. (2002). Motivational interviewing to improve insight and treatment adherence in schizophrenia. *Psychiatric Rehabilitation Journal, 26*, 23–32.

Santos, C. O., Caeiro, L., Ferro, J. M., Albuquerque, R. & Luisa Figueira, M. (2006). Anger, hostility and aggression in the first days of acute stroke. *European Journal of Neurology, 13*, 351–8.

Schacter, D. L. (1990). Toward a cognitive neuropsychology of awareness: implicit knowledge and anosognosia. *Journal of Clinical and Experimental Neuropsychology, 12*, 155–78.

Schaechter, J. D., Moore, C. I., Connell, B. D., Rosen, B. R. & Dijkhuizen, R. M. (2006). Structural and functional plasticity in the somatosensory cortex of chronic stroke patients. *Brain, 129*, 2722–33.

Shad, M. U., Muddasani, S. & Keshavan, M. S. (2006). Prefrontal subregions and dimensions of insight in first-episode schizophrenia–a pilot study. *Psychiatry Research, 146*, 35–42.

Shad, M. U., Muddasani, S., Prasad, K., Sweeney, J. A. & Keshavan, M. S. (2004). Insight and prefrontal cortex in first-episode schizophrenia. *NeuroImage, 22*, 1315–20.

Sherer, M., Bergloff, P., Boake, C., High, W. J. r. & Levin, E. (1998). The Awareness Questionnaire: factor structure and internal consistency. *Brain Injury, 12*, 63–8.

Sherer, M., Hart, T. & Nick, T. G. (2003). Measurement of impaired self-awareness after traumatic brain injury: a comparison of the Patient Competency Rating Scale and the awareness questionnaire. *Brain Injury, 17*, 25–37.

Spalletta, G. & Caltagirone, C. (2008). Depression and other neuropsychiatric complications. In J. Stein, R. Zorowitz, R. Harvey, R. Macko, & C. Winstein (Eds), *Stroke recovery and rehabilitation*, (pp. 453–67). New York, NY: Demos Medical Publishing.

Spalletta, G., Guida, G., De Angelis, D. & Caltagirone, C. (2002). Predictors of cognitive level and depression severity are different in patients with left and right hemispheric stroke within the first year of illness. *Journal of Neurology, 249,* 1541–51.

Spalletta, G., Pasini, A., Costa, A., De Angelis, D., Ramundo, N., Paolucci, S., et al. (2001). Alexithymic features in stroke: effects of laterality and gender. *Psychosomatic Medicine, 63,* 944–50.

Spalletta, G., Ripa, A., Bria, P., Caltagirone, C. & Robinson, R. G. (2006). Response of emotional unawareness after stroke to antidepressant treatment. *Americal Journal Geriatric Psychiatry, 14,* 220–7.

Spalletta, G., Ripa, A. & Caltagirone, C. (2005). Symptom profile of DSM-IV major and minor depressive disorders in first-ever stroke patients. *American Journal Geriatric Psychiatry, 13,* 108–15.

Spalletta, G., Serra, L., Fadda, L., Ripa, A., Bria, P. & Caltagirone, C. (2007). Unawareness of motor impairment and emotions in right hemispheric stroke: a preliminary investigation. *International Journal of Geriatric Psychiatry, 22,* 1241–6.

Spalletta, G., Tomaiuolo, F., Di Paola, M., Trequattrini, A., Bria, P., Macaluso, E., et al. (2008). The Neuroanatomy of Verbal Working Memory in Schizophrenia: A Voxel-Based Morphometry Study. *Clinical Schizophrenia & Related Psychoses, 2,* 79–87.

Spielberger, C. D. (1988). *State-Trait Anger Expression Inventory, Research Edition. Professional Manual.* Odessa, Florida: Psychological Assessment Resources.

Spielberger, C. D., Gorsuch, R. L. & Lurshene, R. E. (1970). *Test Manual for the State-Trait Anxiety Inventory.* Palo Alto, CA: Consulting Psychologists Press.

Spinazzola, L., Pia, L., Folegatti, A., Marchetti, C. & Berti, A. (2008). Modular structure of awareness for sensorimotor disorders: evidence from anosognosia for hemiplegia and anosognosia for hemianaesthesia. *Neuropsychologia, 46,* 915–26.

Starkstein, S. E., Fedoroff, J. P., Price, T. R., Leiguarda, R. & Robinson, R. G. (1992). Anosognosia in patients with cerebrovascular lesions. A study of causative factors. *Stroke, 23,* 1446–53.

Subotnik, K. L., Nuechterlain, K. H., Irzhevsky, V., Kitchen, C. M., Woo, S. M. & Mintz, J. (2005). Is unawareness of psychotic disorder a neurocognitive or psychological defensiveness problem? *Schizophrenia Research, 75,* 147–157.

Synofzik, M., Vosgerau, G. & Newen, A. (2008). I move, therefore I am: a new theoretical framework to investigate agency and ownership. *Consciousness and Cognition, 17,* 411–24.

Vallar, G. & Ronchi, R. (2006). Anosognosia for motor and sensory deficits after unilateral brain damage: a review. *Restorative Neurology and Neuroscience, 24,* 247–57.

Vallar, G., Sterzi, R., Bottini, G., Cappa, S. & Rusconi, M. L. (1990). Temporary remission of left hemianesthesia after vestibular stimulation. A sensory neglect phenomenon. *Cortex, 26,* 123–31.

Vuilleumier, P. (2004). Anosognosia: the neurology of beliefs and uncertainties. *Cortex, 40,* 9–17.

Wechsler, D. (1981). *WAIS-R: Manual: Wechsler Adult Intelligence Scale—Revised.* San Antonio, TX: The Psychological Corporation.

Weinstein, E. A. & Kahn, R. L. (1955). *Denial of illness. Symbolic and physiological aspects.* Springfield, IL: Charles C. Thomas.

VII

Anosognosia and Visual Loss

20

Anton's Syndrome and Unawareness of Partial or Complete Blindness

George P. Prigatano and Thomas R. Wolf

Given that Anton's syndrome was one of the first classical neurological descriptions of anosognosia (Prigatano, Chapter 1, this volume), discussion of this syndrome and related disorders toward the end of this volume may appear unusual. While several case reports have appeared that document the phenomenon of anosognosia for cortical blindness, no experimental studies have emerged to help further reveal the underlying mechanisms responsible for this phenomenon. Thus, scientific advances in understanding anosognosia for cortical blindness secondary to bilateral occipital lesions (i.e., Anton's syndrome) have been limited. Nevertheless, a review of various case reports raises important observations that are relevant to our final discussion. Consequently, a discussion of Anton's syndrome and unawareness of partial or complete blindness secondary to a variety of causes will now be considered.

Anton's Clinical Observations

Förstl, Owen, and David (1993) have provided students of anosognosia with a historically valuable translation of Gabriel Anton's (1898) paper: "On focal diseases of the brain which are not perceived by the patient." Anton's clinical reports are outstanding and clearly demonstrate the reality that a patient can have lost vision, hearing, and movement and be unaware of his or her losses. This can occur in the absence of dementia or acute confusional states. While his description of anosognosia for deafness is equally impressive as his description of anosognosia for blindness, it is the latter phenomenon for which his name is attached.

Anton emphasized that a loss of neurological function may not be perceived by the person if: *(1)* the brain lesions occur in a region known to be important for that function (e.g., occipital lobe for vision, temporal lobe for hearing, etc.); *(2)* they are associated with bilateral cortical lesions that are "almost symmetrical" (Förstl et al., 1993, p. 5); and *(3)* the patient disregards or discounts any objective evidence that he or she has lost his or her functional capacity. In addition *(4)* the patient does not appear to be demented or show significant cognitive impairment that would result in a failure to evaluate his or her present functional capacity.

Case Reports of Anton's Syndrome

Hécaen and Albert (1978) note that before Anton's (1898) report, Dejerine and Vialet (1893) and von Monakow (1897) described cases of cortical blindness in which the blindness was "denied." Following Anton's (1898) description, however, several other case reports replicated Anton's observations (e.g., Abdulqawi, Ashawesh, & Ahmad, 2008; Bergman, 1957; Cusumano, Fletcher, & Patel, 1981; Della Sala & Spinnler, 1988; Galetovic, Karlica, Bojic, & Znaor, 2005; Krovvidi & Bhattacharjee, 2008; Misra, Rath, & Mohanty, 1989; Silverberg & Wilnsky, 1978). The case report of Della Salla and Spinnler (1988) demonstrates the essential features of a "true" Anton's syndrome. First, the patient is completely blind secondary to cortical damage in the occipital regions of the brain. Second, these lesions are bilateral. Third, the patient is not only unaware of her blindness; she rejects any objective evidence of blindness. Fourth, the patient offers plausible, but at times confabulatory responses to explain away any possible evidence of her failure to see (e.g., "The room is dark," or "I don't have my glasses, therefore how can I see?"). Fifth, the patient has an apparent lack of concern (or anosodiaphoria) over her neurological condition.

The natural course of Anton's syndrome has not been extensively reported (Bergman, 1957). We do not know how these patients may or may not change with the passage of time. There are, however, impressive case studies of "reversible" Anton's syndrome that are informative (e.g., Argenta & Morgan, 1998; Roos, Tuite, Below, & Pascuzzi, 1990; Yilmazlar, Taskapilioglu, & Askoy, 2003). Various neurological conditions can compromise bilateral cerebral blood flow within the posterior cerebral arteries, producing localized cortical ischemia (with associated electroencephalogram [EEG] abnormalities). In some instances, the condition is reversed with time and/or treatment. Argenta and Morgan (1998) describe a case of a 19-year-old woman who developed Anton's syndrome following obstetric hemorrhage. The patient developed all of the classical signs associated with Anton's syndrome. Magnetic resonance imaging (MRI) of the brain at that time demonstrated minimal cortical enhancement over the occipital regions during the time she was anosognostic for her blindness.

Her vision eventually returned. She was diagnosed with transient cortical blindness secondary to hypoperfusion of the occipital cortex.

Roos et al. (1990) provide evidence of bilateral occipital EEG abnormalities in a 50-year-old woman who developed Anton's syndrome. At the time MRI revealed small hyperdense lesions in bilateral occipital regions. As her Anton's syndrome abated, the abnormal electrical discharges in the occipital regions resolved.

Abutalebi et al. (2007) present a case of Anton's syndrome following a ruptured aneurysm in the left posterior cerebral artery (PCA). This patient also had widespread vasospasm. The patient was unaware of her visual loss and strongly denied any blindness. While imaging studies of the brain initially suggested that a unilateral lesion may produce Anton's syndrome, a single photon emission computed tomography (SPECT) imaging study revealed hypoperfusion, not only in the left cerebral hemisphere, but in the right as well. This interesting case study again supports the notion that bilateral cerebral dysfunction may be necessary for Anton's syndrome. Structural neuroimaging studies of the brain may underestimate the degree of bilateral cerebral involvement in some cases of anosognosia.

Neuro-ophthalmology of Anton's Syndrome

Blumenfeld (2002) provides a useful review of the visual system from the level of the eye and retina to the neocortex. Three parallel channels of visual information processing are identified and specifically relate to the perception of color, form, and motion. Lesions throughout the cerebral hemispheres yield very predictable forms of visual loss.

Most patients with cortically based visual loss subjectively experience "some" disturbance in their visual capacity, although they may not be precise in describing the nature of their visual loss. An area of considerable interest has been the study of patients presenting with visual recognition disorders primarily from retrochiasmal pathology. These patients have been described as having a visual agnosia (Bauer & Demery, 2003). Visual agnosia can be subdivided into various subtypes, including a failure of the patient to identify words and letters (alexic agnosia), faces (prosopagnosia), and colors (color agnosia). Agnostic disturbances have been further described as "associative" versus "apperceptive" in nature. Associative agnosia refers to a deficit in the ability to recognize a visual object while one can demonstrate a preserved capacity to "see" the object, as demonstrated by the patient's ability to copy, or at least match, the same visual stimuli. In contrast, apperceptive agnosia refers to a broad spectrum of visual perceptual difficulties in which the higher order levels of perception/recognition have been compromised, but the elementary sensory functions appear relatively stable (Bauer & Demery, 2003). The various forms of visual object recognition deficits have been repeatedly associated with either unilateral or bilateral cortical lesions.

Clinically, however, these patients appear aware of their failure at recognition when given appropriate feedback. This is in stark contrast to Anton's syndrome.

Patients with Anton's syndrome "deny" any visual loss or impairment, despite the fact that one can demonstrate that they literally cannot see. It is not uncommon for subacute insidious processes such as a slow-growing neoplasm, or progressive bilateral posterior artery infarction (Verslegers, DeDeyn, Saerens, Marien, Appel, Pickut, & Lowenthal, 1991) to cause visual field loss, as well as visual neglect, that may be initially without conscious awareness on the part of the patient. These patients may be initially misdiagnosed as having Anton's syndrome, but they are quickly correctly identified when it is shown that these patients acknowledge their loss once it has been demonstrated to them. In Anton's syndrome, the "denial" persists with frequent confabulation of details of their visual environment, at times with credible near accuracy.

The visual anosognostic patient, therefore, is unable to see/perceive, refuses to admit to blindness, and acts as though vision is intact, persisting in this behavior despite all evidence to the contrary. Carefully documented cases, however, are rare. Many published cases have been criticized for a lack of detailed assessment of the visual system prior to concluding that lesions at the level of the visual cortex were responsible for the syndrome.

Various brain insults can disturb primary striate visual cortex functioning. They include vasculitis, hemorrhagic or ischemic stroke, carbon monoxide poisoning, embolization or hypoxia during cardiac surgery or following cardiac arrest, hypertensive or pre-eclamptic posterior reversible encephalopathy syndrome (PRES), and brain trauma. Recovery from vascular ischemia is often rapid, whereas after trauma, quite slow. Most of these etiologies involve loss of the primary visual cortex, but rarely peripheral ocular disease in isolation has been implicated.

Some patients with cortical blindness may experience various visual hallucinations (Suzuki, Endo, Yamadori, & Fujii, 1977), reinforcing their "denial" of visual loss. These hallucinations are considered a form of release phenomenon, giving rise to visual images that they can see for a period of time. Polyopsia (multiple repetitive images of the same object spread across the blind field), palinopsia (persistence of after images in the blind field), or Riddoch phenomenon (visual perception of image movement in a blind visual field) have been reported by Cogan (1973), Lance (1976), and Brust & Behrens (1977). These are more frequent with unilateral lesions but may involve bilateral primary cortical insult. Flint, Loh, and Brust (2005) presented a case with neuroimaging and EEG correlates. FLAIR MRI demonstrated subtle signs of ischemic infarction of the left occipital pole, T1 imaging with gadolinium showed gyriform enhancement in the same region, and SPECT scans showed focal hypoperfusion. Electroencephalogram was normal except for borderline slowing in the left occipital region. They concluded that the hallucinations reported by their patient may have resulted from infarction and disinhibition of the primary visual cortex. The prolonged symptoms, normal EEG, and SPECT evidence for hypoperfusion argue against an epileptiform etiology.

These hallucinations typically result after damage to the primary (ventral stream) visual cortex, which contains high-resolution visual acuity information carried from the foveal retina ganglion cells via the classical lateral geniculocalcarine radiations, and ultimately processed in areas of the inferior temporal cortex. A lesion in this location releases or disinhibits the secondary dorsal vision stream, which carries visual motion detection or action perception from the mid to far peripheral retina ganglion cell axons via optic nerve-chiasm-tract to superior-colliculus and then to pulvinar/thalamus, terminating at the posterior parietal cortex association areas (Swartz & Brust, 1984). This intact, but limited perception of visual motion in a perceptually blind visual field has been termed "blindsight." These are the two main vision streams out of many other retino-fugal pathways discussed recently by Rizzolatti and Matelli (2003).

Two additional anatomic areas that are in close proximity to these major vision streams may have dual system roles. The inferior parietal lobule (IPL) and superior temporal gyrus (STG) are situated near both the dorsal and ventral visual system pathways. Recent work favors a combined joint role allowing overlap involvement with both systems (Shapiro, Hillstrom, & Husain, 2002). Findings from functional imaging, electrophysiological, and lesion studies suggest that these regions allow for flexible reconfiguration of behavior between these two alternative pathways and operation. Damage to the right IPL leads to deficits in both maintaining visual attention and also responding to hemineglect, the classical syndrome that follows lesions of this region (Shapiro et al., 2002). These intermediate structures between the dorsal and ventral visual anatomic pathways may be able to change their predominant action depending on other nearby lesions of the visual system.

Compared to the symmetric cortical representation of the primary ventral vision system, lesions involving the dorsal secondary system may have a built-in asymmetry as demonstrated by poor visual recognition of familiar faces, places, and prosopagnosia secondary to mainly nondominant right hemisphere dorsal pathway lesions. Another asymmetry is suggested by visuomotor optic ataxia seen in Balint's syndrome, with abnormal right hand reaching for visual targets from dominant left hemisphere lesions, not seen in nondominant hemisphere pathology (Goodale & Milner, 2004). Degenerative conditions, including parkinsonism and Alzheimer's disease, often are accompanied by these release hallucinations, but none have been described with the denial in Anton's syndrome.

Research on "Anton-Like" Syndromes

Case reports of Anton's syndrome have also appeared in which there is no evidence of occipital pathology. These rare patients have prechiasmal lesions. Not uncommonly, these patients are in a state of "cognitive confusion," with possible frontal lobe involvement. As their cognitive impairment notably improves, they often verbally report recognition of their visual loss. These cases might best be described as individuals with "Anton-like" syndrome.

Swartz and Brust (1984) report on a 60-year-old man who had a history of longstanding ethanol abuse who had complete loss of vision secondary to trauma to both eyes. During a period of "alcohol hallucinosis," he showed anosognosia for his complete blindness. As his acute confusional state and associated confabulations disappeared, he reportedly was aware of his visual loss. As discussed in Chapter 12 of this volume, McDaniel and McDaniel (1991) describe anosognosia for blindness following a self-inflicted gunshot wound to the head, which severed the optic nerves and produced profound frontal lobe dysfunction. During the period of post-traumatic amnesia (or confusion), this patient "denied" her blindness. As her cognitive functioning greatly improved, she began to acknowledge her blindness. Wessling, Simosono, Escosa-Bagé, and de Las Heras-Echeverria (2006) report the case of a 29-year-old male with chronic psychiatric disabilities and history of probable mental retardation. The patient suffered from a seizure disorder and had a progressive deterioration of his vision. The patient verbally denied any visual difficulties. A computed tomography (CT) scan of the brain revealed a "giant extra-axial bifrontal mass with compression and displacement of both frontal lobes, the ventricular system, the falx, and part of the corpus callosum" (p. 673). The neuroimaging findings were dramatic in light of the extensive bilateral frontal lobe pathology that was present. It remained unclear if his significant cognitive impairments secondary to massive frontal lobe dysfunction were at the basis of his imperception.

Other case studies report on patients that have no subjective recognition of loss of vision, but again, these patients have widespread diffuse brain disorders with associated severe cognitive impairment (e.g., Alemdar et al., 2007; Burns et al., 1997; Davis, Sewell, Levy, Price, & Cunningham, 2009; Jaeckle, 1982). As such, they do not meet the traditional criteria for true Anton's syndrome.

Research on Unawareness of Hemianopia

Various brain disorders can produce loss of vision in one-half of each visual field (i.e., hemianopia). Bisiach and Geminiani (1991) noted that "unawareness of hemianopia may . . . range from imperception of the deficit until it is revealed by the examiner to incorrigible denial" (p. 20). Bisiach and Geminiani (1991) also noted that the typical asymmetry of anosognosia for hemiplegia (right being greater than left) is not as clear for anosognosia for hemianopia. They further note no association of unawareness of hemianopia and unilateral neglect (p. 23).

Unfortunately, studies have not appeared that clarify which patients tend to show persistent "incorrigible denial" of their hemianopia once it has been demonstrated to them. Spontaneous recovery of homonymous hemianopia for some patients is well recognized. When it occurs, the majority of patients show improvement within the first month after injury (Zhang, Kedra, Lynn, Newman, & Biousse, 2006). In clinical practice, it is common for many post-acute patients with hemianopia not to immediately recognize a dramatic change in their vision, although they do note that they are having "some problems seeing." When it is demonstrated to them that they have a clear visual field cut or when they discover it on their own (e.g., Kolb, 1990), they accept that there is indeed a loss of vision present. These patients do not reject the evidence. There is also no confabulatory reaction to explain diminished vision. They are motivated to engage in various rehabilitation strategies to try and improve their vision (Schofield & Leff, 2009).

True anosognosia for hemianopia in post-acute patients is not commonly reported. When anosognosia is reported in patients with hemianopia following stroke, it is often seen in patients who suffer very large strokes and who are described as disoriented and confused when examined. Such anosognostic patients also tend to have a higher percentage of premorbid dementia (Pederson, Henrik, Nakayama, Raaschou, & Olsen, 1996). While they can be separated from patients who show neglect, it is more likely that anosognosia for hemianopia is seen in patients who do show neglect (Bisiach, Vallar, Perani, Papagno, & Berti, 1986; Welman, 1969). It remains unclear as to whether their severe attentional disturbances are at the basis of their anosognostic behavior. In light of these observations, a proposed terminology for describing anosognosia or unawareness of visual impairments is suggested.

Proposed Terminology in Describing Anosognosia for Visual Impairments

The term *Anton's syndrome* should be applied to those patients who have lost vision in both visual fields and are described as "completely blind" and are unaware of their blindness. These patients have demonstrated bilateral occipital cortical involvement. They do not show clinical signs of diffuse brain dysfunction. By definition, they should not have a dementia or be in an acute confusional state.

The term *Anton-like syndrome* should be applied to those individuals who are also completely blind, but whose blindness is caused by either injury to the orbit or to the optic nerve. These patients have a brain disorder, but one that is of such a nature as to produce significant cognitive impairment. The individual appears to have difficulty interpreting or recognizing sensory loss secondary to his or her cognitive state. These patients do not have focal lesions in the occipital cortex. In this patient group, there is often a recognition of loss of vision as the acute confusional state disappears.

A third group of patients consists of those who are unaware of a hemianopia (UHEM). By definition, these patients have lesions that disrupt the visual projection areas in parietal, temporal, and/or occipital regions. Their visual loss is

Table 20.1 Proposed Terminology for Describing Patient Groups Who Have Complete or Partial Loss of Vision, a Brain Disorder, and Are Unaware of Their Visual Loss

Terminology	Clinical Phenomenon	Neuroimaging and/or Neuropathological Findings
Anton's syndrome	1. Complete loss of vision and unaware of the loss 2. Orbits and optic nerve are intact 3. Disregards evidence for their blindness 4. Appears unconcerned	Bilateral occipital lobe lesions No widespread brain lesions with associated diffuse cognitive impairment
"Anton-like" syndrome	1. Complete loss of vision and unaware of the loss 2. Orbits and/or optic nerve are damaged 3. Disregard evidence for their blindness 4. Appears unconcerned, but often disoriented or showing confusion	Occipital lobes appear to be intact, but other brain lesions are present which seem to be at the basis of the significant cognitive impairment observed in this group. They do not show signs of purely focal brain dysfunction.
Unawareness of hemianopia (UHEM)	1. Partial loss of vision and unaware of the loss 2. Orbits and optic nerve intact 3. Optic pathways damaged unilaterally 4. Acknowledges objective evidence of visual loss when presented to them 5. May not "notice" restricted vision in everyday life	Damage to visual projection areas can be correlated with parietal, temporal, and/or occipital lesions unilaterally. There is no evidence of bilateral occipital damage and no evidence of an acute confusional state.

limited to part of their visual field, but directly attributed to a brain lesion. They do not show widespread cognitive impairment. They are unaware of their visual loss until it is demonstrated to them. Unlike true anosognostic patients, they acknowledge and remember their visual loss when it is demonstrated to them. In everyday life they may not be consciously aware of visual impairments, but they seem to automatically accommodate for those impairments. This third group may deny their hemianopia when they are in the acute stage, and obviously disoriented or confused. They may also report no visual defects if they have severe unilateral neglect. Table 20.1 attempts to summarize these three groups of patients.

Anton's Syndrome in Children

Two case reports of Anton's syndrome in children have appeared. Trifiletti, Syed, Hayes-Rosen, Parano, and Pavone (2007) reported on a 6-year-old boy who was diagnosed with early-stage cerebral adrenoleukodystrophy. The child initially presented with academic difficulties, but it was noted that he had abnormal eye movements and progressive difficulties with his gait. As the disease progressed, his vision worsened. Visual acuity was measured at less than 20/200, even with correction. The child repeatedly stated that there was nothing wrong with his vision. He was described as "jocular" and unconcerned. An MRI of the brain "confirmed the presence of a leukodystrophy, with involvement of the geniculate body and brainstem . . ." (p. 12). An MRI scan also revealed extreme deep white matter signal changes in parietal and occipital lobes bilaterally. Eventually, the child lost complete vision with no evidence of light perception. He remained unaware of his visual loss.

Yilmazlar et al. (2003) reported cortical blindness and unawareness of that blindness in a 13-year-old boy following TBI. A CT scan of the brain "revealed bilateral occipital epidural hematomas" (p. 157). Evacuation of the hematoma resulted in the reversal of the blindness and associated anosognosia.

These two case studies suggest that anosognosia can exist in children. In both cases, their unawareness could not be explained on the basis of cognitive impairment. In both cases there was unconcern for their clinical condition. In both cases there was evidence of bilateral occipital lobe involvement.

Why Have Group Studies Not Appeared on Anton's Syndrome?

Despite the several case reports that have appeared in the literature over the last 20 years, no group studies on this phenomenon could be located. This most likely is due to the fact that Anton's syndrome is indeed a rare condition. Even in large neurological settings, accumulating a number of cases over a short period of time has proven to be problematic. Yet it is important to study these patients as a group and to monitor their changes or lack of changes over an extended period of time. Perhaps in the future group studies that try to understand the underlying similarities and differences in patients who show true Anton's syndrome versus unawareness of other types of visual impairments will appear.

A Comment on the Neuroanatomical Substrates of Blindsight versus Anton's Syndrome

The phenomenon of blindsight (as described by Weiskrantz, 1997) in some ways is a mirror image of Anton's syndrome. In this case, the patient has limited preserved vision in a hemianopic field, even though the patient is unaware of that preserved vision. Blumenfeld (2002) states, "Blindsight apparently depends on information transmitted to association cortex by extrageniculate visual pathways . . . bypassing the lateral geniculate nucleus and primary visual cortex. Some studies have also demonstrated small islands of preserved vision in the blind hemifield measuring only a few minutes of degree that are not able to support conscious vision but may influence behavior" (p. 855). The implication of these statements is that the cortex is necessary for conscious awareness. Some "threshold" or minimal amount of cortical integrity must be present in order for conscious experience to emerge when a sensory input is delivered to primary visual cortex.

When there are bilateral lesions that are "nearly symmetrical" in primary visual cortical or association areas, there may not be an "adequate amount" of cortical representation to allow consciousness to emerge. When only one hemisphere is affected, then the so-called unaffected hemisphere may detect or recognize visual loss that the damaged or affected hemisphere cannot. This may be why nonconfused individuals often do not show true anosognosia for hemianopia.

David, Owen, and Förstl (1993) summarize post-mortem findings that were initially described by Anton in one of his patients. The findings are significant for the following words: ". . . no severe atrophy . . . cystic necrosis primarily affecting white matter of the left and right occipital lobes" (p. 269). David et al. (1993) correctly point out that disruption of white matter tracks in this region may indirectly affect other brain regions in nonobservable ways. Further neuropathological studies are needed to precisely define the type and extent of cortical and possible subcortical involvement that may be necessary to produce Anton's syndrome. The case studies summarized in this chapter, however, highlight neuroradiographic and EEG correlates of bilateral occipital involvement in true Anton's syndrome. The primary visual cortex (Area 17) and the visual association cortices (Areas 18 and 19) appear to be adversely affected in Anton's syndrome. Whether other brain areas are also necessary to produce this classic syndrome awaits further investigation.

Summary

Limited research has appeared on Anton's syndrome since it was first described in the late 1800s. A recent review of the literature provides ample case studies replicating Anton's early observations. No experimental studies could be identified that provide insight as to the precise mechanism responsible for this form of anosognosia. Case studies do report, however, the phenomenon in children, something frequently not observed in other forms of anosognosia. Some confusion exists in the literature as to what is a true Anton's syndrome versus what has been described as an "Anton-like" syndrome. The study of these patients, however, and those who have partial loss of vision but who are aware of it, strongly supports Anton's earlier observations and impressions. For anosognosia to exist, the brain lesion must occur in a region known to be important for that function. In addition, bilateral cortical lesions that are "almost symmetrical" in nature may be necessary for some syndromes of ano-sognosia. Perhaps recovery of function is seen when either both areas return to normal physiological activity, or the so-called unaffected hemisphere actually regains normal physiological activity, thereby allowing the patient to discover or recognize that indeed an impairment in neurological or neuropsychological function exists.

Acknowledgments

We are grateful to Anthony S. David, M.D. for his helpful review of an earlier version of this chapter.

References

Abdulqawi, R., Ashawesh, K., & Ahmad, S. (2008). Medical image. Anton's syndrome secondary to cerebral vasculitis. *New Zealand Medical Journal, 121*, 89–90.

Abutalebi, J., Arcari, C., Rocca, M. A., Rossi, P., Comola, M., Comi, G. C., Rovaris, M., & Filippi, M. (2007). Anton's syndrome following callosal disconnection. *Behavioural Neurology, 18*, 183–186.

Alemdar, M., Iseri, P., Selekler, M., Budak, F., Demirci, A., & Komsuoglu, S. S. (2007). MELAS presented with status epilepticus and Anton-Babinski syndrome; Value of ADC mapping in MELAS. *The Journal of Neuropsychiatry and Clinical Neurosciences, 19*, 482–483.

Anton, G. (1898). Ueber Herderkrankungen des Gehirnes, welche von Patienten selbst nicht wahrgenommen warden. *Wiener Klinische Wochenschrift, 11*, 227–229.

Argenta, P. A., & Morgan, M. A. (1998). Cortical blindness and Anton syndrome in a patient with obstetric hemorrhage. *Obstetrics and Gynecology, 91*, 810–812.

Bauer, R. M. & Demery, J. A. (2003). *Agnosia*. In K. M. Heilman & E. Valenstein (Eds.), *Clinical Neuropsychology* (4th edition). New York: Oxford University Press.

Bergman, P. S. (1957). Cerebral blindness: An analysis of twelve cases with a special reference to the electroencephalogram and patterns of recovery. *Archives of Neurology and Psychiatry, 78*, 568–584.

Bisiach, E., & Geminiani, G. (1991). Anosognosia related to hemiplegia and hemianopia. In G. P. Prigatano & R. L. Schacter (Eds.), *Awareness of deficit after brain injury: Clinical and theoretical issues* (pp. 17–39). New York: Oxford University Press.

Bisiach, E., Vallar, G., Perani, D., Papagno, C. & Berti, A. (1986). Unawareness of disease following lesions of the right hemisphere: Anosognosia for hemiplegia and anosognosia for hemianopia. *Neuropsychologia, 24*(4), 471–482.

Blumenfeld, H. (2002). *Neuroanatomy through clinical cases*. Sunderland, MA: Sinauer Associates, Inc.

Brust, J. C. M., & Behrens, M. M. (1977). "Release hallucinations" as the major symptom of posterior cerebral artery occlusion: A report of two cases. *Annals of Neurology, 2*, 432–436.

Burns, B. T., Katner, H. P., Couch, D. A., Smith, M. U., Bhutta, T., & Stephens, J. (1997). Atypical presentations of progressive multifocal leukoencephalopathy (PML): Aseptic meningitis and Anton's syndrome. *AIDS Patient Care and STDS, 11*, 71–75.

Cogan, D. G. (1973). Visual hallucinations as release phenomena. *Graefe's Archive for Clinical and Experimental Ophthalmology, 188*(2), 139–150.

Cusumano, J. V., Fletcher, J. W., & Patel, B. K. (1981). Scintigraphic appearance of Anton's syndrome. *Journal of the American Medical Association, 245*, 1248–1249.

David, A., Owen, A. M., & Forstl, H. (1993). An annotated summary and translation of "on the self-awareness of focal brain diseases by the patient in cortical blindness and cortical deafness" by Gabriel Anton. *Cognitive Neuropsychology, 10*, 263–272.

Davis, G. P., Sewell, R. A., Levy, B., Price, B. H., & Cunningham, M. G. (2009). An atypical presentation of Anton syndrome in a patient with preserved cognition despite multiple cerebral infarcts: A case report. *CNS Spectrums, 14*, 15–18.

Dejerine, J. J., & Vialet, N. (1893). Sur un cas de cécité corticale. *Comptes Rendus Hebdomadaire des Séances et Mémoires de la Société de Biolgoié, 11*, 983.

Della Sala, S., & Spinnler, H. (1988). Anton's (-Redlich-Babinski's) syndrome associated with Dide-Botcazo's syndrome: A case report of denial of cortical blindness and amnesia. *Schweizer Archiv für Neurologie und Psychiatrie, 139*, 5–15.

Flint, A. C., Loh, J. P., & Brust, J. C. (2005). Vivid visual hallucinations from occipital lobe infarction. *Neurology, 65*(5), 756.

Förstl. H., Owen, A. M., & David. A. S. (1993). Gabriel Anton and "Anton's symptom" On focal diseases of the brain which are not perceived by the patient (1898). *Neuropsychiatry, Neuropsychology, and Behavioral Neurology, 6*(1), 1–8.

Galetović, D., Karlica, D., Bojić, L., & Znaor, L. (2005). Bilateral cortical blindness— Anton syndrome: Case report. *Collegium Antropologicum, 29*, 145–147.

Goodale, M. A., & Milner, A. D. (2004). *Sight unseen: An exploration of conscious and unconscious vision.* Oxford, England: Oxford University Press.

Hécaen, H., & Albert, M. L. (1978). *Human neuropsychology.* New York: John Wiley & Sons.

Jaeckle, K. A. (1982). Cerebrospinal fluid cytomorphology in systemic lupus erythematosus with Anton's syndrome. *Acta Cytologica, 26*, 532–536.

Kolb, B. (1990). Recovery from occipital stroke: A self-report and an inquiry into visual processes. *Canadian Journal of Psychology, 44*, 130–147.

Krovvidi, H., & Bhattacharjee, A. (2008). Anton's syndrome in a patient with type-2 heparin-induced thrombocytopaenia (HIT). *Acta Anaesthesiological Scandinavica, 52*, 1029–1030.

Lance, J. W. (1976). Simple formed hallucinations confined to the area of a specific visual field defect. *Brain, 99*(4), 719–734.

McDaniel, K. D. & McDaniel, L. D. (1991). Anton's syndrome in a patient with posttraumatic optic neuropathy and bifrontal contusions. *Archives of Neurology, 48*, 101–105.

Misra, M., Rath, S., & Mohanty, A. B. (1989). Anton syndrome and cortical blindness due to bilateral occipital infarction. *Indian Journal of Ophthalmology, 37*, 196.

Pedersen, P. M., Henrik, S. J., Nakayama, H., Raaschou, H. O., & Olsen, T. S. (1996). Frequency, determinants, and consequences of anosognosia in acute stroke. *Journal of Neurological Rehabilitation, 10*(4), 243–250.

Rizzolatti, G., & Matelli, M. (2003). Two different streams from the dorsal visual system: Anatomy and functions. *Experimental Brain Research, 153*(2), 146–157.

Roos, K. L., Tuite, P. J., Below, M. E., & Pascuzzi, R. M. (1990). Reversible cortical blindness (Anton's syndrome) associated with bilateral occipital EEG abnormalities. *Clinical Electroencephalography, 21*, 104–109.

Schofield, T. M., & Leff, A. P. (2009). Rehabilitation of hemianopia. *Current Opinion in Neurology, 22*, 36–40.

Shapiro, K., Hillstrom, A. P., & Husain, M. (2002). Control of visuotemporal attention by inferior parietal and superior temporal cortex. *Current Biology, 12*, 1320–1325.

Silverberg, S., & Wilansky, D. L. (1978). Scintigram in cortical blindness (Anton's syndrome). *Clinical Nuclear Medicine, 3*, 349–350.

Suzuki, K., Endo, M., Yamadori, A., & Fujii, T. (1997). Hemispatial neglect in the visual hallucination of a patient with Anton's syndrome. *European Neurology, 37*, 63–64.

Swartz, B. E., & Brust, J. C. (1984). Anton's syndrome accompanying withdrawal hallucinosis in a blind alcoholic. *Neurology, 34*, 969–973.

Trifiletti, R. R., Syed, E. H., Hayes-Rosen, C., Parano, E., & Pavone, P. (2007). Anton-Babinski syndrome in a child with early-stage adrenoleukodystrophy. *European Journal of Neurology, 14*, e11–12.

Verslegers, W., De Deyn, P. P., Saerens, J., Marien, P., Appel, B., Pickut, B. A., & Lowenthal, A. (1991). Slow progressive bilateral posterior artery infarction presenting as agitated delirium, complicated with Anton's syndrome. *European Neurology, 31*, 216–219.

von Monakow, C. (1897). *Gehirnpathologie*. Vienna: Nothnagel.

Welman, A. J. (1969). Right-sided unilateral visual spatial agnosia, asomatognosia and anosognosia with left hemisphere lesions. *Brain, 92*, 571–580.

Weiskrantz, L. (1997). *Consciousness Lost and Found: Neuropsychological exploration*. New York: Oxford University Press.

Wessling, H., Simosono, C. L., Escosa-Bagé, M., & de Las Heras-Echeverría, P. (2006). Anton's syndrome due to a giant anterior fossa meningioma. The problem of routine use of advanced diagnostic imaging in psychiatric care. *Acta Neurochirurgica (Wien), 148*, 673–675.

Yilmazlar, S., Taskapilioglu, O., & Aksoy, K. (2003). Transient Anton's syndrome: A presenting feature of acute epidural hematoma at the confluens sinuum. *Pediatric Neurosurgery, 38*, 156–159.

Zhang, X., Kedar, S., Lynn, M. J., Newman, N. J., & Biousse, V. (2006). Natural history of homonymous hemianopia. *Neurology, 66*, 901–905.

VIII

Advances in the Study of Anosognosia

21

A Progress Report on the Study of Anosognosia

George P. Prigatano

Progress in the scientific understanding of anosognosia has been steady, but slow. The study of anosognosia, however, has never been boring. The phenomenon is inherently interesting to us as human beings because it reflects a disturbance in brain function that is crucial for our survival and quality of life. Understanding this phenomenon holds much promise for revealing important insights into the organizational components of brain activity that allow human consciousness and self-awareness to emerge.

In retrospect, the seminal observations of Anton (1898) and Babinski (1914) continue to dominate our study of anosognosia. More recently, the findings of Bisiach et al. (1986) greatly influenced this area of study by demonstrating that one could disassociate anosognosia for hemiplegia (AHP) from anosognosia for hemianopia in the same patient. Later investigators further showed one could separate AHP from neglect (Berti et al., 2005) and AHP from aphasia (Breier et al., 1995). These important clinical observations suggested the possibility that conscious awareness of a function, or lack of it, may be organized according to a modularity principle (Bisiach & Geminiani, 1991). It brought to light an important problem for neurologists and neuropsychologists. How is it that we can be aware of ourselves and conscious of our environment and not aware of a dramatic loss of a specific neurological/neuropsychological function? Somehow the organizational activities of the brain allow for both a generalized, integrated conscious awareness of the self while still at the same time relying on a basic modular organizational principle by which awareness of different aspects of the self are made possible.

This book has been dedicated to summarizing the advances that have occurred in the study of anosognosia over the last 20 years, and placing those advances into a historically meaningful context. This progress report reflects my own interpretation of progress that has been made. The other clinicians and investigators who have written chapters in this book may well have emphasized different observations and come to different conclusions. It should be clear that the opinions expressed are my own and are not necessarily endorsed by any of the preceding authors. My comments will attempt to address several of the questions raised in Chapter 1. Those questions not addressed will be considered in the next chapter.

Advances in Clinical Observations

Table 21.1 lists several advances in clinical observations that have relevance to the study of anosognosia and ultimately rehabilitation of patients who show anosognosia. First, two case studies have reported the presence of Anton's

Table 21.1 Advances in Clinical Observations

- Anton's syndrome has been reported in school-age children (see Chapter 20, this volume).
  Implication: Anosognosia is not a purely "adult" disorder. It can occur in the developing brain.
- Anton's syndrome is potentially reversible with appropriate medical treatment (see Chapter 20, this volume).
- The caloric vestibular stimulation (CVS) effect of briefly abolishing anosognosia for hemiplegia (AHP), hemi-neglect (N), and hemi-anesthesia is readily seen with left ear stimulation in right brain–damaged subjects, but not with right ear stimulation in left brain–damaged patients.
  Implication: The right (nondominant) cerebral hemisphere has a special role to play in body representation or body schema (see Chapter 2, this volume).
- The CVS effect observed in a patient with severe left neglect and anosognosia for hemiplegia (Ramachandran, 1994) suggests that the patient may have had implicit knowledge of her impairments during the time she verbally denied her hemiplegia.
  Implication: This suggests that in a given patient there may be a dissociation between implicit versus explicit awareness of an impaired neurological function (for further discussion of this important point, see Chapter 17, this volume).
- While AHP and N are frequently seen together in most patients following right cerebral hemisphere stroke, they can be "disassociated" in rare cases (Berti et al., 2005; see Chapter 2, this volume).
  Implication: Further evidence for the "modularity" of human impaired awareness of different neurological disturbances.
- Chronic anosognosia for hemiplegia after severe traumatic brain injury (TBI) in which bilateral cerebral damage is documented can be briefly overcome by behavioral manipulations, but it is resistant to permanent improvement (Cocchini et al., 2002).
  Implication: Permanence of AHP may depend on bilateral brain dysfunction in regions that support awareness of motor control. In addition, multiple neuropsychological disturbances (such as neglect and profound memory impairment) may interfere with recovery (see Chapters 12 and 17, this volume).
- The clinical picture of recovery appears different for different patients with AHP (see Chapter 17, this volume).
  Implication: Understanding mechanisms of change (recovery) in individual patients may provide insight into mechanisms responsible for these "overlapping" disturbances associated with AHP.

---

syndrome in school-age children. One study also suggests impaired self awareness in school age children with severe TBI (see Prigatano, Chapter 12, this volume). These observations suggest that anosognosia is not a purely "adult" disorder. It can exist in children and may well impact their overall recovery. Second, with timely medical treatment, Anton's syndrome has been shown to be potentially reversible in some patients. This may be true for other forms of anosognosia.

A third finding is that the caloric vestibular stimulation (CVS) effect is mainly observed when cold water is placed in the left ear of right brain–damaged patients who show AHP, hemi-neglect, and hemi-anesthesia. Injecting cold water in the right ear of left brain–damaged patients who show hemi-anesthesia does not produce such dramatic effects. The implication of this clinical observation is that the right hemisphere appears to play a special role in body representation or body schema. As Critchley (1953) noted AHP may reflect an underlying disorder of body schema. It may be for this reason that right hemisphere lesions have been commonly implicated in AHP.

A fourth clinical observation was made by Ramachandran (1994), which is of relevance for future studies. He presents an interesting case of an elderly lady who, after suffering a right hemisphere stroke, showed a left neglect and AHP. Following caloric stimulation of the left ear, the patient was able to report that she was aware of her hemiplegia/hemiparesis before the stimulation effect occurred. That is, during the time in which she verbally or explicitly denied any impairment in her motor functioning, she now reports she did have a sense that she could not move her left arm. This clinical observation suggests that there may be different neural networks associated with implicit versus explicit (i.e., verbally reported conscious) awareness in anosognostic patients (see Vocat & Vuilleumier, Chapter 17, this volume). Further case studies are necessary to support this rather interesting and intriguing hypothesis.

A fifth observation is that AHP and neglect in fact can be separated (Berti et al., 2005), as noted above. While these two phenomena are very frequently observed together (see Pedersen, Jorgensen, Nakayama, Raaschou, & Olsen, 1996), Berti et al. (2005) report a single patient who was anosognostic for hemiplegia but did not show neglect. Understanding the neuroanatomical correlates of these two phenomena and where they overlap and do not overlap may provide important insights as to brain regions involved in AHP.

A sixth clinical observation has relevance to the field of rehabilitation. Cocchini, Beschin, and Della Sala (2002) provided an informative case study of a young man who showed persistent anosognosia for hemiplegia and neglect several years post severe traumatic brain injury. This patient had bilateral cerebral dysfunction. While the investigators were able to overcome the patient's unawareness for his hemiplegia for a brief period of time, the behavioral manipulations did not result in any persistent improvement in his awareness. The authors provide a theoretical explanation for this phenomenon, which includes the notion that multiple neuropsychological deficits, including neglect and severe memory loss, may perpetuate the existence of AHP. While not specifically a focus of their discussion, their case study also suggests that when there is bilateral cerebral dysfunction in homologous areas of both sides of the brain underlying a certain function, recovery from anosognosia may be difficult, if not impossible. A similar conclusion can be drawn from studies of adults and children who demonstrate Anton's syndrome.

A seventh clinical observation, which is not new, but needs to be repeated, is that recovery patterns following AHP may be different across patients (Vocat & Vuilleumier, Chapter 17, this volume). Understanding how various symptoms resolve and over what time course following AHP may give insights into the various mechanisms responsible for AHP and associated disorders.

Advances in Empirical Findings

Many new empirical findings have been reported on anosognosia and impairment in self-awareness (ISA) over the last 20 years. Table 21.2 lists a few of the more recent findings that appear to hold considerable theoretical importance. The preceding chapters document those advances in more detail.

It has been recognized that the anatomical correlates of AHP typically involve frontal-parietal and frontal-temporal-parietal cortices. There is also growing evidence that many of these patients have subcortical lesions (see Pia et al., 2004). More recent studies, however, have argued for the special role of the dorsal prefrontal cortex of the right hemisphere and the right insular cortex. The right insular cortex has been shown to play an important role in subjective feeling states (see Craig, Chapter 4, this volume) and has been repeatedly found to be adversely affected in patients with AHP (see Bottini et al., Chapter 2; Karnath & Baier, Chapter 3; and Vocat & Vuilleumier, Chapter 17, this volume). Thus, a new empirical finding is that the insular cortex as well as the dorsal premotor cortex may be especially important in AHP and related phenomena.

While AHP has been repeatedly shown to relate to large lesions of the right hemisphere, particularly secondary to a disruption of blood flow from the right middle cerebral artery (see Bottini et al., Chapter 2; Karnath & Baier, Chapter 3; and Vocat & Vuilleumier, Chapter 17, this volume), recent research suggests that there may be different anatomical correlates of AHP during the very acute stages in contrast to subacute and post-acute stages (see Vocat & Vuilleumier, Chapter 17, this volume). This suggests that when the patient is studied, the symptoms that are present at that time may relate to different neuroimaging findings, and therefore, imply different neuroanatomical correlates/mechanisms.

Despite these advances, however, no single anatomical location or neuropsychological mechanism has been identified to account for AHP in all patients (see Heilman & Harciarek, Chapter 5, this volume). What can be said, however, is

Table 21.2 Advances in Empirical Findings

- Anatomical correlates of anosognosia for hemiplegia (AHP) have been linked to lesions involving the frontal-parietal or frontal-temporal-parietal cortices with involvement of subcortical structures (e.g., thalamus and/or basal ganglia) of the right hemisphere (see Pia et al., 2004, and Chapter 2, this volume).
- Recent studies have now argued that the right dorsal premotor cortex and insula may be especially important in these phenomena, which was not previously recognized (see Chapters 2, 3, 4, and 17, this volume).
- Recent neuroimaging findings suggest that the anatomical correlates of AHP may change with the passage of time since lesion onset (see Chapter 17, this volume).
- No single anatomical location or neuropsychological mechanism has been identified to account for AHP in all patients (see Chapter 5, this volume).
- Large lesions of the right cerebral hemisphere are frequently observed in AHP. A parallel finding is that persistent impaired self-awareness (ISA) after traumatic brain injury (TBI) is often associated with severe injuries in which there is bilateral cerebral dysfunction involving large areas of the frontal and temporal regions (see Chapter 12, this volume).
- Hysterical sensorimotor loss correlates with hypometabolic activity in subcortical regions, particularly the thalamus and basal ganglia, but not the cortex (see Chapter 17, this volume).
- ISA in dementia of the Alzheimer's type (Chapter 10, this volume), mild cognitive impairment (Chapter 18, this volume), and severe TBI (see Chapters 12 and 18, this volume) have been repeatedly associated with right frontal (typically dorsal) cortical lesions.
- "Milder" forms of ISA have been now reported in a wide range of patient groups, including Huntington's disease, nondemented, nondepressed Parkinson patients, patients with mild cognitive impairment, TBI, dementia of the Alzheimer's type, and frontal temporal dementia.
- Anosognosia for motor and language deficits has been identified in left hemisphere–damaged patients (see Chapter 7, this volume).

---

that large lesions within a given hemisphere or bilateral cerebral dysfunction is often associated with some form of anosognosia.

An additional important observation is that hysterical sensorimotor loss has been correlated with functional neuroimaging changes at the level of the thalamus and basal ganglia versus at the level of the cortex (see Vocat & Vuilleumier, Chapter 17, this volume). While previous studies suggest that post-acute anosognosia is correlated with cortical dysfunction (including the "fifth cortical lobe," i.e., the insula), hysterical sensorimotor loss has been correlated with subcortical changes. A future area of inquiry should explore the possibility that post-acute anosognosia is primarily a "cortical disorder," whereas hysterical sensorimotor loss may be a functional disturbance at the subcortical level.

A sixth empirical finding is that it has been repeatedly suggested that disruption of the right frontal (typically dorsal) cortex is associated with ISA in various patient groups. This has been reported in patients with dementia of the

Alzheimer's type (Starkstein & Power, Chapter 10, this volume), mild cognitive impairment (Johnson & Ries, Chapter 18, this volume), and in cases of severe traumatic brain injury (Prigatano, Chapter 12; Johnson & Ries, Chapter 18, this volume).

As several chapters of this textbook document, "milder" forms of anosognosia may be seen in diverse patient groups, including those who have Huntington's disease (Tranel et al., Chapter 8, this volume), nondemented Parkinson's disease (Prigatano et al., Chapter 9, this volume), TBI (Prigatano, Chapter 12, this volume), and schizophrenia (Gilleen et al., Chapter 13, this volume). Finally, with the advent of new behavioral methodology, one can now clearly demonstrate anosognosia of aphasia and motor impairments in left hemisphere stroke patients (Cocchini & Della Sala, Chapter 7, this volume).

Advances in Methodology

Table 21.3 lists several advances in the behavioral and/or clinical assessment of patients with anosognosia or ISA. Table 21.4 lists advances that have occurred primarily in the field of neuroimaging. Innovative questions or tasks have been presented to anosognostic patients to determine whether there is implicit awareness of their deficits, even though the patient may verbally explicitly "deny" any hemiparesis. Ramachandran (1994), for example, asked patients if they would

Table 21.3 Advances in Methodology: Behavioral/Clinical

- Novel tasks for anosognosia for hemiplegia (AHP) patients have been developed to detect possible implicit awareness of hemiplegia when there is verbal explicit "denial" of the hemiparesis (e.g., will the patient choose to conduct a bimanual task if the reward is greater than carrying out a unimanual task; Ramachandran, 1994).
- AHP patients are asked to carry out motor tasks with the "unaffected" hand to detect if there is evidence of bilateral cerebral dysfunction despite neuroimaging findings (Prigatano et al., in preparation).
- Assessing AHP in aphasic patients via the use of a visual analog test (Chapter 7, this volume).
- Using self versus other reports on a variety of questionnaires, impaired self-awareness (ISA) of affective changes following brain disorders can now be identified (see Chapters 14 and 16, this volume).
- Using structured interviews and questionnaire methods, ISA for mental illness can be identified in various neuropsychiatric disorders, including schizophrenia (see Chapter 13, this volume).
- Self-reports of the capacity to carry out a variety of motor tasks (walking, standing, hand-finger movements) in an effort to copy what an examiner has just performed help reveal subtle signs of ISA in patient groups thought not to show anosognosia for their motor deficits (see Chapter 9, this volume).

Table 21.4 Advances in Methodology: Medical and Neuroimaging

- Use of the Wada procedure to detect awareness of hemiplegia and aphasia following right versus left brain anesthesia (see Chapter 5, this volume)
- Use of standard magnetic resonance imaging (MRI) scans of the brain to identify neuroimaging (i.e., anatomical) correlates of anosognosia for hemiplegia (AHP) at different time frames (see Chapters 2, 3, and 17, this volume)
- Use of voxelwise lesion-behavioral mapping (VLBM) techniques with MRI scans of the brain to more precisely identify neuroanatomical correlates of AHP (see Chapter 3, this volume)
- Use of positron emission tomography (PET) to identify neural substrates of anosognosia of cognitive impairment in Alzheimer's disease (see Chapter 10, this volume)
- Use of single photon emission computerized tomography (SPECT) to detect decreases in regional cerebral blood flow in patients with hysterical sensorimotor loss (see Chapter 17, this volume) and in Anton's syndrome (see Chapter 20, this volume)
- Use of fMRI to study correlates of "normal" self-reflective thought and impaired self-awareness (ISA) in patients with mild cognitive impairment as well as severe traumatic brain injury (TBI) (see Chapter 18, this volume)

prefer to carry out a task that typically involved bimanual responses versus unimanual tasks that required a single hand to carry out the task. The rewards were greater for carrying out the bimanual task and the goal was to determine whether with such rewards the patient would still prefer to carry out a unimodal task, suggesting that at some level they have awareness of their motor limitations. This type of behavioral investigation approaches an important theoretical issue in the study of anosognosia. Further behavioral methodology needs to be developed to test both the explicit and implicit awareness that may exist in patients at different stages of their recovery following AHP and other related disorders.

A second behavioral advance has been to measure motor skills in the so-called unaffected hand in AHP patients (Prigatano et al., in preparation). Patients who show anosognosia for left hemiplegia may, in fact, show impaired motor performance in the so-called unaffected hand (Prigatano et al., in preparation; also see Prigatano & Altman, 1990). These behavioral measures suggest that there may, in fact, be bilateral cerebral dysfunction, even when neuroimaging only identifies a lesion in a single hemisphere. One can demonstrate that there may be hypometabolic activity in both cerebral hemispheres, even though standard computed tomography (CT) or magnetic resonance imaging (MRI) may show a stroke in one hemisphere. This has been specifically reported in one case of Anton's syndrome (see Prigatano & Wolf, Chapter 20, this volume).

As noted earlier, aphasic patients are now able to answer questions concerning their language and motor abilities based on new behavioral methodology. Cocchini and Della Sala (Chapter 7, this volume) have introduced an innovative visual analog test to assess awareness of motor and language deficits in aphasic patients. This is an important breakthrough and should allow for more systematic assessment of AHP in aphasic patients.

The development of numerous self-report questionnaires has allowed for the assessment of ISA for a wide variety of cognitive dysfunctions, which have been summarized by Orfei and colleagues (Chapter 19, this volume). This methodology has also allowed us to assess possible unawareness of changes in personality or the individual's affective state (Rankin, Chapter 14; Jorge, Chapter 16, this volume). The study of anosognosia suggests that it can exist for cognitive, perceptual, motor, and affective disturbances.

Behavioral methodologies have emphasized the importance of using multiple approaches in order to obtain reliable estimates of ISA, particularly in complicated disorders such as schizophrenia (Gilleen et al., Chapter 13, this volume). No single behavioral methodology has yet achieved universal acceptance.

An additional behavioral approach has been to ask patients to mimic a series of motor tasks that are first conducted by the examiner. The patient is then asked to immediately make judgments about whether he or she had any difficulty performing the motor tasks. This type of methodology may help reveal subtle ISA for motor deficits in Parkinson's disease patients (Prigatano et al., Chapter 9, this volume).

While innovative behavioral assessments have occurred, the most dramatic changes in methodology have appeared in the field of neuroimaging. These technological advances have greatly improved our understanding of possible neuroanatomical correlates of AHP and other forms of anosognosia. As Table 21.4 illustrates, over the last 20 years, standard MRI scans have been repeatedly used to correlate AHP with specific lesion locations and at different times during the recovery course. The new methodology using voxelwise lesion-behavior mapping has led to greater precision in correlating lesion location with AHP. Metabolic imaging techniques (SPECT and PET) also have helped us better understand the correlates of Anton's syndrome, as well as ISA in Alzheimer's disease patients, and in patients with hysterical sensorimotor loss. For example, Salmon and colleagues' (2006) research shows bilateral temporoparietal hypometabolic changes in patients with dementia of the Alzheimer's type who have poor self-awareness of their cognitive limitations when compared to relative's reports. Bilateral frontal hypometabolic suppression was observed when the patient made self-reflective statements regarding his or her strengths and limitations. Finally, the use of fMRI has provided interesting findings regarding brain structures that are involved in normal self-reflective thought, as well as areas that seem to be activated when the patient shows good versus poor awareness of cognitive or behavioral limitations (see Johnson & Ries, Chapter 18, this volume).

The studies initiated by Heilman and colleagues (Chapter 5, this volume) also utilize the Wada procedure to systematically assess the role of right versus left cerebral hemisphere dysfunction in anosognosia for hemiplegia versus aphasia.

Table 21.5 Advances in New Models/Hypotheses

- Anosognosia is a multifaceted phenomenon that may be caused by multiple component dysfunction (see Chapter 17, this volume). Therefore, several models/ predictions have appeared to explain anosognosia for hemiplegia (AHP) (see Chapters 2, 3, 5, and 17, this volume). No single model, however, has been universally accepted.
- The insular cortex (the fifth lobe) plays a crucial role in the phenomenon of subjective awareness (see Chapter 4, this volume).
- Damage to the insular cortex plays a more important role in AHP than had been previously recognized (see Chapter 3, this volume).
- The neuroanatomical (i.e., neuroimaging) and neuropsychological correlates of AHP change with time (see Chapter 17, this volume).
- The patient with anosognosia may be oriented and communicate in a logical manner, but still be unable to evaluate the evidence that a neurological or neuropsychological function has been severely compromised.
- The neuroanatomical (and, therefore, neurological and neuropsychological) mechanisms responsible for AHP are different than what is observed in hysterical sensorimotor loss (see Chapter 17, this volume).
- Anosodiaphoria, a common feature of AHP, may also be due to several mechanisms, but damage to the right frontal lobe may be an important neural correlate of this disturbance (see Chapter 5, this volume).
- A common, if not crucial feature of AHP is a disturbed sense of limb ownership (see Chapter 3, this volume). Damage to the insular cortex may be especially important in this phenomenon (see Chapter 3, this volume), but several studies have also implicated the importance of the parietal cortex in producing this phenomenon (Critchley, 1953; Ramachandran, 1994).
- Psychological denial clearly cannot explain AHP (see Chapters 5 and 17, this volume).
- Persistent anosognosia for a lost neurological or neuropsychological function may be due to bilateral, nearly asymmetrical lesions underlying that functional impairment. A corollary of this hypothesis is that recovery from anosognosia will be associated not only with a return to normal function in temporarily disturbed brain areas producing the syndrome (for example, reversal of Anton's syndrome, Chapter 20, this volume), but it may well show improvement in the so-called nonlesioned or "unaffected" hemisphere.
- The neurocircuits involved in self-reflective thought may differ from those involved in accurate self-reporting (awareness) of how one is functioning in different domains.

Advances in New Models/Hypotheses

Anosognosia is ultimately a disturbance in the subjective experience of one's self caused by a brain disorder. Subjective experience or awareness can be altered for many reasons. Thus, there is not a single set of neurological or neuropsychological "causes" that will always produce anosognosia in its various forms. This being said, the study of anosognosia has revealed several interesting findings that lead to different theoretical perspectives.

While Babinski (1914) introduced the term *anosognosia* to describe a disturbance of subjective awareness of hemiplegia following stroke, Anton's (1898) early reports help explain from an empirical perspective the cause of anosognosia. As reviewed in the previous chapter, Anton (1898) emphasized that a loss of neurological (and neuropsychological) function may not be (subjectively) perceived (or experienced) by the person if the brain lesions occur in a region known to be important for that function (e.g., occipital lobe for vision, temporal lobe for hearing, etc.). For anosognosia to occur when the patient is completely blind, bilateral cortical lesions that are "almost symmetrical" need to be present.

A key feature of anosognosia is that the patient "disregards or discounts any objective evidence that they have lost their functional capacity." This "discounting of the evidence" must occur in a patient who *appears* to have the capacity to objectively evaluate the evidence (i.e., they are not demented or show severe cognitive impairment).

These are the necessary conditions for the diagnosis of anosognosia. If one utilizes this basic model, it is easy to see why debates continue to emerge regarding the causes of AHP. The brain anatomy and physiology that allow for the initiation of a motor response, the actual performance of the motor act, the monitoring and control of the motor act while it is being performed, and the recognition that the "goal" of the act has or has not been achieved are not fully understood (Frith, Blakemore, & Wolpert, 2000). Thus, the first condition: the brain lesion(s) must be in an area known to be important for that function cannot be specified for AHP. With more complicated neuropsychological functions such as memory or social judgment, the underlying brain regions are much less understood. It is for this reason that by simply looking at an MRI scan of the brain, one cannot predict whether anosognosia will or will not be present for a given individual. Also, the organization of the higher integrative functions may show some variability across individuals, making the task even more difficult.

The patient's discounting of the evidence while apparently having the capacity to evaluate the evidence forms a crucial problem for the study of anosognosia. Could it be that the patient actually does not have the underlying brain capacity to evaluate the evidence? This is essentially the model of Bisiach, Vallar, Perani, Papagno, and Berti (1986). While the patient is not so cognitively impaired that they cannot communicate or follow a logical argument, the actual subcomponents of a functional system that allow for conscious awareness to emerge are, by their nature, compromised. Thus, the clinician gets the false impression that the patient can actually evaluate the evidence. In reality, they may not be able to evaluate the evidence, because the functional representation of a given ability has been seriously compromised.

A failure to consider this possibility has led to the debate as to whether the "discounting of the evidence" is motivated (i.e., a form of psychological denial) or represents a disturbance of that neurological or neuropsychological function at its highest levels (Bisiach et al., 1986; Bisiach & Geminiani, 1991). The creative work of Vocat and Vuilleumier (Chapter 17, this volume) continues to suggest that the personality of the patient and his or her emotional state cannot explain AHP.

Yet case reports continue to surface that do suggest that at some level denial may, in fact, be present for some patients who show AHP (Ramachandran, 1994).

Karnath and Baier (Chapter 3, this volume) have demonstrated that AHP, and particularly somatoparaphrenia, may be specifically related to lesions of the insular cortex (Karnath & Baier, Chapter 3, this volume). There is a growing and impressive literature that the insular cortex (Craig, Chapter 4, this volume) may, in fact, play a key role in subjective awareness of bodily states and subjective, conscious experiences of the "self." Goldstein (1952) was one of the first to note that changes in personality following brain injury often involves the insular cortex. The changes in personality were also thought to reflect a disturbance in the patient's abstract reasoning capacity. This appears to be an oversimplified view. Exactly how damage to the insular cortex affects feeling states and "personality" awaits further investigation. Also, its role in AHP needs to be further assessed.

The work of Vocat and Vuilleumier (Chapter 17, this volume) provides an impressive set of data that demonstrates that AHP does not occur in isolation of other neurocognitive disturbances. Thus, to understand AHP, one must also understand how these other neurocognitive disturbances are changing with time. This may give important clues as to how to differentiate AHP from hysterical reactions (also see the work of House & Hodges, 1988).

Anosodiaphoria, which is also commonly associated with AHP, may be especially related to significant right hemisphere dysfunction. It has been suggested that disturbance of the right frontal region may play an especially important role in anosodiaphoria (Heilman & Harciarek, Chapter 5, this volume).

Before leaving the discussion on new models or hypotheses regarding AHP, it should be noted that several models have appeared since 1988. Many of these models are reviewed in some detail in this volume (see Bottini et al., Chapter 2; Karnath & Baier, Chapter 3; Heilman & Harciarek, Chapter 5; and Vocat & Vuilleumier, Chapter 17), along with their limitations. Furthermore, several chapters specifically consider Levine's "discovery" theory, Geschwind's disconnection hypothesis, Schacter's "conscious aware-ness system," Heilman's feed-forward theory, Frith's feedback theory, Vuilleumier's ABC model, and Bisiach's modality-specific monitoring systems. Each model clearly has value and has explained certain features observed in some AHP patients. Depending on the lesion location and the time the patient is examined, different symptoms can be explained by different models. However, given the variability of different symptoms over time in AHP patients, no model has been universally accepted.

Research on the neuroimaging correlates of self-reflection also raises inter-esting questions/hypotheses. Johnson and Ries (Chapter 18, this volume) suggest that a certain neural network is important in self-reflection. That network includes the mesial prefrontal cortex, the posterior cingulate, and the thalamus. In patients who have impaired self-awareness (MCI and severe TBI), this basic neural circuit seems to be activated when the patient is involved in self-reflective activities. Different versions of this basic pattern were seen in patients with MCI and severe TBI. However, regions that are known to be important in accurate self-reflection, particularly as it relates to one's social self (the dorsal frontal region) may be compromised when the patient has poor self-awareness. Thus, there may be one set of neural circuits involved in self-reflection and diverse neural circuits involved in actual accurate self-reporting of how one is functioning. This rather broad hypothesis needs to be further evaluated.

While certain regions of the brain play a key role in various neuropsychological functions (Heilman & Valenstein, 2003), neuroimaging studies have repeatedly shown that both cerebral hemispheres are often involved in carrying out many neuropsychological tasks. It may come as no surprise, therefore, that in the study of anosognosia or ISA in various patient groups, evidence of bilateral cerebral dysfunction repeatedly has been reported. This leads to the hypothesis that bilateral cerebral dysfunction may be common in many forms of anosognosia.

In light of these observations, we will now address some unanswered questions.

Are We Closer to a Scientific Definition of Anosognosia?

The answer is yes. Anosognosia can be defined as a lack of conscious representation (i.e., subjective awareness) of a neurological/neuropsychological dysfunction caused by damage to or temporary disruption of neural networks that are crucial for the operation of that function. Thus, the damage occurs in an area known to be important for that function (Anton, 1898). It appears that there is an interaction between lesion location and a certain "critical" mass of brain tissue loss or disruption that alters the threshold of neural activity that interferes with the emergence of conscious representation.

While the size and precise distribution of this "critical" mass have not been identified, different syndromes of ISA, or anosognosia, have been shown to relate to disturbances in different neural networks. Thus, AHP is associated with different neural network disturbances than anosognosia for complete cortical blindness. The list can be expanded, depending on the neurological/ neuropsychological functional system that is the focus of investigation.

If a given neurological/neuropsychological function requires bilateral cerebral activation, then anosognosia will be present when crucial bilateral brain regions are damaged or temporarily disrupted (e.g., Anton's syndrome). If the function can emerge within the context of a single cerebral hemisphere, then damage to a single hemisphere may produce anosognosia. This appears to be the case of anosognosia for jargonistic output in aphasic patients.

An important corollary of this definition is that if a disturbed neurological/ neuropsychological function can be detected by the so-called unaffected cerebral hemisphere (that has a separate consciousness; see Sperry, 1974), the patient may be guided to become aware of or self-discover an impaired neurological/neuropsychological function without being truly anosognostic. This appears to occur when the person becomes aware of a homonymous hemianopsia with the help of a neuro-ophthalmological examination. In "true" anosognosia, the patient has the phenomenological experience of functioning normally, because brain regions crucial for evaluating faulty perceptions are, by definition, compromised.

The degree and type of unawareness observed in different brain dysfunctional patients will be correlated with the underlying brain pathology responsible for the neurological/neuropsychological disturbances. Neuronal loss or disruption versus primarily "white matter" lesions seems to play an important role in the emergence of anosognosia. For example, in severe traumatic brain injury, the individual often has a lack of awareness of their socially inappropriate behaviors (see Prigatano, Chapter 12, this volume). These individuals frequently show significant bilateral frontal lobe contusions affecting both the cortex and underlying white matter. Since the frontal lobes are crucial for the ability to monitor one's behavior and to interpret the social cues and reactions of others (Stuss & Knight, 2002), damage to these bilateral regions often produces a permanent ISA for socially inappropriate comments or behavior. In contrast, patients who have very focal frontal lobe dysfunction or deep white matter lesions only may be accurate in their judgments regarding their social behaviors and overall functional capacity.

It appears highly unlikely that premorbid personality plays any role in anosognosia for hemiplegia, as noted above (see Vocat & Vuilleumier, Chapter 17, this volume). The premorbid personality, however, may influence the type of confabulatory response that an individual makes when trying to explain to others the discrepancy of his or her view regarding his or her own functioning versus others' view. Cultural factors also will clearly influence how brain dysfunctional patients report their disturbances and how family members report the patient's limitations (see Prigatano, Chapter 12, this volume).

A key issue in the study of anosognosia is to determine the type and region of neural network disturbance that is necessary to produce anosognosia for a given patient. At this point, there is clear consensus, however, that "large" versus "small" neural network disturbances are responsible for anosognosia for hemiplegia and cortical blindness (see Bottini et al., Chapter 2; Karnath & Baier, Chapter 3; Heilman & Harciarek, Chapter 5; Vocat & Vuilleumier, Chapter 17; and Prigatano & Wolf, Chapter 20, this volume).

What Has Been Revealed about the Mechanisms Responsible for Anosognosia for Hemiplegia?

Several chapters in this volume document that overlapping neural networks appear to be associated with anosognosia for hemiplegia (see Bottini et al.,

Chapter 2; Karnath & Baier, Chapter 3; Heilman & Harciarek, Chapter 5; and Vocat & Vuilleumier, Chapter 17, this volume). Those neural networks appear to include the right frontal lobe, the right parietal lobe, the cingulate gyrus, the insular cortex, and the thalamus. These networks appears to mediate the conscious representation of feeling states (insula), the capacity to maintain alertness and perceive sensory inputs (the thalamus and parietal lobes), the ability to attend to relevant, emotionally significant stimuli (cingulate), and to imagine, to monitor, and to initiate an "intended" or "planned" action (right dorsal frontal lobe in conjunction with other cortical, e.g., parietal, and subcortical structures involved in carrying out voluntary movement). Knowing where the arm and leg are in space and being able to "feel" these appendages may also play an important role (the parietal cortex). The role of memory disturbance in AHP is more debatable. An AHP patient may eventually become aware of his or her hemiparesis but still show persistent memory difficulties (Vocat & Vuilleumier, Chapter 17, this volume). Thus, AHP is hypothesized to be the result of disturbances in several overlapping neural networks that normally function together for conscious representation to occur.

Variations in the neural network systems that are disturbed may help explain why there is variability in the clinical features associated with AHP. For example, individuals who show AHP often show signs of unilateral neglect (Bisiach et al., 1986; Pedersen et al., 1996). Some patients with AHP have significant frontal lobe pathology and may not intend to move their arm (see Heilman & Harciarek, Chapter 5, this volume) or have the capacity to imagine their arm in motion (Frith et al., 2000). Therefore, they may not receive feedback that their arm cannot properly function. Many, if not all, patients may experience that the arm does not "feel like theirs" (see Karnath & Baier, Chapter 3, this volume). This may be directly related to lesions of the right insular cortex or the parietal cortex. Finally, most patients with AHP show a restriction of their emotional reactions to whatever neurological or neuropsychological disturbances can be momentarily demonstrated to them. These patients may have widespread lesions affecting multiple areas of the right hemisphere. The variability of lesion sites, particularly after stroke, helps explain the variability in symptoms that clinical investigators have seen over the years. That is, no two patients are alike as it relates to the exact features of their AHP. This does not, however, rule out a scientific definition or explanation of AHP.

A clinical feature that is often not discussed regarding CVA patients who have AHP is their tendency to be hypoaroused. Many of these patients will sit in their wheelchair with their head turned away from the left side of space (presumably secondary to neglect phenomenon) and bent forward, suggesting a hypoaroused state. How does one explain this latter clinical phenomenon in light of the definition that has been provided? There is a large research literature that argues for the importance of an "ascending arousal system of the brain," which allows for an adequate arousal component to be present in order for conscious representation to occur. Damage to the upper brain stem, hypothalamus, and thalamus may disturb the cholinergic and monoaminergic inputs, among other neurotransmitter functions, thereby undercutting the basic biological foundation that makes arousal a necessary, but insufficient condition for complex human consciousness (Posner, Saper, Schiff, & Plum, 2007). Caloric stimulation of the inner ear of some patients who have AHP allows them to temporarily overcome their anosognosia because of heightened arousal. Many of these patients, however, will quickly fall back into a state of anosognosia once the caloric stimulation effect has been minimized (Bottini et al., Chapter 2, this volume).

These observations are compatible with the Jacksonian notion that there are layers upon layers of neural organization that allow higher integrative functions to emerge (Luria, 1966). Damage at different levels of these layers of organization will potentially produce variations in disturbances in self-awareness, and ultimately, different syndromes of anosognosia. Given these observations, we can only restate what Heilman and Harciarek note (Heilman & Harciarek, Chapter 5, this volume): *"we have not identified a single mechanism that can entirely account for anosognosia for hemiplegia in all patients"* (p. 122, italics added).

Vocat and Vuilleumier (Chapter 17, this volume) provide further information as to the neural correlates of AHP at different time periods following stroke. During the early stage (3 days post stroke), lesions of the anterior insula, the anterior part of the claustrum and putamen, the anterior internal capsule, the head of the caudate, and the anterior periventricular white matter within the right hemisphere are identified. Patients who continued to show AHP into a second week also have evidence that their stroke extended into several other regions of the right hemisphere, including the prefrontal cortex, the temporoparietal junction, the frontal white matter, and the anterior internal capsule, as well as the hippocampus and amygdala.

Anosognosia for Aphasia

Lesions involving the supramarginal gyrus and the angular gyrus of the left, language-dominant hemisphere can produce language disturbances for which the patient appears to be unaware. Jargon aphasia is the most common and readily available example of anosognosia for aphasia (Rubens & Garrett, 1991). Kertesz (Chapter 6, this volume) points out that jargon aphasics who appear unaware of their aphasic output appear to have lesions limited to the left hemisphere. This may be an example of the proposed hypothesis that if a neuropsychological function (i.e., monitoring of linguistic output) is mediated by a single hemisphere, then damage to crucial regions in that hemisphere by itself may produce anosognosia. Unfortunately, the study of anosognosia in aphasia has not led to greater insights as to the underlying mechanism or mechanisms responsible for this condition.

Anosognosia for Complete Cortical Blindness or Anton's Syndrome

A series of case reports continues to document the reality of Anton's syndrome and associated characteristics (Prigatano & Wolf, Chapter 20, this volume). These case reports repeatedly find that bilateral occipital lesions involving the primary visual cortex and associated visual cortex seem to underlie this syndrome. There are a few case studies of Anton's syndrome that have "reversed" when posterior cerebral artery perfusion has improved.

As is noted by Prigatano and Wolf (Chapter 20, this volume) and reported by Förstl, Owen, & David (1993), Anton described anosognosia not only for visual loss, but for hearing or word deafness. To date, studies have not appeared that help explain the underlying mechanism for anosognosia of central hearing loss associated with bilateral temporal lobe damage. Case reports in which thalamic lesions may alter auditory perceptual skills with the individual not recognizing their disturbances have been limited.

Why Don't All Brain-Dysfunctional Patients Show Anosognosia or Impaired Self-Awareness?

An interesting question that emerges is why do some brain dysfunctional patients show anosognosia or ISA and others apparently do not? The answer must be tentative. Three factors seem to influence whether ISA is present. The first is whether the size of neuronal network disturbances reaches some critical point to compromise the individual's sense of self-awareness. Second, the speed at which the central nervous system is altered or changed may be important. For example, anosognosia for hemiplegia is most noted following stroke. It may be less likely in patients who show slow-growing tumors. Third, actual compromise of gray matter may be important. In this regard, patients with multiple sclerosis who have primarily white matter lesions may show relatively good self-awareness of impaired functioning until the disease progresses to the point at which cortical (i.e., neuronal) networks are disturbed.

Given this analysis, we can also approach the question: Is anosognosia a purely cognitive/perceptual dysfunction, or do emotions or feeling states play an important role? The answer appears to be related to the function that has been lost. The patient's indifference over his or her lost neurological or neuropsychological functioning should not be taken as evidence that some disruption of emotional or motivational circuits have necessarily been compromised. If the individual has no conscious representation of a disturbance, he or she understandably would not have any emotional reaction, since he or she has no knowledge of what has occurred. The work of Jorge (Chapter 16, this volume) also emphasizes that the patient may be unaware of a feeling state after traumatic brain injury, and it remains unclear to what degree cognitive difficulties relate to this unawareness. One must simply answer at the present time that no definitive statement can be made about this question. Clinically, however, it appears that anosognosia for classic syndromes does involve some disruption of both cognitive and feeling processes that are normally integrated in the intact brain.

What Role Do Neurotransmitters Play in Impaired Self-Awareness or Frank Anosognosia?

Traditional research on ISA and anosognosia has attempted to relate specific regional areas of brain dysfunction to the various manifestations of ISA and anosognosia. The underlying neurotransmitter disturbances that may correlate with ISA and anosognosia have for the most part been neglected. The study of patients with traumatic brain injury, however, emphasizes that a key component to ISA in this group may be a disruption in the arousal-maintaining systems of the brain. Disturbances of a number of neurotransmitter functions may impair arousal levels to the degree that the individual cannot effectively attend to environmental inputs and, therefore, perceive disturbances in function (see Prigatano, Chapter 12, this volume). The study of ISA of motor abnormalities in Parkinson patients raises the interesting possibility that disturbances of the dopaminergic system are important for their form of ISA (see Prigatano et al., Chapter 9, this volume).

If specific neurotransmitter disturbances are associated with different forms of anosognosia, this leads to a second very interesting question. Are there any genetic predispositions for anosognosia following various brain disorders? This is an area that has not been investigated to date but deserves attention in future research (also see Robertson, Chapter 15, this volume).

Neuroimaging/Neuroanatomical, Neurophysiological, and Neuropsychological Changes Associated with Hysterical Sensorimotor Loss: Are They Different from Anosognosia for Hemiplegia?

Vocat and Vuilleumier (Chapter 17, this volume) address the neuroimaging/ neuroanatomical and neurophysiological changes associated with hysterical sensorimotor loss. They review a variety of studies which suggest that the correlates are different for hysterical sensorimotor loss versus AHP. Their own experimental findings suggest that thalamic and basal ganglia hypometabolic activities may be especially associated with hysterical sensorimotor loss. In their patient group, disturbances of neural networks at the cortical level did not appear to be compromised.

In an experimental model of repression or motivated forgetting, Anderson et al. (2004) asked students to learn a series of paired associated words and then attempt to suppress their recall of certain associations. Their findings included a suppression of activation bilaterally in the hippocampus. However, there was also reduced activation in cortical regions, including the frontal lobes, the insular cortex, and the left parietal cortex, as well as the bilateral cuneus. The magnitude of the changes was modest, but nevertheless, reduction in activation was noted in a complex neurocircuitry involving both cortical and subcortical regions.

In clinical practice, it is not uncommon that patients who seem to be using denial and repression as a method of coping report significant cognitive limitations. Prigatano and Kirlin (2009) noted, for example, that patients with nonepileptic seizure disorders often report significant cognitive sequelae. Objective neuropsychological assessment of these patients suggests, however, that their cognitive complaints are not paralleled with objectively poor performance on a variety of cognitive tasks (this is especially true for word-finding difficulties). Rather, measures of anxiety and depression strongly correlate with their cognitive complaints. This suggests that brain regions involved in affect control and expression may be especially compromised in patients who present with some form of dissociative disorder in which the phenomenon of denial is common.

Are Disturbances in Self-Awareness Observed in Certain Psychiatric Populations Related to Impaired Brain (i.e., Neuropsychological) Functions?

Gilleen and colleagues (Chapter 13, this volume) provide a scholarly summary of various studies that have attempted to answer this question for schizophrenic patients. While the answer appears to be "yes," they note that the relationships documented by some researchers have not been found consistently by others. It appears, however, that in psychotic disorders, ISA may well reflect underlying brain pathology. Whether this is true in neurotic disorders or in character disorders remains to be studied.

How Is It Possible That a Patient Can Retain Consciousness, Be Oriented to Time and Place, and Remember What Is Being Said, and Still Be Unaware of a Neurological or Neuropsychological Impairment/Disturbance?

While this question was briefly considered in the introductory comments of this chapter, more should be said about it. If we could answer this question, we would have both a scientific definition of anosognosia and an explanation as to the nature of consciousness, which includes subjective awareness of the self in the "here and now." Obviously, we have neither, and therefore, our answer to this question also will be quite limited. Based on clinical observation of persons with AHP, as well as individuals who have suffered severe TBI and have persistent ISA several years post trauma, the following comments are offered.

Human consciousness and self-awareness have evolved over thousands of years, as have other brain functions. Our phenomenological experiences suggest that there are three major divisions of consciousness (Zeman, 2001; also see Prigatano & Johnson, 2003). The first has to do with the basic sleep-wake cycle. The most rudimentary form of consciousness allows us to be "awake" and be aware of the "here and now." It depends on the intactness of brainstem, hypothalamic, and thalamic structures. The cholinergic system is crucial for this type of awareness. Severe disturbances of these brain structures and the cholinergic system can produce coma, delirium, or place the person in an obtunded state in which he or she cannot meaningfully respond to the environment. During this time, however, the person may have some minimal awareness of themselves and of the environment. This basic dimension of consciousness, therefore , is quite robust and is organized according to specific neural pathways (Posner et al., 2007). It allows us the most rudimentary sense of the "I" or "me" experience. This dimension may be maintained even when other dimensions of consciousness are disturbed.

As the cerebral hemispheres develop (including the insular cortex), the experience of subjective awareness undergoes greater development and with it, greater monitoring of one's internal and external environment. We can now make finer discriminations about ourselves. We are not only awake, but acutely aware of ourselves and any internal or external environmental changes that are important to adapt to. When there is damage to primary sensory (e.g., vision) and/or sensorimotor functions (e.g., tactile perception and movement), the person may be aware that something is "wrong" if the crucial structures responsible for those functions are not completely compromised. If they are completely compromised, as described by Anton (1898), the individual may maintain some rudimentary sense of self, but have a clear loss of subjective awareness of a specific neurological and/or neuropsychological dysfunction. This is, of course, the classic syndrome of anosognosia.

In day-to-day life and clinical practice, a third aspect of conscious awareness can be observed. Many patients with severe traumatic brain injury regain consciousness but have a limited awareness of their own disturbed neuropsychological functioning. In addition, they may appear selfish, immature, or childlike. When probing further for the causes of these behavioral characteristics, it appears that many of these individuals are unable to perceive the phenomenological world of another and therefore fail to develop what might be broadly called an empathetic response. They appear to have difficulty subjectively being aware of another person's "mind." This third "level" of consciousness may be a result of complex disturbance in the first two layers, or some disruption of what has been referred to as the "mirror-neuron system" (see Rizzolatti & Craighero, 2004; Rizzolatti & Sinigaglia, 2008).

Obviously, this analysis is rudimentary and does not explain how conscious awareness of the self actually emerges from brain activity. This is the central mind–body problem for which no one has an answer to date. While several theorists have approached this problem (Laureys & Tononi, 2009), the Nobel laureate Gerald Edelman (1989) has proposed an interesting model on how consciousness and memory functions are interconnected. Ivanitsky (2000) has attempted to further test and refine that model. Ivanitsky (2000) presents psychophysiological data that suggests that sensory information received in the occipital regions is projected to hippocampal and hypothalamic centers, which in turn project back to the primary visual cortex. This "loop" allows for synthesis of what is "seen now" and how it compares with "what was seen in the past." At the same time, the motivational relevance of that sensory (visual) input is evaluated. This "recurring loop" somehow allows consciousness to emerge. Ivanitsky (2000) also notes that the frontal cortex is crucial in evaluating the significance of the emerging conscious representations and is the basis for decision making that has adaptive value. If accurate, this broad model also resonates with Sperry's (1969) assertion that human consciousness actually influences underlying brain systems that allow it to occur in the first place.

Concluding Comments

The study of anosognosia has revealed important findings as to the neuroanatomical and neuropsychological correlates associated with the different forms of anosognosia. The study of anosognosia has been driven by the development of new methods of assessment, as well as clinical observations and theoretical propositions. The measurement of anosognosia has to be individualized as Bisiach and Geminiani (1991) emphasized, while at the same time encompassing objective assessments of various symptoms that change with time and/or treatment. It also requires the use of innovative neuroimaging techniques to help explain the changing symptom picture. Numerous chapters in this text have outlined assessment techniques that are helpful in assessing different forms of anosognosia and associated symptoms.

A key issue is understanding the natural course of anosognosia or impaired self-awareness in different patient groups and adjusting the assessment techniques according to the extent and nature of anosognosia that is observed. Innovative case reports also continue to force theorists to develop models or concepts that are more precise in their prediction, but yet broad in their scope of symptom explanation.

In the twenty-first century, Anton begins to emerge as perhaps the most prominent figure because he not only described anosognosia but also presented ideas that help explain it today. Babinski, who is also an important figure, provided a clear description of AHP and provided a word that allowed that phenomenon to become a focus of study in neurology and neuropsychology. The question now emerges: Is there anything that can be done to effectively manage or treat patients who show anosognosia or impaired self-awareness after brain injury? The final chapter of this volume, Chapter 22, will address this and related questions.

Acknowledgments

I am grateful to Daniel Tranel, Ph.D. for his helpful review of an earlier version of this chapter.

References

Anderson, M. C., Ochsner, K. N., Kuhl, B., Cooper, J., Robertson, E., Gabrieli, S. W., Glover, G. H., & Gabrieli, J. D. E. (2004). Neural systems underlying the suppression of unwanted memories. *Science, 303*, 232–235.

Anton, G. (1898). Ueber Herderkrankungen des Gehirnes, welche von Patienten selbst nicht wahrgenommen warden. *Wiener Klinische Wochenschrift, 11*, 227–229.

Babinski, J. (1914). Contribution à l'etude des troubles mentaux dans l'hémiplégie organique cérébrale (Anosognosie). *Revue Neurologique, 27*, 845–847.

Berti, A., Bottini, G., Gandola, M., Pia, L., Smania, N., Stracciari, A., et al. (2005). Shared cortical anatomy for motor awareness and motor control. *Science, 309*(5733), 488–491.

Bisiach, E., & Geminiani, G. (1991). Anosognosia related to hemiplegia and hemianopia. In G. P. Prigatano & R. L. Schacter (Eds.), *Awareness of deficit after brain injury: Clinical and theoretical issues* (pp. 17–39). New York: Oxford University Press.

Bisiach, E., Vallar, G., Perani, D., Papagno, C., & Berti, A. (1986). Unawareness of disease following lesions of the right hemisphere: Anosognosia for hemiplegia and anosognosia for hemianopia. *Neuropsychologia, 24*(4), 471–481.

Breier, J. I., Adair, J. C., Gold, M., Fennell, E. B., Gilmore, R. L., & Heilman, K. M. (1995). Dissociation of anosognosia for hemiplegia and aphasia during left-hemisphere anesthesia. *Neurology, 45*(1), 65–67.

Cocchini, G., Beschin, N., & Sala, S. D. (2002). Chronic anosognosia: A case report and theoretical account. *Neuropsychologia, 40*, 2030–2038.

Critchley, M. (1953). *The parietal lobes.* New York: Hafner Press.

Edelman, G. M. (1989). *The remembered present: A biological theory of consciousness.* New York: Basic Books.

Förstl, H., Owen, A. M., & David. A. S. (1993). Gabriel Anton and "Anton's symptom": On focal diseases of the brain which are not perceived by the patient (1898). *Neuropsychiatry, Neuropsychology, and Behavioral Neurology, 6*(1), 1–8.

Frith, C. D., Blakemore, S. J., & Wolpert, D. M. (2000). Abnormalities in the awareness and control of action. *Philosophical Transactions of the Royal Society of London B Biological Sciences, 355*(1404), 1771–1788.

Goldstein, K. (1952). The effect of brain damage on the personality. *Psychiatry, 15,* 245–260.

Heilman, K. M., & Valenstein, E. (Eds.) (2003). *Clinical Neuropsychology* (4th edition). New York: Oxford University Press.

House, A., & Hodges, J. (1988). Persistent denial of handicap after infarction of the right basal ganglia: A case study. *Journal of Neurology, Neurosurgery, and Psychiatry, 51,* 112–115.

Ivanitsky, A. M. (2000). Informational synthesis in crucial cortical areas, as the brain basis of the subjective experience. In R. Miller, A. M. Ivanitsky, & P. M. Balaban (Eds). *Complex brain functions: Conceptual advances in Russian neuroscience* (pp. 73–96). Reading, MA: Harwood Academic Publishers.

Laureys, S., & Tononi G. (Eds.) (2009). *The neurology of consciousness.* London: Elsevier-Academic Press.

Luria, A. R. (1966). *Higher cortical functions in man.* New York and London: Basic Books and Plenum Press.

Pia, L., Neppi-Modona, M., Ricci, R., & Berti, A. (2004). The anatomy of anosognosia for hemiplegia: A meta-analysis. *Cortex 40*(2), 367–377.

Pedersen, P. N., Jorgensen, H. S., Nakayama, H., Raaschou, H. O., & Olsen, T. S. (1996). Frequency, determinants, and consequences of anosognosia in acute stroke. *Journal of Neurological Rehabilitation, 10,* 243–250.

Posner, J. B., Saper, C. B., Schiff, N. D., & Plum, F. (Eds.). (2007). *Plum and Posner's diagnosis of stupor and coma* (4th edition). New York: Oxford University Press.

Prigatano, G. P. (1999). *Principles of neuropsychological rehabilitation.* New York: Oxford University Press.

Prigatano, G. P., & Altman, I. M. (1990). Impaired awareness of behavioral limitations after traumatic brain injury. *Archives of Physical Medicine and Rehabilitation, 71,* 1058–1064.

Prigatano, G. P., & Johnson, S. C. (2003). The three vectors of consciousness and their disturbances after brain injury. *Neuropsychological Rehabilitation, 13*(1/2), 13–29.

Prigatano, G. P., & Kirlin, K. A. (2009). Self appraisal and objective assessment of cognitive and affective functions in persons with epileptic and nonepileptic seizures. *Epilepsy & Behavior, 14,* 387–392.

Ramachandron, V. S. (1994). Phantom limbs, neglect syndromes, repressed memories, and Freudian Psychology. *International Review of Neurobiology, 37,* 291–372.

Rizzolatti, G., & Craighero, L. (2004). The mirror-neuron system, *Annual Review of Neuroscience, 27,* 169–192.

Rizzolatti, G., & Sinigaglia, C. (2008). *Mirrors in the brain.* New York: Oxford University Press.

Rubens, A. B., & Garrett, M. F. (1991). Anosognosia of linguistic deficits in patients with neurological deficits. In G. P. Prigatano & D. L. Schacter (Eds.), *Awareness of deficit after brain injury: Clinical and theoretical implications* (pp. 40–52). Oxford, England: Oxford University Press.

Salmon, E., Perani, D., Herholz, K., Marique, P., Kalbe, E., Holthoff, V., et al. (2006). Neural correlates of anosognosia for cognitive impairment in Alzheimer's disease. *Human Brain Mapping, 27,* 588–597.

Sperry, R. W. (1969). A modified concept of consciousness. *Psychological Review*, 76(6), 532–536.

Sperry, R. W. (1974). Lateral specialization in the surgically separated hemispheres. In F. O. Schmitt & F. G. Worden (Eds.), *The Neurosciences* (pp. 5–19). Cambridge, MA: MIT Press.

Stuss, D. T., & Knight, R. T. (Eds.) (2002). *Principles of frontal lobe function.* Oxford, England: Oxford University Press.

Zeman, A. (2001). Invited review. Consciousness. *Brain, 124,* 1263–1289.

22

Management and Rehabilitation of Persons with Anosognosia and Impaired Self-Awareness

George P. Prigatano and Jeannine Morrone-Strupinsky

The management and rehabilitation of persons with anosognosia can range from a simple series of preventive steps aimed at avoiding complications as the patient "spontaneously" recovers, to a series of interventions dictated by the patient's neurological and neuropsychological characteristics, as well as possible psychiatric comorbidities. Clinically, we have adapted a simple model for classifying disturbances in self-awareness after various brain disorders that guides our interventions.

A Model for Classifying Disorders of Self-Awareness Associated with Brain Disorders

Disorders of self-awareness are observed in various patient populations and can range from "mild" to "severe." When the patient has a complete unawareness of a lost neurological and/or neuropsychological function, the term *anosognosia* is used. This is readily seen in cases of anosognosia for hemiplegia (AHP) and Anton's syndrome. With time and/or treatment, the person can progress from a complete syndrome of unawareness (i.e., anosognosia) to a partial syndrome of unawareness. We have used the term *impaired self-awareness (ISA)* to describe a partial syndrome of unawareness of the disturbed function. In cases of ISA, patients have "some" awareness of their impairments and can use both non-defensive (from a psychological perspective) and defensive methods of coping with their limited awareness of an impaired neurological (e.g., a homonymous hemianopia) or a neuropsychological function (e.g., memory impairment) (Prigatano, 1999). It is important to determine whether ISA is associated with denial of disability (DD). When denial is present, it can complicate the

495

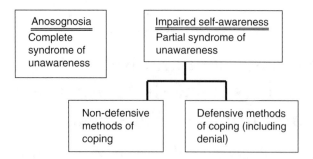

Figure 22.1 A clinical model for classifying disorders of self-awareness associated with brain disorders. (Adapted from Prigatano, 1999.)

management of the patient. Figure 22.1 provides a summary of this model. Before attempting to demonstrate the clinical application of this model, a discussion of what is meant by the term *denial* is necessary.

A Definition of *Denial*

Denial is a term used to describe one psychological method of coping with a loss or threat of a loss that has personal significance to the individual. From a psychiatric perspective, denial is a defense against anxiety and emotionally painful experiences (Freedman, Kaplan, & Sadock, 1976). Denial is considered by some psychiatrists as a "negation of reality by means of fantasy" (Paredes, 1974, p. 24). It transforms reality to suit the purposes and wishes of the individual. Characteristically, this process exists side by side with the capacity to test reality.

Denial is a common method of coping for most human beings, especially when they find it difficult to change their behavior or wishes. Sometimes the denial is quick and reflexive, but readily gives way to reality. For example, upon hearing the news of a death of a loved one, a person may say, "No" in a low, but forceful manner. The response is clearly a wish that something had not happened. When faced with the facts, however, the person may now become quiet, tearful, and eventually accept the reality of the loss. At the other end of the continuum, denial may persist for years and serve as a way of reducing anxiety. Ultimately, however, the consequences of denial may penetrate this "defense system" and the individual eventually faces a problem that he or she had not wanted to face previously. This is commonly seen in individuals with alcohol addiction. While they may drink daily in an uncontrolled fashion, they do not consider themselves to have a "drinking problem." They will state that they could stop drinking anytime they want to, but they do not wish to stop drinking. When they eventually lose several jobs, a spouse, and/or family, they may momentarily come to the possibility that they are denying their alcoholism.

Not uncommonly during this time, however, they will blame others for the losses. When finally they have a seizure secondary to alcohol withdrawal, the reality of the addiction now becomes clearer.

It is difficult to measure and treat denial. Clinically, denial is observed by interacting with a person over a lengthy period of time. It is treated within the context of a trusting (psychotherapeutic) relationship in which the patient begins to observe and understand his or her behavior and its negative consequences. Clinicians, working with psychiatric and brain-dysfunctional patients, frequently see many signs of denial. It is characterized by refusal to face certain facts about themselves. It is an attempt to mitigate or reduce anxiety, as noted above. When evidence for a behavioral limitation is brought to his or her attention, it is not uncommon for the individual to give it momentary recognition, but then provide an explanation that discounts the value of the feedback. Sentences that begin as: "Yes, but. . ." are common in patients who use denial (Prigatano & Klonoff, 1998).

Since denial can range from a normal method of coping to an unadaptive psychological defense, it is logical that it can coexist with ISA following a brain disorder. There may be, however, behavioral indications that separate the neuropsychological signs of ISA from denial of disability (DD).

Prigatano and Klonoff (1998) proposed a Clinician's Rating Scale to help separate these two phenomena in brain-dysfunctional patients. The scale was based on clinical judgment, and it has not been externally validated. Persons who show ISA often are perplexed when given feedback about their impairments. They do not have a negative or positive reaction, but seem to be neutral or unclear as to what the feedback is saying. When they discover through various forms of cognitive rehabilitation that they may, in fact, have greater neuropsychological difficulty than they previously perceived, they may momentarily stop and try to clarify their misunderstanding. Even during such times, however, it is not uncommon for their affect to be rather bland, which suggests a mild form of anosodiaphoria.

This is in striking contrast to individuals who have DD in the presence or absence of ISA. These individuals often become irritated, if not agitated, when given feedback. They often discount the feedback. They are emotionally vigilant of others' reactions to them. They are quick to provide a logical argument to counteract any unpleasant perceptions about themselves. At times, simple tasks that reflect bilateral cerebral dysfunction, such as the Halstead Finger Tapping Test, may help identify TBI patients who have ISA versus patients with no known neurological disorders, but who have DD (Prigatano, 1998).

Clinical Variability in Patients Who Present with Anosognosia and Impaired Self-Awareness

If there is a single consensus that can be found in the ideas expressed in the preceding chapters, it is that anosognosia for different neurological and neuropsychological deficits can be produced by a variety of interconnected, but different brain dysfunctions. The phenomenon clearly is "multifactorial" in nature (see Vocat & Vuilleumier, Chapter 17; Orfei et al., Chapter 19, this volume). Thus, one can only begin to discuss strategies for managing and rehabilitating persons with anosognosia by describing specific case examples. Individual case examples reveal common features, as well as those that are unique to individual patients. Both need to be kept in mind when considering how to manage and rehabilitate such patients (also see Prigatano, 2008a).

Three case vignettes of patients who present with AHP will first be described. This will be followed by a discussion of three patients who have persistent ISA associated with severe traumatic brain injury (TBI). One of these three TBI patients showed behavioral indications of both ISA and DD. Then two patients who have been diagnosed with early stages of a dementing condition—one with probable vascular dementia, the other with probable dementia of the Alzheimer's type—will be presented. The first patient showed signs of ISA and DD. The second patient showed only signs of ISA.

Anosognosia for Hemiplegia: Three Cases

Case 1

Case 1 was a 51-year-old, right-handed female who suffered a rupture of an arteriovenous malformation in the right parietal lobe. Unfortunately, this was followed by later strokes in the distribution of the middle cerebral artery (MCA) and the posterior cerebral arteries (PCA). This led to bilateral lesions in the posterior region of the cerebral hemispheres, but spared the primary visual cortex. The patient presented with a dense left hemiparesis, for which she was completely unaware (i.e., AHP). She also showed severe neglect and hemi-anesthesia on the left side. She was completely blind, but became aware of her blindness within a few hours of her stroke. Visual evoked potentials following her most recent stroke revealed a pattern compatible with complete cortical blindness (Prigatano et al., in preparation).

When first examined, the patient sat in a wheelchair with her head and neck deviated to the right. When asked if she had any difficulty moving her two arms and hands, she reported none. When asked to clap her hands, she raised her right hand and moved it in a clapping motion, but the left hand was motionless. When asked again if there was anything wrong with her left hand, she responded, "Not that I'm aware of."

During this time, her speech and language skills were grossly within the normal range. She understood questions that were asked of her and as noted above, freely reported there was a loss of vision. She expressed a desire that her vision would return, but was not observed to be overly upset or depressed when discussing the loss of her vision. At other times, however, she did report being despondent.

This patient "spontaneously" recovered from her AHP and was considered not anosognostic 15 days after she entered neurorehabilitation (approximately 3 weeks post onset of her hemiplegia). When asked about her motor functioning at that time, she freely admitted that she had difficulty moving her left arm and leg. She would also spontaneously note, however, she was not sure where her left arm or leg was in space. As she continued to recover, she had the distinct sense that her left arm was not her left arm. She noted that it "got in the way." Initially she thought it was the arm of her sister, but then later recognized it was her own arm. With time, the left arm "no longer got in the way," but it did not feel like her arm. She would repeatedly report that it felt like someone else's arm was within her arm. It appears that somatoparaphrenia persisted, even after AHP resolved.

Her clinical course was characterized by a resolution of AHP, followed by a paralleled reduction, but not elimination, of left hemi-neglect. There were no specific rehabilitation activities for AHP, but she did receive standard occupational therapies, which included tactile recognition and movement exercises.

Case 2

Cocchini, Beschin, and Della Sala (2002) present a case study of a 27-year-old man with 16 years of education who suffered a severe TBI. The following is a brief synopsis of that extensive report. One year post TBI, this patient continued to show AHP and clear signs of left extrapersonal neglect in daily activities and on formal testing. It was noted that the patient was "overly agnostic on his motor and cognitive deficits." While the authors were able to momentarily overcome his anosognosia and demonstrate to him that he could not use his left arm, this did not result in a resolution of his AHP. They explained the persistence of his AHP on the basis of neglect and severe memory impairment. This case study suggests that in some instances AHP may be permanent. Long-term management of these patients is seldom, if ever, discussed.

Case 3

Fotopoulou, Rudd, Holmes, and Kopelman (2009) report a case of a 67-year-old woman who had AHP secondary to a large infarction in the right middle cerebral artery. Neurological examination also revealed mild dysarthria, lower left facial weakness, left hemi-spatial neglect, left homonymous hemianopia, left hemi-anesthesia, and right gaze deviation.

As was true of Case 1, this patient was quite verbal and seemed to understand all questions posed to her. When testing motor functions, she appeared to be unaware of her motor deficits on the left side. This condition was noted 22 days post onset of her neurological problems. The authors reportedly played back to the patient a video of her attempting to carry out a variety of motor activities.

They indicated that the patient "recovered instantly and permanently when viewing herself in a video replay" (Fotopoulou et al., 2009, p. 1256).

Their interpretation of this startling finding was that some individuals who have AHP may be unable to observe themselves from "outside" (i.e., take the third person's perspective). This intriguing hypothesis needs to be replicated in other individual cases. It is an unexpected finding, since a defining characteristic of AHP has been the fact that the patient discounts all evidence concerning his or her motor impairments. In this case, the patient seemed to be quite impressed with the evidence. Perhaps the method of presenting the information was responsible for the change in her perceptions. As will be discussed below, however, videotaping has been used in the neuropsychological rehabilitation of TBI patients who have ISA without such a dramatic effect (Prigatano et al., 1986). In each of these cases of anosognosia, there was no clinical evidence of denial.

Persons with Impaired Self-Awareness after Severe Traumatic Brain Injury

The next three cases to be presented all had prolonged loss of consciousness and admitting Glasgow Coma Scale (GCS) scores equal to or less than 8 following TBI. Each individual showed unequivocal, bilateral frontal contusions using computed tomography (CT) or magnetic resonance imaging (MRI) of the brain secondary to TBI. Case 4 is reported in more detail in Prigatano et al. (1986) and Case 6 in Prigatano and Maier (2008). Case 5 has not been previously reported. Each of these patients had undergone an extensive neuropsychological examination, and two of them were followed and treated within the context of a holistic neuropsychological rehabilitation program (Cases 4 and 5). The sixth case had been followed for 8 years (Case 6).

Case 4

Case 4 was a 21-year-old man who fell from a bridge while smoking marijuana. He was cooperative, but showed little outward signs of emotion. When he was involved in rehabilitation activities, however, he clearly was not apathetic. He eagerly engaged in all tasks that were presented to him. His ideas about himself were unrealistic, and his assessment of his own limitations suggested ISA. He would recognize some cognitive limitations, but never at a level that reflected others' perceptions, including the therapists, his attending physicians, and his family members.

With extensive cognitive rehabilitation and psychotherapy, he began to "accept" that his neuropsychological impairments may have been more severe than he thought, but he would never spontaneously voice this opinion. He would agree to it when comparison findings were presented. He never seemed, however, convinced by the feedback provided by others. He was, however, guided by such feedback. There was no resistance to the feedback.

While receiving cognitive rehabilitation, he was videotaped as he attempted a variety of cognitive tasks that reflected his neuropsychological deficits. Reviewing those videotapes made him pause in his perception of himself, but never substantially changed his perception. He would momentarily agree that perhaps he had greater limitations than he had thought, but by the next day would return to his previous assessment of himself. He was followed for several years. He acknowledged that he had "some" deficits, but repeatedly reported less impaired functioning than what other attentive individuals reported. He expressed normal sadness over his life situation, with persistent ISA.

Case 5

Case 5 was a 40-year-old man who fell from a ladder. During his post-acute phase, he was hyperverbal, tangential, and showed many signs of "frontal lobe" dysfunction, including poor judgment and reduced abstract reasoning abilities. He would often report that he could go back to work as an electrician. He did not feel there were any significant neurocognitive problems, despite overwhelming evidence that such impairments were, in fact, present.

He was trustful of his wife who emphasized to him that he was having difficulties that he did not fully recognize. She emphasized the importance of following the guidelines of the therapists, which he did. While he never fully believed that he could not go back to his old work, he was guided to accept limited work responsibilities with extensive counseling and cognitive rehabilitation. He showed no defensiveness when given feedback about his limitations, nor did he show any signs of anxiety or irritation. If anything, he described simple frustration in his inability to function at his old job.

Case 6

Case 6 was a 28-year-old gentleman who suffered a TBI secondary to a motor vehicle accident. This gentleman did not undergo neuropsychological rehabilitation but had been seen over an 8-year period of time with repeated neuropsychological assessments. When the neuropsychological examination findings were presented to him, he would discount the findings and, at times, give out a loud laugh. The laugh did not seem to reflect a sense of humor, but disbelief in what was being said to him. He repeatedly insisted that he could go back to work and regain all of his physical functioning if only given an opportunity to do so.

He and his mother, however, did not pursue neuropsychological rehabilita-tion. Consequently he received no such services. He simply stayed at home and began to deteriorate from a psychiatric point of view. He ultimately developed paranoid ideation, which reached psychotic proportions. It is unclear if the persistent impaired awareness contributed to the paranoid ideation, but it did appear probable (Prigatano, 1988). This patient often had an explanation for why neuropsychological test findings did not have any relevance to his day-to-day functioning. Unlike the other two patients, he insisted, with some agitation in his voice, that he was better than what the test scores reflected. His "resistance" to "hearing the feedback" was clear.

Persons with Early Dementia Who Show Impaired Self-Awareness

The next two cases presented with neuropsychological characteristics of a beginning dementing condition. As described below, both had significant memory difficulties, but differed considerably in how they experienced their memory impairments.

Case 7

Case 7 was an 83-year-old woman who was followed for approximately 5 years. She reported that her memory function was not as "bad" as her husband reported. She noted occasional problems with memory, but attributed this to the normal aging process. On neuropsychological testing, her intelligence was within the normal range, but her memory function was clearly impaired relative to age and IQ estimates. She also showed slight difficulties with orientation to time and place. Language function was intact. She reported absolutely no difficulties in any area of memory functioning. Her husband reported consider-able difficulties on day-to-day memory tasks.

As the patient was followed, a consistent picture emerged in which there was a subtle, but continuous decline in memory function associated with decline in visuospatial problem-solving skills and ability to shift her cognitive set. She became more and more dependent on her husband and insisted that he be with her, attending to her needs literally 24 hours a day, 7 days a week.

When it was suggested that her husband needed some form of respite care and that she might benefit from instruction in memory compensation techniques, she was adamant in stating that she did not want to do either. She saw her husband as being the person who had the responsibility of caring for her. She denied any substantial memory difficulties. When her memory difficulties and her husband's needs were discussed with her, she would make it quite clear she was displeased with the feedback. She appeared to show not only ISA, but DD.

Case 8

Case 8 is a 70-year-old, right-handed male who presented with memory difficulties. He has been followed for 6 years. When initially examined, he reported minimal difficulties with memory. His wife reported moderate to severe difficulties. Unlike the previous patient, he did not state that his memory was better than what his spouse said. He simply felt that there was a difference of opinion.

Despite the fact that he had been a successful business owner for many years, his IQ scores were in the low average range. He showed difficulties with verbal reasoning and visuospatial problem solving, something that would not be expected, given his professional achievements. The patient was subsequently evaluated on a yearly basis. He has shown a progressive decline in his memory functioning and now meets criteria for dementia of the Alzheimer's type.

His wife has repeatedly noted a decline in her husband's functioning, particularly his failure to understand what is being said to him and to follow instructions. While this patient wished to have his spouse care for him on a 24-hour, 7-day basis, he was not belligerent or in any way negative when given feedback concerning his difficulties or his wife's needs. He made comments to the effect, however, that he felt humiliated by his performance on neuropsychological tests.

He repeatedly reported that his level of memory impairment was substantially less severe than what his wife reported. As he showed a progressive deterioration in his memory and related cognitive functioning, he was comforted by the guidance of his wife. He recognized her needs and was willing to allow her to have appropriate respite care. Similar to the previous patient, he had a childlike, demanding quality to any unmet needs. Unlike the previous patient, however, he was not hostile or angry when the logic behind a decision was explained to him.

Clinical Issues That These Vignettes Bring to Light

Each of the patients discussed had unequivocal brain dysfunction. Each patient demonstrated a lack of awareness of his or her physical and/or cognitive limitations. Beyond that, there were notable differences. Some patients spontaneously improved with time; others did not. Some seemed to benefit from rehabilitation exercises; others did not. Some showed a flat affect and perhaps anosodiaphoria when confronted with their deficits; others did not. The patients came from different backgrounds and were of different ages and sociocultural status. Their underlying brain pathologies varied according to diagnostic category. Their therapies had to be modified according to who they were before the onset of their particular brain disorder, as well as the deficits they presented with when examined. As illustrated in Figure 22.2, some were getting "better" with the passage of time, and others were deteriorating. How should these patients be approached in their clinical management and rehabilitation?

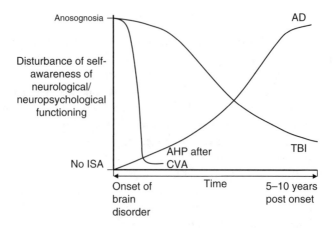

Figure 22.2 An oversimplified representation of the relationship between severity of disturbances in self-awareness and the passage of time in various brain disorders. AD, Alzheimer's disease; AHP, anosognosia for hemiplegia; CVA, cerebrovascular accident; ISA, impaired self-awareness; TBI, traumatic brain injury.

Clinical Guidelines in Management and Rehabilitation of Persons with Anosognosia and Impaired Self-Awareness

The first step in the management and rehabilitation of persons who have anosognosia or ISA is to determine the extent (severity) of the unawareness of the patient. The second step is to determine if nondefensive or defensive methods of coping are present in the ISA condition. We believe that in cases of "true" anosognosia, by definition, there is no defensive reaction. Different strategies of intervention are utilized when there is ISA and defensive methods of coping versus nondefensive methods of coping (as briefly described below).

The third step is to determine the chronicity of the anosognosia or ISA and the likelihood of it "spontaneously" improving with time. Related to this is the need to determine the presence or absence of associated neurological or neuropsychological disturbances that may underlie or contribute to the impaired awareness (the fourth step). This information helps guide the rehabilitation exercises/ activities for the patient.

The fifth step is to form a working alliance with the patient, and if possible, the patient's family members. Establishing a working alliance with patients who show anosognosia or ISA appears to relate to a positive rehabilitation outcome (Klonoff, Lamb, & Henderson, 2001; Prigatano et al., 1994; Schönberger, Humle, & Teasdale, 2006a; Schönberger, Humle, Zeeman, & Teasdale, 2006b). This process requires time and effort on the part of the clinician. If possible, the patient should be seen on a daily basis while being on an inpatient unit. Detailed records of how symptoms are or are not changing with time and/or treatment need to be carefully documented (Bisiach & Geminiani, 1991). This gives the clinician an early view of what brain mechanisms most likely underlie the complete or partial awareness syndromes. It also provides useful information that can be applied in the long-term care of patients.

The sixth step is to develop an individual neuropsychological rehabilitation plan (INRP) that considers *(a)* how the symptom picture is or is not changing with time and treatment; *(b)* the preserved and disturbed neurological and neuropsychological functions associated with anosognosia or ISA; and *(c)* the level of awareness that is present for different functional capacities. This latter information is used to develop a hierarchical treatment plan that moves from "simple" awareness tasks to "more complex" awareness tasks. The task must be interesting to the patient (seventh step) and not be too easy or too difficult for him or her. Various reinforcers are needed for the successful engagement and completion of tasks by the person who has anosognosia or ISA.

The final step (eighth step) is that the INRP needs to persist until the person recovers lost awareness of a neurological or neuropsychological function, or shows substantial improvement. At times, the clinician and/or treating therapist may be discouraged and feel that they need to give up on this task. This is understandable, given the limits of our knowledge. However, it should be kept in mind that the clinician's creativity should constantly be at work to develop and design new programs of intervention. While financial and logistic issues will also limit what can be done, a responsible, ethical treatment of these patients requires extensive interventions for as long as it is feasible. Table 22.1 summarizes these eight steps.

Table 22.1 Clinical Guidelines in the Management and Rehabilitation of Persons with Anosognosia and Impaired Self-Awareness

1. Determine the extent (severity) of the unawareness: A complete or partial syndrome?
2. Determine in cases of ISA (a partial syndrome) if defensive and/or nondefensive methods of coping are present.
3. Determine the chronicity of anosognosia or ISA: Will it likely improve with time? Stay the same? Or "get worse?"
4. Determine the associated neurological and neuropsychological disturbances that may underlie or contribute to the anosognosia or ISA.
5. Establish a working alliance with the patient (and family, if possible). Requires time and effort.
6. Develop an individual neuropsychological rehabilitation plan (INRP)
   a. Detailed records of the anosognosia or ISA and how the symptom picture changes or does not change with time and/or intervention
   b. Documented preserved and disturbed neurological and neuropsychological functions associated with anosognosia or ISA over time
   c. Determine level of awareness for different functional activities
   d. Develop a hierarchical treatment plan
7. Make the rehabilitation task interesting to the patient.
8. Extend the training program as long as there is some "hope" of improving awareness of impaired neurological and neuropsychological functions.

ISA, impaired self-awareness.

Hierarchical Treatment Plan for Anosognosia for Hemiplegia

The three clinical vignettes of AHP that were described earlier illustrate different clinical courses and outcomes. Given that frontal, parietal, and insular cortical lesions are commonly associated with AHP (see Bottini et al., Chapter 2; Karnath & Baier, Chapter 3; Craig, Chapter 4; Heilman & Harciarek, Chapter 5; Vocat & Vuilleumier, Chapter 17, this volume), a hierarchical treatment plan may begin with basic discriminations of temperature and pressure in both hands (and possibly legs). This should be followed by a series of tasks that focus on basic tactile recognition (i.e., round, square, etc.), as well as finger recognition, and ultimately, object recognition. This should be done bilaterally. It should be followed by a series of right-left orientation commands to help the individual recognize difficulties he or she may have in identifying where various body parts are in space. It is interesting, for example, that some patients can readily identify where a left affected limb is with their right hand, but have notable difficulties finding the unaffected right hand with the affected left hand. Clinical ingenuity determines the variety of tasks that can be utilized in order to help with these basic perceptions of internal feeling states and basic tactile perceptions that help identify and reconstruct the body schema.

As is noted in earlier chapters, neglect and AHP are commonly associated (Karnath, Baier, & Nägele, 2005). When they are associated, the rehabilitation of AHP requires also working at improving the hemi-neglect. There are many different strategies that have been proposed to do this (Robertson & Halligan, 1999; Singh-Curry & Husain, 2008). An important aspect in the rehabilitation of these patients is to utilize their interest patterns in order to help demonstrate that, in fact, they have difficulties attending to one side of space. Leonard Diller (1974) showed a convincing videotape of how this could be done.

The patient was a physician who had suffered a stroke and had an associated left unilateral neglect. The physician repeatedly reported he had no difficulties looking to the left or detecting objects on the left. It was well-known that this physician enjoyed earning large sums of money in his practice prior to his neurological illness. In order to help this patient, Dr. Diller and colleagues performed the following task. The patient was asked to sit in front of a table where various denominations of money had been previously placed. For example, $20, $50, and $100 bills were placed in both the right and left hemispaces. The patient was then told that he could have all of the money that he picked up. The physician eagerly picked up as many currency notes that he could find; all, of course, being on the right side of space. After he had done so, the therapist asked the physician whether all of the money had been picked up off the table. The physician said indeed it had. The therapist then asked the physician to double-check. Again, the physician insisted that all of the money on the table had been successfully picked up. The therapist then gently brought into his right visual field the fact that a $50 bill and a $100 bill were not detected. When

Table 22.2 Hierarchical Interventions with Patients with Anosognosia for Hemiplegia

1. Detection of hot vs. cold; right vs. left side
2. Detection of presence or absence of tactile stimulation; right vs. left side
3. Detection of degree of pressure of tactile stimulation; "light" vs. "hard"; right vs. left side
4. Detection of location of tactile stimulation (including finger recognition) and tactile recognition of objects; right vs. left side
5. Right–left orientation responses.
   a. Identify body parts and locations in space with the "affected" and "nonaffected" hands
6. Detection of the presence of neglect (yes or no)
7. Behavioral strategies to improve hemi-inattention or frank neglect if present (see Robertson & Halligan, 1999; Singh-Curry & Husain, 2008)
8. Application of traditional OT and PT services for patients with hemiplegia
9. Long-term monitoring of awareness of one's limitations and its impact on ADLs
10. Assessment of the patient's emotional/motivational status and the ability to be guided by the working alliance with the therapists/physicians

ADLs, activities of daily living.

the physician recognized that he had lost the opportunity to pick up this money, he had an emotional reaction and never again forgot his problems with inattention.

As the neglect resolves, oftentimes AHP resolves, as noted above. In cases where AHP does not resolve as the neglect resolves, other techniques are needed to help the patient. Requests to carry out a series of bimanual tasks may be used in conjunction with traditional occupational and physical therapy activities. Once the individual is aware of his motor difficulties, the occupational and physical therapists should continue to work on a variety of cognitive rehabilitation therapies. It is well-known that patients with AHP may, in fact, have a less favorable functional outcome than patients who have hemiplegia without AHP (Jehkonen, Ahonen, Dastidar, Laippala, & Vilkki, 2000; Pedersen, Jorgensen, Nakayama, Raaschou, & Olsen, 1996). Table 22.2 provides a suggested hierarchical system of intervention for patients with AHP.

Hierarchical Treatment Plan for Impaired Self-Awareness after Severe Traumatic Brain Injury

After severe TBI, disturbances of consciousness can occur at three levels (Prigatano & Johnson, 2003). There may be a disturbance of the sleep-wake cycle with persistent difficulties in sustaining an adequate arousal level. There may be disturbances in self-awareness of neuropsychological and/or neurological functioning. Finally, there may be disturbances in awareness of the others' phenomenological state. Table 22.3 lists one possible hierarchical treatment plan to consider for persons who have ISA after severe TBI.

Table 22.3 Hierarchical Intervention Plan for Impaired Self-Awareness after Severe Traumatic Brain Injury

1. Arousal/sleep-wake cycle disturbances are first addressed.
   a. Self-monitoring sleep (e.g., how many hours did you sleep last night? Did you dream? Do you remember your dreams? What did you dream?)
   b. Self-monitoring energy level throughout the day (e.g., rate from 0 to 10 level of fatigue on an hourly basis; 0 means not tired at all, 10 means severe. Count the number of yawns throughout the course of a day and how they change with time).
   c. Self-monitor internal physiological state (e.g., have the patient walk on a treadmill or pedal on an exercise bicycle and record heart rate. After varying intervals of time, have the patient judge what his or her heart rate presently is. Measure the patient's heart rate at that time and provide feedback. This feedback loop may help the patient better subjectively experience and then predict what his or her heart rate level is as exercise continues at various time intervals).
2. Self-awareness of one's neuropsychological functioning in the here and now is then addressed.
   a. Individual activities at self-monitoring cognitive performance are begun (e.g., have the patient do digit-symbol coding tasks for 60 seconds. Score responses and have the patient predict what he or she will do on the next trial. Provide feedback as to the accuracy of predictions and continue this process to help patients gain insight into possible errors in their judgment. Word-search tasks and memory for words tasks can be utilized using the same procedure).
   b. Cognitive group activities (see Prigatano et al., 1986)
   c. Psychotherapy group activities (see Prigatano et al., 1986)
   d. Social/business group activities—milieu and feedback from others (see Prigatano et al., 1986)
3. Self-awareness of the other's phenomenological state now addressed (e.g., role playing, watching television and identifying the feelings and intentions of others, and listening to music and identifying the feelings generated by the music in self and others).
4. Writing of one's own life history—the integration of these "Three Vectors of Consciousness" and how they underlie disturbances of self-awareness after traumatic brain injury.

Table 22.4 Hierarchical Interventions for Patients Who Are Developing Impaired Self-Awareness and/or Anosognosia Associated with the Early Stage of Dementing Conditions

1. Self-monitoring of internal bodily states
   a. The patient scans his or her body for areas of tension in order to become more aware of bodily sensations. The patient subsequently rates the level of tension and tracks whether it correlates with memory or other functional lapses.
   b. The patient learns how to control tension in his or her body through two methods:
      1) Using a motor or implicit/procedural memory skill, such as progressive muscle relaxation.
      2) Controlling his breath (i.e., diaphragmatic breathing).
2. Self-monitoring of old and new "emotional" memories:

(continued)

Table 22.4 (Continued)

    a. The patient listens to and dances to songs from when he or she was a young adult, or views photographs or personal belongings from different periods of his or her life. The patient and therapist proceed from the distant past up to the present and create a timeline of memories of meaningful events in the patient's personal history.

    b. The patient attends the symphony or goes to a local museum. Meeting after such outings and discussing what was viewed/experienced could highlight gaps in short-term memory, but in a supportive environment. The experience could be used as a teaching moment to illustrate the difference between long-term and short-term memory.

3. Self-monitoring of ability to recall objects in space:

    a. The therapist and patient participate in route-finding tasks that are motivating to the patient. Afterward, the therapist and patient process the level of difficulty the patient had in completing the task and discuss what this might mean in a more general sense (i.e., route-finding while driving).

    b. Coupons for things the patient likes could be hidden in the therapist's office with the patient observing. After a certain time period, the patient is given several minutes to look for the coupons. The patient's emotional reaction is discussed if he or she can or cannot find the coupons. The impact of emotion on memory is discussed.

4. Self-monitoring of "higher-order" cognitive processes:

    a. Judgment-of-learning (JOL) and feeling-of-knowing (FOK) tasks are methods to evaluate self-monitoring processes. The patient with Alzheimer's disease (AD) is more likely to be distressed by inaccurate assessment of one's performance if the topic is something in which he or she is interested. To increase the likelihood the patient will be able to generalize what he or she learned about his or her memory skills, the patient and therapist chart performance over time on JOL tasks.

    b. The therapist and patient participate in activities of personal and social awareness/perspective taking. This is best conducted in a group setting.

      1) Fellow group members rate other members' progress in different areas.

      2) Watching films about AD may help stimulate discussion regarding the impact of the disease on the self and on close relationships.

The goal of this hierarchical treatment plan is to help individuals first become more aware of their level of arousal and degree of fatigue. After this is done, the individuals are involved in a series of individual and cognitive retraining tasks that help them perceive their awareness of their neuropsychological capabilities/ deficits and how it influences their functioning in interpersonal (group) interaction (Prigatano et al., 1986; Prigatano, 1999). Also, under this level of intervention is a variety of activities aimed at having them become aware of their feeling states, and finally, how they function within social business activities.

Following this training, the individual may work at a variety of activities that help improve his or her perceptions of other persons' psychological states (i.e., entering the other's phenomenological field). Role playing, watching movies, and relating to musical choices of others can all be useful ways of stimulating this form of awareness.

Hierarchical Treatment Plan for Impaired
Self-Awareness in Patients with Early Dementia

Unlike patients who suffer a stroke or severe TBI, persons who are in the early stages of a dementia slowly develop their disturbances in self-awareness (Clare, 2004). Moreover, many show a progressive decline (not recovery) of this impaired brain function over time (see Fig. 22.2). As Pietrini, Salmon, and Nichelli (2009) have noted, dementia often results in the "brain losing itself."

This patient group is perhaps the most difficult to approach and manage from a neuropsychological rehabilitation point of view because of their prognosis. Clinically, we have found that both a neuropsychologically oriented model of rehabilitation, as well as appropriately timed psychotherapeutic interventions, may be necessary to help this patient group and their families. As is true with other forms of intervention, when anosognosia or ISA is present, one must begin with an understanding of the neuropathological changes that most likely underlie the ISA.

In Alzheimer's disease (AD), the medial temporal lobe, parietal lobe, and posterior cingulate/precuneus often show reduced metabolic activity early in the course of the disease (Minoshima et al., 1997). Medial frontal and orbitofrontal cortices also deteriorate as the disease progresses. This may contribute to reductions in awareness of one's own functioning and social comportment (Salmon et al., 2006). Furthermore, Starkstein, Sabe, Chemerinski, Jason, and Leiguarda (1996) were able to dissociate elements of cognitive versus behavioral unawareness in patients with AD. Cognitive unawareness is associated with greater intellectual decline, a higher frequency of delusions, significant apathy, and lower depression. Behavioral unawareness is related to higher disinhibition scores and pathological laughing. Any hierarchical treatment plan must keep these two dimensions in mind.

Generally speaking, however, when working with patients who show early signs of dementia, the management and rehabilitation activities must be dictated by the severity of their neurocognitive impairments and their associated disruption of self-awareness. Since the posterior cingulate shows hypometabolism early in the course of the disease, rehabilitation activities aimed at functions known to be mediated by this region may be a useful starting point. The posterior cingulate is involved in the integration of interoceptive and exteroceptive information required for conscious/controlled processing (Salmon et al., 2005), as well as orientation to time and place in individuals with AD (Hirono et al., 1998). As Table 22.4 suggests, the first set of tasks may focus on identifying internal and external sources of stress. The interventions may begin with asking patients to scan their bodies for tension, in order to help them become more aware of internal bodily sensations. Subsequently, the therapist may teach patients how to control tension in their bodies through a motor or implicit memory skill, such as progressive muscle relaxation. Procedural learning/ memory remains relatively intact early in the course of the disease. Indeed, Suhr, Anderson, and Tranel (1999) showed the benefits of progressive muscle relaxation in individuals with AD. Starting treatment in this manner is non-threatening and can help build trust in the therapeutic relationship, which may improve patients' willingness to follow through on recommendations made by their therapist and family members.

The next level in the treatment hierarchy is to focus on functions mediated in part by the medial temporal lobes. These regions are important for the "memory/ emotion" interface and provide an area of rehabilitation that is interesting to many patients. The arts are particularly effective at tapping into emotions. Listening to and dancing to songs from when patients were young adults can generate very deeply felt emotions. With the aid of family members (both to bring in items to stimulate discussion and verify the veracity of patients' recall), showing pictures or personal belongings from different time periods of patients' lives can aid with reminiscence, which could proceed from the distant past up to the present.

A local institute has an arts program in which small groups of patients with AD go to the symphony or the art museum. Meeting after such outings and discussing what was viewed/experienced could highlight gaps in short-term memory, but in a supportive environment. These exercises could help clarify the distinction between long-term memory and short-term memory, and they should help patients understand that the latter is affected in AD. In a similar vein, encouraging patients to schedule pleasurable activities can help to counteract apathy, which is correlated with reduced awareness (Aalten, Van Valen, Clare, Kenny, & Verhey, 2005). This can be done in concert with teaching patients how to use simple calendars as memory aids.

Disturbances of parietal lobe function are common in AD patients. Consequently, rehabilitation activities should include engaging the patient in route-finding tasks. These tasks must be crafted to be motivating to the patient. For example, the therapist can request that the patient locate the cafeteria or the Starbucks coffee stand at the hospital. The therapist may offer to purchase a cup of coffee for the patient upon arrival at the destination. The therapist and patient can then discuss the level of difficulty the patient experienced when attempting to complete the task. This may help the patient obtain better insight into issues related to other important areas of functioning, such as driving a car.

Other tasks that may reflect both parietal and medial temporal lobe dysfunction should be considered. Analogous to the task Dr. Diller did with the physician with neglect who was motivated by money, many elderly patients are interested in obtaining coupons. Coupons can be hidden in the therapist's office with the patient watching. After a certain time period, the patient can be given several minutes to look for the coupons and keep what he or she finds. Like the physician who had neglect, patients with AD may experience an emotional reaction if they cannot find many of the coupons they initially were interested in obtaining.

Moving up the treatment hierarchy, tasks involving presumed frontal lobe functioning may also help the therapist bring the patient's challenges to light. Judgment-of-learning (JOL) and feeling-of-knowing (FOK) tasks are methods used to evaluate monitoring processes. Judgment-of-learning tasks require subjects to predict, at the time information is being studied, the likelihood of subsequently recalling recently studied items. Feeling-of-knowing tasks involve making judgments, after the recall phase of a memory task, about the likelihood of subsequently recognizing nonrecalled semantic information or episodic information (Cosentino & Stern, 2005). Again, information to be learned should be interesting to the patient in order to motivate him or her to do well. Furthermore, the patient is more likely to be distressed by poor performance if the topic is something he or she is interested in (e.g., current baseball statistics/players).

A challenge, however, is that although the patient's immediate awareness of deficits may be improved, his sustained awareness may remain impaired. For example, patients may overpredict their performance prior to the first learning trial, but subsequently update post-trial estimates based on performance. After a 20-minute delay, patients may again overpredict performance, suggesting that they cannot not permanently (or generally) update their beliefs about their own memory based on poor task performance (Cosentino & Stern, 2005). To increase the likelihood patients will be able to generalize what they learned about their memory skills, simple worksheets could be used on which patients and therapists chart performance over time. These activities are aimed at helping patients self-monitor their behavior and performance.

At the highest level of the hierarchy, therapists and patients should work on tasks of personal and social awareness/perspective taking (Cosentino & Stern, 2005; Salmon et al., 2006). This is best conducted in a group setting (Prigatano et al., 1986). Fellow group members can rate other members' progress in different areas. This requires a cohesive group of members who have grown to trust each other. These neuropsychological tasks are aimed at providing patients with ISA who are in the early stages of a dementia an opportunity to self-discover (via graded training techniques) disturbances in higher cerebral functioning of which they may be only partially aware. Doing so in a respectful manner is crucial. It can only be done in the context of a good working alliance with the patient that takes into consideration his or her emotional state and how he or she faces a loss of functioning. It requires a psychotherapeutic approach to the patient.

Such an approach, when working with various brain-dysfunctional patients, necessitates that the treating clinician seriously consider the psychological makeup of the person and how it interacts with the effects of brain injury to produce the symptom picture (Prigatano, 1999). We will now briefly consider working with brain-dysfunctional patients who present with both ISA and DD.

Neuropsychological Rehabilitation of Brain-Dysfunctional Patients Who Have Both Impaired Self-Awareness and Denial of Disability

Patients who present with DD and ISA require more than systematic cognitive rehabilitation to help them have a realistic view of their disabilities and to learn to make choices that are important for their physical and psychological state of well-being. A key feature of DD is *resistance*; not perplexity as a response to feedback regarding their neurological/neuropsychological limitations. While different models might be utilized to help deal with resistance, psychodynamic models represent an approach to thinking about the patient's life situation that may be especially helpful (Prigatano, 2008b). These models emphasize that past experiences and modes of thinking and behaving clearly influence the patient's present behavior. They further assume that the patient may not be fully aware of feeling states and accompanying motivations that guide his or her interpretation of a social or interpersonal situation, irrespective of the effects of a brain disorder. It furthermore emphasizes the importance of knowing what the patient experiences as an important starting point for any form of psychotherapeutic intervention.

This model suggests that the dialogue with the patient that is predicated on an understanding of the complexities of the doctor–patient interaction will lead to greater treatment compliance (Ciechanowski, Katon, Russo, & Walker, 2001) and ultimately greater insight for both parties as to the type of decisions that are made in dealing with life's problems. These ingredients form the basis of a psychodynamically oriented psychotherapeutic relationship, which can be helpful when working with brain-dysfunctional patients (Prigatano, 2008b).

It is beyond the scope of this chapter to discuss in detail the psychotherapeutic management of persons who demonstrate DD and ISA after brain injuries. However, one clinical vignette is described to clarify how this process can unfold when it is successful. A 20-year-old man suffered anoxic brain injury secondary to cardiac arrest. He became densely amnestic, but slowly improved. Severe memory impairment, however, has been noted now for more than 18 years. He passively engaged in a holistic form of a neuropsychological rehabilitation program for several months following the acute onset of his illness (Prigatano, 1999). At the end of that time, he was partially aware (i.e., ISA) of his memory difficulties and his limited capacities to successfully complete his academic studies. When data were presented regarding his diminished capacities, he acknowledged it, but discounted its impact. He returned back to his academic studies, but unfortunately failed to successfully complete them. He subsequently developed severe headaches and panic attacks. He reported no connection between his academic failure and his somatic/psychiatric symptoms.

Over the course of several years, he was guided to seek out a lower level of education and occupational goals. While resistant, he ultimately was able to discuss the reasons for his resistance within the context of psychotherapy. He had experienced the psychotherapist as being extremely supportive of him during the time he was engaged in neuropsychological rehabilitation. The psychotherapist, who was aware of the interpersonal dynamics between this young man and his father, used this information to help guide the therapist's reactions to the patient's choices. Ultimately the patient drew a connection between his poor choices in dealing with his present life issues and conflicts that *predated* his cognitive impairments. This "self-discovery" (with the aid of the therapist) helped the patient make decisions that were now in his best interest. With better decisions, his somatic and affective disturbances gradually disappeared. While he had limited self-awareness, he also presented with DD. The DD, however, was successfully managed within the context of the psychotherapeutic relationship.

Summary Comments

The study of anosognosia and ISA has led to a greater understanding of this important set of disturbances in higher integrative brain functioning. The application of this new knowledge, in conjunction with principles of neuropsychological rehabilitation (Prigatano, 1999), promises to help us be more effective in managing and rehabilitating patients with brain dysfunction. Much more work is, of course, needed in this area. In this last chapter, however, we have attempted to provide a few guidelines to aid this process, while focusing on a variety of clinical issues that are encountered in doing this work.

References

Aalten, P., Van Valen, E., Clare, L., Kenny, G., & Verhey, F. (2005). Awareness in dementia: A review of clinical correlates. *Aging & Mental Health, 9*(5), 414–422.

Bisiach, E., & Geminiani, G. (1991). Anosognosia related to hemiplegia and hemianopia. In G. P. Prigatano & D. L. Schacter (Eds.), *Awareness of deficit after brain injury: Clinical and theoretical issues* (pp. 17–39). New York: Oxford University Press.

Ciechanowski, P. A., Katon, W. J., Russo, J. E., & Walker, E. A. (2001). The patient–provider relationship: Attachment theory and adherence to treatment in diabetes. *American Journal of Psychiatry, 158*, 29–35.

Clare, L. (2004). Awareness in early-stage Alzheimer's disease: A review of methods and evidence. *British Journal of Clinical Psychology, 43*, 177–196.

Cocchini, G., Beschin, N., & Della Sala, S. (2002). Chronic anosognosia: A case report and theoretical account. *Neuropsychologia, 40*, 2030–2038.

Cosentino, S., & Stern, Y. (2005). Metacognitive theory and assessment in dementia: Do we recognize our areas of weakness? *Journal of the International Neuropsychological Society, 11*, 910–919.

Diller, L. (1974). Studies in scanning behavior in hemiplegics. *Rehabilitation Monograph No. 50: Studies in cognition and rehabilitation in hemiplegia*. New York: New York University Medical Center.

Fotopoulou, A., Rudd, A., Holmes, P., & Kopelman, M. (2009). Self-observation reinstates motor awareness in anosognosia for hemiplegia. *Neuropsychologia, 47,* 1256–1260.

Freedman, A. M., Kaplan, H. I., & Sadock, B. J. (Eds.) (1976). *Modern synopsis of comprehensive textbook of psychiatry/II* (2nd edition). Baltimore: The Williams & Wilkins Co.

Hirono, N., Mori, E., Ishii, K., Ikejiri, Y., Imamura, T., Shimomura, T., Hashimoto, M., Yamashita, H., & Sasaki, M. (1998). Hypofunction in the posterior cingulate gyrus correlates with disorientation for time and place in Alzheimer's disease. *Journal of Neurology, Neurosurgery, and Psychiatry, 64,* 552–554.

Jehkonen, M., Ahonen, J.-P., Dastidar, P., Laippala, P., & Vilkki, J. (2000). Unawareness of deficits after right hemisphere stroke: Double-dissociations of anosognosias. *Acta Neurologica Scandinavica, 102,* 378–384.

Karnath, H. -O., Baier, B., & Nägele, T. (2005). Awareness of the functioning of one's own limbs mediated by the insular cortex? *The Journal of Neuroscience, 25*(31), 7134–7138.

Klonoff, P. S., Lamb, D. G., & Henderson, S. W. (2001). Outcomes from milieu-based neurorehabilitation at up to 11 years post discharge. *Brain Injury, 15*(5), 413–428.

Minoshima, S., Giordani, B., Berent, S., Frey, K. F., Foster, N. L., & Kuhl, D. E. (1997). Metabolic reduction in the posterior cingulate cortex in very early Alzheimer's disease. *Annals of Neurology, 42,* 85–94.

Paredes, A. (1974). Denial, deceptive maneuvers, and consistency in the behavior of alcoholics. In F. Seixas & R. Cadoret (Eds.), *The person with alcoholism* (pp. 23–33). New York: Academy of Sciences.

Pedersen, P. N., Jorgensen, H. S., Nakayama, H., Raaschou, H. O., & Olsen, T. S. (1996). Frequency, determinants, and consequences of anosognosia in acute stroke. *Journal of Neurological Rehabilitation, 10,* 243–250.

Pietrini, P., Salmon, E., & Nichelli, P. (2009). Consciousness and dementia: How the brain loses its self. In S. Laureys & G. Tononi (Eds.), *The neurology of consciousness: Cognitive neuroscience and neuropathology* (pp. 204–216). New York: Academic Press.

Prigatano, G. P. (1988). Anosognosia, delusions, and altered self-awareness after brain injury. *BNI Quarterly, 4*(3), 40–48.

Prigatano, G. P. (1998). Disorders of behavior and self awareness. In P. Azzoui & B. Bussel (Eds.), *Syndrome frontal: Evaluation et réducation, Actes des 11 Entretiens de l'Institut Garches* (pp. 77–84). Paris: Arnette Publishers.

Prigatano, G. P. (1999). *Principles of neuropsychological rehabilitation*. New York: Oxford University Press.

Prigatano, G. P. (2008a). Anosognosia and the process and outcome of neurorehabilitation. In D. T. Stuss, G. Winocur, and I. H. Robertson (Eds.), *Cognitive neurorehabilitation: Evidence and application* (2nd edition, pp. 218–231). Cambridge, England: Cambridge University Press.

Prigatano, G. P. (2008b). Neuropsychological rehabilitation and psychodynamic psychotherapy. In J. Morgan and J. Ricker (Eds.), *Textbook of clinical neuropsychology* (pp. 985–995). New York: Taylor & Francis.

Prigatano, G. P., Fordyce, D. J., Zeiner, H. K., Roueche, J. R., Pepping, M., & Wood, B. C. (1986). *Neuropsychological rehabilitation after brain injury.* Baltimore: Johns Hopkins University Press.

Prigatano, G. P., & Johnson, S. C. (2003). The three vectors of consciousness and their disturbances after brain injury. *Neuropsychological Rehabilitation, 13*(1/2), 13–29.

Prigatano, G. P., & Klonoff, P. S. (1998). A clinician's rating scale for evaluating impaired self-awareness and denial of disability after brain injury. *The Clinical Neuropsychologist, 12*(1), 56–67.

Prigatano, G. P., Klonoff, P. S., O'Brien, K. P., Altman, I., Amin, K., Chiapello, D. A., Shepherd, J., Cunningham, M., & Mora, M. (1994). Productivity after neuropsychologically oriented, milieu rehabilitation. *The Journal of Head Trauma Rehabilitation, 9*(1), 91–102.

Prigatano, G. P., & Maier, F. (2008). Neuropsychiatric, psychiatric, and behavioral disorders associated with traumatic brain injury. In I. Grant & K. Adams (Eds.), *Neuropsychological assessment of neuropsychiatric disorders* (3rd edition, pp. 618–631). New York: Oxford University Press.

Robertson, I. H., & Halligan, P. W. (1999). *Spatial neglect: A clinical handbook for diagnosis and treatment.* Hove, England: Psychology Press.

Salmon, E., Perani, D., Herholz, K., Marique, P., Kalbe, E., Holthoff, V., Delbeuck, X., Beuthien-Baumann, B., Pelati, O., Lespagnard, S., Collette, F., & Garraux, G. (2006). Neural correlates of anosognosia for cognitive impairment in Alzheimer's disease. *Human Brain Mapping, 27,* 588–596.

Salmon, E., Ruby, P., Perani, D., Kalbe, E., Laureys, S., Adam, S., & Collette, F. (2005). Two aspects of impaired consciousness in Alzheimer's disease. In S. Laureys (Ed.), *Progress in brain research* (pp. 287–298). New York: Elsevier.

Schönberger, M., Humle, F., & Teasdale, T. W. (2006a). The development of the therapeutic working alliance, patients' awareness and their compliance during the process of brain injury rehabilitation. *Brain Injury, 20,* 445–454.

Schönberger, M., Humle, F., Zeeman, P., & Teasdale, T. W. (2006b). Working alliance and patient compliance in brain injury rehabilitation and their relation to psychosocial outcome. *Neuropsychological Rehabilitation, 16,* 298–314.

Singh-Curry, V., & Husain, M. (2008). Rehabilitation of neglect. In D. Stuss, G. Winocur, & I. H. Robertson (Eds.), *Cognitive neurorehabilitation* (2nd edition): *Evidence and application* (pp. 449–463). Cambridge, England: Cambridge University Press.

Starkstein, S. E., Sabe, L., Chemerinski, E., Jason, L., & Leiguarda, R. (1996). Two domains of anosognosia in Alzheimer's disease. *Journal of Neurology, Neurosurgery, and Psychiatry, 61,* 485–490.

Suhr, J., Anderson, S., & Tranel, D. (1999). Progressive muscle relaxation in the management of behavioural disturbance in Alzheimer's disease. *Neuropsychological Rehabilitation, 9*(1), 31–44.

Author Index

Subject Index